CLINICAL GUIDE TO
ULTRASONOGRAPHY

CLINICAL GUIDE TO
ULTRASONOGRAPHY

CHARLOTTE HENNINGSEN, MS, RT, RDMS, RVT
Chair and Professor
Diagnostic Medical Sonography Department
Florida Hospital College of Health Sciences
Orlando, Florida

With a foreword by
LENNARD D. GREENBAUM, MD

With more than 1100 illustrations and 36 color plates

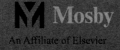 Mosby
An Affiliate of Elsevier

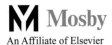

An Affiliate of Elsevier

11830 Westline Industrial Drive
St. Louis, Missouri 63146

NOTICE

Ultrasonography is an ever-changing field. Standard safety precautions must be followed, but as new
research and clinical experience broaden our knowledge, changes in treatment and drug therapy may
become necessary or appropriate. Readers are advised to check the most current product information
provided by the manufacturer of each drug to be administered to verify the recommended dose, the
method and duration of administration, and contraindications. It is the responsibility of the
licensed health care provider, relying on experience and knowledge of the patient, to determine
dosages and the best treatment for each individual patient. Neither the publisher nor the author
assumes any liability for any injury and/or damage to persons or property arising from this
publication.

Library of Congress Cataloging-in-Publication Data

Henningsen, Charlotte.
    Clinical guide to ultrasonography / Charlote Henningsen.
        p. ; cm.
    Includes bibliographical references and index.
    ISBN 0-323-01938-2
        1. Diagnosis, Ultrasonic–Case studies.   I. Title.
        [DNLM: 1. Ultrasonography–methods–Case Report. WN 208 H517c 2004]
    RC78.7.U4H467 2004
    616.07'543–dc22

                                                                    2003066610

Publisher: Andrew Allen
Editor: Jeanne Wilke
Senior Developmental Editor: Linda Woodard
Publishing Services Manager: Patricia Tannian
Senior Project Manager: Anne Altepeter
Book Design Manager: Gail Morey Hudson

Printed in the United States of America
Last digit is the print number: 9   8   7   6   5   4   3   2   1

Contributors

AHMED AL-MALT, MD
Perinatologist
Fetal Diagnostic Center of Orlando
Orlando, Florida

KATHI KEATON BOROK, BS, RDMS, RDCS
Clinical Coordinator
Florida Hospital College of Health Sciences
Orlando, Florida

FRANKLYN C. CHRISTENSEN, MD
Attending Physician, Maternal-Fetal Medicine
Maternal Fetal Specialists, Northside Hospital
Atlanta, Georgia

GARY E. CLAGETT, BS, RVT, RDMT, RT(R)
Chief Technologist
Centura-Penrose St. Francis Health System
Colorado Springs, Colorado

KIMBERLY EISEN, BS, RT, RDMS
Ultrasound Supervisor
Florida Hospital
Orlando, Florida

ARMANDO FUENTES, MD
Perinatologist
Maternal Fetal Center at Florida Hospital
Orlando, Florida

LENNARD D. GREENBAUM, MD, FACR
Chief, Section of Diagnostic Ultrasound
Department of Radiology
Orlando Regional Healthcare System
Orlando, Florida

JOYCE GRUBE, MS, RDMS
Clinical Coordinator
Kettering College of Medical Arts
Kettering, Ohio

SANDRA HAGEN-ANSERT, MS, RDMS, RDCS
Non-Invasive Cardiac Sonographer
Medical University of South Carolina
Charleston, South Carolina

MICHAEL HARTMAN, MS, RDMS, RVT, RT(R)
Program Director, Diagnostic Medical Sonography and
Cardiovascular Technology, Thomas Jefferson University
Philadelphia, Pennsylvania

JILL HERZOG, BS, RT (R), RDMS, RVT
Instructor, Diagnostic Medical Sonography
Mercy College of Health Sciences
Des Moines, Iowa

D. ASHLEY HILL, MD
Associate Director, Department of Obstetrics/Gynecology
Florida Hospital
Orlando, Florida

FELICIA JONES, BS, RDMS, RVT
Program Director
Tidewater Community College
Virginia Beach, Virginia

KATHRYN M. KUNTZ, BS, RT, RDMS, RVT
Assistant Professor of Radiology
Diagnostic Medical Sonography Program Director
Mayo Clinic
Rochester, Minnesota

GREGORY LOGSDON, MD
Radiologist
Florida Hospital/Orlando Diagnostic Radiology Department
Orlando, Florida

ROBERT MAGNER, RDMS, RVT, BA, R (R, CT)
Ultrasound Supervisor
United States Air Force Academy
USAFA, Colorado

LISA MULLEE, MS, RDMS, RDCS, RVT
Assistant Professor of Cardiovascular Laboratory
Tallahassee Memorial Hospital
Tallahassee, Florida

LEIF PENROSE, BA, RDMS, RVT, RT(R, CT)
Director, Ultrasound Program
Coosa Valley Technical College
Rome, Georgia

CHRISTOPHER MICHAEL RICKETTS, MD
Obstetrics Fellow
Department of Family Medicine, Florida Hospital
Orlando, Florida

DANA SALMONS, BS, RT, RDMS
Sonographer
Florida Hospital
Orlando, Florida

TAMARA SALSGIVER, AAS, RT(R), RDMS, RVT
Program Director,
Diagnostic Medical Sonography
Greenville Technical College
Greenville, South Carolina

REGINA SWEARENGIN, BS, RDMS
Program Coordinator
Austin Community College
Austin, Texas

PAMELA A. KUNAU SZCZESNIAK, BA, BS, RDMS
Lead Sonographer
Florida Hospital Medical Center
Orlando, Florida

MSGT CHERYL A. VANCE, MA, RT, RDMS, RVT
Program Director, Diagnostic Ultrasound Course
United States Air Force
Sheppard AFB, Texas

JOHN W. VAN WERT, MD
Board Certified Obstetrician/Gynecologist
Managing Partner
Premier Obstetrics and Gynecology of Orlando, P.A.
Maitland, Florida

KIMBERLY WATTS, BS, RT(R), CNMT, RDMS
Director of Sonography Program
Caldwell Community College & Technical Institute
Hudson, North Carolina

KERRY WEINBERG, MPA, RDMS, RDCS
Director, Diagnostic Medical Sonography Program
New York University
New York, New York

JOSEPH YEE, MD
Clinical Associate Professor of Radiology
New York University School of Medicine
New York, New York

Reviewers

GINA M. AUGUSTINE, MLS, RT(R)
Coordinator, Advanced Level Radiographic Externship
    Program
St. Francis Hospital of New Castle
New Castle, Pennsylvania

HEATHER ANNE BERKEY, BS, RDMS, BS, RT(R)
Unit Coordinator, Perinatal Ultrasound
Thomas Jefferson University
Philadelphia, Pennsylvania

KENT BLEVINS JR., MM, RT(R), RDMS, RVT
Academic Clinical Coordinator, DMS Program
Oregon Institute of Technology
Klamath Falls, Oregon

**ADELIA THAL BULLINS, RDMS, RVT, BS, AAS, CNMT,
    RT(N)**
Clinical Coordinator
Forsyth Technical Community College
Winston Salem, North Carolina

DIANE BURDA, RT, RDMS, RVT, RDCS
Ultrasound Specialist
Lakeland, Florida

MARY K. HENNE, BS, CNMT, RDMS
Instructor and Sonographer
Columbia — St. Mary's Hospital
Milwaukee, Wisconsin

RUBEN MARTINEZ, BS, RDCS, RVT
Ultrasound Instructor
Florida Hospital College of Health Sciences
Orlando, Florida

JOSEPH B. MORTON III, AS, BS, MBA, RT(R), RDMS
Sonographer
St. Mary's Hospital — Milwaukee
Milwaukee, Wisconsin

SUSANNA LYNN OVEL, RT(R), RDMS, RVT
Senior Sonographer and Trainer
Radiological Associates
Sacramento, California

CRAIG F. PENEFF, BSAS, RDMS, RVT
Assistant Professor and Program Director
Diagnostic Medical Sonography
Lorain County Community College
Elyria, Ohio

ROSY SILVERMAN, RDMS, MPH
Director
Femwell Diagnostic Center
Miami, Florida

LISA M. STROHL, BS, RT(R), RDMS, RVT
Continuing Medical Education Manager
American Institute of Ultrasound in Medicine
Laurel, Maryland

MATTIE J. TABRON, EdD, RT(R)(T), FASRT
Associate Professor and Chairman
Department of Radiation Therapy
Howard University
Washington, DC

CHERYL ZELINSKY, MM, RT(R), RDMS
Director, Diagnostic Medical Sonography Program
Oregon Institute of Technology
Klamath Falls, Oregon

To my husband
PETE
for the love, patience, and understanding that he showed
while I sat at my computer writing for hours on end.

And for his computer expertise, upon which I relied heavily,
especially through that hated hard drive crash.

His unwavering support and timely humor are the reasons
that I dedicate this book to him.

Foreword

Many books about ultrasound have been written based on an organ system approach, with a standard format of normal anatomy, benign disease, and then malignant disease. Charlotte Henningsen has taken a different approach in her *Clinical Guide to Ultrasonography*. Almost all of the chapters are based on how patients present clinically for their ultrasound examination. This fact makes the book a "real world" reference for the practicing sonographer. It is not meant to replace any of the excellent ultrasound texts that may be in your library, but I believe that it is a worthy addition because it is a practical, concise, pathology-based reference that sonographers can use daily during their busy work schedules. Topics are covered succinctly, providing the sonographer with pertinent information he or she needs to produce an optimally diagnostic examination. Charlotte has drawn on her years of experience as both a practicing sonographer and an educator to present the information in a format that should be useful to the sonographer who is already in the workplace.

I have had the pleasure of working closely with sonographers for almost 30 years. There is a partnership between the physician who reads the sonogram and the sonographer who produces the images. The more the sonographer understands the anatomy in question, the significance of the patient's clinical presentation, and the possible disease processes that may be causing that presentation, the better the study he or she produces. Good sonographers are continuously thinking and modifying their patient examinations based on their moment-to-moment interpretation of real-time scanning and the images they are producing. If the sonographer does not recognize an abnormality and record or image it, there is no way that even the best sonologist can make the diagnosis. This book should help sonographers understand and recognize disease processes better and, therefore, improve the quality of their examinations.

Lennard D. Greenbaum, MD

Preface

Clinical Guide to Ultrasonography is a pathology-focused ultrasound textbook that presents the abnormalities encountered with sonography from a clinical perspective. This text is not intended to replace comprehensive texts, which also focus on basic anatomy and imaging techniques, but will partner with those texts as a ready reference for sonographic pathology or enhance discussion of clinical case studies. *Clinical Guide to Ultrasonography* is a practical resource for students and sonographers as they consider patient symptoms with possible findings and diagnoses.

CONTENT AND ORGANIZATION

The book is organized into four major parts: abdomen, gynecology, obstetrics, and superficial structures. A few miscellaneous topics are covered in a separate part. Chapters are organized by patient symptom or clinical presentation to correlate with the patient history that the sonographer or sonography student may encounter in the clinical environment.

Hundreds of ultrasound images, including color Doppler and power imaging, assist the sonographer in visualizing the pathologic conditions described. Many of the chapters are enhanced with illustrations that demonstrate relevant anatomic information. The text also includes pediatric and vascular imaging, subjects that are not always covered in other clinical textbooks.

FEATURES

Every chapter contains an opening clinical scenario that sets up a realistic situation for the student to use as a frame of reference. These clinical scenarios heighten reader interest, facilitate applying information in the clinical setting, and encourage the critical thinking skills necessary for a sonographer to be more than a picture taker. Normal anatomy is then briefly reviewed, with the remainder of the chapter focused on the pathology associated with the titular symptom. Summary tables and glossaries provide quick references to covered material. Additional case studies and study questions close each chapter and are designed to develop and enhance critical thinking skills and measure comprehension of the material. Answers to case studies and study questions are provided in an appendix to provide opportunity for discussion before seeking the answers.

ELECTRONIC IMAGE COLLECTION

An electronic image collection on CD-ROM that includes the images from the book is available for those teaching a course with the text, providing an easy-to-use and cost-effective alternative to traditional pathology slide sets.

EVOLVE—ONLINE COURSE MANAGEMENT

Evolve is an interactive learning environment designed to work in coordination with *Clinical Guide to Ultrasonography*. Instructors may use Evolve to provide an Internet-based course component that reinforces and expands on the concepts delivered in class. Evolve may be used to publish the class syllabus, outlines, and lecture notes; set up "virtual office hours" and e-mail communication; share important dates and information through the online class Calendar; and encourage student participation through Chat Rooms and Discussion Boards. Evolve allows instructors to post examinations and manage their grade book online. For more information, visit http://www.evolve.elsevier.com or contact an Elsevier sales representative.

This textbook is designed to provide realistic clinical applications of sonography to the sonography student and the sonographer. Identification of pathology by the sonographer is the key to a correct diagnosis. I hope this book inspires you to embrace the knowledge necessary to be a valuable member of a diagnostic imaging team.

Charlotte Henningsen

Acknowledgments

I would like to express gratitude and appreciation to all of the individuals who have assisted in my career development and who have been a source of encouragement and inspiration.

I would like to express my gratitude to the employees of Florida Hospital College of Health Sciences who have celebrated this process every step of the way. Thanks to the college administration, Dr. David Greenlaw and Dr. Don Williams, for allowing me the time and resources I required and for their continuing encouragement; the library staff, especially Beck Hutchinson, Consuelo Saulo, Jenny Alleyne, and Marley Soper, for diligently and expertly gathering research and for cheering me along; the IT team, especially Steve Roche and Tony Conley, for being so attentive to my needs; my secretary, Anita Spry, for her smile and for keeping me sane; and the faculty of the sonography department, Kathi Borok and Ruben Martinez, for taking on extra tasks and for their enthusiasm.

I must acknowledge Dr. Gregory Logsdon, Dr. Armando Fuentes, Dr. Diane Kawamura, Sandy Hagen-Ansert, and Susan Magee, individuals who have significantly contributed to and encouraged my professional development. I would like to thank the many sonographers with whom I have worked over the years who have shared their knowledge with me and my students, especially the sonographers of Florida Hospital and the Maternal Fetal Center. I thank the students that I have taught over the years for inspiring and challenging me. Their enthusiasm for the profession is contagious!

Thanks to my contributors who worked diligently to meet their deadlines and produce chapters of excellence.

I would like to thank my family and friends, who have been extremely supportive and understanding—especially my parents, for understanding why the vacations were cut short.

Finally, I would like to recognize the very supportive and able staff at Elsevier who have guided me through this process: Jeanne Wilke for providing the opportunity and allowing me to stretch my creativity, Linda Woodard for holding my hand throughout the process while offering her expertise and friendship, and Anne Altepeter for helping to put it all together in the end. Their encouragement never waned.

Charlotte Henningsen

Contents

PART I
ABDOMEN

1 Right Upper Quadrant Pain, 3

Gallbladder, 4
Biliary Tract Disease, 9
Liver, 11

2 Liver Mass, 20

Liver, 21
Benign Neoplasms, 21
Malignant Neoplasms, 24

3 Diffuse Liver Disease, 33

Hepatocellular Disease, 35

4 Epigastric Pain, 49

Pancreas, 51
Pancreatitis, 52
Pancreatic Neoplasms, 53

5 Hematuria, 58

Genitourinary System, 60
Urolithiasis, 60
Benign Neoplasms, 62
Malignant Neoplasms, 65

6 Rule Out Renal Failure, 76

Hydronephrosis, 77
Acute Glomerulonephritis, 78
Papillary Necrosis, 79
Renal Failure, 79
Renal Artery Stenosis, 80
Acute Tubular Necrosis, 81
Renal Infection, 82

7 Cystic Versus Solid Renal Mass, 92

Renal Cysts, 93
Renal Cystic Disease, 96

8 Left Upper Quadrant Pain, 104

Spleen, 105
Congenital Variants, 105
Splenomegaly, 106
Cysts, 107
Abscesses, 107
Infarct, 108
Benign Neoplasms, 108
Malignant Neoplasms, 109
Trauma, 110

9 Pediatric Mass, 116

Biliary, 117
Liver, 118
Adrenal, 119
Renal, 120

10 Pulsatile Abdominal Mass, 134

Abdominal Aortic Aneurysm, 135
Ruptured Aneurysm, 137
Aortic Dissection, 137

11 Gastrointestinal Imaging, 143

Appendicitis, 145
Pyloric Stenosis, 150
Intussusception, 153

12 Retroperitoneum, 161

Lymphadenopathy, 162
Adrenal Mass, 162
Retroperitoneal Fibrosis, 165

PART II
GYNECOLOGY

13 Abnormal Uterine Bleeding, 173

Normal Uterine Anatomy, 175
Uterine Physiology, 175
Leiomyoma, 176
Adenomyosis, 180
Adenomyomas, 181
Endometrial Hyperplasia and Carcinoma, 183

Endometrial Polyps, 186
Sonohysterography, 188

14 Lost Intrauterine Device, 197

Sonographic Appearance of an Intrauterine
Device, 198
Intrauterine Device Complications, 199

15 Pelvic Inflammatory Disease, 206

Sonographic Findings, 208

16 Infertility, 216

Endometriosis, 217
Polycystic Ovarian Disease, 217
Congenital Uterine Anomaly, 219

17 Ovarian Mass, 227

Normal Ovarian Anatomy, 229
Ovarian Cysts, 229
Cystic/Complex Neoplasms, 232
Solid Neoplasms, 239

PART III
OBSTETRICS

18 Uncertain Last Menstrual Period, 249

First-Trimester Biometry, 250
Second- and Third-Trimester Biometry, 255

19 Size Greater than Dates, 264

Excessive Fetal Growth, 265
Increased Fundal Height, 267

20 Size Less than Dates, 276

Oligohydramnios, 277
Fetal Renal Anomalies, 278
Intrauterine Growth Restriction, 282
Premature Rupture of Membranes, 284

21 Bleeding with Pregnancy, 291

First-Trimester Bleeding, 292
Second-Trimester Bleeding, 297
Postpartum Bleeding, 301

22 Multifetal Gestation, 307

Imaging Protocol, 309
Embryology of Twinning, 311
Complications, 313
Abnormal Twinning, 314
Maternal Complications, 316

23 Elevated Alpha Fetoprotein, 323

Neural Tube Defects, 325
Abdominal Wall Defects, 328
Amniotic Band Syndrome, 331
Ectopia Cordis, 331

24 Genetic Testing, 338

Maternal Serum Screening, 339
Genetic Testing, 340
Chromosomal Anomalies, 341

25 Fetal Anomaly, 354

Fetal Brain, 355
Fetal Face, 359
Fetal Thorax, 360
Fetal Abdomen, 362
Fetal Skeleton, 365
VACTERL Association, 370

26 Abnormal Fetal Echocardiography, 376

Risk Factors That Indicate Fetal
Echocardiography, 377
Fetal Rhythm Irregularities, 378
Congenital Heart Anomalies, 380

PART IV
SUPERFICIAL STRUCTURES

27 Breast Mass, 393

Breast, 395
Cystic Masses, 398
Benign Neoplasms, 401
Breast Cancer, 403
Metastases, 407
Augmentation, 408
Inflammation, 408
Hematoma, 411
Male Breast Diseases, 411

28 Scrotal Mass, 419

Scrotum, 420
Extratesticular Mass, 421
Cysts of the Scrotum, 421
Calcifications, 424
Intratesticular Mass, 426
Testicular Trauma, 430

29 Neck Mass, 439

Thyroid Gland, 440
Parathyroid Gland, 444

Lymph Nodes, 445
Other Neck Masses, 446

30 Elevated Prostate Specific Antigen, 451

Prostate, 452

PART V
MISCELLANEOUS

31 Hip Dysplasia, 461

Anatomy of the Hip, 462
Developmental Dysplasis of the Hip, 462
Sonographic Evaluation of Infant Hips, 463
Treatment, 467

32 Neonatal Neurosonography, 470

Neonatal Head, 471
Intracranial Hemorrhage, 472
Periventricular Leukomalacia, 474
Cerebral Edema, 475
Hydrocephalus, 476
Congenital Malformations, 477
Infant Spine, 482
Tethered Cord, 484

33 Carotid Artery Disease, 491

Normal Anatomy, 492
Sonographic Imaging Techniques, 492
Doppler Imaging: Spectral Analysis, 494
Color Doppler, 494
Carotid Artery Stenosis, 495
Carotid Artery Occlusion, 497
Subclavian Steal, 498
Carotid Dissection, 498
Fibromuscular Dysplasia, 499

34 Leg Pain, 502

Normal Vascular Anatomy, 504
Arterial Disease, 506
Other Arterial Occlusive Diseases, 509
Venous Disease, 509

Answers to Case Studies, 516

I

ABDOMEN

Right Upper Quadrant Pain

CHARLOTTE HENNINGSEN and GREGORY LOGSDON

CLINICAL SCENARIO

◼ A 72-year-old man is seen by his physician with right upper quadrant pain, nausea and vomiting, and unexplained weight loss. The patient has a positive Murphy's sign on clinical examination, and a right upper quadrant ultrasound is ordered. The sonographic examination results reveal a thick-walled gallbladder with a 3.5-cm cauliflower-shaped mass projecting into the gallbladder in the fundal region (Fig. 1-1, *A* and *B*). A layering of low-level echoes also is identified in the dependent portion of the gallbladder and moves slowly with a change in patient position. The common bile duct measures 4 mm. The sonographer also identifies two hyperechoic lesions in the liver (Fig. 1-1, *C*). What is the most likely diagnosis for this patient?

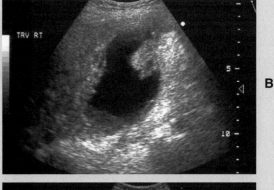

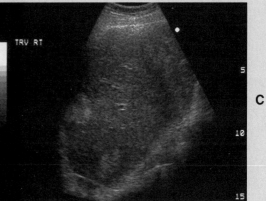

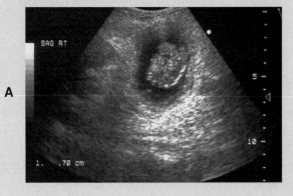

Fig. 1-1 **A,** Cauliflower-shaped mass protrudes from, **B,** fundus of gallbladder. **C,** In addition, two hyperechoic lesions are identified in liver.

OBJECTIVES

◼ Describe the sonographic appearance of common gallbladder disease.

◼ List the risk factors associated with gallbladder disease.

◼ Identify laboratory values specific to gallbladder disease.

◼ Describe the sonographic appearance of liver cysts and abscesses.

◼ List the most common causes of abscess development in the liver.

◼ Describe the sonographic appearance of hematomas of the liver.

Right upper quadrant pain is a common clinical problem. The causes of right upper quadrant pain include cholelithiasis and other gallbladder diseases, although liver diseases and neoplasms (see Chapters 2 and 3) may also be seen with similar symptoms. A thorough clinical examination, laboratory tests, and a right upper quadrant ultrasound may be used to reveal the source of the discomfort. When gallbladder and liver diseases are suspected, the sonographer should take note of specific laboratory findings including bilirubin levels, liver function test results, and white blood cell counts.

In addition to the conditions discussed in this chapter, right-sided pain may also be associated with diseases of the kidney (see Chapters 5, 6, and 7), the pancreas (see Chapter 4), and the gastrointestinal (GI) tract.

GALLBLADDER
Normal Sonographic Anatomy

The gallbladder is a teardrop-shaped structure that is responsible for the concentration and storage of bile. The normal gallbladder is 7 to 10 cm in length and 3 to 4 cm in diameter. The lumen of the gallbladder is anechoic in normal circumstances, and the gallbladder wall appears thin and smooth, with a measurement of less than 3 mm in thickness (Fig. 1-2).[1] A sonographic evaluation of the gallbladder should also include an evaluation of the bile ducts. The common bile duct (Fig. 1-3, *A*) should measure 6 mm, and the common hepatic duct should measure less than 4 mm. The common bile duct size may be increased in patients who have undergone a cholecystectomy and in older individuals.[1]

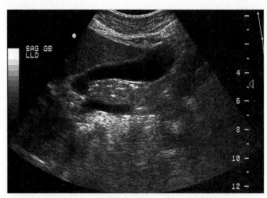

Fig. 1-2   Normal gallbladder is identified in 30-year-old woman with epigastric pain.

Cholelithiasis

Cholelithiasis, also known as *gallstones*, is the most common disease of the gallbladder. Gallstones are usually composed of cholesterol, although stones may be made up of pigment or a mixed composition. A predisposition for gallstone formation is seen in patients with impaired gallbladder motility and bile stasis. The typical patient has the five *f*s: fat, female, forty, fertile, and flatulent. Other risk factors that predispose the patient to the development of gallstones include diet-induced weight loss, pregnancy (Fig. 1-4), **total parenteral nutrition** (TPN), **diabetes,** estrogen use, oral contraceptive use, hemolytic diseases, and white or Hispanic race. Cholelithiasis has also been identified in both genders, in childhood, and in the fetus. Furthermore, a decrease in gallbladder symptoms has been associated with coffee consumption because coffee stimulates the release of cholecystokinin,

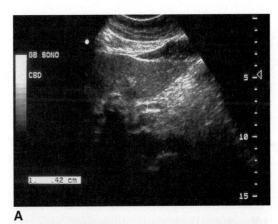

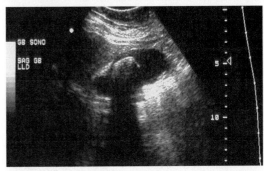

Fig. 1-3 In 40-year-old woman with pain after eating, **A,** common bile duct is within normal limits, but, **B,** gallbladder contains multiple large gallstones.

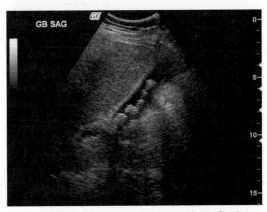

Fig. 1-4 Multiple gallstones are identified in pregnant patient with right upper quadrant pain. (Courtesy Lori Davis and Natalie Cauffman, Florida Hospital Deland.)

encourages the contractility of the gallbladder, and may increase the motility of the colon.[2]

Most individuals with cholelithiasis are asymptomatic. Symptoms of cholelithiasis include right upper quadrant pain, especially after meals (Fig. 1-3, *B*), and patients may also have increased symptoms after a meal high in fat. Other symptoms include epigastric pain,

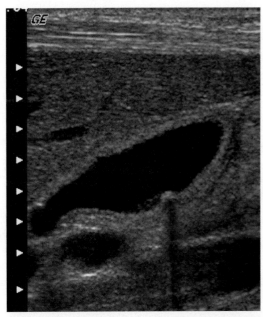

Fig. 1-5 Small echogenic focus with shadowing is noted in gallbladder. (Courtesy GE Medical Systems.)

nausea and vomiting, and pain that radiates to the shoulder.

Sonographic Findings. Gallstones appear sonographically as an echogenic focus (Fig. 1-5) or as multiple echogenic foci that shadow and move. The imaging protocol should include two patient positions (i.e., supine and decubitus) to document the movement of the stones.

Sludge

Sludge, also referred to as *echogenic bile,* frequently occurs from bile stasis. This condition can occur with prolonged fasting or hyperalimentation therapy and with obstruction of the gallbladder. The clinical significance of this finding is unclear.

Sonographic Findings. The sonographic appearance of sludge is that of low- to medium-level echoes within the gallbladder (Fig. 1-6) that are nonshadowing, layer, and move slowly with a change in patient position from the viscous nature. Sludge may be identified in conjunction with cholelithiasis, cholecystitis, and other biliary diseases, including gallbladder carcinoma.

Cholecystitis

Cholecystitis is an inflammation of the gallbladder that can have many forms: acute or chronic, calculous or acalculous.

Acute Cholecystitis. The most common cause of acute cholecystitis is cholelithiasis that creates a cystic

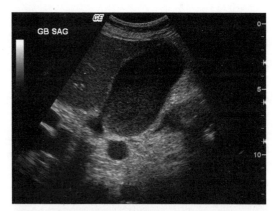

Fig. 1-6 Gallbladder is filled with sludge. (Courtesy Lori Davis and Natalie Cauffman, Florida Hospital Deland.)

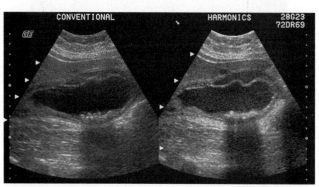

Fig. 1-8 Note thickened gallbladder wall, sludge, and cholelithisis identified in patient with acute cholecystitis. (Courtesy GE Medical Systems.)

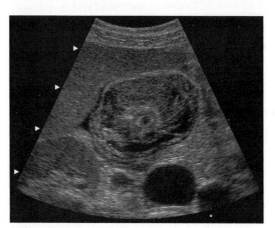

Fig. 1-7 Patient with acute cholecystitis had grossly thickened gallbladder wall and pericholecystic fluid. (Courtesy GE Medical Systems.)

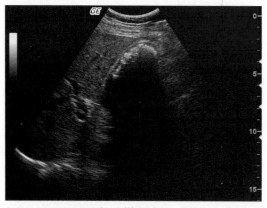

Fig. 1-9 Contracted gallbladder filled with stones. (Courtesy Lori Davis and Natalie Cauffman, Florida Hospital Deland.)

duct obstruction.[3] Because of the high prevalence of associated cholelithiasis, acute cholecystitis is more common in female patients. Clinical symptoms include right upper quadrant pain, fever, and **leukocytosis.** Serious complications can occur in patients with acute cholecystitis, including empyema, gangrenous cholecystitis, emphysematous cholecystitis, and gallbladder rupture.

Acalculous cholecystitis (ACC) is an acute inflammation of the gallbladder in the absence of cholelithiasis (Fig. 1-7). The etiology is multifactorial, and patients include those with TPN, postoperative patients, and trauma and burn patients. ACC is more common in male patients.[4]

Sonographic findings. The sonographic findings (Fig. 1-8) associated with acute cholecystitis usually include cholelithiasis. Other findings include a thickened gallbladder wall, a sonographic **Murphy's sign,** sludge, pericholecystic fluid, and an enlarged gallbladder.

Chronic Cholecystitis. Chronic cholecystitis occurs from multiple attacks of acute cholecystitis and results in fibrosis across the gallbladder wall. Patients may have transient biliary colic but usually lack the acute tenderness identified in patients with acute cholecystitis.

Sonographic findings. The sonographic findings suggestive of chronic cholecystitis include gallbladder wall thickening and cholelithiasis. The WES sign (Wall, Echo, Shadow) is described as a contracted gallbladder and the presence of gallstones (Fig. 1-9) and may be identified in association with chronic cholecystitis and cholelithiasis.

Emphysematous Cholecystitis. Emphysematous cholecystitis is a complication of acute cholecystitis in which gas invades the gallbladder wall and lumen and may also be present in the biliary ducts. Emphysematous cholecystitis occurs with ischemia of the gallbladder wall and subsequent bacterial invasion. As many as 50% of patients with acute emphysematous

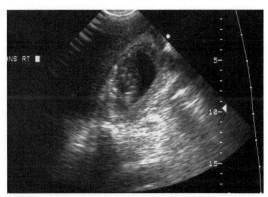

Fig. 1-10 Comet-tail artifacts emanate from lumen and wall of emphysematous gallbladder.

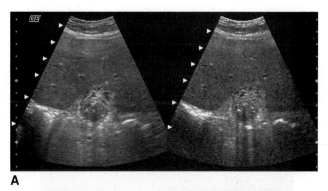

A

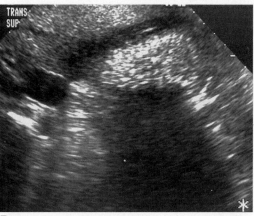

B

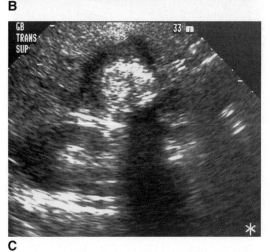

C

Fig. 1-11 **A,** Grossly abnormal gallbladder is seen in patient with gangrenous cholecystitis. **B** and **C,** This 34-year-old woman had gangrenous cholecystitis develop after severe attack of acute cholecystitis precipitated by cholelithiasis. Longitudinal and transverse images show grossly edematous gallbladder wall, intraluminal echoes, and shadowing. (**A** Courtesy GE Medical Systems.)

cholecystitis have diabetes, and 50% or less have cholelithiasis.[5] Complications of emphysematous cholecystitis include the development of gangrene of the gallbladder and gallbladder rupture.

Sonographic findings. The ultrasound appearance of emphysematous cholecystitis includes air in the gallbladder wall and lumen (Fig. 1-10). Air may be seen as increased echogenicity with or without reverberation artifact.

Gangrenous Cholecystitis. Another complication of acute cholecystitis is gangrenous cholecystitis (Fig. 1-11), which carries an increase in morbidity and mortality and may lead to gallbladder perforation. The gallbladder wall is thickened and edematous, with focal areas of **exudate,** hemorrhage, and necrosis. Patients more commonly have generalized abdominal pain rather than a positive Murphy's sign.[6]

Sonographic findings. The sonographic appearance of gangrenous cholecystitis includes focal thickening of the gallbladder wall, striations across the gallbladder wall (Fig. 1-12), intraluminal echoes, and intraluminal membranes. Pericholecystic fluid may be present, as may cholelithiasis, which is often associated with gangrenous cholecystitis.

Gallbladder Perforation. Gallbladder perforation is a complication of acute cholecystitis that may develop within a few days to several weeks after the onset of the symptoms of the acute gallbladder inflammation. Perforation usually occurs in the gallbladder fundus after cystic duct obstruction, gallbladder distention, and resultant ischemia and necrosis.[7]

Risk factors for gallbladder rupture include gallstones, infection, diabetes, trauma, malignant disease, drugs, **angiitis,** and **atherosclerosis.** Clinical presentation may reveal abdominal pain, leukocytosis, and fever, and the mortality rate is as high as 24%.[7]

Sonographic findings. The sonographic findings of gallbladder perforation may include cholelithiasis, gallbladder wall thickening, intraluminal debris, and ascites. In addition, sonographic visualization of the

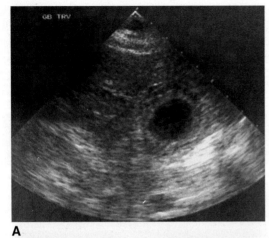

A

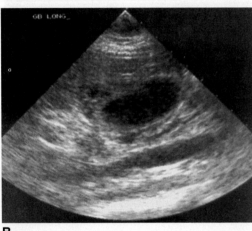

B

Fig. 1-12 **A** and **B,** Note striated, thickened gallbladder wall and low-level echoes shown within gallbladder lumen.

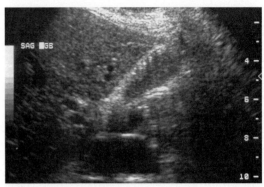

Fig. 1-13 Comet-tail artifacts are seen emanating from gallbladder wall. Lack of comet-tail artifact from within lumen differentiates hyperplastic cholecystosis from emphysematous cholecystitis.

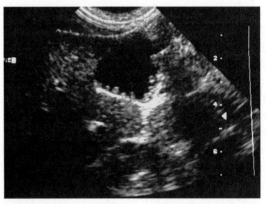

Fig. 1-14 Note multiple polypoid lesions in gallbladder wall, an incidental finding in patient for renal ultrasound.

gallbladder may reveal the actual perforation site in the gallbladder wall (described as the "hole sign"), pericholecystic abscess, and gallstones free-floating in ascites that surrounds the liver.[7]

Hyperplastic Cholecystosis

Hyperplastic cholecystosis describes a group of proliferative and degenerative conditions that affect the gallbladder. The incidence of hyperplastic cholecystosis is increased in female patients. These benign conditions include adenomyomatosis and cholesterolosis.

Adenomyomatosis. Adenomyomatosis of the gallbladder occurs with diffuse or localized hyperplasia of the gallbladder mucosa that extends into the muscular layer and results in mucosal diverticula, known as Rokitansky-Aschoff sinuses.[8] Adenomyomatosis may be asymptomatic or may be seen with symptoms similar to those of gallstones.

Sonographic findings. Adenomyomatosis may appear sonographically as anechoic or echogenic foci within the gallbladder wall corresponding with the Rokitansky-Aschoff sinuses. Shadowing or comet-tail artifact (Fig. 1-13) may be seen emanating from the diverticula, and gallbladder wall thickening may also be noted. Adenomyomatosis may also be seen in association with cholelithiasis.[9]

Cholesterolosis. Cholesterolosis is characterized by the deposition of cholesterol across the gallbladder wall and is also referred to as a *strawberry gallbladder* because of the appearance of the cholesterol deposits within the gallbladder mucosa. This condition may be localized or diffuse and is associated with cholelithiasis.

Sonographic findings. Cholesterolosis may present sonographically as multiple small cholesterol polyps that arise from the gallbladder wall (Fig. 1-14). These polypoid lesions do not shadow or move with variation in patient position. Comet-tail artifacts may also be identified emanating from the cholesterol polyps and may be indistinguishable sonographically from adenomyomatosis. **Gallbladder polyps** may also occur in isolation, and when they are small, they are insignificant.

Gallbladder Carcinoma

Carcinoma of the gallbladder is the most common cancer of the biliary tract, and most tumors occur in the gallbladder fundus. Most gallbladder cancers are classified as adenocarcinoma. The etiology is unclear; however, risk factors include gallstones, chronic cholecystitis, **porcelain gallbladder,** exposure to carcinogens, and some blood groups. Gallbladder carcinoma is also more common in female patients and in older persons.

The clinical symptoms are nonspecific in the early stages and may mimic benign gallbladder disease. Patients may have weight loss, **anorexia,** right upper quadrant pain, jaundice, nausea and vomiting, and hepatomegaly. Late diagnosis is more common, which speaks to the poor prognosis of this malignant disease for which the mean survival rate is 6 months.[10]

Sonographic Findings. The sonographic findings of gallbladder carcinoma (Fig. 1-15) include an inhomogeneous, polypoid lesion with irregular margins; localized wall thickening; a mass that replaces the gallbladder; and calcification of the gallbladder wall. Associated gallstones may be visualized as may metastatic lesions within the liver, ascites, and intraductal biliary dilation. Color Doppler imaging may be used to differentiate biliary sludge, which is avascular, from a hypoechoic mass, which would show flow.[11]

See Table 1-1 for a listing of gallbladder pathology, symptoms, and sonographic findings.

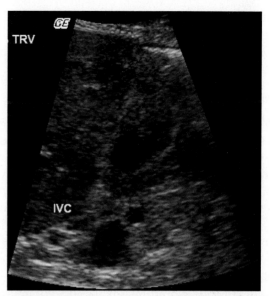

Fig. 1-15 Irregular mass is seen in gallbladder fundus. (Courtesy Lori Davis and Natalie Cauffman, Florida Hospital Deland.)

BILIARY TRACT DISEASE
Choledocholithiasis

Choledocholithiasis describes stones that are located in the bile ducts. This condition usually occurs with the migration of gallstones into the common duct. When obstruction of the duct occurs, the patient has jaundice and an elevated bilirubin level. Patients may also have right upper quadrant pain.

Table 1-1	*Diseases of the Gallbladder*	
Pathology	**Symptoms**	**Sonographic Findings**
Cholelithiasis	Asymptomatic, right upper quadrant pain, pain after fatty meals, epigastric pain, nausea and vomiting	Echogenic foci that shadow and move
Cholecystitis	Right upper quadrant pain, fever	Thickened gallbladder wall; gallstones and sludge may be seen; WES sign
Adenomyomatosis	Asymptomatic, right upper quadrant pain	Anechoic or echogenic foci in gallbladder wall; wall thickening or comet-tail or shadow artifacts may be seen
Cholesterolosis	Asymptomatic, right upper quadrant pain	Multiple polypoid lesions in gallbladder wall; comet-tail artifact may be seen
Adenocarcinoma	Right upper quadrant pain, weight loss, anorexia, jaundice, nausea and vomiting, hepatomegaly	Irregular polypoid mass, localized wall thickening, calcification of gallbladder wall

Sonographic Findings. The sonographic findings of choledocholithiasis include echogenic foci that shadow within the duct (Fig. 1-16, *A*) with or without ductal dilation (Fig. 1-16, *B*).

Cholangiocarcinoma

Cholangiocarcinoma is a rare malignant disease that can occur anywhere along the biliary tract, although it most commonly occurs in the perihilar region (Klatskin's tumor). In the United States, cholangiocarcinoma occurs in 1 in 100,000 and increases in frequency with increasing age. Cholangiocarcinoma is classified as adenocarcinoma in 95% of cases.[12] Risk factors include exposure to radionuclides and chemical carcinogens and some biliary tract diseases, including sclerosing cholangitis and choledochal cyst.

The clinical symptoms of cholangiocarcinoma include painless jaundice, which is the most common presentation, and **pruritus**, abdominal pain, anorexia, malaise, and weight loss. Gallstones and intrahepatic stones may also be identified with cholangiocarcinoma.

Pertinent laboratory findings include elevated bilirubin level, abnormal liver function test results, and a positive **carcinoembryonic antigen** (CEA). Many patients are not candidates for surgical resection at the time of diagnosis because of extensive vascular involvement, and treatment may only be **palliative** and may focus on relief of obstruction. The prognosis depends on the stage of the disease at the time of diagnosis but overall is considered poor.[12]

Sonographic Findings. The sonographic evaluation of cholangiocarcinoma may reveal a liver mass or a mass arising from within the ducts (Fig. 1-17). Intrahepatic biliary tract dilation may also be identified in the absence of extrahepatic dilation. Sonographic imaging may show a mass disrupting the union of the right and left hepatic ducts (Fig. 1-18), and the gallbladder may be collapsed.

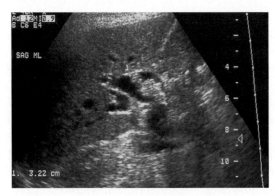

Fig. 1-17 Irregular, echogenic mass is arising within common bile duct of 95-year-old woman with prior history of cholecystectomy and current history of jaundice. Intrahepatic ductal dilation was also identified.

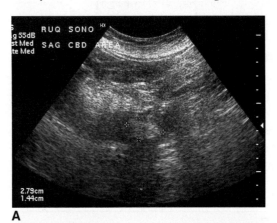

A

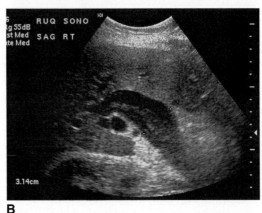

B

Fig. 1-16 Echogenic focus, with, **A,** shadowing, is visualized within, **B,** dilated common bile duct (CBD) of patient with history of cholecystectomy and right upper quadrant pain. Biliary sludge is also seen layering within dilated CBD.

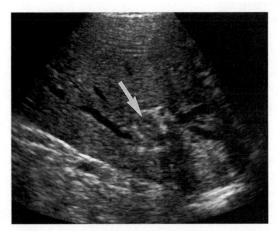

Fig. 1-18 Cholangiocarcinoma. Transverse scan at level of porta hepatis reveals intrahepatic dilation of right and left bile ducts. Poorly defined isoechoic mass *(arrow)* is causing obstruction.

Cholangitis

Cholangitis is defined as inflammation of the bile ducts. Cholangitis may be classified as Oriental cholangitis, which may be identified in the United States with increasing immigration; sclerosing cholangitis, which may be associated with ulcerative colitis; AIDS cholangitis; and acute obstructive suppurative cholangitis. Depending on the type of cholangitis, the cause may be ductal strictures, parasitic infestation, bacterial infection, stones, or neoplasm. Clinical symptoms include fever, abdominal pain, and jaundice.

Sonographic Findings. The sonographic findings of cholangitis (Fig. 1-19, *A* and *B*) include biliary duct dilation and thickening of the walls of the ducts.

See Table 1-2 for a listing of biliary tract pathology, symptoms, and sonographic findings.

LIVER
Normal Sonographic Anatomy

The liver is located in the right upper quadrant and extends partially into the left upper quadrant. Normal liver parenchyma should appear homogeneous and display midlevel echogenicity (Fig. 1-20, *A*). When compared with the renal parenchyma, normal liver parenchyma appears hyperechoic or isoechoic (Fig. 1-20, *B*), and when compared with the pancreas, the liver appears hypoechoic or isoechoic. Within the parenchyma, tubular structures corresponding to veins, arteries, and ducts can also be visualized. The normal size of the liver is 15 to 20 cm in length at the midclavicular line.[1]

Abscess

Liver abscess is associated with an increased incidence of morbidity and mortality. Hepatic abscess may be bacterial (pyogenic) in origin or the result of a parasite. In addition, the candidal fungus can also affect the liver, especially in patients with immunocompromised conditions.

The liver may also be infected by the *Echinococcus* tapeworm, which is more common where sheep herding is prevalent. Hepatic echinococcosis is an inflammatory cystic reaction that may present as a cystic or complex

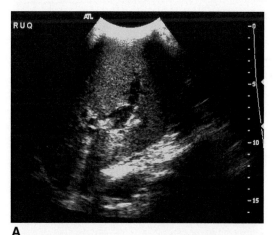

A

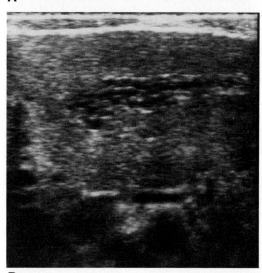

B

Fig. 1-19   A, Ultrasound findings of dilated ducts with thickened walls and intraductal stones in 67-year-old man with history of sclerosing cholangitis and, **B,** AIDS cholangitis. Transverse scan through left lobe of liver shows irregular thickening of walls of intrahepatic bile ducts.

Table 1-2	*Diseases of the Biliary Tract*	
Pathology	**Symptoms**	**Sonographic Findings**
Choledocholithiasis	Right upper quadrant pain, jaundice	Echogenic foci that shadow in ducts; with or without ductal dilation
Cholangiocarcinoma	Painless jaundice, pruritus, abdominal pain, anorexia, malaise, weight loss	Liver mass, mass within ducts, intrahepatic ductal dilation
Cholangitis	Fever, abdominal pain, jaundice	Biliary ductal dilation, thickening of ductal walls

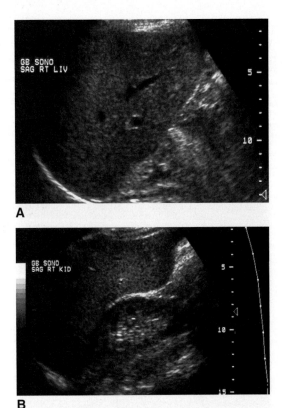

A

B

Fig. 1-20 Normal liver shows, **A,** typical homogeneous texture and, **B,** comparative echogenicity of liver to kidney, which may be hyperechoic or isoechoic to the kidney.

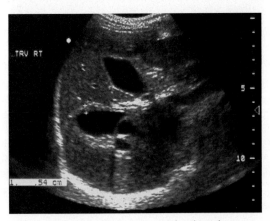

Fig. 1-21 Thick-walled cyst with daughter cysts is identified in patient with abdominal pain.

lesion (Fig. 1-21). Some causes of inflammatory reactions of the liver, including amebiasis and *Echinococcus*, are not endemic to the United States; however, patients who have traveled to affected areas and immigrants from endemic populations may have these uncommon lesions.

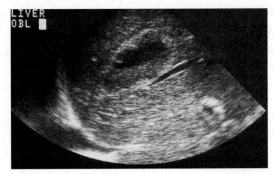

Fig. 1-22 Thick-walled abscess shows fluid-debris level.

Pyogenic Abscess. Pyogenic abscess or bacterial abscess is responsible for 8 to 20 of 100,000 hospitalizations each year.[13] These pus-containing lesions are most commonly the result of biliary tract disease but are also associated with spread from an infection via the hepatic artery or portal vein and with trauma or surgery. Cirrhosis, neoplasm, and sickle cell anemia can also predispose a patient to abscess formation. The most common organisms identified in pyogenic abscesses are *Escherichia coli* and *Klebsiella pneumoniae*.[13]

Pyogenic abscesses are multiple in approximately 50% of patients. A solitary hepatic abscess is more common in the right lobe of the liver, but multiple abscesses may be identified in both lobes.[14] Symptoms include fever, jaundice, and right upper quadrant pain. Patients may also have nausea and vomiting, anorexia, and fatigue. Liver function test results are usually elevated but nonspecific, and most patients will have leukocytosis. Diagnostic procedures may include aspiration of the purulent material for microscopic evaluation that may be performed with ultrasound guidance. Prompt diagnosis and treatment is essential because untreated pyogenic abscesses are virtually uniformly lethal.[13]

Sonographic findings. The sonographic appearances of abscesses are variable in size, number, and appearance. They can appear complex or hypoechoic and can show a fluid-debris level (Fig. 1-22). They are typically round or ovoid with irregular walls. Artifacts of enhancement or shadowing (if gas is present) may also be identified.

Amebic Abscess. Amebiasis is caused by the protozoan parasite *Entamoeba histolytica*, which is endemic to parts of Mexico, Central America, South America, India, and Africa. Amebiasis most commonly involves the GI tract and may be asymptomatic. Dissemination outside the GI tract most commonly involves the liver through the portal vein, where ischemia and resultant hepatic necrosis lead to abscess formation; however, spread to the brain and lungs may also occur.[15]

The clinical presentation of hepatic amebic abscess includes right upper quadrant pain, hepatomegaly, fever, and diarrhea. Liver function test results are nonspecific, and laboratory test results may also reveal leukocytosis. Amebic abscesses are more common in male patients and are more commonly identified in the right lobe of the liver.[15] Amebiasis is usually treated medically with metronidazole; however, chloroquine and iodoquinol may also be administered. Aspiration for diagnostic and therapeutic purposes may be used in those patients with resistance to medical treatment. The mortality rate without treatment is high because of abscess rupture.[15]

Sonographic findings. The sonographic evaluation of hepatic amebiasis may reveal multiple, hypoechoic lesions (Fig. 1-23). The lesions may be round or oval with irregular walls (Fig. 1-24). Fluid-debris levels and acoustic enhancement may also be seen. Amebic abscess may not be differentiated sonographically from pyogenic abscess, echinococcal cysts, or necrotic neoplasm; therefore, clinical correlation is paramount in an accurate diagnosis.

Cysts

Hepatic cysts of the liver may be congenital or acquired. Congenital cysts of the liver are lined with epithelium and are ductal in origin. Autosomal dominant polycystic kidney disease (ADPKD) is an inherited disorder that leads to renal failure. Liver cysts are frequently identified in addition to the renal findings in patients with ADPKD; however, these liver cysts do not affect liver function.

Acquired cysts of the liver are not true cysts and may be the result of trauma, parasitic or pyogenic abscesses, or necrotic neoplasm.

Sonographic Findings. The ultrasound diagnosis of a simple cyst rests on certain criteria. The cyst should be anechoic, smooth walled, and round or oval and have posterior enhancement (Fig. 1-25, *A*). Cysts may be solitary or multiple (especially when associated with ADPKD) and vary greatly in size (Fig. 1-25, *B*). Cysts of the liver are commonly asymptomatic and incidental findings.

Hematoma

Hematomas of the liver may be classified as subcapsular or intrahepatic and are usually the result of trauma. Hematomas may result from hemorrhage within a neoplasm and may also be a rare complication of pregnancy associated with preeclampsia and hemolysis, elevated liver enzymes, and low platelet count (HELLP) syndrome. Patients with hematomas of the liver may

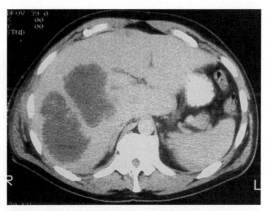

Fig. 1-23   Multiple, amebic abscesses appeared iso-echoic to liver on sonographic examination. Computed tomographic scan fully shows extensiveness of abscess formation.

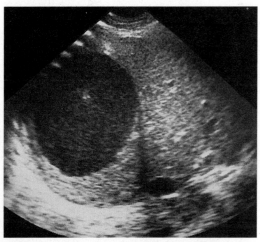

Fig. 1-24   Amebic liver abscess—classic morphology. Transverse sonogram shows well-defined oval subdiaphragmatic mass increased through transmission. Uniform low-level internal echoes and absence of well-defined wall are seen.

have hepatomegaly and right upper quadrant pain. Hypotension and a decreased hematocrit may indicate a severe hemorrhage.[16]

Sonographic Findings. The ultrasound appearance of hematomas (Fig. 1-26) varies depending on the age of the bleed. An acute process will usually be echogenic in appearance and will eventually become cystic, although septations may be visualized in a resolving hematoma. A subcapsular hematoma may also have varying echogenicity and will usually be comma shaped. Serial ultrasounds may be used to show resolution of these lesions.

See Table 1-3 for a listing of liver lesion pathology, symptoms, and sonographic findings.

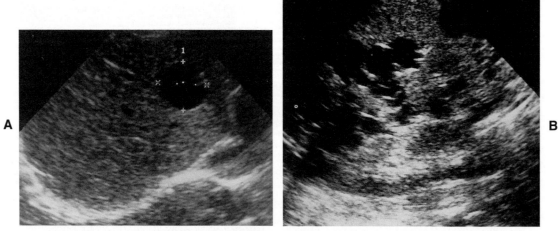

Fig. 1-25 **A,** Simple hepatic cyst shows smooth, uniform borders and no internal echoes (anechoic). **B,** Polycystic liver disease shows multiple cysts throughout liver and kidney.

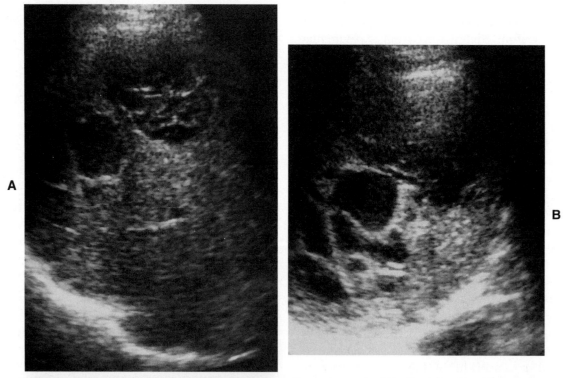

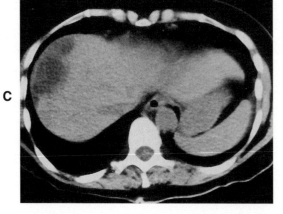

Fig. 1-26 Hepatic trauma. **A** and **B,** Complex mass was found in right lobe of liver in patient who had been in car accident. **C,** Computed tomographic scan of 54-year-old woman shows collection of blood in right lateral border of liver.

Table 1-3	*Lesions of the Liver*	
Pathology	Symptoms	Sonographic Findings
Abscess	Right upper quadrant pain, fever, jaundice, nausea and vomiting, anorexia, fatigue	Round or oval; hypoechoic lesion; fluid-debris level; complex, irregular wall; with or without enhancement
Cysts	Asymptomatic, pain when cysts are large	Round or oval; anechoic, thin-walled, posterior enhancement
Hematoma	Right upper quadrant pain, hepatomegaly	Echogenic to cystic, septations

SUMMARY

Multiple causes exist for right upper quadrant pain, including a variety of diseases of the liver and gallbladder. Clinical examination, laboratory tests, and imaging procedures, including ultrasound, can assist with an accurate diagnosis so that an appropriate treatment plan can be implemented.

CLINICAL SCENARIO—DIAGNOSIS

■ The large, irregular polypoid mass suggests gallbladder cancer. The echogenic lesions in the liver further cement the diagnosis and point to metastatic disease. Sludge is also seen within the gallbladder, and the normal common bile duct confirms that the malignant disease does not obstruct the biliary tract.

CASE STUDIES FOR DISCUSSION

1. A 45-year-old man is seen with epigastric pain of 3 weeks' duration. A right upper quadrant ultrasound reveals multiple, small, polypoid lesions that arise from the gallbladder wall (Fig. 1-27, *A* and *B*). The remainder of the sonographic examination is unremarkable. Subsequent investigation of the GI tract reveals gastroenteritis. What is the most likely diagnosis for the finding in the gallbladder?

2. A 68-year-old woman is seen with right upper quadrant pain. The ultrasound examination reveals a distended gallbladder with a wall thickness of 1.8 mm. The gallbladder contains low-level echoes that layer and are gravity dependent and multiple, small echogenic foci that shadow (Fig. 1-28, *A* and *B*). The common bile duct measures 10 mm and also contains a small echogenic focus (Fig. 1-28, *C*) in its distal aspect. What is the most likely diagnosis?

3. A 49-year-old woman is seen at an emergency room with epigastric pain of 1 day's duration, nausea and vomiting, and an elevated temperature. The sonographic examination reveals a thick-walled gallbladder and evidence of gallstones (Fig. 1-29, *A* and *B*). What is the most likely diagnosis?

4. A 36-year-old man is seen with right upper quadrant pain, diarrhea, and fever. Interrogation of history and symptoms reveals that the patient recently returned from a 2-week

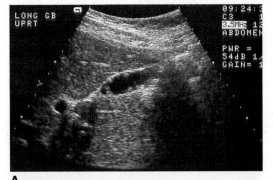

A

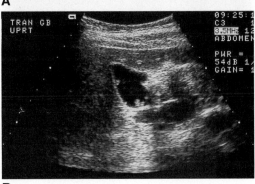

B

Fig. 1-27   Multiple polypoid lesions arising from gallbladder wall are shown in, **A,** longitudinal and, **B,** transverse images.

CASE STUDIES FOR DISCUSSION—cont'd

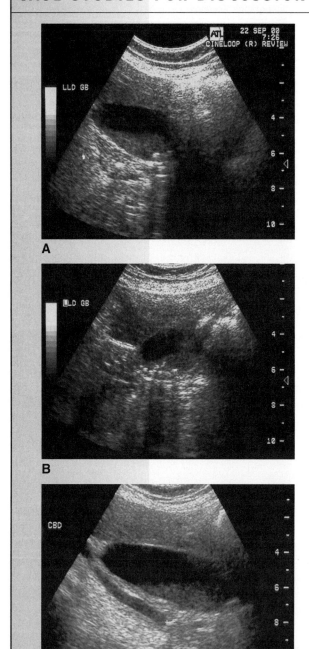

A

B

C

Fig. 1-28 **A,** Longitudinal and, **B,** transverse images of gallbladder show low-level echoes that layer and are gravity dependent in addition to multiple echogenic foci that shadow. **C,** Common bile duct also shows small echogenic focus with shadowing.

business trip in South America. A sonographic examination of the right upper quadrant reveals a 3-cm mass in the right lobe of the liver that appears to be isoechoic to the liver, with a surrounding hypoechoic halo. Acoustic enhancement posterior to the mass is also shown (Fig. 1-30, *A* and *B*). What is the most likely diagnosis?

5. A 64-year-old man undergoes an ultrasound for right-sided pain to rule out gallbladder disease. The patient also has a history of ADPKD and bilateral nephrectomy. Sonographic examination of the right upper quadrant reveals a normal gallbladder and multiple thin-walled, anechoic structures within the liver (Fig. 1-31). This would be most consistent with what diagnosis?

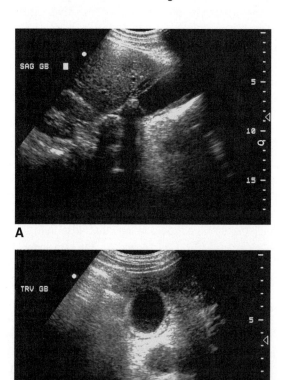

A

B

Fig. 1-29 Thickened gallbladder wall and multiple echogenic foci with shadowing are shown in the longitudinal image **(A)**. The transverse image **(B)** also demonstrates the thickened wall.

CASE STUDIES FOR DISCUSSION—cont'd

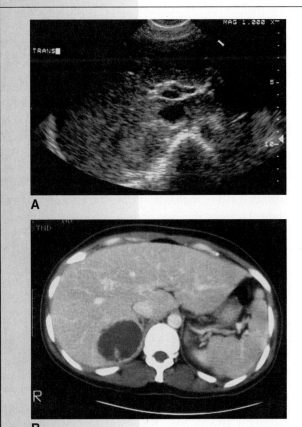

A

B

Fig. 1-30 Sonographic findings are shown in, **A,** right lobe of liver, and, **B,** correlating computed tomographic image also shows lesion.

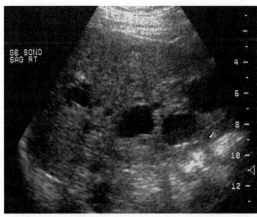

Fig. 1-31 Sonographic findings identified in patient with history of autosomal dominant polycystic kidney disease.

STUDY QUESTIONS

1. A 40-year-old obese woman undergoes an ultrasound examination of the right upper quadrant. The patient has right upper quadrant pain after a lunch of a hamburger and fries. Sonographic investigation reveals two echogenic foci within the gallbladder that shadow and are gravity dependent. What is the most likely diagnosis?
   a. cholecystitis
   b. cholelithiasis
   c. cholesterolosis
   d. gallbladder carcinoma
   e. sludge

2. A 73-year-old woman has right upper quadrant pain, nausea and vomiting, and weight loss. Her physician also notes that the whites of her eyes are yellow and orders an ultrasound of the gallbladder to rule out which of the following?
   a. amebiasis
   b. adenomyomatosis
   c. choledocholithiasis
   d. cholelithiasis
   e. gallbladder carcinoma

3. A 52-year-old man with diabetes is seen with signs and symptoms of severe, acute cholecystitis. The ultrasound findings reveal a gallbladder devoid of stones. The gallbladder wall is thickened, and multiple comet-tail artifacts are identified emanating from the wall. The gallbladder lumen contains low-level echoes from which comet-tail artifacts are also seen. What is the most likely diagnosis?
   a. acute cholecystitis
   b. adenomyomatosis

  c. chronic cholecystitis
  d. emphysematous cholecystitis
  e. gallbladder perforation

4. A 33-year-old man with AIDS undergoes an ultrasound for abdominal pain, fever, and jaundice. Sonographic findings reveal dilation of the bile ducts and thickening of the bile duct walls. Based on the patient history, what is the most likely diagnosis?
  a. abscess
  b. acute cholecystitis
  c. cholangitis
  d. gallbladder carcinoma
  e. hematoma

5. A 55-year-old woman is seen with severe right upper quadrant pain and fever and a history of biliary tract disease. Laboratory values reveal elevated liver function tests and leukocytosis. A right upper quadrant ultrasound examination reveals a solitary, hypoechoic lesion in the right lobe of the liver that measures 4.5 cm at its largest diameter. The walls of the lesion appear thickened, and acoustic enhancement is identified posterior to the lesion. This is most consistent with which of the following?
  a. amebic abscess
  b. hemorrhagic cyst
  c. hematoma
  d. hepatoma
  e. pyogenic abscess

6. A solitary, anechoic lesion is identified in the right lobe of a 50-year-old woman. The lesion is 2.5 cm with smooth walls and acoustic enhancement. The patient has mild epigastric pain, especially with spicy foods, and the remainder of the ultrasound examination is unremarkable. The anechoic lesion most likely represents which of the following?
  a. abscess
  b. cholecystitis
  c. hematoma
  d. hepatoma
  e. liver cyst

7. A 32-year-old woman with intermittent pain in the right upper quadrant is seen for an abdominal ultrasound. The ultrasound examination reveals a gallbladder with multiple comet-tail artifacts emanating from the gallbladder wall. The lumen of the gallbladder is anechoic, and the remainder of the examination is unremarkable. This most likely represents which of the following?
  a. adenomyomatosis
  b. cholangitis
  c. cholecystitis
  d. cholelithiasis
  e. cholesterosis

8. A renal ultrasound is ordered for a patient in intensive care with renal failure, TPN, and a long history of hospitalization. During imaging of the right kidney, the sonographer notices that the gallbladder contains low-level echoes that layer and are gravity dependent. This is most consistent with which of the following?
  a. abscess
  b. cholecystitis
  c. cholelithiasis
  d. emphysematous cholecystitis
  e. sludge

9. A 35-year-old man with a history of hepatitis A undergoes an ultrasound of the liver. The ultrasound reveals a hypoechoic liver and hepatomegaly. In addition, multiple, small echogenic foci that shadow and move are seen in the gallbladder. This incidental gallbladder finding is most consistent with which of the following?
  a. adenomyomatosis
  b. cholangitis
  c. cholecystitis
  d. cholelithiasis
  e. cholesterolosis

10. A 74-year-old woman is seen with right upper quadrant pain, jaundice, and nausea and vomiting. Ultrasound of the gallbladder reveals cholelithiasis. In addition, a 3-cm, cauliflower-shaped mass is seen arising from a stalk within the gallbladder fundus. This is most suggestive of which of the following?
  a. abscess
  b. cholecystitis
  c. gallbladder carcinoma
  d. gallbladder perforation
  e. gangrenous cholecystitis

REFERENCES

1. Hagen-Ansert SL: *Textbook of diagnostic ultrasonography*, vol 1, ed 5, St Louis, 2001, Mosby.
2. Leitzmann MF et al: A prospective study of coffee consumption and the risk of symptomatic gallstone disease in men, *JAMA* 281:2106-2112, 1999.
3. Park MS et al: Acute cholecystitis: comparison of MR cholangiography and US, *Radiology* 209:781-785, 1998.
4. Hatada T et al: Acute acalculous cholecystitis in a patient on total parenteral nutrition: case report and review of the Japanese literature, *Hepato-Gastroenterology* 46:2208-2211, 1999.
5. Wu CS, Yao WJ, Hsiao CH: Effervescent gallbladder: sonographic findings in emphysematous cholecystitis, *J Clin Ultrasound* 26:272-275, 1998.
6. Rumack CM, Wilson SR, Charboneau JW: *Diagnostic ultrasound*, vol 1, ed 2, St Louis, 1998, Mosby.
7. Neimatullah MA, Rasuli P, Ashour M et al: Sonographic diagnosis of gallbladder perforation, *J Ultrasound Med* 17:389-391, 1998.
8. Ishizuka D, Shirai Y, Tsukada K et al: Gallbladder cancer with intratumoral anechoic foci: a mimic of adenomyomatosis, *Hepato-Gastroenterology* 45:927-929, 1998.
9. Alberti D, Callea F, Camoni G et al: Adenomyomatosis of the gallbladder in childhood, *J Pediatr Surg* 33:1411-1412, 1998.
10. Szarnecki GM, Karol IG, Khalil H: Gallbladder, carcinoma, http://www.emedicine.com/radio/topic 289.htm, retrieved March 21, 2002.
11. Pandey M et al: Carcinoma of the gallbladder: role of sonography in the diagnosis and staging, *J Clin Ultrasound* 28:227-232, 2000.
12. Ahrendt SA, Nakeeb A, Pitt HA: Cholangiocarcinoma, *Clin Liver Dis* 5:191-218, 2001.
13. Johannsen EC, Sifri CD, Madoff LC: Pyogenic liver abscesses, *Infect Dis Clin North Am* 14:547-563, 2000.
14. Verbanck J, Ponette J, Verbanck M et al: Sonographic detection of multiple *Staphylococcus aureus* hepatic microabscesses mimicking *Candida* abscesses, *J Clin Ultrasound* 27:478-481, 1999.
15. Hoffner RJ, Kilaghbian T, Esekogwu VI et al: Common presentations of amebic liver abscess, *Ann Emerg Med* 34:351-355, 1999.
16. Chan ADS, Gerscovich EO: Imaging of subcapsular hepatic and renal hematomas in pregnancy complicated by preeclampsia and the HELLP syndrome, *J Clin Ultrasound* 27:35-40, 1999.

BIBLIOGRAPHY

Mouratidis B, Antonio G: Sonographic diagnosis of subcapsular liver hematoma mimicking tumor in a neonate, *J Clin Ultrasound* 28:53-57, 2000.

Liver Mass

CHARLOTTE HENNINGSEN

CLINICAL SCENARIO

■ A 35-year-old woman is seen for an ultrasound of the liver. The patient is a sonography student in whom two liver lesions were identified during an abdominal Doppler lab. The patient is in good health, with a history of a hysterectomy 1 year ago for uterine **leiomyomata** and previous long-term use of oral contraceptives.

A right upper quadrant ultrasound reveals a well-defined, echogenic lesion (Fig. 2-1, *A*) in the posterior right lobe of the liver that measures 1.5 cm at the greatest diameter. Also noted is a 5-cm isoechoic, homogeneous lesion in the anterior right lobe (Fig. 2-1) that shows a central vascular scar. What are the possible diagnoses for these lesions

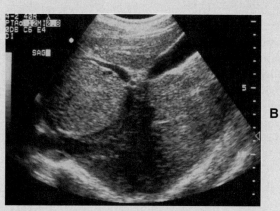

Fig. 2-1 **A** and **B**, A 5-cm isoechoic lesion is identified. Note also, **A**, 1.5-cm hyperechoic lesion seen.

OBJECTIVES

■ Describe the sonographic appearance of the more common benign neoplasms of the liver.

■ Describe the sonographic appearance of the more common malignant neoplasms of the liver.

■ Differentiate the Doppler findings in a variety of neoplasms of the liver.

■ List the risk factors associated with various lesions of the liver.

■ Identify pertinent laboratory values associated with specific neoplasms of the liver.

GLOSSARY OF TERMS

Aflatoxin: a carcinogenic fungus found in grains (corn, wheat) and peanuts

Angiomyolipoma: a tumor comprised of fat, vessels, and muscle tissue that is frequently identified in the kidneys and occurs rarely in the liver

Angiosarcoma: the most common malignant disease of mesenchymal origin in the liver

Anorexia: loss of appetite

Budd-Chiari syndrome: a rare syndrome characterized by the occlusion of the hepatic veins or the inferior vena cava or both

Cholelithiasis: gallstones

Cystadenoma: rare cystic tumor comprised of biliary epithelial cells that may undergo malignant transformation

Diabetes mellitus: a disorder marked by a decrease or lack of secretion of insulin by the pancreas

Epithelioid hemangioendothelioma: a rare malignant vascular tumor of endothelial origin that sonographically appears as multiple hypoechoic lesions in the periphery of the liver

Fibrolamellar carcinoma: a rare malignant neoplasm; occurs in younger patients than does hepatocellular carcinoma; is of hepatocellular origin, although distinct from hepatocellular carcinoma; serum alpha-fetoprotein level is usually normal

Hepatocytes: cells in the parenchyma of the liver that perform the metabolic functions

Kupffer's cells: phagocytic cells in the parenchyma of the liver

Leiomyomata: benign, smooth muscle tumors frequently seen in the uterus; also known as *fibroids*

Lymphangioma: a mass comprised of dilated lymph vessels

Lymphoma: a neoplasm of lymphoid tissue; the liver may be a primary site

Neoplasm: abnormal tissue growth, malignant or benign

Nodular regenerative hyperplasia: a rare benign process of diffuse liver involvement by nodules comprised of hyperplastic hepatocytes; associated with portal hypertension

Tuberous sclerosis: disorder characterized by mental retardation, seizures, and skin lesions; associated with the development of lesions in multiple systems within the body

Von Gierke's disease: an autosomal recessive disease marked by excessive storage of glycogen in the liver, kidneys, and intestinal tract

A sonographic examination of the abdomen that reveals a liver mass may be ordered for many reasons based on patient symptoms and clinical findings. Many benign liver lesions are asymptomatic and are discovered incidentally by the sonographer. The mass may be palpable on clinical examination or present with clinical findings of hepatomegaly, or abnormal laboratory values may warrant further investigation of the liver. Patients may have right upper quadrant pain that, when coupled with symptoms such as weight loss and fever, suggests malignant disease.

In addition to neoplasms of the liver, patients with pain or palpable mass in the right upper quadrant may have biliary disease (see Chapter 1) or a mass in the kidney or adrenal gland (see Chapters 5, 6, 7, and 12). Based on the patient's history and clinical presentation, a thorough sonographic examination of the patient's right upper quadrant should aid in the identification of the origin of the symptom.

LIVER

Normal Sonographic Anatomy

The liver is located in the right upper quadrant and extends partially into the left upper quadrant. Normal liver parenchyma should appear homogeneous and display midlevel echogenicity (Fig. 2-2). When compared with the renal parenchyma, normal liver parenchyma appears hyperechoic or isoechoic, and when compared with the pancreas, the liver appears hypoechoic or isoechoic. Within the parenchyma, tubular structures corresponding to veins, arteries, and ducts can also be visualized. The normal size of the liver is 15 to 20 cm in length at the midclavicular line.[1]

BENIGN NEOPLASMS

Hemangioma

Cavernous hemangioma is the most common benign tumor of the liver. Blood-filled channels comprise these

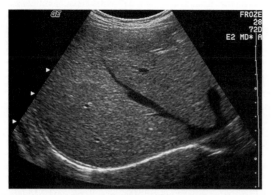

Fig. 2-2 Transverse image of normal liver shows homogeneous texture and hepatic veins. (Courtesy GE Medical Systems.)

well-defined vascular lesions. Hemangiomas occur in approximately 4% of the population,[2] although they have been reported in as many as 20% in an autopsy series.[3] A female prevalence over males of 5:1 exists, and hemangiomas can occur in all age groups.[2,3] Patients are usually asymptomatic, although right upper quadrant pain can occur with hemorrhage or rupture.

Sonographic Findings. The most common appearance of a hemangioma is a well-defined, hyperechoic mass that may be round, oval, or lobulated (Fig. 2-3, *A* and *B*). Acoustic enhancement is frequently seen because of the vascular nature of this lesion. The sonographic appearance of hemangiomas may also be of variable echogenicity dependent on the size of the lesion and the amount of fibrosis and degeneration. Hemangiomas may appear anechoic to echogenic (Fig. 2-3, *C* and *D*) and homogeneous, heterogeneous, or complex and may contain calcifications.[1,3] Color

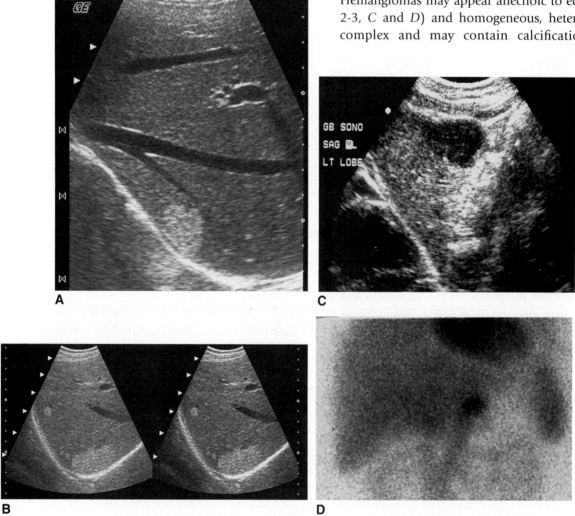

Fig. 2-3 Hemangiomas are usually echogenic. When located near diaphragm, they may be demonstrated in, **A,** mirror artifacts that frequently are seen in this region. **B,** Hemangiomas may be multiple and may enhance. **C,** This hemangioma was hypoechoic to liver, and diagnosis was confirmed with other imaging methods, including, **D,** nuclear medicine examination that showed vascular nature of tumor. (**A** and **B** Courtesy GE Medical Systems.)

Doppler and power Doppler have been of little use in the characterization of hemangiomas.[4,5]

Liver Cell Adenoma

Liver cell adenoma, also known *hepatocellular adenoma*, is a rare tumor, although its incidence has increased since the introduction of oral contraceptives. Liver cell adenoma has also been associated with the use of anabolic steroids and with metabolic diseases, such as type I glycogen storage disease **(von Gierke's disease)** and **diabetes mellitus.** This lesion can also occur as a spontaneous event.[3]

Liver cell adenoma is usually a solitary lesion comprised of hepatocytes that contain fat and glycogen. Large subcapsular vessels increase the chance of a significant hemorrhage, which can lead to death. Patients may have right upper quadrant pain from rupture and bleeding in the tumor. Liver cell adenoma also has a slight potential for malignant transformation.[3]

Sonographic Findings. The most common appearance for a liver cell adenoma (Fig. 2-4) is that of an encapsulated, well-defined lesion that is hyperechoic from the fat content in this tumor. Hemorrhage within the lesion may appear anechoic, hypoechoic, or hyper-

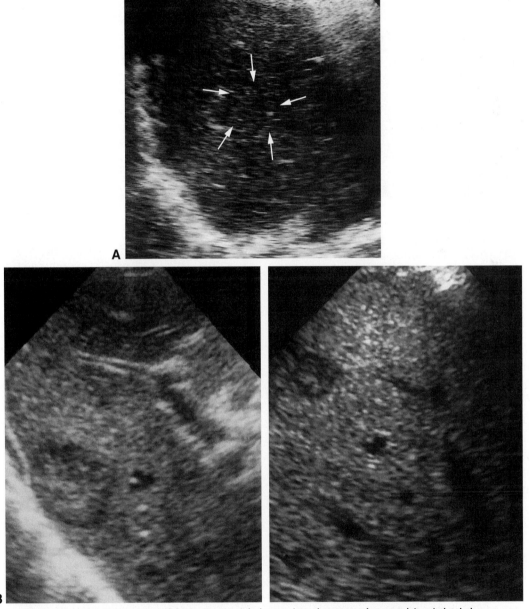

Fig. 2-4   A, A 31-year-old woman with hepatic adenoma *(arrows)* in right lobe. **B,** Hepatic adenoma appears as well-defined lesion with central hyperechoic area surrounded by halo.

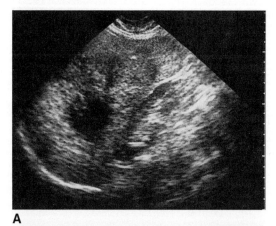

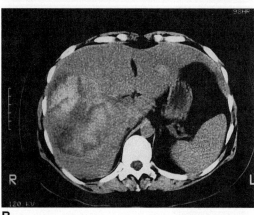

Fig. 2-5 Hemorrhagic adenoma in young woman taking birth control pills with severe right upper quadrant pain. **A,** Sagittal sonogram shows complex, inhomogeneous large right lobe liver mass. Hypoechoic center suggests partial fluid content. **B,** Unenhanced computed tomographic scan confirms large mass and also presence of high-density blood within mass.

echoic (Fig. 2-5). Color Doppler imaging may show the significant peripheral vasculature of this lesion.[3]

Focal Nodular Hyperplasia

Focal nodular hyperplasia (FNH) is the second most common benign liver **neoplasm** after hemangioma.[3] FNH is composed of **hepatocytes, Kupffer's cells,** and bile ductules in a tumorous organization that is well defined and without a true capsule.[3,6] Within this tumor is a central fibrous scar that contains vessels that extend outward in a radial pattern.

Typically identified as a solitary tumor, FNH is seen most commonly in women younger than 40 years and is associated with the use of oral contraceptives.[1] FNH has also been identified in association with hemangiomas.[6] FNH is commonly asymptomatic, and the tumor may be discovered as an incidental finding; however, patients may have right upper quadrant pain.

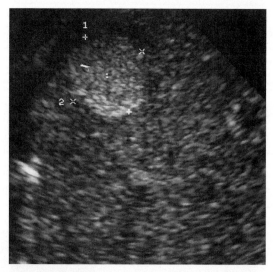

Fig. 2-6 Focal nodular hyperplasia appears as well-defined lesion with hyperechoic internal texture.

Sonographic Findings. Sonographically, FNH may appear isoechoic, hypoechoic, or hyperechoic (Fig. 2-6). These lesions are often homogeneous. The central fibrous scar, when identified, appears as a hyperechoic band. Color Doppler or power Doppler imaging techniques are useful in identification of the prominent vascularity (Fig. 2-7) of the central scar.[3,6]

Lipoma

Lipomas of the liver are rare fatty tumors that lack a capsule. Patients are usually asymptomatic. An association is found between lipomas, renal **angiomyolipomas,** and **tuberous sclerosis.**[1,2]

Sonographic Findings. Lipomas are highly echogenic lesions. A distinguishing feature is a propagation speed error that may be noted because of the slower speed of sound through fatty tissues than through the adjacent liver parenchyma (Fig. 2-8, *A* and *B*). This feature may be identified by noting that structures deep to the lipoma are displaced.[1,2]

Other Benign Neoplasms

In addition to those benign neoplasms discussed previously, other benign neoplasms infrequently occur in the liver. These include the angiomyolipoma, **cystadenoma, lymphangioma,** and **nodular regenerative hyperplasia.**

MALIGNANT NEOPLASMS
Hepatocellular Carcinoma

Hepatocellular carcinoma (HCC) is the most common, primary malignant neoplasm of the liver. HCC is composed of epithelial cells. The prevalence varies

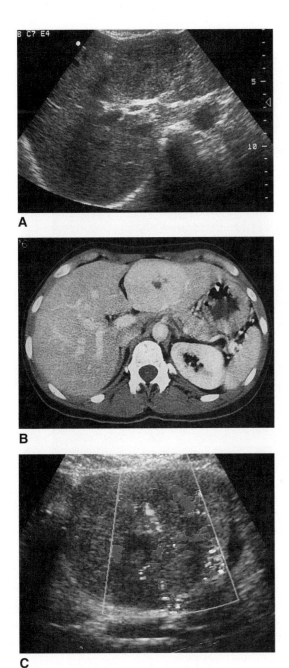

A

B

C

Fig. 2-7 Focal nodular hyperplasia. **A,** Transverse sonogram shows subtle isoechoic mass with contour abnormality and central hypoechoic scar in lateral segment of left lobe of liver. **B,** Contrast-enhanced computed tomographic scan confirms vascular enhancing scar neoplasm with contour bulge. **C,** Magnified color Doppler image shows profuse vascularity typical of this disease. Perilesional and intralesional blood flow frequently creates spoke-wheel appearance.

worldwide, dependent on predisposing factors such as hepatitis B and **aflatoxin** exposure, which contributes to the high frequency of HCC in Africa and southeast Asia. The incidence of HCC in the United States is low,

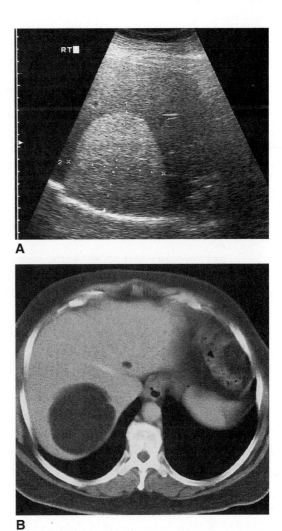

A

B

Fig. 2-8 Hepatic lipoma mimicking hemangioma. **A,** Sonogram shows focal, highly echogenic, solid liver mass. Discontinuity of diaphragm from altered rate of sound transmission is clue to correct diagnosis. **B,** Confirmatory computed tomographic scan shows fat density of mass.

occurring in 3 to 7 of 100,000 of the population, with a male predominance.[7] The development of HCC is seen in most cases in patients with preexisting cirrhosis.

Patients with HCC may have a palpable mass, hepatomegaly, fever, and the signs of cirrhosis. In addition to the abnormal liver function test results related to cirrhosis, patients may also have elevated serum alpha-fetoprotein levels. The tumor may invade the hepatic veins and cause **Budd-Chiari syndrome** or may invade the portal venous system. Patients often have the advanced stages of the disease at the time of diagnosis, which negatively affects the survival rate of approximately 1% at 5 years.[8]

Sonographic Findings. The sonographic appearance of HCC is variable. Small discrete lesions are usually

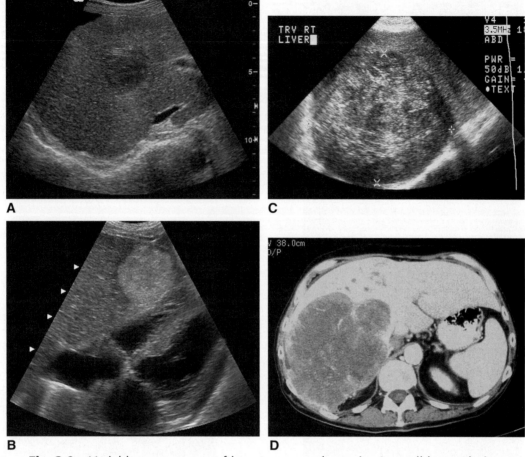

Fig. 2-9 Variable appearances of hepatoma are shown in, **A**, small hypoechoic lesion, **B**, hyperechoic lesion, and, **C**, heterogeneous lesion that is seen with ultrasound and, **D**, computed tomography. (**A** and **B** Courtesy GE Medical Systems.)

hypoechoic (Fig. 2-9, *A*), and larger lesions that are greater than 3 cm are commonly hyperechoic and heterogeneous (Fig. 2-9, *B* to *D*). HCC may also appear as isoechoic lesions or as a diffuse parenchymal pattern of inhomogeneity. Lesions may have a hypoechoic halo, and small lesions may acoustically enhance. Doppler imaging is useful in showing tumor invasion in the hepatic veins, inferior vena cava (IVC), or portal veins (Fig. 2-10, *A* and *B*). In addition, color and power Doppler may show flow within and surrounding the tumor.[7]

Metastases

Metastatic liver disease is the process by which tumor cells from a primary carcinoma travel to the liver via lymphatic channels or blood vessels. In the United States, metastasis to the liver is 18 to 20 times more common than primary malignant disease in the liver.[1,2] The most common primary carcinomas to metastasize to the liver are colon, breast, and lung. The prognosis is dependent on the type of primary carcinoma and the extent of metastatic disease, with an overall 5-year survival rate of 5%.[2,8] Carcinomas with survival rates of less than a year after discovery of liver metastasis include malignant diseases of the pancreas, stomach, and esophagus, whereas malignant disease of the colon has a greater survival rate.[2]

Patients with liver metastasis may have symptoms of jaundice, pain, weight loss, and **anorexia.** They also have abnormal liver function tests and hepatomegaly. A history of a primary malignant disease may help to confirm the diagnosis of metastatic disease when lesions of the liver are discovered.

Sonographic Findings. Metastatic disease of the liver may have variable appearances, and multiple lesions are more commonly seen than are solitary lesions. The sonographic appearance of the lesion does not definitively correlate with the type of primary malignant disease. Metastatic lesions may appear hyperechoic, hypoechoic, or isoechoic to the liver parenchyma (Fig. 2-11). A hypoechoic halo surrounding the lesion is frequently

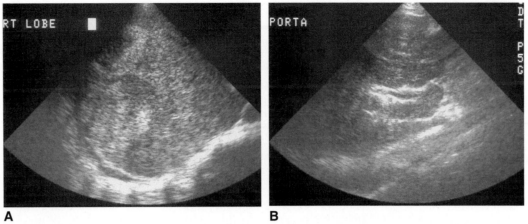

Fig. 2-10   **A,** Large hepatoma was identified in 45-year-old woman with long history of chronic active hepatitis. **B,** Portal vein thrombosis was also identified.

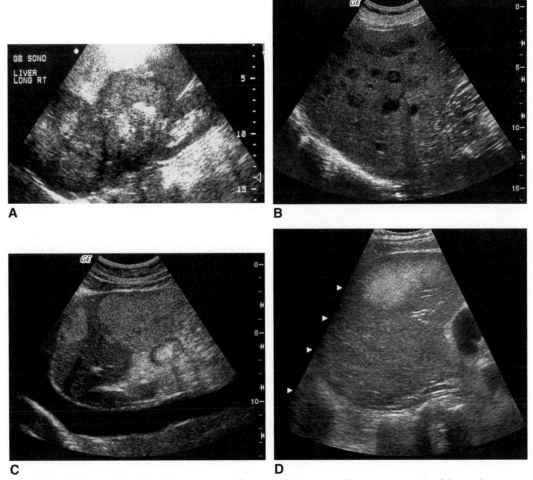

Fig. 2-11   Variable appearances of, **A,** metastasis to liver are seen in this patient with history of colon cancer and in, **B, C,** and **D,** liver metastasis. (**B** to **D** Courtesy GE Medical Systems.)

Table 2-1	*Lesions of the Liver*	
Pathology	Symptoms	Sonographic Findings
Hemangioma	Asymptomatic, right upper quadrant pain	Round or oval, well-defined, hyperechoic; may enhance
Adenoma	Right upper quadrant pain	Encapsulated, well-defined, hyperechoic lesion; peripheral vasculature with Doppler scan
Focal nodular hyperplasia	Usually asymptomatic	Isoechoic, hyperechoic, or hypoechoic lesion; homogeneous, central vascular scar with Doppler scan
Lipoma	Usually asymptomatic	Highly echogenic lesion; propagation speed artifact
Hepatocellular carcinoma	Palpable mass, hepatomegaly, fever, signs of cirrhosis	Hypoechoic mass when small; hyperechoic and inhomogeneous when large, diffuse inhomogeneity; peripheral and intratumoral flow with Doppler scan
Metastasis	Jaundice, pain, weight loss, anorexia	Multiple lesions, variable echogenicity; diffuse inhomogeneity

seen. Lesions may have a target (bulls-eye) appearance, contain calcifications, and appear heterogeneous or complex. Anechoic lesions are uncommon presentations for metastatic disease and will frequently contain low-level echoes and have thick walls. Metastasis to the liver may also present as a diffuse process with an overall inhomogeneous parenchymal pattern.

Other Malignant Neoplasms

In addition to those malignant neoplasms discussed previously, other malignant neoplasms infrequently occur in the liver. These include the **angiosarcoma,** cystadenocarcinoma, **fibrolamellar carcinoma, epithelioid hemangioendothelioma,** and **lymphoma** (see Chapter 3).

SUMMARY

Sonographic examination of the liver can assist in the identification of liver masses (Table 2-1). Characterization of the sonographic appearance coupled with patient history can lead to diagnosis and proper patient management. Biopsy is the most definitive method of tumor diagnosis; however, it may not always be indicated, in which case imaging methods may serve as the final diagnostic tools.

CLINICAL SCENARIO—DIAGNOSIS

◼ Because of the young age and good health of our patient, a malignant neoplasm would be highly unlikely. The sonographic appearance of the small, echogenic lesion is consistent with a hemangioma. The history of oral contraceptives suggests that the larger lesion could be a liver cell adenoma or FNH. The sonographic appearance of this mass, in addition to the vascularity shown with Doppler, suggests an FNH. The patient also underwent magnetic resonance imaging to confirm the diagnosis and is being followed periodically with ultrasound.

CASE STUDIES FOR DISCUSSION

1. A 62-year-old woman with a history of right upper quadrant pain is seen for an abdominal ultrasound. The patient also reveals a history of breast cancer and confirms a recent weight loss. Ultrasound examination reveals multiple lesions (Fig. 2-12, *A* and *B*) throughout the parenchyma of the liver. What is the most likely diagnosis?

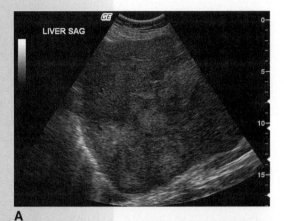

A

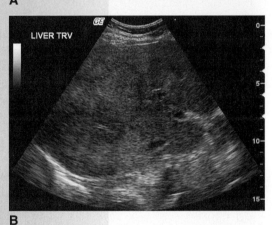

B

Fig. 2-12 Diffusely inhomogeneous liver is shown with multiple lesions identified throughout liver parenchyma as identified in the longitudinal **(A)** and transverse **(B)** images. (Courtesy Lori Davis and Natalie Cauffman, Florida Hospital Deland.)

2. A 54-year-old woman has a recent diagnosis of endometrial carcinoma, and a hysterectomy has been performed. An ultrasound is ordered to rule out gallstones and reveals a hyperechoic lesion in the liver (Fig. 2-13). What are the possible diagnoses?

3. A 27-year-old woman is seen for an ultrasound of the liver after a cesarean section. The obstetrician reported palpation of a "hard liver mass" at the time of the surgery.

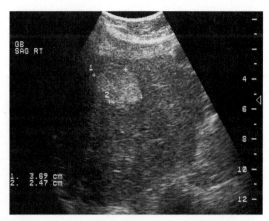

Fig. 2-13 Hyperechoic lesion is identified in the liver.

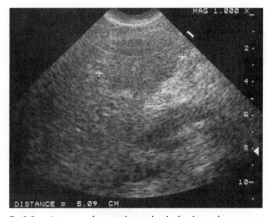

Fig. 2-14 Image shows isoechoic lesion demarcated by calipers.

The ultrasound shows an isoechoic mass in the left lobe of the liver that is relatively homogeneous (Fig. 2-14). The patient states that she was taking oral contraceptives for 7 years before her pregnancy. What is the most likely diagnosis?

4. A 77-year-old man with a history of cirrhosis and a gastrointestinal bleed is seen for an abdominal ultrasound. The ultrasound revealed thrombosis of the portal vein and splenomegaly (Fig. 2-15, *A*). In the anterior segment of the right lobe of the liver, a poorly defined, hypoechoic mass was identified that measured 7.7 cm × 3.2 cm × 7.7 cm (Fig. 2-15, *B* and *C*). **Cholelithiasis** (Fig. 2-15, *D*) was also noted. What is the most likely diagnosis for the liver mass?

5. A 69-year-old woman is seen for an ultrasound of the gallbladder because of right upper quadrant pain. The patient also states that she has been having back pain and underwent treatment for colon cancer 4 years ago. The

CASE STUDIES FOR DISCUSSION—cont'd

ultrasound reveals a "target" lesion (Fig. 2-16, *A*) in the left lobe of the liver and the possibility of two subtle lesions in the right lobe (Fig. 2-16, *B*). The gallbladder appears normal. What is the most likely diagnosis?

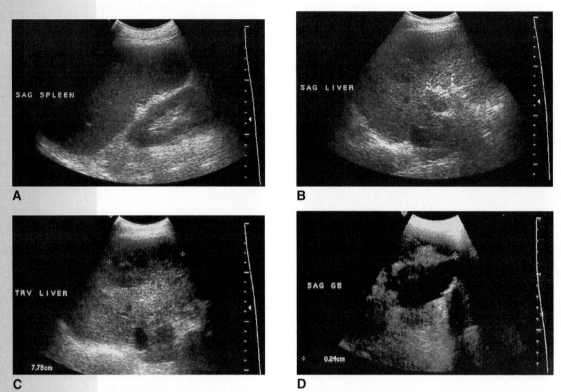

Fig. 2-15 **A,** Splenomegaly is seen in this patient with history of cirrhosis. Hypoechoic lesion is identified in, **B** and **C,** liver and, **D,** gallstones.

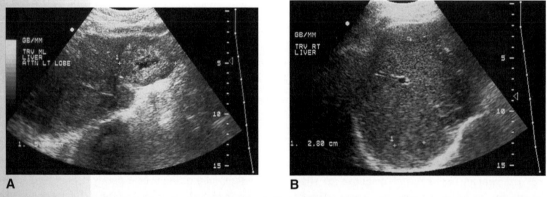

Fig. 2-16 **A,** Target lesion is identified in left lobe. **B,** One of subtle lesions identified in posterior right lobe.

STUDY QUESTIONS

1. A 65-year old man with a history of chronic active hepatitis is seen with abdominal pain. Laboratory values reveal abnormal liver function test results and an elevated serum alpha-fetoprotein level. Ultrasound reveals a lobulated, hypoechoic mass in the posterior segment of the right lobe of the liver. Color Doppler imaging shows a mosaic flow pattern within the mass. This is most suggestive of which of the following?
   a. focal nodular hyperplasia
   b. hemangioma
   c. hepatocellular carcinoma
   d. liver cell adenoma
   e. metastasis

2. A 32-year-old woman with a history of right upper quadrant pain with fatty foods is seen for ultrasound. The ultrasound reveals the presence of gallstones and in addition, a 3-cm isoechoic mass in the liver. Power Doppler investigation of the lesion shows a "spoke-wheel" pattern of flow. What is the most likely diagnosis?
   a. focal nodular hyperplasia
   b. hemangioma
   c. hepatocellular carcinoma
   d. liver cell adenoma
   e. metastasis

3. A 24-year-old woman is seen for a renal ultrasound because of a recently diagnosed congenital uterine anomaly. The renal ultrasound is unremarkable. Incidentally noted is a 1.5-cm echogenic mass in the right lobe of the liver. This most likely represents which of the following?
   a. focal nodular hyperplasia
   b. hemangioma
   c. hepatocellular carcinoma
   d. liver cell adenoma
   e. metastasis

4. A 38-year-old woman with a history of von Gierke's disease is seen for an abdominal ultrasound because of right upper quadrant pain. Two hyperechoic lesions are identified in the liver. Doppler reveals flow around the periphery of each of the lesions. This would be most consistent with which of the following?
   a. focal nodular hyperplasia
   b. hemangioma

c. hepatocellular carcinoma
d. liver cell adenoma
e. metastasis

5. A 45-year-old man with a history of hepatitis is seen for ultrasound examination of the abdomen. The sonographer identifies a 6-cm complex mass in the liver. This would be suspicious for which of the following tumors?
   a. cystadenoma
   b. hemangioma
   c. hepatocellular carcinoma
   d. liver cell adenoma
   e. metastasis

6. A 70-year-old woman is seen for malaise and wasting. The clinician orders an abdominal ultrasound because of the patient's history of colon cancer and elevated liver function tests. The sonographer notes multiple hyperechoic lesions within the liver and hepatomegaly. This is suggestive of:
   a. angiosarcoma
   b. hemangioma
   c. hepatocellular adenoma
   d. hepatocellular carcinoma
   e. metastatic disease

7. A 32-year-old obese woman is seen for a right upper quadrant ultrasound to rule out gallstones. The sonographer's inquiry into the patient's symptoms reveal a fatty food intolerance. Ultrasound examination of the abdomen reveals cholelithiasis and a 1.5-cm echogenic lesion in the liver. The most likely diagnosis for the liver lesion is:
   a. focal nodular hyperplasia
   b. hemangioma
   c. liver cell adenoma
   d. nodular regenerative hyperplasia
   e. solitary metastatic lesion

8. A 59-year-old woman with a history of ovarian cancer and increasing abdominal girth is seen for an abdominal ultrasound. The ultrasound reveals ascites and multiple hypoechoic lesions in the right and left lobes of the liver. This is consistent with:
   a. angiosarcoma
   b. epithelioid hemangioendothelioma
   c. hepatocellular carcinoma
   d. metastasis
   e. nodular regenerative hyperplasia

9. A 50-year-old African immigrant with right upper quadrant pain and weight loss is seen for ultrasound. The patient states that he worked in the fields growing and harvesting a variety of grains for 30 years. Laboratory results reveal an elevated serum alpha-fetoprotein level. Ultrasound examination shows a 4-cm heterogeneous lesion in the liver and a small amount of ascites. This would suggest which of the following?
   a. angiosarcoma
   b. cystadenocarcinoma
   c. epithelioid hemangioendothelioma
   d. hepatocellular carcinoma
   e. metastasis

10. A 47-year-old woman with a history of pancreatic carcinoma who is undergoing chemotherapy is seen. Previous ultrasound examination performed 3 months ago showed a normal-appearing liver. The current ultrasound examination reveals two echogenic lesions in the right lobe of the liver. This would be most consistent with which diagnosis?
    a. hemangioma
    b. hepatocellular carcinoma
    c. focal nodular hyperplasia
    d. liver cell adenoma
    e. metastasis

REFERENCES

1. Hagen-Ansert SL: *Textbook of diagnostic ultrasonography*, vol 1, ed 5, St Louis, 2001, Mosby.
2. Rumack CM, Wilson SR, Charboneau JW: *Diagnostic ultrasound*, vol 1, ed 2, St Louis, 1998, Mosby.
3. Mergo PJ, Ros PR: Benign lesions of the liver, *Radiol Clin North Am* 36:319-331, 1998.
4. Perkins AB, Imam K, Smith WJ et al: Color and power Doppler sonography of liver hemangiomas: a dream unfulfilled? *J Clin Ultrasound* 28:159-165, 2000.
5. Young LK, Yang WT, Chan KW et al: Hepatic hemangioma: quantitative color power US angiography–facts and fallacies, *Radiology* 207:51-57, 1998.
6. Uggowitzer MM et al: Echo-enhanced Doppler sonography of focal nodular hyperplasia of the liver, *J Ultrasound Med* 18:445-451, 1999.
7. Fernandez MP, Redvanly RD: Primary hepatic malignant neoplasms, *Radiol Clin North Am* 36:333-348, 1998.
8. Kawamura DM: *Abdomen and superficial structures*, ed 2, Philadelphia, 1997, Lippincott.

BIBLIOGRAPHY

Anderson KN, Anderson LE, Glanze WD: *Mosby's medical, nursing, & allied health dictionary*, ed 5, St Louis, 1998, Mosby.
Chiaramonte M et al: Rate of incidence of hepatocellular carcinoma in patients with compensated viral cirrhosis, *Cancer* 85:2132-2137, 1999.
Ding H et al: Hepatocellular carcinoma: depiction of tumor parenchymal flow with intermittent harmonic power Doppler US during the early arterial phase in dual-display mode, *Radiology* 220:349-356, 2001.

3 Diffuse Liver Disease

FELICIA JONES

CLINICAL SCENARIO

■ A 51-year-old man is seen at the radiology department for an abdominal ultrasound. He has elevated aspartate aminotransferase and alanine aminotransferase levels and increasing abdominal girth. No previous films are available for comparison. History included cholecystectomy complicated by biliary obstruction 5 years previously.

The abdominal ultrasound reveals a homogeneous liver with increased echogenicity. No distinct solid or cystic masses are noted, but free fluid is noted within the abdomen (Fig. 3-1). The hepatic vasculature is difficult to evaluate, and the hepatic parenchyma is difficult to penetrate. What are the possible diagnoses for this patient?

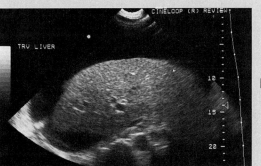

Fig. 3-1 **A,** Sagittal image of right lobe of liver. Visualization and evaluation of border of liver is possible because of free fluid within abdominal cavity. **B,** Transverse image of right lobe of liver. Echogenicity of liver is difficult to evaluate because of increased enhancement from surrounding free fluid.

OBJECTIVES

■ Define the processes that cause and affect diffuse liver disease.

■ Define and describe hepatocellular diseases and their sonographic findings.

■ Compare and contrast the varying diffuse liver diseases and their sonographic appearances.

■ Understand and describe the accompanying laboratory value changes associated with diffuse liver diseases.

■ Describe the Doppler changes that accompany diffuse liver diseases.

■ Define and describe the sonographic findings associated with the conditions caused by diffuse liver diseases.

GLOSSARY OF TERMS

Acute hepatitis: hepatitis that resolves within 4 months after the initial infection

Albumin: byproduct of protein metabolism that decreases with parenchymal liver disease

Alcoholic hepatitis: see cirrhosis

Alpha fetoprotein: plasma protein produced in the fetal liver and by hepatocellular carcinomas; elevated levels may also be seen in cirrhosis and hepatitis

Alanine aminotransferase: a liver enzyme formerly referred to as serum glutamic-pyruvic transaminase

Ascites: an accumulation of serous fluid within the potential spaces of the abdomen

Aspartate aminotransferase: a liver enzyme formerly referred to as serum glutamic-oxaloacetic transaminase

Bilirubin: end product of red blood cell metabolism that is stored in the liver and used to help metabolize fatty foods

Chronic hepatitis: persistence of changes associated with hepatitis for more than 6 months

Cirrhosis: degenerative disease of the liver in which the hepatocytes are gradually replaced with fibrous and fatty tissues

Cruveilhier-Baumgarten syndrome: the development of paraumbilical collateral flow in cases of portal hypertension

Direct bilirubin: bilirubin that has been absorbed by the hepatocytes and is then water-soluble; also known as *conjugated bilirubin*

Esophageal veins: common collateral pathway for the hepatic circulation in cases of portal hypertension

Fat sparing: areas of normal liver parenchyma not replaced with fatty tissues occasionally seen in patients with fatty liver disease

Fatty liver disease: the accumulation of fat within hepatic parenchyma that is often associated with alcoholism, obesity, and diabetes

Gamma-glutamyl transpeptidase: aids in the transport of amino acids across cell membranes; elevates in cases of parenchymal liver disease and is especially sensitive to alcohol-related liver disease; often parallels alkaline phosphatase (ALP)

Hepatitis: an inflammatory condition of the liver caused by a viral infection or a reaction to drugs or alcohol

Hepatocellular disease: dysfunction of the hepatocytes

Hepatofugal: portal vein blood flow away from the liver

Hepatoma: primary liver carcinoma or hepatocellular carcinoma

Hepatopetal: portal vein blood flow toward the liver

Hodgkin's lymphoma, or Hodgkin's disease: painless enlargement of the lymph nodes and lymphoid tissues of the body

Indirect bilirubin: bilirubin present in the blood stream and not yet absorbed by the hepatocytes; water-insoluble; also known as *unconjugated bilirubin*

Levovist: an ultrasound contrast agent

Lymphadenopathy: diseases of the lymph nodes

Lymphoma: neoplastic disease of lymphoid tissues

Lymphosarcoma: diffuse lymphoma

Mesocaval shunt: blood is shunted from the superior mesenteric vein directly into the inferior vena cava

Morison's pouch: the potential space located between the liver and the right kidney

Non-Hodgkin's lymphoma: malignant lymphoma arising from lymphoid tissues of the immune system

Optison: an intravenously administered ultrasound contrast agent

Periportal cuffing: thickening of the portal vein walls

Portacaval shunt: shunts blood from the main portal vein at the confluence of the superior mesenteric vein and splenic vein directly into the inferior vena cava

Portal hypertension: increased size and pressure within the portal venous system often leading to collateral vessels and reversed flow within the portal vein

Prothrombin time: determines the time necessary for blood clotting to occur; increases in cases of parenchymal liver disease or vitamin K deficiency

Recanalized umbilical vein: opening of the potential space located within the ligament of teres left by the fetal umbilical vein

Sarcoma: malignant tumor of the connective tissues or lymphoid tissues

Splenorenal shunt: blood is shunted from the splenic vein into the left renal vein

Subphrenic spaces: the potential spaces located between the liver and the diaphragm

---

GLOSSARY OF TERMS—cont'd ▰

Transjugular intrahepatic portosystemic shunt: A procedure that involves the placement of a shunt to direct blood past the hypertensive portal venous system or venous varices and aid in the return of venous blood to general circulation

Venous collateral flow: alternative circulatory pathways that develop after pathologic changes prevent normal vascular pathways from serving as an adequate source of blood to an organ

---

Diseases that affect the functional cells of the liver, the hepatocytes, are referred to as *hepatocellular*.[1-3] These diseases are treated medically rather than surgically. **Hepatocellular disease** occurs as the hepatocytes are damaged and liver function decreases.[1,4] Disease processes that affect the liver diffusely occur because of neoplasms, infections, fatty infiltration, or liver fibrosis.[4,5] The sonographic appearance of the liver varies depending on the disease involved. The sonographic appearance of the liver will also change as the disease persists from an acute phase into a more long-standing chronic illness.

Patients with diffuse liver diseases often have elevated liver enzyme levels, especially **aspartate aminotransferase** (AST) and **alanine aminiotransferase** (ALT) levels that elevate as cellular function decreases as a result of the diffuse changes to the hepatocytes.[2,5] Although both ALT and AST levels are sensitive to liver diseases, AST levels may also elevate in patients with diseases of the bone or muscular systems.

Laboratory values, such as **gamma-glutamyl transpeptidase** (GGT) and **albumin,** may be helpful in determination of the nature of the liver disease.[3-5] These protein levels are likely to increase in cases of hepatic cellular damage, although acute damage to liver cells where these proteins are processed may lead to a decrease in albumin levels.[6]

Increased white blood cell (WBC) levels often indicate infection and should alert the sonographer to suspect abscesses or infectious processes. **Prothrombin time** (PTT) is a liver enzyme that functions in blood clotting and often increases in cases of hepatic cellular damage.[2,4,5,7,8]

Bilirubin is produced by the breakdown of hemoglobin. That process begins in the spleen and continues in the liver. Bilirubin that has been absorbed by the hepatocytes is referred to as *direct,* or *conjugated,* bilirubin. Levels of direct bilirubin are likely to increase in cases of biliary obstruction and liver cellular diseases. *Indirect,* or *unconjugated,* bilirubin levels may increase in cases of anemia or other diseases that lead to increased breakdown of red blood cells.[2,4,5,7,8]

Because many laboratory values are likely to increase from a wide variety of diseases, the examination of more than one laboratory value is always helpful in determination of a definitive diagnosis. A good clinical history is imperative in a thorough assessment with ultrasound. Table 3-1 is provided as a guide to laboratory values related to diffuse liver diseases.

HEPATOCELLULAR DISEASE

The liver may be enlarged, especially in acute stages of disease change, but in some diseases, such as hepatitis, the acute sonographic findings may be subtle and difficult to detect.[3] Often the liver becomes atrophied as pathologic changes become more chronic and the hepatocytes are replaced either by fat cells or fibrous tissues. Replacement of the hepatocytes by fat and fibrous components leads to decreased liver function and a general increase in liver enzymes over time.[1,6,7] Liver cells regenerate, and this process may be accompanied by the development of regenerating liver nodules. The presence of these nodules further complicates the sonographer's ability to evaluate liver parenchyma and assess the liver for possible masses.[2]

As damage to the hepatocytes increases, liver function decreases, which will affect the liver's ability to conjugate bilirubin[1,9] and to receive blood from the portal venous system. Damage to the liver can lead to jaundice as the bilirubin accumulates in the interstitial fluids as it leaks from the hepatocytes. The type of bilirubin with an elevated level will help determine the disease present. Direct or conjugated bilirubin levels become elevated as the hepatocytes become damaged. **Direct bilirubin** levels also increase in cases of biliary obstruction. Indirect or unconjugated bilirubin levels usually are elevated in cases of increased destruction of red blood cells. Damage to the hepatocytes can lead to an increase in both direct and **indirect bilirubin** levels.[1,2]

Table 3-1	*Liver-Related Laboratory Values*
Test	**Significance of Change**
Alkaline phosphatase	↑ in liver disease
Ammonia	↑ in liver disease and diabetes mellitus
Bile and bilirubin	↑ during obstruction of bile ducts
Glucose	↑ in diabetes mellitus and liver disease
Hematocrit	↓ in cirrhosis of liver
Hemoglobin	↓ in cirrhosis of liver
Iron	↑ in liver disease
Lactic dehydrogenase (LDH)	↑ in liver disease

Lipids: total
  Cholesterol: total
    HDL
    LDL
  Triglycerides
  Phospholipids
  Fatty acids
	↑ (cholesterol) in chronic hepatitis
	↑ (cholesterol) in acute hepatitis

Platelet count	↑ in cirrhosis of liver
Transaminase	↑ in liver disease
Urea	↑ in some liver diseases ↓ during obstruction of bile ducts

HDL, High density lipoprotein; *LDL,* low density lipoprotein.

The hepatocytes become unable to perform their normal functions because of fibrous and fatty replacement, which eventually may also lead to portal hypertension.[1,10] The increased pressure within the portal vein causes it to become enlarged and tortuous. The spleen is forced to store the excess blood the liver is unable to receive and also enlarges. As this process worsens, varices or collateral channels form to provide the portal vein with a means of bypassing the liver. **Ascites,** the accumulation of free fluid within the abdominal cavity, may develop as pressures within the liver increase and serous fluids leak from the remaining hepatocytes and into the surrounding peritoneal cavity.[1,11]

When associated with chronic diffuse liver diseases, the accumulation of serous fluid within the potential spaces of the abdomen occurs as a result of severe hepatocyte damage and liver failure. This may be because of hypoalbuminemia or severe **portal hypertension.** The increased pressure within the liver causes the fluids to leak from the liver sinuses and into the hepatic

lymphatics. When the pressures are high enough, some fluids will leak directly into the peritoneal cavity.

The increasing pressure within the portal venous system may prevent blood from flowing in its normal direction, toward the liver. This normal flow is referred to as *hepatopetal.* Doppler scan examination of these patients may detect **hepatofugal,** or reverse, portal flow in the portal and splenic veins. These patients may have vascular collateral channels develop to supply the liver with blood. These patients may also undergo surgical intervention with the placement of shunts, such as **transjugular intrahepatic portosystemic shunt** (TIPS) catheters, to help return portal blood back into systemic circulation.[2] A comparison of **hepatitis, cirrhosis,** and **hepatoma** is provided in Table 3-2.

Fatty Liver Disease

Fatty liver disease is an acquired and reversible disorder that results from the accumulation of triglycerides within the hepatocytes.[1,5] Alcoholism, obesity, and diabetes are the most common causes of fatty liver

Table 3-2	*Liver Function Tests for Diffuse Liver Diseases*					
	ALT	AST	ALP	Direct Bilirubin	Indirect Bilirubin	AFP
Hepatitis	↑↑↑	↑↑	↑	↑↑↑		
Cirrhosis	↑	↑	↑	↑↑↑		
Hepatoma	↑	↑	↑↑			↑↑↑

disease.[1] Fatty infiltration occurs, depending on the sonographic appearance, in the following three grades: mild, moderate, and severe.

Sonographic Findings. The fatty replaced liver usually has increased echogenicity with increased attenuation.[2] The liver is difficult to penetrate, and the vascular structures are often difficult to visualize, especially the hepatic veins (Fig. 3-2, *A* and *B*). Areas of the liver may be spared from fatty infiltration. These fat spared areas appear as localized regions of decreased echogenicity within the more echogenic liver (Fig. 3-2, *C* and *D*).[3] This **fat sparing** most often is seen anterior to the gallbladder and the right portal vein or within the left lobe.[2,5] Fatty infiltration of the liver varies in severity from mild to severe.

Because fat increases the attenuation within liver parenchyma, use of a lower frequency transducer may helpful in the imaging of patient anatomy. Care must be taken to keep in mind the loss of resolution that will accompany a lower frequency transducer. Harmonic imaging if available can be another useful tool in evaluation of the dense liver. The frame rate of the image may become degraded on certain machines with this option.

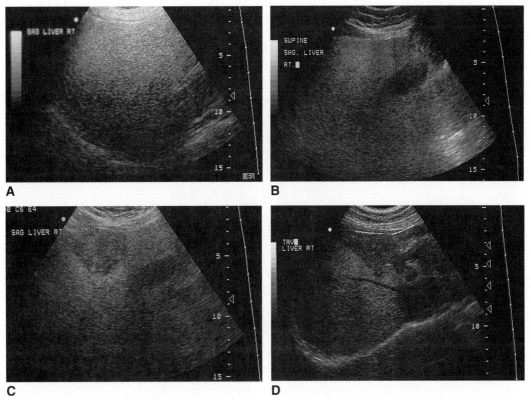

Fig. 3-2 **A,** Moderate fatty liver disease. Replacement of normal hepatocytes by fat cells leads to increase in echogenicity and smooth texture to liver. Liver becomes dense and difficult to penetrate sonographically. Diaphragm is visualized, but increased attenuation of liver parenchyma is seen. **B,** Severe fatty liver disease. Fatty liver appears smooth in echo texture and hyperechoic anteriorly, although sound cannot penetrate to posterior margin of liver and diaphragm is not visualized. **C** and **D,** Hypoechoic mass in liver represents normal hepatic parenchyma. Remaining liver parenchyma has been infiltrated by fat cells and is hyperechoic compared with normal parenchymal texture. Determination of presence of fat, normal parenchyma, or neoplasm is difficult without biopsy results.

Table 3-3   Types of Hepatitis

Findings	Hepatitis A	Hepatitis B	Hepatitis C	Hepatitis D	Hepatitis E	Hepatitis F	Hepatitis G
	Treated with bed rest	Increased risk for development of cirrhosis and hepatoma	Increased risk for development of cirrhosis and hepatoma; leading cause of liver failure and transplantation in United States	Only occurs in patients with hepatitis B infection	Mostly found in Asia and South America	Similar to hepatitis C; uncertain whether it is separate virus yet	Similar to hepatitis C
Acute versus chronic	Mostly acute and resolved within 6 months	Becomes chronic in up to 10% of newly infected people each year	Becomes chronic in up to 85% of newly infected people each year	Severity of infection worsens with coinfection	Mostly acute and resolved within 6 months		
Mechanisms of contraction	Infected food or drinking water	Blood and body fluid contact	Blood and body fluid contact	Blood and body fluid contact	Infected food or drinking water	Blood and body fluid contact	Blood and body fluid contact
Vaccine available?	Yes	Yes	No				

Hepatitis

The multiple variations of this disease (hepatitis A to G) vary in severity and sonographic findings (Table 3-3).[5] The two most common forms of hepatitis are A and B. Type A infections are generally spread via fecal contaminated materials. Type B infections are typically spread via blood contamination.[2,5,6] Occupational Safety and Health Administration (OSHA) considers hepatitis B one of the most serious threats to healthcare workers. Healthcare workers have a risk factor for hepatitis B that is three to five times greater than the general population. Each year approximately 100 deaths are caused by hepatitis B, which is generally contracted via needle sticks from infected patients.[12] Hepatitis C is a rapidly growing concern to healthcare workers. OSHA estimates that as many as 1000 workers per year are contaminated with hepatitis C. These contaminations generally occur through needle stick exposures to contaminated blood. Hepatitis C is now the leading cause of liver transplantation in the United States.[12]

Acutely, damage to the liver may vary from mild to severe. Liver cells are damaged, healed by the reticuloendothelial system, and then regenerated. Symptoms include nausea, vomiting, and fatigue and can progress to liver failure depending on the patients' immune response.

Patients are seen with flu-like symptoms. The liver is often slightly enlarged, and splenomegaly may be present. AST and ALT levels are usually markedly elevated.[1,5] Uncomplicated **acute hepatitis** generally resolves itself within 4 months of the infection and is most often associated with type A hepatitis.

Sonographic Findings. The liver may be enlarged and may show decreased echogenicity, although often the liver appears normal in echo texture (Fig. 3-3).[3,5,13] Because of an accumulation of fluid within the hepato-

cytes, the walls of the gallbladder may thicken and appear prominent.[2,5] **Periportal cuffing,** or thickening of the portal vein walls, may be noted, and the walls of the portal veins may appear more hyperechoic than normal,[2,13] which may be referred to as the "starry sky" appearance.[4]

Hepatitis that persists for more than 6 months is considered chronic. Most often this occurs with hepatitis B and sometimes with hepatitis C but not with hepatitis A or E,[1,2] which resolve spontaneously. In **chronic hepatitis,** the liver texture becomes coarse and hyperechoic.[2] Chronic hepatitis is difficult to distinguish from fatty infiltration of the liver on the basis of sonographic appearances only. The walls of the portal veins may become more difficult to assess and appear hypoechoic because of fibrosis.[4,5]

Cirrhosis

Cirrhosis is hepatocellular disease that leads to liver necrosis, fibrosis, and regeneration.[1,13] The liver becomes atrophied and dense. Cirrhotic liver changes are often associated with and start as fatty liver replacement, but that is not always the case. Cirrhosis is among the top five most common causes of death in the United States.[2,6] Cirrhosis may develop from the abuse of alcohol, the use of certain drugs, chemical reactions, biliary obstruction, and cardiac disease.[1,5,6] Patients with cirrhosis have hepatomegaly, jaundice, and ascites.[3,8] Acute cirrhosis may have a normal sonographic appearance or may have an appearance similar to that of fatty infiltration. The caudate lobe and the lateral segment of the left lobe are most commonly hypertrophied, with a caudate to right lobe ratio greater then 0.65 considered abnormal, and the right lobe and medial segment of the left lobe frequently display focal atrophy.[2]

Sonographic Findings. The cirrhotic liver is often described as coarse with a nodular surface.[9,13] The surface of the liver is often scalloped (Fig. 3-4, A). Regenerating nodules form on a micronodular or macronodular level, depending on the severity of the disease. However, these nodules are not often seen sonographically because of their small size.[3] If seen sonographically, regenerating nodules are hypoechoic compared with the surrounding liver.[2,3,13]

Because of the replacement of hepatocytes by fibrotic tissues, the liver is often described as "bright" and the hepatic vasculature is often difficult to visualize sonographically (Fig. 3-4, B).[9] The caudate lobe is often spared from this process. Chronically, patients have hepatosplenomegaly, ascites, and a nodular liver surface.[2,5,6,9]

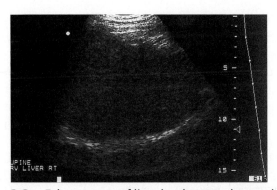

Fig. 3-3 Echo texture of liver has become hypoechoic in acute hepatitis. Liver texture may remain normal in appearance.

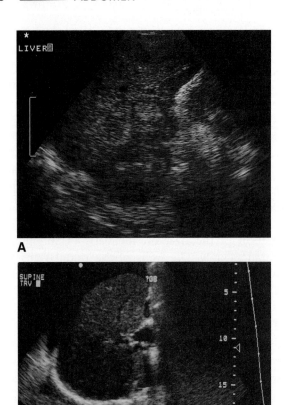

A

B

Fig. 3-4 **A,** Liver parenchyma becomes coarse, heterogeneous, and hyperechoic as hepatocytes are replaced with fibrous tissues, are damaged, and are regenerated. **B,** As hepatocytes are damaged, fluids leak and accumulate in peritoneal cavity. Border of liver becomes visible, and nodular irregularities may be noted.

The changes associated with liver fibrosis are irreversible,[9] and patient symptomology includes nausea, anorexia, weight loss, and the development of varicosities. Cirrhosis will progress to liver failure and portal hypertension.[4] Patients with cirrhosis are at increased risk for hepatocellular carcinoma (HCC).[2,5,9]

Portal Hypertension

Portal hypertension is defined as an increase in portal venous pressure exceeding 12 mm Hg.[1] Damaged hepatocytes impede the flow of blood into the liver and thereby cause an increase in portal vein pressure. Portal veins are considered enlarged at greater than 13 mm in diameter.[10,13]

The most common cause of portal hypertension in North America is cirrhosis.[10] Patients with portal hypertension have enlarged portal veins that show decreasing respiratory variations with steady, monophasic spectral

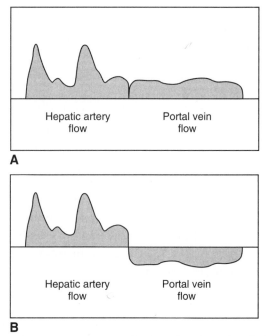

A

B

Fig. 3-5 **A,** Hepatopetal portal vein blood flow. **B,** Hepatofugal portal vein blood flow.

tracings. Normal blood flow within the liver is hepatopetal or toward the liver (Fig. 3-5, *A*). Hepatofugal blood flow (blood flow away from the liver) may be present as **venous collateral flow** and splenomegaly develops (Fig. 3-5, *B*).[5,6] Contrast sonography may be helpful in detection of collateral and low velocity portal vein flow by increasing the reflectivity of the red blood cells within the circulation.[14,15]

As blood pools, unable to enter the hepatic circulation, the risk of portal vein thrombosis increases. Thrombi will vary in appearance with age. New thrombus is hyperechoic, and older thrombus is hypoechoic. Chronic thrombus associated with recanalization of the portal vein is referred to as *cavernous transformation of the portal vein.*[2,11,13]

Varices are veins that dilate because of increased pressure in the portal venous system. Collateral veins redirect blood to alternative pathways to reenter the main venous circulation. Examples of portal venous collateral pathways can be seen in Fig. 3-6. The most common varice is the splenorenal. Blood is diverted from the splenic vein into the left renal vein. From there, blood enters the inferior vena cava (IVC).[10]

The second pathway is through the paraumbilical vein and is often referred to as a *recanalized umbilical vein.* The fetal umbilical vein lies in the potential space occupied by the ligament of teres and becomes patent when the pressure in the liver elevates to allow for a

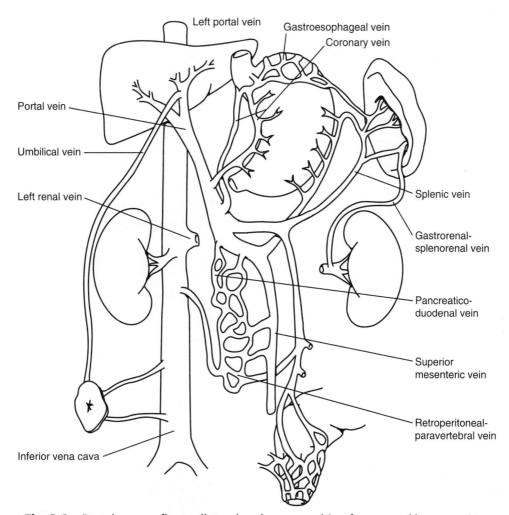

Left portal vein

Gastroesophageal vein

Coronary vein

Portal vein

Umbilical vein

Left renal vein

Splenic vein

Gastrorenal-splenorenal vein

Pancreatico-duodenal vein

Superior mesenteric vein

Retroperitoneal-paravertebral vein

Inferior vena cava

Fig. 3-6   Portal venous flow collateral pathways resulting from portal hypertension.

collateral pathway of blood to bypass the damaged hepatocytes. The remnant of the fetal umbilical vein becomes patent once again and can be visualized within the potential space occupied by the ligament of teres. Blood is diverted into the IVC via this pathway.[6,10,13] The development of collaterals via this pathway is referred to as *Cruveilhier-Baumgarten syndrome,*[13,16] and some authors say that these patients are at a lesser risk of development of **esophageal vein** varices and gastro-intestinal bleeding.

The third pathway is through the left gastric or coronary vein. In these cases, blood is diverted from the portal vein to the esophagus. This pathway may be present in as many as 80% of patients with cirrhosis[2] and puts the patient at great risk because the varices in the distal esophagus are fragile and subject to hemorrhage.[10] These patients have gastrointestinal bleeds develop and are at risk of bleeding to death quickly.[1,6,10]

Shunts may be placed surgically to reduce the build-up of pressure within the portal venous system. Common

shunts include the **portacaval shunt,** in which blood is redirected from the main portal vein at the confluence of the superior mesenteric vein directly into the IVC; the **splenorenal shunt,** in which blood is shunted from the splenic vein into the left renal vein; and the **mesocaval shunt,** in which blood is shunted from the superior mesenteric vein directly into the IVC.[6]

Another common surgical shunt is a TIPS catheter. A TIPS catheter is a catheter that is placed through the jugular vein into the right atrium. From the right atrium, the catheter enters a hepatic vein (Fig. 3-7), usually the right hepatic vein. The needle is then forced into the nearby portal vein, generally the right portal vein. This establishes a pathway through which blood can bypass the liver and return directly to the IVC.[9,10,13]

Sonographic Findings. A TIPS catheter will have strong echogenic walls and an anechoic lumen (Fig. 3-8, *A*). Doppler examination of a TIPS catheter should show flow toward the IVC with an average velocity between 100 and 190 cm/s.[13] Flow with a velocity of less

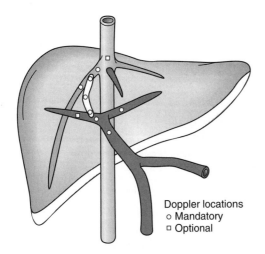

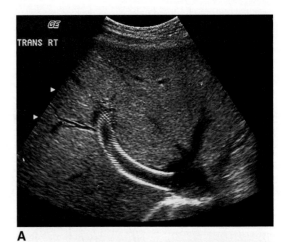

A

Fig. 3-7 Diagram of TIPS catheter placement.

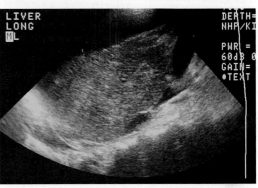

B

than 90 cm/s indicates decreased flow through the stent and may be the result of thrombosis (Fig. 3-8, *B* and *C*) or stenosis within the stent. Flow velocities of more than 190 cm/s indicate high-grade stenosis within the stent.[4,6,13]

Hepatoma

Patients with a history of long-standing hepatitis or cirrhosis are at greater risk for development of HCC or hepatoma. As many as 80% of patients with cirrhosis will develop HCC.[2,5,17] The presence of HCC rarely affects liver enzymes, although it may produce an increase in **alpha fetoprotein** (AFP) levels.[7]

Sonographic Findings. HCC can appear as diffuse texture changes throughout the liver or focal masses. Masses can be either hypoechoic or hyperechoic (Fig. 3-9) and often have a peripheral halo surrounding them.[2,3,7] Distinguishing between HCC and liver metastases or fatty liver infiltration without biopsy results and a strong patient history may be impossible. Portal veins or hepatic veins may be invaded by tumor infiltration. Doppler and color Doppler can be used to help rule out tumor invasion into these vessels.

Ultrasound contrast imaging has been shown to be effective in documenting small lesions within the liver. Contrast agents are administered intravenously before ultrasound examination and enhance the detection of blood flow and parenchymal variations. Contrast enhanced harmonic imaging with microbubble contrast agents generally causes hepatic lesions to appear hypervascular.[6,13-15] Small hypoechoic lesions such as hepatomas show enhanced border and parenchymal differentiation after contrast administration.[14-16]

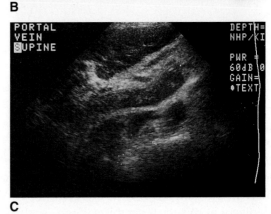

C

Fig. 3-8 **A,** To help alleviate problems associated with increasing pressure within liver cells, shunts may be placed surgically. TIPS catheter (seen as hyperechoic tube) allows blood to drain from portal vein into hepatic veins and then back into circulation through IVC. **B,** Liver is small with heterogeneous parenchyma. Parenchymal changes are from ischemia caused by lack of blood supply because of thrombosed portal vein. Ascites is noted within abdominal cavity. **C,** Portal vein is enlarged and filled with hypoechoic echoes indicative of portal vein thrombosis. (**A** Courtesy GE Medical Systems.)

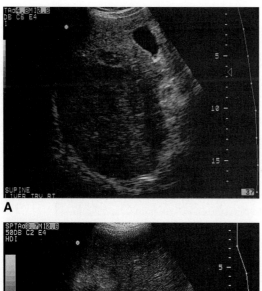

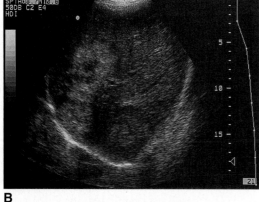

Fig. 3-9 **A,** Hepatoma seen as large hypoechoic mass occupying right posterior lobe of liver. **B,** Hepatoma seen as focal hyperechoic mass with peripheral halo surrounding edges of mass.

Contrast agents detect these changes with enhancement of the acoustic properties of the parenchyma. The contrast agents are eventually removed from the body by the reticuloendothelial system. Hepatic imaging must occur within 15 minutes after contrast administration but may last longer.

Examples of contrast agents used in ultrasound imaging include **Levovist** (not available in the United States at this time), **Optison,** Definity (not available in the United States at this time except for cardiac imaging), SonoVue (not available in the United States at this time), and Sonazoid (not available in the United States at this time). The ability of contrast-enhanced ultrasound to detect small lesions may prevent patients from undergoing the more expensive computed tomographic (CT) or magnetic resonance imaging (MRI) examinations.[15] Unlike CT contrast agents, sonographic contrast agents do not cause adjacent tissues to resonate and can be administered in patients with renal failure.[14]

Lymphoma

Although **lymphoma** is not a disease related directly to the hepatocytes and their function, it may diffusely affect the echo texture of the liver. When multiple organs contain lymphoma, the disease is referred to as *lymphosarcoma*, or *sarcoma*. When just the lymph nodes are affected pathologically, the disease is referred to as *lymphadenopathy*.[1]

Sonographic Findings. Patients with lymphoma will have hepatomegaly and possibly splenomegaly. **Hodgkin's lymphoma** within the liver may appear as heterogeneous parenchyma (Fig. 3-10, *A*) or focal hypoechoic masses (Fig. 3-10, *B*).[2] **Non-Hodgkin's lymphomas** tend to be more echogenic in sonographic appearance. Lymphomas are often anechoic and may be mistaken for cystic masses (Fig. 3-10, *C*). A true cyst has well-defined borders, good posterior enhancement, and no internal echoes. Lymphomas usually lack well-defined borders.[16]

Table 3-4 is a summary of the pathology, symptoms, and sonographic findings of diffuse liver disease.

SUMMARY

Sonographic evaluation of liver parenchyma can help in the diagnostic process of diffuse liver diseases. Patient history and laboratory values are extremely important in a differential diagnosis, and a definitive diagnosis is often not possible without a biopsy. The diagnostic process is dependant on sonographers making careful note of sonographic findings and reporting them concisely and correctly.

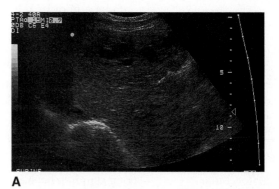

Fig. 3-10 **A,** Lymphoma can have anechoic echo texture and may be mistaken for cystic mass unless borders and posterior enhancement are carefully evaluated. *Continued*

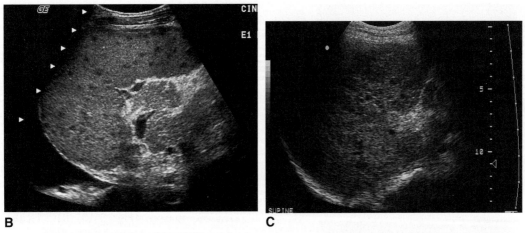

B   C

Fig. 3-10, *cont'd*   **B,** Lymphoma often shows multiple hypoechoic masses within organ parenchyma. (Courtesy GE Medical Systems.) **C,** Lymphoma of liver shows heterogeneous hypoechoic changes to liver parenchyma.

Table 3-4	*Summary of Diffuse Liver Disease Pathologies*	
Pathology	**Symptoms**	**Sonographic Findings**
Fatty liver	Usually asymptomatic; jaundice, nausea, vomiting, pain, abdominal tenderness	Increased echogenicity, increased attenuation, decreased penetration, difficulty visualizing vascular structures
Fat sparing	Asymptomatic	Decreased echogenic regions within hyperechoic liver, often anterior to right portal vein or within left lobe
Hepatitis, acute	Flu-like symptoms; nausea, vomiting, fatigue	Normal appearance, enlarged liver with decreased echogenicity, prominent portal vasculature
Hepatitis, chronic	Flu-like symptoms; nausea, vomiting, fatigue, liver failure	Coarse and hyperechoic liver parenchyma, poorly visualized vasculature
Cirrhosis, acute	Asymptomatic, peripheral edema, ascites, fatigue, abnormal liver enzymes	Normal appearance, caudate lobe and left lateral lobe hypertrophied (caudate to right lobe ratio > 0.65), right and left medial lobes often atrophy
Cirrhosis, chronic	Nausea, anorexia, weight loss, tremors, jaundice, dark urine, fatigue, varicosities; may progress to liver failure and portal hypertension	Coarse parenchyma, decreased size, nodular surface, free fluid in Morison's pouch, extensive ascites
Portal hypertension	Asymptomatic, cirrhosis, ascites, varices	Enlarged portal veins, monophasic spectral tracings, hepatofugal blood flow, portal varices, ascites, splenomegaly
Hepatocellular carcinoma	Long-standing hepatitis or cirrhosis, abdominal pain, weight loss, palpable mass, fever, jaundice	Diffuse parenchymal changes, focal masses (either hypoechoic or hyperechoic), often with peripheral hypoechoic halo
Lymphoma	Enlarged, nontender lymph nodes; fever, fatigue, night sweats, weight loss, bone pain, abdominal mass	Diffuse parenchymal changes, focal hypoechoic masses, focal hyperechoic masses (more commonly associated with non-Hodgkin's lymphomas), no posterior enhancement noted

CLINICAL SCENARIO—DIAGNOSIS

■ Based on the elevated laboratory values, the change in liver echogenicity without distinct masses noted, and the poorly defined hepatic vasculature, several possibilities exist. Because the liver parenchyma remains homogeneous, we can rule out hepatoma, focal fatty liver disease, and lymphoma. Hepatitis is rarely a diagnosis made on the basis of ultrasound alone and is not associated with free fluid unless it is a chronic disease process.

A more thorough patient history would help us in this process. If the patient were obese, we might suspect fatty

liver disease, or if the patient had a history of alcohol abuse, we might suspect cirrhosis initially. We would not expect fatty liver disease to be associated with free fluid within the peritoneal cavity.

The patient's history of cholecystectomy complicated by biliary obstruction makes biliary cirrhosis a likely choice, and this patient does indeed have cirrhosis. The presence of free fluid makes this diagnosis most likely. The final diagnosis was made on the basis of the results of a liver biopsy.

CASE STUDIES FOR DISCUSSION ▬▬▬▬▬

1. A 31-year-old woman is seen for an ultrasound. The patient is moderately obese and has vague peptic discomfort. She has no history of cancer, nausea, or vomiting. The ultrasound is ordered to rule out biliary disease. Ultrasound reveals a hypoechoic liver that is difficult to penetrate (Fig. 3-11, *A* and *B*). Vasculature is poorly imaged (see Fig. 3-11, *A*). What is the most likely diagnosis?

2. A 27-year-old man undergoes a right upper quadrant ultrasound in the emergency room. The patient has right upper quadrant pain and a history of drug abuse. Ultrasound reveals a hypoechoic liver with no distinct masses seen (Fig. 3-12). What is the best diagnosis?

3. A 64-year-old man undergoes an ultrasound to rule out liver mass (Fig. 3-13). He has right upper quadrant pain, elevated liver enzyme levels, and a long history of alcohol

abuse. The ultrasound shows a diffusely inhomogeneous liver. What is the best diagnosis?

4. A 55-year-old man undergoes an ultrasound to rule out a mass. The patient has increasing abdominal girth, vague discomfort, and anorexia. AST and ALT levels are elevated. No distinct masses are noted, but the liver is hyperechoic and free fluid is noted within the abdominal cavity (Fig. 3-14). The border of the liver shows nodular irregularities. What is the best diagnosis?

5. A 41-year-old woman undergoes an ultrasound to assess a TIPS catheter. The patient has liver failure and is seen for a 6-month follow-up on the TIPS catheter. At the time of the initial examination, the velocity within the catheter was noted to be 75 cm/s. The catheter is patent and shows forward flow (Fig. 3-15). Flow velocity within the catheter is noted to be 80 cm/s. What is the best diagnosis?

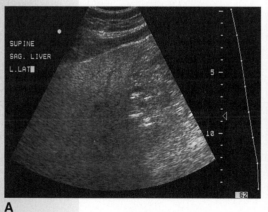
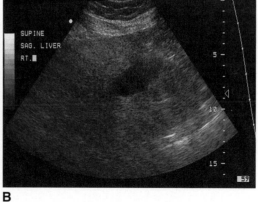

A **B**

Fig. 3-11 **A,** Sagittal image of liver. Notice poor definition of hepatic vessels and smooth hepatic echo texture. **B,** Sagittal image of liver. Note hypoechoic echo texture and poor visualization of hepatic vasculature.

CASE STUDIES FOR DISCUSSION—cont'd

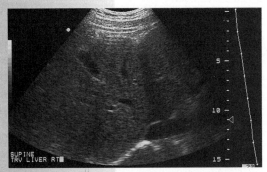

Fig. 3-12 Transverse image of right lobe of liver. Note hypoechoic echo texture of liver parenchyma.

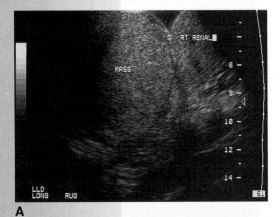

A

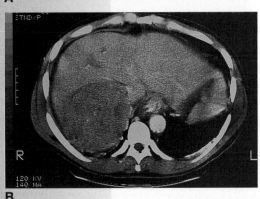

B

Fig. 3-13 **A,** Sagittal image of kidney liver interface documenting large mass superior to right kidney. **B,** Computed tomographic image shows large mass in right posterior lobe of liver.

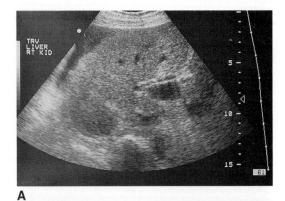

A

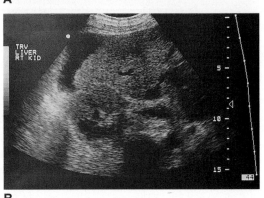

B

Fig. 3-14 **A,** Transverse image of liver. Note free fluid and scalloped borders of liver. **B,** Transverse image of liver and right kidney.

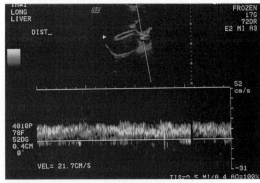

Fig. 3-15 Doppler tracing from TIPS catheter shows forward flow.

STUDY QUESTIONS

1. A 51-year-old man undergoes an ultrasound of the right upper quadrant. Pertinent history includes multiple previous ultrasound examinations that document a small liver that is difficult to penetrate. Liver enzyme levels (AST, ALT, GGT, PTT, and albumin) are elevated. The patient is very thin, with a slightly protruding abdomen. The liver remains small and difficult to penetrate, with poorly documented hepatic vasculature. No specific masses are noted. Free fluid is noted within Morison's pouch (the right subhepatic space) and the right subphrenic space. The anterior border of the liver is noted to have a scalloped appearance. Which of the following is the most likely diagnosis?
   a. acute hepatitis
   b. chronic hepatitis
   c. hepatoma
   d. cirrhosis
   e. fatty infiltration

2. A 43-year-old woman undergoes an ultrasound to rule out gallstones. No laboratory values are available. She is moderately obese. The gallbladder contains a single stone, which produces a clean posterior shadow. The liver is hyperechoic, but hepatic vasculature is poorly seen. No distinct masses are noted. Based on her history and the findings described, which of the following is the most likely diagnosis?
   a. acute hepatitis
   b. chronic hepatitis
   c. hepatoma
   d. cirrhosis
   e. fatty infiltration

3. A 21-year-old man undergoes a right upper quadrant ultrasound in the emergency room. AST and ALT levels are elevated. The liver appears normal in echo texture without masses noted. The right posterior lobe extends inferiorly beyond the lower pole of the right kidney. Which of the following is the most likely diagnosis?
   a. acute hepatitis
   b. chronic hepatitis
   c. hepatoma
   d. cirrhosis
   e. fatty infiltration

4. A 52-year-old man with long-standing cirrhosis undergoes an abdominal ultrasound scan. AST, ALT,

and GGT levels are elevated . The liver is small and difficult to penetrate. Doppler examination reveals hepatofugal blood flow in the main portal vein. Which of the following is the most likely diagnosis based on these findings?
   a. acute hepatitis
   b. portal hypertension
   c. recannalized umbilical vein
   d. hepatoma

5. A 41-year-old woman with long-standing cirrhosis undergoes an abdominal ultrasound scan. AST, ALT, and GGT levels are elevated. The liver is small and difficult to penetrate. A sonolucent area is noted between the left lateral and medial lobes and shows flow with color Doppler. Based on these findings, what is the most likely diagnosis?
   a. portal hypertension
   b. fatty infiltration
   c. recannalized umbilical vein
   d. hepatoma
   e. both a and c

6. A 62-year-old man with long-standing cirrhosis undergoes an abdominal ultrasound scan. AST, ALT, and GGT levels are elevated. The patient has long-standing portal venous hypertension that has been managed with the placement of a TIPS catheter. Ultrasound has been requested to assess the shunt for patency and size. The velocity within the TIPS catheter was documented at 150 cm/s on the previous study of 6 months ago. Current flow is documented at 200 cm/s. What is most likely on the basis of the provided information?
   a. catheter stenosis
   b. shunt thrombosis
   c. normal flow characteristics noted
   d. worsening liver function

7. A 31-year-old woman undergoes a right upper quadrant ultrasound scan. She is obese and has right upper quadrant pain. Liver enzyme levels are normal. The gallbladder is normal in appearance. The liver is noted to be hyperechoic, and hepatic vasculature is difficult to define. One hypoechoic area is noted anterior to the right portal vein near the porta hepatus. On the basis of these findings, what is the most likely diagnosis?
   a. acute hepatitis
   b. portal hypertension
   c. fatty infiltration

   d. fat sparing
   e. cirrhosis
   f. both c and d

8. A 36-year-old woman undergoes a right upper quadrant ultrasound. AST and ALT levels are elevated. The liver appears hyperechoic in appearance. The portal veins appear prominent, with thick walls noted. The gallbladder shows a thick wall without internal inclusions. Based on the findings noted, which of the following is the most likely diagnosis?
   a. acute hepatitis
   b. chronic hepatitis
   c. hepatoma
   d. cirrhosis
   e. fatty infiltration

9. A 54-year-old man with fatigue is seen in the ultrasound department. Liver enzyme levels are slightly elevated. The liver is heterogeneous in echo texture. Based on the findings noted, what is the best diagnosis?
   a. cirrhosis
   b. hepatoma
   c. acute hepatitis
   d. lymphoma

10. A patient is seen in the ultrasound department with a long-standing history of cirrhosis and a recent surgical intervention of portal hypertension. Sonographically, a tubular structure is noted within the right lobe of the liver that shows blood flow within it. Based on the history and the sonographic findings, which of the following is the most likely diagnosis?
   a. mesocaval shunt
   b. portacaval shunt
   c. splenorenal shunt
   d. TIPS catheter

REFERENCES

1. Beers MH, Berkow R: *The Merck manual*, ed 17, Whitehouse Station, NJ, 2001, Merck & Co, Inc.
2. Hagen-Ansert SL: *Textbook of diagnostic ultrasonography*, vol 1, ed 5, St Louis, 2001, Mosby.
3. Zwiebel WJ, Sohaey R: *Introduction to ultrasound*, Philadelphia, 1998, WB Saunders.
4. Hickey J, Goldberg F: *Ultrasound review of the abdomen, male pelvis and small parts*, Philadelphia, 1999, Lippincott.
5. Kawamura DM: *Diagnostic medical sonography: a guide to clinical practice*, vol III, Philadelphia, 1992, Lippincott.
6. Gill KA: *Abdominal ultrasound: a reactionary's guide*, Philadelphia, 2001, WB Saunders.
7. Kim CK, Lim JH, Lee WJ: Detection of hepatocellular carcinomas and dysplastic nodules in cirrhotic liver, *J Ultrasound Med* 20:99-124, 2001.
8. Thibodeau GA, Patton KT: *The human body in health and disease*, St Louis, 1997, Mosby.
9. Bates JA: *Abdominal ultrasound: how, why and when.* Leeds, United Kingdom, 1999, Churchill Livingstone.
10. Andrew A: Portal hypertension: a review, *J Diagn Med Sonography* 17:193-200, 2001.
11. Miller BF: *Miller-Keane encyclopedia and dictionary of medicine, nursing and allied health*, ed 6, Philadelphia, 1997, WB Saunders.
12. US Department of Labor: *Occupational Safety and Health Administration. Safer needle devices: protecting health care workers,* http://www.osha.gov/SLTC/needlestick/safer needledevices/saferneedledevices.html, retrieved June 22, 2003.
13. Rumack CM, Wilson SB, Charboneau JW: *Diagnostic ultrasound*, vol 1, ed 2, St Louis, 1998, Mosby.
14. Numata K et al: Contrast-enhanced wide-band harmonic gray scale imaging of hepatocellular carcinoma: correlation with helical computed tomographic findings. *J Diagn Med Sonography* 20:89-97, 2001.
15. Merton DA: Contrast enhanced hepatic sonography. *J Ultrasound Med* 18:5-15, 2002.
16. Lawson TL: *Diagnostic ultrasonography test and syllabus.* 1994, American College of Radiology, Reston, Virginia.
17. Fishman EK: *Current concepts in the diagnosis and management of patients with parenchymal liver disease. Role of spiral and multidetector CT,.* http://www.ctisus.org/multidetector/syllabus/liver_disease.html, retrieved June 22, 2003.

4 Epigastric Pain

JOYCE GRUBE

CLINICAL SCENARIO

■ A 62-year-old man is seen with epigastric pain and nausea for 2 weeks. He has a history of smoking 1½ packs of cigarettes a day for more than 40 years. He has tried to quit smoking several times, to no avail. In the past 4 months he has had a weight loss of 26 pounds, without an intentional change in his diet. On physical examination, a palpable mass is found in the right upper quadrant. His physician notices early signs of jaundice and orders a complete blood workup. Because of his suspicions, the physician also orders an abdominal sonographic examination.

Sonographic images reveal an enlarged gallbladder with no evidence of gallstones (Fig. 4-1, *A*). The wall of the gallbladder appears normal, with no signs of inflammation. The common bile duct measures 1.3 cm at its maximum diameter, which is abnormal (Fig. 4-1, *B*). In the head of the pancreas, an ill-defined, predominantly hypoechoic lesion is noted (Fig. 4-1, *C*). What is the likely diagnosis?

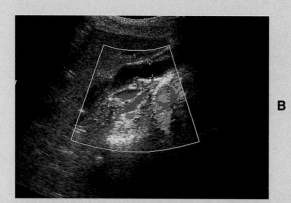

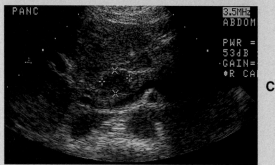

Fig. 4-1 **A,** Sonographic image of gallbladder. **B,** Sonographic image of dilated common bile duct. **C,** Sonographic image of head of pancreas.

OBJECTIVES

- List several causes of epigastric pain not associated with pancreatic disease.
- Describe the normal sonographic appearance of the pancreas and surrounding structures.
- Describe the sonographic appearance of the more common inflammations of the pancreas.
- Describe the sonographic appearance of the more common benign and malignant neoplasms of the pancreas.

- List the risk factors associated with various diseases of the pancreas.
- Identify pertinent laboratory values associated with specific diseases of the pancreas.

GLOSSARY OF TERMS

Acini: smallest cells of the pancreas that comprise the exocrine portion

Amylase: a pancreas enzyme that converts starches to carbohydrates

Choledocholithiasis: presence of biliary stones in the common bile duct

Cholelithiasis: presence of stones in the gallbladder

Courvoisier's gallbladder: enlargement of the gallbladder caused by a slow progressive obstruction of the distal common bile duct (as in adenocarcinoma of the head of the pancreas)

Cystic fibrosis: a hereditary disease that causes excessive production of thick mucus by the endocrine glands

Diverticulitis: inflammation of pouchlike herniations of the bowel wall

Endoscopic retrograde cholangiopancreatogram: an imaging procedure used to evaluate bile ducts and pancreatic ducts

Esophagitis: inflammation of the mucosal lining of the esophagus

Fatty infiltration: accumulation of fat within the cells of a structure or organ

Gastric reflux: an abnormal backward flow of gastric fluids into the esophagus

Harmonics: frequencies that are integral multiples of a fundamental or original frequency

Hippel-Lindau disease: a hereditary disease characterized by neoplasms or cysts that form in a variety of organs, including the pancreas

Hypoglycemic episode: a decreased amount of glucose in the blood caused by increased insulin

Islets of Langerhans: small cells that compose the endocrine portion of the pancreas

Leukocytosis: an abnormal increase in white blood cells caused by infections

Lipase: a pancreas enzyme that breaks down fat

Lymphoma: a malignant neoplasm that arises from the lymphoid tissues

Obstructive jaundice: excessive bilirubin in the bloodstream caused by an obstruction of bile flow from the liver; characterized by a yellow discoloration of the sclera of the eye, skin, and mucous membranes

Oral contrast agent: cellulose suspended in a liquid form, consumed by a patient to enhance gastrointestinal structures during sonographic examination

Polycystic disease: multiple cysts of the pancreas that originate from polycystic renal disease

Pseudocyst: a space or cavity that contains fluid but has no lining membrane

---

Initial sonographic evaluation of the patient with epigastric pain may reveal a broad spectrum of findings. If the pancreas appears normal, the clinician must include inflammation of the pancreas and other non–pancreas-related pathology among the differential diagnoses. Diagnoses not specific to the pancreas may include gastric or duodenal ulcer disease, **gastric reflux** disease or **esophagitis, diverticulitis** of the transverse colon, biliary disease, liver abscess, heart disease, or aortic dissection. Diseases that cause epigastric pain specific to the pancreas are included in the scope of this chapter.

Although computed tomographic (CT) scan plays a primary role in evaluation of the pancreas for disease, sonography is more readily available, more cost effective, and offers a nonradiation alternative for the evaluation of epigastric pain.[1] The pancreas is often thought of as the most difficult organ in the abdomen to image. Sonographers may improve visualization of the pancreas with a variety of techniques including (1) a complete understanding of the surrounding anatomy and gastrointestinal structures, (2) persistence while scanning, (3) image optimization, and (4) the use of **oral contrast agents.**[1] Nonetheless, sonography plays a significant role in the evaluation of the patient with jaundice, the serial examination of inflammatory processes, and needle guidance for interventional procedures of the pancreas.

PANCREAS
Normal Sonographic Anatomy

The pancreas is a retroperitoneal organ that lies in the anterior pararenal space of the epigastrium. The entire pancreas is contained between the C-loop of the duodenum and the splenic hilum. The different

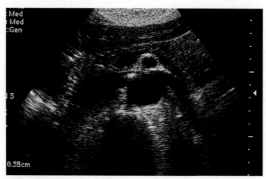

Fig. 4-2   Normal pancreas and surrounding vasculature in mid epigastrium on sonography.

portions of the pancreas include the head, uncinate process, neck, body, and tail. The normal adult pancreas is approximately 12 to 15 cm in length.[2] The normal pancreatic duct may be visualized at a measurement of 2 mm or less.[3]

The echogenicity of the pancreas is isoechoic to hyperechoic compared with the liver and may increase with age and obesity because of **fatty infiltration.**[2] In children, the pancreas may appear hypoechoic to isoechoic compared with the liver because of less fat composition.

The lie of the pancreas in the epigastrium is transverse yet slightly oblique, with the head located more inferior than the tail. The pancreas is a nonencapsulated organ, so the borders are somewhat indistinct on sonography. Therefore, the sonographer must have a thorough understanding of the surrounding vasculature to aid in the detection of the pancreatic boundaries (Fig. 4-2).

The sonographer must also appreciate the portions of the gastrointestinal tract that surround the pancreas and make visualization difficult. The fundus of the stomach lies superior to the pancreatic tail. The body of the stomach lies anterior to the pancreatic tail. The pylorus lies anterior to the pancreatic body and neck. The superior duodenum (first portion) lies anterior to the pancreatic neck and superior to the head of the pancreas. The descending duodenum (second portion) lies lateral to the head. The horizontal duodenum (third portion) lies inferior to the pancreatic head. The ascending duodenum (fourth portion) lies inferior to the body of the pancreas. The transverse colon lies anterior and inferior to the entire length of the pancreas (Fig. 4-3). Identification of the various portions of the gastrointestinal tract during scanning will allow the sonographer to change the patient position to move obscuring bowel away from the pancreas.

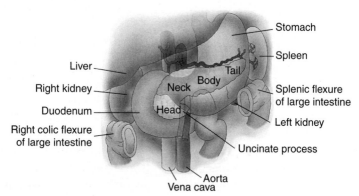

Fig. 4-3   Relationship of stomach, duodenum, and transverse colon with pancreas.

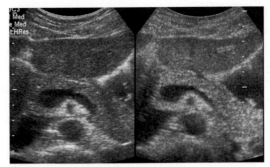

Fig. 4-4 Conventional transverse image of normal pancreas on *left*. Same pancreatic view with tissue harmonic imaging on *right*. Note improved clarity and detail of anatomic structures with harmonics.

Harmonics may enable the sonographer to optimize visualization of the pancreas, especially in technically difficult cases. Harmonic imaging is based on the concept that an ultrasound pulse interacts with tissue and echoes are created at the original or fundamental frequency along with echoes at multiples of the original frequency (i.e., a 2-MHz pulse will generate echoes at 2 MHz, 4 MHz [second harmonic], 6 MHz, [third harmonic], 8 MHz [fourth harmonic]). Conventional ultrasound listens to the fundamental frequency and ignores the harmonic frequencies. Tissue harmonic imaging uses the second harmonic frequency for image clarity. Harmonic imaging in the abdomen may also reduce image artifacts, haze, and clutter and significantly improve contrast resolution (Fig. 4-4).

If the pancreatic tail is the primary area of interest, the sonographer or physician may elect to use an oral contrast agent to complement the study. The cellulose suspension should remain in the stomach for an adequate period to provide an acoustic window for better visualization of the pancreatic tail (Fig. 4-5).[1]

PANCREATITIS
Acute Pancreatitis

Acute pancreatitis is characterized by the escape of toxic pancreatic juices into the parenchymal tissues of the gland. These digestive enzymes cause destruction of the acini, ducts, small blood vessels, and fat and may extend beyond the gland to peripancreatic tissues. Acute inflammation of the pancreas is generally caused by one of two factors: biliary disease and alcoholism. Other sources may include trauma, pregnancy, peptic ulcer disease, medications, hereditary factors, systemic infections, posttransplant complications, and iatrogenic causes (e.g., **endoscopic retrograde cholangiopancreatogram [ERCP]**, endoscopy).[2] Patients with acute

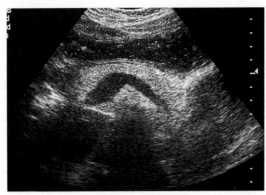

Fig. 4-5 Normal transverse pancreas image after patient ingestion of oral contrast agent. Note superior visualization of pancreatic tail immediately posterior to suspended contrast in stomach.

pancreatitis have a sudden onset of persistent mid-epigastric pain that may be moderate to severe and that often radiates to the patient's mid back. Fever and **leukocytosis** accompany the attack. Classically, serum **amylase** levels increase within 24 hours of onset and **lipase** levels increase within 72 hours.

Sonographic Findings. The pancreas may appear normal in the early stage of acute pancreatitis, with no noticeable change in the size or echogenicity of the gland. Once the changes become evident, acute pancreatitis may have a diffuse or focal appearance on sonographic examination. The pancreatic duct may be enlarged in either presentation. Diffuse disease causes an increase in size and a decrease in echogenicity from swelling and congestion. The borders of the pancreas may appear irregular. Focal inflammation may be seen as enlargement and a hypoechoic appearance to a specific region of the gland. If focal pancreatitis is present in the pancreatic head, biliary dilation and a **Courvoisier's gallbladder** may also be appreciated. The sonographer must carefully evaluate the pancreatic head for adenocarcinoma and the biliary tree for the presence of **cholelithiasis** and **choledocholithiasis** as a possible cause of pancreatitis.

Chronic Pancreatitis

Recurrent attacks of acute inflammation of the pancreas are considered chronic pancreatitis. Further destruction of the pancreatic parenchyma results in atrophy, fibrosis, scarring, and calcification of the gland. Stone formation within the pancreatic duct is common, as is the development of pancreatic pseudocysts in 25% to 40% of patients.[2] Patients generally have progressing epigastric pain. Jaundice may also be seen in patients with a distal biliary duct obstruction.

Sonographic Findings. On ultrasound, the pancreas generally appears smaller than normal and hyperchoic because of scarring and fibrosis. Diffuse calcifications are the classic sonographic feature of chronic pancreatitis and are usually noted throughout the parenchyma, causing a coarse echotexture.[4] Stones may also be visualized within a dilated pancreatic duct. Associated findings include **pseudocyst** formation, cholelithiasis, choledocholithiasis, and portosplenic thrombosis.

Pseudocysts

Pseudocysts are composed of extravasated pancreatic enzymes that escape into the peripancreatic soft tissues. The fluid begins to collect, and eventually a thickened wall of collagen and granulation tissue develops (different from the thin, epithelial cell wall of a true cyst). Pseudocysts may result from acute and chronic pancreatitis or from trauma to the pancreas. Pseudocysts can be singular or multiple. Most often, they arise from the tail of the pancreas and are located in the lesser sac. Less often, they may be located in the right and left anterior pararenal spaces, peritoneum, mesentery, pelvis, groin, or mediastinum. Pseudocysts may be fairly large on initial diagnosis because of late symptoms from compression effects. Aspiration or surgery is necessary in 80% of pancreatic pseudocysts, and 20% resolve spontaneously.

Sonographic Findings. Pancreatic pseudocysts are generally well defined and internally anechoic with posterior acoustic enhancement. Occasionally, they may appear complex with internal echoes from inflammation, hemorrhage, or necrosis. They may also have internal septations or calcified walls. Serial sonographic examination is an excellent method for following spontaneous regression of pseudocysts. In addition, sonography plays a useful role in percutaneous aspiration of pseudocysts.

PANCREATIC NEOPLASMS
Adenocarcinoma

Adenocarcinoma is the most common neoplasm, comprising 95% of all malignant diseases that affect the pancreas.[3] Adenocarcinoma arises from the pancreatic ductal epithelium and rarely from the **acini** and is more common among men after age 60 years. The prognosis for patients with adenocarcinoma is extremely poor; it is the fourth leading cause of death from cancer in the United States.[2,4]

Adenocarcinoma is most commonly found in the head of the pancreas and least commonly in the tail. The most frequently recognized symptom is a persistent, aching pain in the mid epigastrium or mid back. The type and onset of symptoms are also related to the location of the tumor. Tumors that arise from the pancreatic head cause constriction of the distal biliary duct, and, therefore, symptoms are seen fairly early. Patients typically have a palpable gallbladder and **obstructive jaundice.** If the tumor arises from the pancreatic body or tail, symptoms tend to manifest later in the disease and metastasis is likely. Patients may have weight loss, nausea and vomiting, diabetes, and intestinal malabsorption.

The remaining malignant tumors that affect the pancreas include cystadenocarcinoma, malignant islet cell tumors, ampullary carcinoma, squamous cell carcinoma, and **lymphoma.**

Sonographic Findings. The most common sonographic appearance of adenocarcinoma is an irregular hypoechoic mass in the pancreas. Isoechoic tumors may simply be seen as enlargement or an irregular contour of a specific region of the pancreas. If the tumor is large on initial diagnosis, compression or deviation of adjacent structures may be evident. Sonographers must also rely on indirect sonographic features of adenocarcinoma, which may include pancreatic duct dilation, displacement of vasculature surrounding the pancreas, Courvoisier's gallbladder, dilated extrahepatic and intrahepatic bile ducts, biliary sludge, lymphadenopathy, and liver metastasis.

Cystadenomas

Cystadenomas of the pancreas are rare cystic tumors that arise from the pancreatic duct tissues and that typically affect women more often than men. Cystadenomas may be microcystic serous type (cysts measure less than 2 cm) or macrocystic mucinous type (cysts measure greater than 2 cm). The microcystic form is always benign, and the macrocystic form carries suspicion of malignant disease (cystadenocarcinoma). Cystadenomas occur more frequently in the body and tail of the pancreas. They may be unilocular or multilocular and may have internal echoes, septations, papillary projections, and calcifications. Patients may be asymptomatic or have epigastric pain, weight loss, palpable abdominal mass, or jaundice.

Sonographic Findings. Cystadenomas have a variety of sonographic appearances. They generally appear as a single or lobulated anechoic mass with posterior acoustic enhancement. They may have internal septations, thick walls, internal echoes, papillary projections, calcifications, or an overall solid appearance. Differentiation between benign and malignant tumors is not possible without histopathology. Cystadenomas may also appear similar to pseudocysts,[5] **polycystic disease, cystic fibrosis,**[6] and **Hippel-Lindau disease.**[2,4]

Islet Cell Tumors

Islet cell tumors of the pancreas are primary tumors that arise from the **islets of Langerhans.** They are classified as functioning and nonfunctioning based on their potential to secrete hormones. Nonfunctioning islet cell tumors make up approximately 30% of all islet cell tumors and have a tendency to be malignant. Functioning islet cell tumors are more often benign, with the two most common known as *insulinomas* and *gastrinomas*. Patients with insulinomas may have obesity and **hypoglycemic episodes.** Islet cell tumors are slow-growing small tumors that are generally found in the body and tail of the pancreas. Multiple islet cell tumors may be present on diagnosis.

Sonographic Findings. Most islet cell tumors are hypoechoic compared with the surrounding pancreas tissues. Visualization of these tumors is difficult because of their small size. Intraoperative ultrasound has been extremely valuable in the identification and localization of islet cell tumors.[1] Harmonic imaging, as part of image optimization techniques, may also improve the detection of small tumors.[7]

Table 4-1 is a summary of the pathology, location, and sonographic findings of pancreatic masses.

SUMMARY

Sonography assessment of the patient with epigastric pain may be performed to determine initial diagnosis or as a follow-up examination of pancreatic disease. In either case, sonography provides valuable information in differentiation of solid and cystic tumors, assessment of tumor extent, provision of serial evaluation, and performance of interventional treatments of pancreatic diseases. Clinicians should recognize the feasibility of sonography for precise diagnosis and avoidance of unnecessary and costly examinations for the patient.

CLINICAL SCENARIO—DIAGNOSIS

■ Significant weight loss and jaundice are clear warning signs of pancreatic cancer. The identification of an ill-defined hypoechoic lesion in the head of the pancreas of a symptomatic patient is strongly suggestive of adenocarcinoma (see Fig. 4-1, *C*). Sonography also is used to confirm the nature of a palpable mass in the right upper quadrant as a Courvoisier's gallbladder (gallbladder enlargement from a distal common bile duct obstruction; see Fig. 4-1, *A*). A common bile duct that measures 1.3 cm is markedly dilated and correlates with obstructive jaundice (see Fig. 4-1, *B*). After CT scan, this patient had a surgical biopsy that proved ductal adenocarcinoma. The patient lived 82 days after the day of diagnosis.

Table 4-1	*Pancreatic Masses*	
Pathology	**Typical Location**	**Sonographic Findings**
Pseudocyst	Tail	Anechoic, posterior enhancement; may also appear complex with internal septations or calcified walls
Adenocarcinoma	Head	Irregular, hypoechoic mass; may have secondary pancreatic duct dilation, biliary dilation, lymphadenopathy, and liver metastasis
Cystadenoma 　Microcystic 　Macrocystic 　Cystadenocarcinoma	Body and tail	Single or lobulated anechoic mass, posterior enhancement; may have internal septations, thick walls, internal echoes, papillary projections, calcifications, or solid appearance
Islet cell tumor 　Malignant islet cell tumor 　Insulinoma 　Gastrinoma	Body and tail	Hypechoic, small

CASE STUDIES FOR DISCUSSION

1. A moderately overweight 43-year-old woman is seen in the sonography department for an abdominal examination. She states that she has had mild indigestion, nausea, general fatigue, and episodes of low blood sugar. The sonographic examination reveals a normal gallbladder with a common bile duct of 4.3 mm. While imaging the pancreas, the sonographer notices a small, oval, predominantly hypoechoic lesion between the body and tail that measures 1.5 cm (Fig. 4-6). What is the most likely diagnosis?

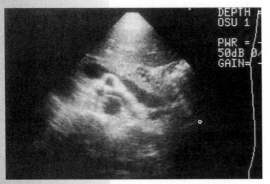

Fig. 4-6   Small hypoechoic mass is visualized between body and tail of pancreas.

2. A 72-year-old man with fatigue and depression from the recent death of his wife reports to the sonography department for an abdominal ultrasound examination. The primary care physician had palpated a pulsatile abdominal mass in the mid abdomen and asked the sonographer to evaluate the aorta for evidence of an aneurysm. The sonographer documents a normal-sized abdominal aorta yet discovers an incidental mass near the tail of the pancreas. The mass measures 3.6 cm and appears hypechoic compared with the normal pancreas tissue. A subsequent CT scan provides no additional information (Fig. 4-7). What are the possible diagnoses?

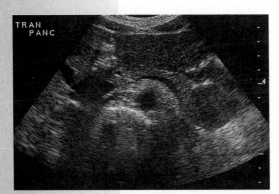

Fig. 4-7   Large hypoechoic mass measuring 3.6 cm was found on sonogram in tail of pancreas.

3. A 50-year-old man with chronic epigastric pain and nausea and vomiting is seen by his physician. The patient is a Vietnam veteran with many years of alcohol abuse who has had recent weight loss, malaise, and loss of appetite. The sonographic examination reveals a hyperechoic, heterogeneous pancreas with a pancreatic duct that measures 0.7 cm. Also noted is a round, 2-cm echogenic structure with posterior shadowing within the body/tail region of the pancreas (Fig. 4-8). What is the most likely diagnosis?

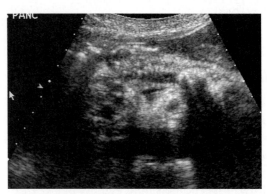

Fig. 4-8   Transverse pancreatic image reveals hyperechoic gland, dilated pancreatic duct, and presence of pancreatic duct stone.

4. A 60-year-old woman in excellent health is seen by her physician with epigastric discomfort for 6 months. The sonographer notices an unusual lesion near the tail of the pancreas. The lesion appears as a multilobulated, cystic mass with posterior acoustic enhancement. A CT scan examination is ordered and confirms the presence and location of the tumor. A surgical biopsy is then performed (Fig. 4-9). What is the most likely diagnosis?

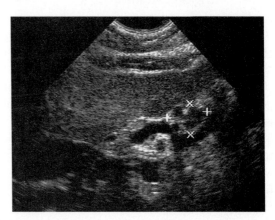

Fig. 4-9   Small multilobulated cystic mass is noted near tail of pancreas.

CASE STUDIES FOR DISCUSSION—cont'd

5. A 31-year-old man is seen in the emergency department with severe midepigastric pain radiating to his back, with nausea and vomiting that he states came on suddenly with a fever 24 hours previously. The laboratory blood work results show an elevated white blood cell count, moderately elevated amylase level, and mildly elevated lipase. With further questioning, the patient admits to an alcoholic binge with old college buddies 2 days previously. An ultrasound examination of the upper abdomen reveals an irregular, hypoechoic region in the tail of the pancreas (Fig. 4-10). What is the likely diagnosis?

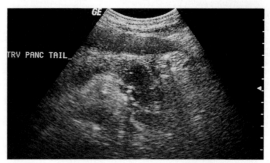

Fig. 4-10 Irregular hypoechoic lesion is noted in tail of pancreas.

STUDY QUESTIONS

1. Which of the following conditions make the pancreas difficult to image for sonography?
   a. its deep location in the mid abdomen
   b. proximity of the stomach and duodenum
   c. proximity of the transverse colon
   d. indistinct borders from absence of a true capsule
   e. all of the above

2. A 69-year-old man with alcoholism is seen with leukocytosis, an elevated amylase level, and a rising lipase level. The entire pancreas appears enlarged and hypoechoic, with ill-defined borders. The most likely diagnosis is which of the following?
   a. acute focal pancreatitis
   b. acute diffuse pancreatitis
   c. chronic pancreatitis
   d. pseudocyst
   e. hemorrhagic pancreatitis

3. A 47-year-old woman with previous cholelithiasis returns to the sonography department after a cholecystectomy 6 months previously. She now has severe epigastric pain and persistent fever. Sonographic results show choledocholithiasis, a dilated pancreatic duct, and fluid collection anterior to the tail of the pancreas. The fluid collection most likely represents which of the following?
   a. acute focal pancreatitis
   b. acute diffuse pancreatitis
   c. chronic pancreatitis
   d. pseudocyst
   e. hemorrhagic pancreatitis

4. A 52-year-old woman is seen in the emergency department with epigastric discomfort and chest pressure. Electrocardiogram results are normal, and a nitroglycerin tablet does not relieve the pain. The laboratory values show an elevated white blood cell count, mildly elevated amylase level, and markedly elevated lipase level. The abdominal sonographic examination reveals a small, hyperechoic pancreas with dilated pancreatic duct. The most likely diagnosis is which of the following?
   a. acute focal pancreatitis
   b. acute diffuse pancreatitis
   c. chronic pancreatitis
   d. pseudocyst
   e. hemorrhagic pancreatitis

5. A 45-year-old woman is seen by her physician with mild epigastric pain, weight loss, and a large palpable abdominal mass. The sonographic examination reveals a 9-cm multilobulated, cystic mass occupying the mid epigastrium. The cysts measure larger than 2 cm, with internal papillary projections and calcifications. CT scan results confirm the mass originates from the pancreatic body. The most likely diagnosis is which of the following?
   a. pseudocyst
   b. microcystic cystadenoma
   c. macrocystic cystadenocarcinoma
   d. islet cell tumor
   e. Hippel-Lindau disease

6. A 56-year-old woman is seen in the sonography department for a renal examination. While scanning

the left kidney, the sonographer notices a multicystic mass in the tail of the pancreas. The patient is asymptomatic for pancreatic disease. CT scan follow-up confirms a multicystic lesion, with cysts that measure less than 2 cm. The most likely diagnosis is which of the following?

a. pseudocyst
b. microcystic cystadenoma
c. macrocystic cystadenocarcinoma
d. adenocarcinoma
e. Hippel-Lindau disease

7. A 39-year-old morbidly obese woman undergoes surgery for a gastric stapling and an abdominal exploratory procedure. She had hormonal imbalances. During surgery, the surgeon notices an irregularity on the anterior surface of the pancreas. Intraoperative sonography reveals two small hypoechoic lesions that measure approximately 1 cm. The most likely diagnosis is which of the following?

a. pseudocysts
b. microcystic cystadenomas
c. adenocarcinomas
d. islet cell tumors
e. Hippel-Lindau disease

8. Visualization of which of the following structures is most improved with oral contrast during pancreatic sonography?

a. head of the pancreas
b. tail of the pancreas
c. peripancreatic tissues
d. pancreatic duct
e. uncinate process of the pancreas

9. Because of difficulty in examination of the pancreas, sonographers must rely on indirect features of adenocarcinoma. These may include all of the following except:

a. Courvoisier's gallbladder
b. pancreatic duct dilation
c. dilated bile ducts
d. fluid-filled stomach
e. liver metastasis

10. Image-optimizing techniques that are useful for improvement of visualization of the pancreas may include all of the following except:

a. decreasing transducer frequency for thin patients
b. color or power Doppler
c. harmonic imaging
d. oral contrast agents
e. variable focusing capabilities

REFERENCES

1. McGahan JP, Goldberg BB: *Diagnostic ultrasound: a logical approach*, Philadelphia, 1998, Lippincott.
2. Rumack CM, Wilson SR, Charboneau JW: *Diagnostic ultrasound*, vol 1, ed 2, St Louis, 1998, Mosby.
3. Hagen-Ansert SL: *Textbook of diagnostic ultrasonography*, vol 1, ed 5, St Louis, 2001, Mosby.
4. Kurtz AB, Middleton WD: *Ultrasound: the requisites*, St Louis, 1996, Mosby.
5. Scott J et al: Mucinous cystic neoplasms of the pancreas: imaging features and diagnostic difficulties, *Clin Radiol* 55:187-192, 2000.
6. Kawamura DM: *Abdomen and superficial structures*, ed 2, Philadelphia, 1997, Lippincott.
7. Ding H et al: Sonographic diagnosis of pancreatic islet cell tumor: value of intermittent harmonic imaging, *J Clin Ultrasound* 29:411-416, 2001.

BIBLIOGRAPHY

Anderson KN, Anderson LE, Glanze WD: *Mosby's medical, nursing, & allied health dictionary*, ed 5, St Louis, 1998, Mosby.

Lundstedt C, Dawiskiba S: Serous and mucinous cystadenoma/cystadenocarcinoma of the pancreas, *Abdom Imaging* 25:201, 2000.

Nocente R et al: An apparent idiopathic case of relapsing acute pancreatitis, *Hepato-Gastroenterology,* 48:572-573, 2001.

Kullavanijaya P et al: Adenocarcinoma of the pancreas: the clinical experience of 45 histopathologically proven patients, a 6 year study, *J Med Assoc Thailand* 84:640-647, 2001.

5

Hematuria

KERRY WEINBERG and JOSEPH YEE

CLINICAL SCENARIO

■ An abdominal ultrasound is ordered for a woman who is almost 60 years old and has a history of lung carcinoma. Multiple abdominal lesions were identified previously on a computed tomographic (CT) scan. The patient is now seen in the sonography department with flank pain and hematuria.

Bilateral solid hypoechoic masses are identified—one in the right lower pole and one in the left renal parenchyma at the level of the mid to upper pole. Increased cortical blood flow is also seen. No hydronephrosis is identified in either kidney, and the urinary bladder is empty. What is the most likely diagnosis?

OBJECTIVES

■ Describe the sonographic appearance of the genitourinary system.

■ List the causes of hematuria.

■ Describe the sonographic appearance of urolithiasis.

■ Describe the sonographic appearance of the common benign neoplasms of the kidney.

■ Describe the sonographic appearance of the common malignant neoplasms of the kidney.

■ Describe the clinical signs and symptoms associated with hematuria.

GLOSSARY OF TERMS

Aniridia: absence of the iris

Beckwith-Wiedemann syndrome: an autosomal recessive syndrome that is characterized by an omphalocele, macroglossia, enlarged organs, and neonatal hyperglycemia

Candle sign: low continuous ureteral jet flow that is seen with a partial ureter obstruction or ureterocele

Cystoscopy: use of a lighted tube to see within the urinary bladder

Dysuria: painful or difficult urination

Erythropoietin: a hormone that promotes the formation of red blood cells

Extravasation: forcing of blood or lymph out of the vessel and into the surrounding tissue

Hematoma: a localized walled-off collection of blood that is not in a vessel; the blood is usually clotted

Gross hematuria: blood in the urine that can be seen with the unaided eye

Hematuria: blood in the urine

Hemangioma: a congenital anomaly in which the proliferation of blood vessels forms a mass that may resemble a neoplasm

Hemihypertrophy: a condition in which one side of the body is larger than the other side of the body

Hydroureter: ureter enlarged with fluid

Idiopathic: no known cause

Infundibulum: the funnel-shaped portion of the calyces that joins with the renal pelvis

Intravenous pyelogram: an invasive radiographic procedure in which a contrast agent is injected into a peripheral vein and the kidneys, ureters, and bladder are visualized

Intravenous urogram: see intravenous pyelogram

Leukoplakia: a white patch of oral mucous membrane, not specific to any disease, used as a clinical term without histologic connotation

Lithotripsy: the crushing of stones with sound waves or mechanical force that may be used to break down stones in the renal pelvis, ureter, or urinary bladder

Macroglossia: enlarged tongue

Microscopic hematuria: blood in the urine that is seen only with a microscope

Nephrolithiasis: renal calculi

Renal colic: severe pain caused by a stone obstructing or passing the renal collecting system or ureter

Twinkle sign: a color Doppler artifact in which the color rapidly changes posterior to a urinary tract stone with a comet tail appearance

Tuberous sclerosis: a hereditary disease involving multiple systems in which renal cysts and lesions form in the body; the classic clinical conditions include mental retardation, seizures, and cutaneous lesions

Ureteropelvic junction: the point at which the ureter joins the renal pelvis

Urolithiasis: stone in the urinary system

von Hippel-Lindau disease: an autosomal dominant type of phacomatosis that is primarily associated with hemangiomas or hemangioblastomas of the cerebellumor fourth ventricle and that may also be associated with cysts or hamartomas of the kidneys, adrenal glands, or other organs

---

Hematuria is often the first symptom of a urinary tract problem. The cause of the hematuria may occur anywhere within the urinary system (kidney, ureters, bladder, or urethra). Problems of the lower urinary tract (ureter or bladder) are more likely to have hematuria than are problems of the upper urinary tract (kidney). The amount of blood in the urine can vary from **gross** (visible) **hematuria** to **microscopic hematuria**. No correlation is found between the amount of blood in the urine and the severity of the urinary tract disease. Hematuria is a nonspecific finding, and the most common causes are acute infection (see Chapter 6), tumor, or stones within the urinary tract. Other less common causes include trauma, congenital anomaly, renal vein thrombosis, renal cysts, renal infarction, sickle cell disease, enlarged prostate (see Chapter 30), and bleeding disorders, or the cause may be unknown or undetected.

Urinary tract diseases may not be diagnosed during the early stages when many patients are asymptomatic and do not have urine discoloration unless the amount of red blood cells is significant. The symptoms are primarily related to the cause of the hematuria. Patients with a bladder or kidney tumor, polycystic renal disease, hydronephrosis, benign prostatic hyperplasia, or **urolithiasis** may not have pain. Patients passing a stone have pain or renal colic. Other symptoms patients with hematuria may have include flank pain, fever, vomiting, nausea, fatigue, and **dysuria.**

A urinalysis is performed to confirm the presence of blood in the urine. A culture may also be performed to detect whether bacteria or tumor cells are present in the urine. Once hematuria is detected, a urologic consultation, **cystoscopy, intravenous pyelogram** (IVP), computed tomography (CT), magnetic resonance imaging (MRI), or renal ultrasound examination may be performed to determine the pathology.

GENITOURINARY SYSTEM
Normal Sonographic Anatomy

The kidneys are oval or bean-shaped organs that measure approximately $11 \times 7 \times 3$ cm.[1] They are retroperitoneal and lie anterior to the psoas muscles. The kidneys are paralumbar organs located between the twelfth thoracic vertebra (T12) and the third lumbar vertebra (L3),[1] with the upper poles lying more medial than the lower poles. The liver usually causes the right kidney to be situated slightly lower than the left kidney.

The kidneys have a well-defined border with three layers of protective tissue. The inner, or true, layer is a fibrous capsule that is continuous with the outer layer of the ureters. It protects the kidney from infection. The middle layer is called the *perinephric capsule* and is composed of adipose tissue. It helps hold the kidney in place and protects the kidney from trauma. The outer layer, which surrounds the kidney and adrenal gland, is called *Gerota's fascia.* It consists of fibrous connective tissues that protect and anchor the kidney.

The inner anatomy of the kidney consists of the following three distinct sections: the renal parenchyma (cortex), medullary pyramids (which collect and transport urine to the collecting system), and renal sinus (which contains the collecting system, vessels, fat, and lymphatic tissue). The renal sinus is the echogenic oval region in the mid portion of the kidney, the renal cortex has a midlevel echogenicity, and the medullary pyramids are less echogenic than the cortex. When the renal cortex is compared with the liver, it is hypoechoic (Fig. 5-1, *A* to *E*).

The ureters are not usually imaged on a sonogram unless they are dilated. The ureters exit from the medial aspect of the kidneys and follow a horizontal course anterior to the psoas muscle to the posterior lateral aspect of the urinary bladder. When the ureter is dilated, it appears as a linear anechoic or sonolucent structure.

The urinary bladder is only visualized when it is distended, and then it appears as a fluid-filled, anechoic, thin-walled symmetric structure. Reverberations may be seen in the anterior portion of the fluid-filled urinary bladder.

The urethra is a tubular structure that extends from the base of the urinary bladder to the outside of the body. The urethra in a female is much shorter than that in a male. It is typically not imaged unless an obstruction exists at the urethral level. With sonographic imaging, it appears as a short anechoic or sonolucent tubular structure.

UROLITHIASIS
Nephrolithiasis

Calculi, or stones, can form anywhere within the urinary tract. Most stones originate within the kidney **(nephrolithiasis).** The development of calculi is influenced by hereditary and familial predisposition, high concentrations of stone constituents (uric acid, calcium salts, or a combination of calcium oxalate and calcium phosphate), changes in urine pH, or the presence of bacteria. The development may also be **idiopathic.**[2] Stones are more commonly found in men. The clinical presentation varies depending on the size or location of the stone or whether the stone is being passed. Calculi located in the kidney or proximal portion of the ureter may cause either no pain or dull flank pain, whereas lower back pain radiating down the pelvis may be caused by a stone in the distal ureter or bladder. Severe, sharp pain **(renal colic)** is usually caused by the passage of a stone down the urinary tract. Other clinical symptoms may include nausea, vomiting, fever, chills, and, depending on the presence of obstruction, oliguria. The laboratory findings may consist of hematuria, white blood cells, and bacteria.

A staghorn calculus is a stone that fills the renal pelvis and extends into the **infundibulum** and calyces, causing dilation of the calyces. Stones can cause obstruction of the renal collecting system, or they may pass into the ureter and obstruct it, causing a **hydroureter.** The three most common sites of obstruction are the **ureteropelvic junction** (UPJ), the point at which the ureter crosses over the pelvic brim, or the location at which the ureter enters into the urinary bladder. Stones may also pass into the urinary bladder or, in rare cases, obstruct the urethra.

Sonographic Findings. Calculi appear sonographically as crescent-shaped, echogenic foci. The presence of posterior acoustic shadowing varies according to the

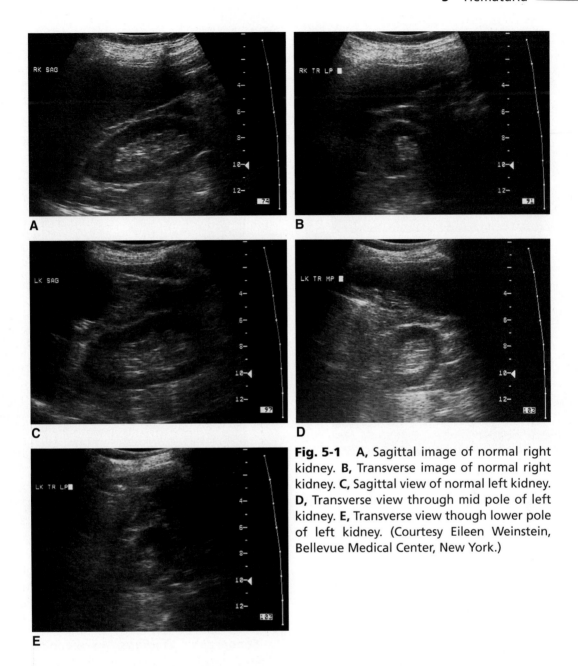

Fig. 5-1 **A,** Sagittal image of normal right kidney. **B,** Transverse image of normal right kidney. **C,** Sagittal view of normal left kidney. **D,** Transverse view through mid pole of left kidney. **E,** Transverse view though lower pole of left kidney. (Courtesy Eileen Weinstein, Bellevue Medical Center, New York.)

size and composition of the stone. Very small stones may not have posterior acoustic shadowing. The use of tissue harmonics when small calculi are suspected increases the chance of seeing posterior acoustic shadowing. Patients with urinary tract calculi who undergo scanning with new-generation equipment may have a color Doppler artifact. The artifact is called a *twinkle sign*, which is imaged as a rapidly changing color posterior to the stone with a comet tail (Fig. 5-2, *A* and *B;* see Color Plate 1 for a color version of Fig. 5-2, *B*).[3,4] A calculus in the kidney may cause obstructive hydronephrosis (see Chapter 6). Stones that pass into the ureter may obstruct it. Absence of a unilateral ureteral jet may occur with complete ureteral

obstruction. A partial ureteral obstruction may cause absence of a ureteral jet or decreased blood flow, which has a pattern that resembles a burning candle **(candle sign)** (Fig. 5-3, *A* and *B*). Sonographic documentation of a ureteral stone is difficult to obtain because of the small size of the calculi, posterior location of the ureter (where the area of interest may not be in the focal zone), lack of fluid surrounding the stone, and adjacent bowel gas (Fig. 5-4, *A* and *B;* see Color Plate 2 for a color version of Fig. 5-4, *B*).

Stones in the urinary bladder appear as echogenic foci that move when patient position is changed. An abdominal radiograph, **an intravenous urogram,** or an antegrade or retrograde study may be used in the

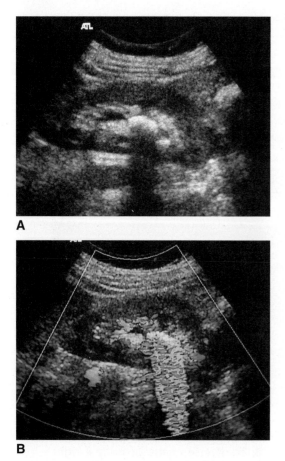

A

B

Fig. 5-2 **A,** Sagittal image of right kidney with large calculi. Posterior shadowing is seen with no renal obstruction. **B,** Sagittal image of right kidney with large calculi. Multiple colors are seen posterior to stone. This is called *twinkle sign*.

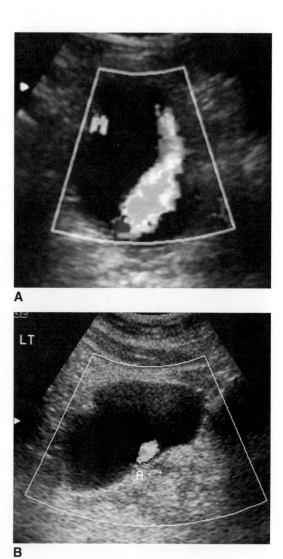

A

B

Fig. 5-3 **A,** Transverse view of normal right ureteral jet. **B,** Stone is causing partial obstruction of left ureter. Low-flow ureteral jet candle sign is seen.

diagnosis of small stones that are not imaged on a sonographic study.

BENIGN NEOPLASMS

Benign neoplasms of the kidney are rare. Any neoplasm of the kidney is assumed to be malignant unless it is proved otherwise.[5]

Adenoma

A renal adenoma is one of the most common benign renal masses.[6,7] Adenomas are small, usually measuring 1 cm or less and rarely larger than 3 cm. They are asymptomatic unless they enlarge.[5] Adenomas arise from tubular epithelial cells and are believed to be the counterpart of malignant renal cell carcinoma (RCC).[8] They are usually located in the renal cortex and are often found as an incidental finding at surgery or autopsy. They may be the cause of painless hematuria.

Sonographic Findings. An adenoma is a well-defined small solid mass usually found in the renal cortex. It may cause bulging of the cortex. It has a similar sonographic appearance to RCC, which tends to be hyperechoic, with areas of calcifications.

Hemangiomas

Hemangiomas of the kidneys are rare benign neoplasms that consist of a mass of blood vessels and that usually occur in the third or fourth decade of life.[6] Patients have hematuria and may have pain. Hemangiomas are difficult to diagnose before surgery.

Sonographic Findings. Hemangiomas are usually small (less than 1 cm), round hyperechoic masses. They may be located at the pelvocalyceal junction or in the inner medulla.

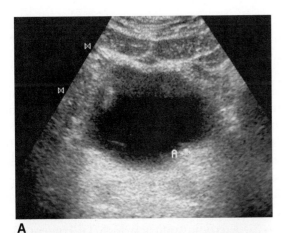

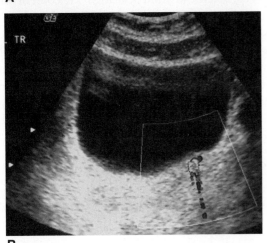

Fig. 5-4 **A,** Small left ureteral stone is measured. **B,** Multiple colors are seen posterior to left ureteral stone. This is called *twinkle sign*.

Hematoma

Hematomas are usually caused by biopsy or trauma in which the kidney becomes lacerated or fractured. One type of renal trauma may be caused by **lithotripsy.** Hematomas may also be caused by the pathologic conditions of RCC, angiomyolipoma (AML), segmental renal infarction, arteriovenous malformation, hemorrhagic cyst, or abscess or have an idiopathic cause.[9] Blood tends to collect either in the perinephric space or below the renal capsule (subcapsular hematoma). Symptoms range from mild abdominal or flank pain to intense pain, depending on the amount of blood that has undergone **extravasation.** Hematocrit levels drop in cases with severe blood loss.

Sonographic Findings. Hematomas vary in sonographic appearance, depending on the age of the patient. Fresh blood (less than 24 hours) may appear anechoic. With a high-resolution transducer, swirling internal echoes may be seen. Hematomas in the acute stages are echogenic. As a clot forms, the hematoma becomes complex, with hypoechoic and echogenic areas. As the blood clot liquefies, the sonographic appearance anechoic. With a chronic hematoma, areas of calcification with posterior acoustic shadowing may be seen within the hematoma. Doppler imaging is used to determine whether the hematoma is actively bleeding.

A subcapsular hematoma is located between the renal capsule and the cortex and may flatten the cortex. Subcapsular hematomas are difficult to visualize sonographically during the acute phase; they may have the same sonographic echogenicity as the renal cortex. A perinephric hematoma may have an elongated shape that follows the contour of the kidney.

Lipoma

Lipomas are composed of fatty tissue and are found more often in females.[10] They are the most common mesenchymal-type tumor. Other mesenchymal-type tumors that are found less often include fibroma, leiomyoma, angiolipoma, and AML.

Sonographic Findings. Lipomas of the kidney appear sonographically as well-defined echogenic masses. They tend to be less than 5 cm in diameter.

Oncocytoma

A renal oncocytoma is a solid epithelial neoplasm with a generally benign course.[11] Renal oncocytomas usually occur in middle to old age, with a male-to-female ratio of 1.7:1. Oncocytomas can range in size from 1.5 to 12 cm.[9] Patients are usually asymptomatic but may have pain and hematuria.[12]

Renal oncocytoma has been difficult to diagnose before surgery, which may account for the 2% to 14% of renal tumors thought to be malignant before surgery.[12] With ultrasound, CT, and MRI, the chance of a preoperative diagnosis increases. A conservative surgical approach can be used instead of nephrectomy, a radical surgical treatment.[12]

Sonographic Findings. The sonographic appearances of renal oncocytomas are nonspecific. They may appear as a well-defined, thin-walled homogeneous mass or lesion less than 5 cm with a central scar or a stellate architecture.[11] The absence of hemorrhage and necrosis along with the presence of a pseudocapsule are characteristics that are used to differentiate an oncocyoma from RCC.[11] Power Doppler may be useful for differential diagnosis of a small, benign, solid renal mass versus a malignant mass (Fig. 5-5, *A* to *C*).

Angiomyolipoma (Hamartoma)

Angiomyolipoma (AML) is a common renal cortex mass that consists mostly of fat cells along with muscle cells and arterial vessels. Large AML is a vascular neoplasm with a tendency to hemorrhage. When hemorrhage occurs, the mass has areas of necrosis, cystic degeneration, and calcification. Solitary AMLs are found more commonly in women ages 40 to 60 years. Bilateral multiple AMLs are more commonly found with tuberous sclerosis.

Patients are usually asymptomatic, unless hemorrhage occurs. When hemorrhage does occur, patients can have flank pain, hematuria, and hypertension.

Sonographic Findings. The most common appearance for an AML is a homogeneous, well-defined lesion that is hyperechoic from the high fat content in the tumor. Increased posterior acoustic enhancement may also be seen. AMLs are found in the renal cortex and are hyperechoic even at low gain settings. If hemorrhage occurs, the bleeding may be within the tumor or extend into the subcapsular or perinephric space. Power Doppler may be useful for differential diagnosis of small solid renal mass. AMLs have slow flow and therefore usually have no color (Fig. 5-6, *A* and *B*).

Other Benign Neoplasms

In addition to those neoplasms discussed previously, other benign neoplasms that seldom occur in the kidney

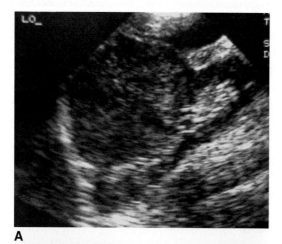

A

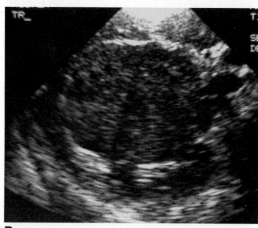

B

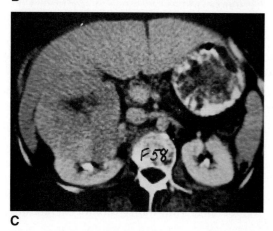

C

Fig. 5-5 **A,** Longitudinal view of right kidney shows large oncocytoma mass. **B,** Transverse image through oncocytoma with compression of right kidney. **C,** Computed tomographic transverse cross section of abdomen at level of right renal oncocytoma shows central scar, which is characteristically used in diagnosis of oncocytoma.

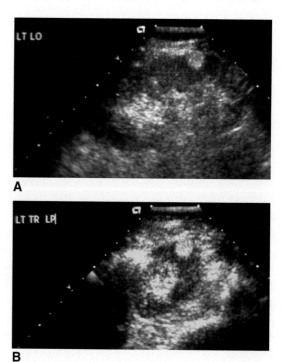

A

B

Fig. 5-6 **A,** Small angiomyolipoma is imaged in lower anterior pole of right kidney as echogenic mass. **B,** Transverse view of lower pole of right kidney shows small angiomyolipoma.

include fibroma, papilloma, myxoma, juxtaglomerular tumor (reninoma), and leiomyoma.

MALIGNANT NEOPLASMS

Renal Cell Carcinoma

Renal cell carcinoma (RCC) is also referred to as *hypernephroma* or *adenocarcinoma*. RCC accounts for 85% of clinically relevant renal tumors[13] and for 1% to 2% of adult cancers.[14] It is twice as common in females as in males and occurs most often in the fifth to sixth decades of life. An increased incidence of RCC is seen in patients with **von Hippel-Lindau disease,** advanced age, adult polycystic kidney disease, **tuberous sclerosis,** and long-term dialysis, or in patients who smoke.

Some patients with RCC have hematuria. Other clinical signs may include a palpable mass, flank pain, weight loss, fever, or hypertension. If the RCC is hormonally related, the patient will have hormone-specific symptoms. In addition, abnormal laboratory findings may be seen, such as **erythropoietin,** red blood cells, white blood cells, and bacteria in the urine and elevated creatinine and blood urea nitrogen (BUN) levels. The tumor may spread throughout the kidney and perinephric fat, invade the renal vein, and travel to the inferior vena cava (IVC). Approximately 30% of patients have metastasis at the time of diagnosis.[12] Metastasis to the regional lymph nodes, lungs, bone, contralateral kidney, liver, adrenal glands, and brain may occur. At the time of diagnosis, 1% of RCCs are bilateral.[15] Prognosis depends on the stage of the disease at diagnosis.

Sonographic Findings. The sonographic appearance of RCC is variable. The most common appearance is a solid hypoechoic parenchymal mass (Fig. 5-7, *A* to *C*). Occasionally, RCC is echogenic and can be confused with an AML. The mass may have calcifications or appear complex, with tumor necrosis or hemorrhage (Figs. 5-8 and 5-9). A cystic appearance is rare, although it can be differentiated from a benign cystic mass when thick septations, wall thickening, or wall irregularities are identified. In addition, the internal blood flow is increased. Doppler and color flow are useful in the identification of invasion of the IVC and renal vein. The renal vein blood flow will have low velocity if the renal vein obstruction is severe.[6]

Nephroblastoma

Nephroblastoma is also called *Wilms' tumor.* Nephroblastoma is the most common solid malignant renal mass in children. It is usually unilateral but may

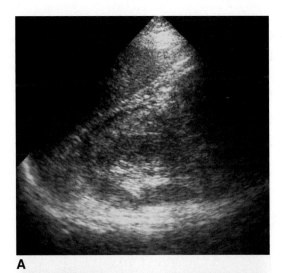

A

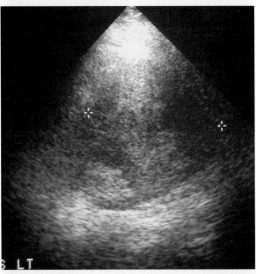

B

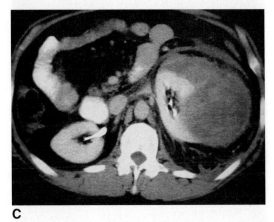

C

Fig. 5-7   Large, left renal, lower pole renal cell carcinoma (RCC). **A,** Longitudinal image of left kidney with lower pole hypoechoic mass. **B,** Transverse view of large RCC. **C,** Abdominal computed tomographic scan at level of kidneys. Left kidney is malrotated and colon is deviated to right side by large left renal mass.

be bilateral. Nephroblastoma usually occurs before age 3 to 4 years and is seldom found after age 8 years. Nephroblastomas are associated with **Beckwith-Wiedemann syndrome**, sporadic **aniridia**, and **hemihypertrophy**.

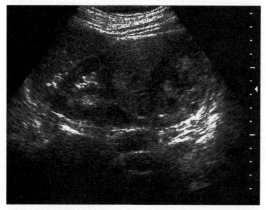

Fig. 5-8 Complex mass involves lower pole of left kidney, renal cell carcinoma. (Courtesy Eileen Weinstein, Bellevue Medical Center, New York.)

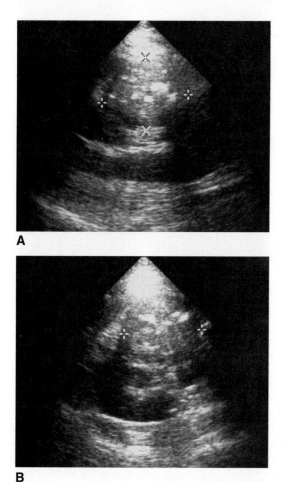

Fig. 5-9 **A,** Solid mass with calcifications in mid pole of right kidney. **B,** Transverse view of solid mass with calcification in mid pole of right kidney.

Malignant involvement can extend into the retroperitoneal nodes and the renal vein and may extend into the heart via the IVC. Metastasis may occur in the liver, lungs, and brain. The most common clinical presentation is a palpable abdominal mass. Other clinical symptoms include pain, malaise and weight loss, nausea, vomiting, hypertension, and gross hematuria. If venous obstruction occurs, leg edema, varicocele, or Budd-Chiari syndrome may also be present.

Sonographic Findings. The sonographic appearance of nephroblastoma is a large, well-defined homogeneous mass that is slightly more echogenic than the liver. Hemorrhagic or necrotic areas that have a sonolucent or cystic appearance may be found in the mass. The mass may distort the renal sinus or cause kidney obstruction (Fig. 5-10, *A* and *B*). The mass may extend beyond the renal capsule and invade the renal vein, IVC, or right atrium of the heart or involve the retroperitoneal nodes.

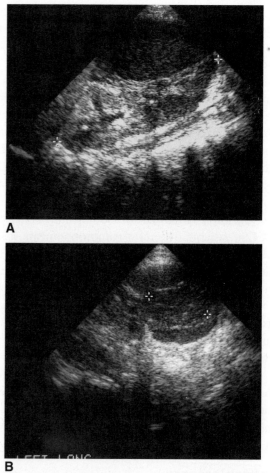

Fig. 5-10 One-month-old infant with bilateral nephroblastomas. **A,** Sagittal view shows right homogeneous mass, nephroblastoma. **B,** Sagittal image of left kidney shows hypoechoic nephroblastoma distorting renal collecting system.

Transitional Cell Carcinoma

More than 90% of malignant diseases that involve the renal pelvis and ureter are transitional cell carcinoma (TCC).[15] TCC of the renal pelvis occurs five to 10 times less frequently than does RCC.[15] TCC most often involves the urinary bladder, and in a percentage of cases, involvement of the kidneys and ureters is seen.

Patients with TCC typically have painless hematuria, but if the lesion involves the collecting system, the patient may have pain and hydronephrosis. Bladder lesions may cause hematuria and blood clots. TCC occurs more often in males than in females, and an increased incidence is seen with age, with 60 years of age as the mean.

Sonographic Findings. The most common sonographic appearance of TCC is a bulky hypoechoic mass in the bladder; many TCCs are flat and not visible. TCC lesions in the kidney found within the renal sinus may cause separation and dilation of the renal collecting system. The renal contour stays preserved, and the internal renal architecture becomes distorted with malignant invasion. Calcifications are rare. Color Doppler is not a helpful evaluation of TCC (Fig. 5-11, *A* to *E*).

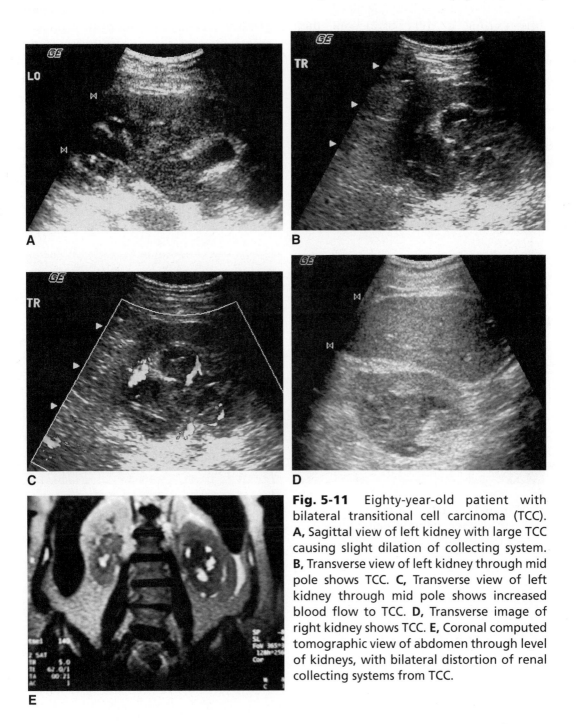

Fig. 5-11 Eighty-year-old patient with bilateral transitional cell carcinoma (TCC). **A,** Sagittal view of left kidney with large TCC causing slight dilation of collecting system. **B,** Transverse view of left kidney through mid pole shows TCC. **C,** Transverse view of left kidney through mid pole shows increased blood flow to TCC. **D,** Transverse image of right kidney shows TCC. **E,** Coronal computed tomographic view of abdomen through level of kidneys, with bilateral distortion of renal collecting systems from TCC.

Squamous Cell Carcinoma

Squamous cell carcinoma (SCC) is a rare tumor that represents 15% of all urothelial tumors.[5] SCC is more invasive than TCC; it invades the renal wall, renal vein, and IVC early, and has a poor prognosis. SCC is typically preceded by chronic irritation from chronic infection, **leukoplakia,** drug use, and urinary calculi.[15] The presentation is the same as with TCC: painless, gross hematuria, and palpable kidney from the hydronephrosis.

Sonographic Findings. The most common appearance of SCC is a large bulky mass in the renal pelvis (Fig. 5-12, *A* and *B*). If renal calculi are identified with hydronephrosis causing a UPJ obstruction, the suggestion of SCC may be made sonographically. CT scan and IVP are typically used to make a preoperative diagnosis.

Other Malignant Masses

In addition to those discussed previously, other malignant neoplasms infrequently occur in the kidney. These include lymphoma (Fig. 5-13), sarcoma (Figs. 5-14 and 5-15, *A* to *D*), adult Wilms' tumor, lymphangioma, and malignant rhabdoid tumor.

Table 5-1 is a summary of the pathology, symptoms, and sonographic findings in hematuria.

SUMMARY

Many renal cortical tumors are discovered with CT, MRI, and ultrasound imaging of the upper abdomen for other reasons. Patients with a history of hematuria and no other clinical symptoms are common. Hematuria may be an early sign of a serious renal disease. Causes of hematuria include congenital anomaly, infection, tumor, or stones. In older men, benign prostatic hyperplasia is a common cause of hematuria. Sonographic examination of the urinary system can aid in the identification of the cause of hematuria. Characterization of the sonographic appearance coupled with the patient history and other tests, urine analysis, cystoscopy, IVP, CT, or MRI can lead to diagnosis and proper patient management. Surgical intervention is typically the treatment for a renal mass, but imaging methods for characterization of the mass as benign versus malignant can assist in the surgical decision to remove the mass versus a total nephrectomy.

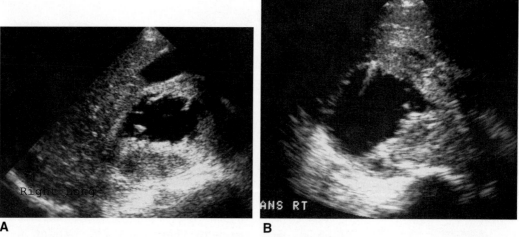

A   **B**

Fig. 5-12 Sixty-year-old patient with metastatic disease. **A,** Sagittal image of right kidney shows irregular-shaped mass filling renal sinus. **B,** Transverse image of the squamous cell carcinoma.

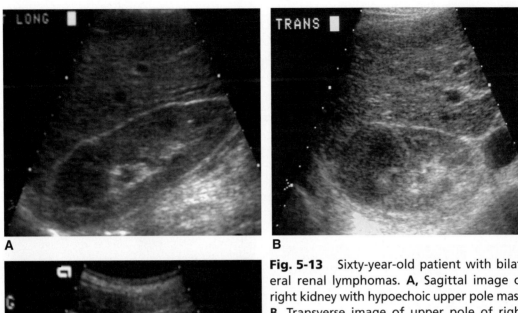

Fig. 5-13 Sixty-year-old patient with bilateral renal lymphomas. **A,** Sagittal image of right kidney with hypoechoic upper pole mass. **B,** Transverse image of upper pole of right kidney with hypoechoic lymphoma. **C,** Transverse view of left kidney with anechoic lymphoma.

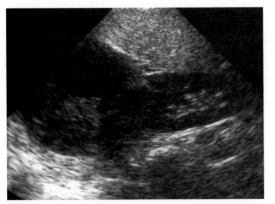

Fig. 5-14 Fifty-one-year-old woman with renal capsular sarcoma.

CLINICAL SCENARIO—DIAGNOSIS

■ The increased cortical blood flow that was noted bilaterally would be consistent with RCC. However, the patient history of a primary carcinoma with metastatic disease suggests that the renal masses are also part of the metastatic process. The patient is undergoing treatment for bilateral metastatic renal disease, although a poor outcome is expected.

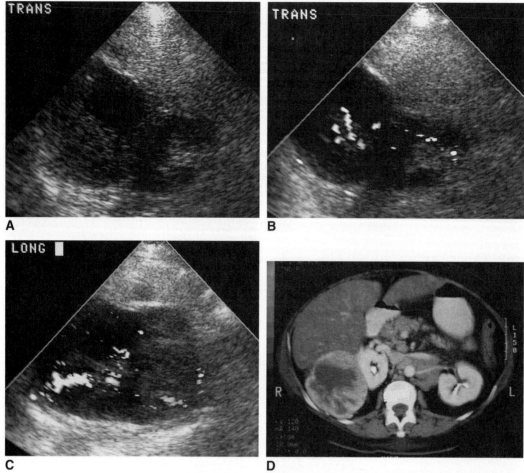

Fig. 5-15 Patient with renal sarcoma. **A,** Transverse view of right kidney with hypoechoic mass with slightly echogenic area. **B,** Documentation of blood flow to renal sarcoma. **C,** Longitudinal image documents upper pole mass (sarcoma) with increased vascularity. **D,** Computed tomographic scan at level of kidneys documents right renal sarcoma.

Table 5-1	*Causes of Hematuria*	
Pathology	**Symptoms**	**Sonographic Findings**
Nephrolithiasis	Pain, nausea, vomiting, fever, chills, hematuria	Echogenic foci with posterior shadowing, with or without hydronephrosis or dilated ureter (decreased ureteral jets)
Adenoma	Asymptomatic, hematuria	Small, solid, well-defined, hyperechoic mass in cortex
Hemangioma	Pain, hematuria possible	Small, hyperechoic, round mass
Hematoma	Usually asymptomatic; hematuria possible	Small, solid, echogenic lesion
Lipoma	Asymptomatic	Echogenic, well-defined mass
Oncocytoma	Asymptomatic; pain and hematuria possible	Well-defined, thin wall, homogeneous lesion; central scar or stellate architecture

Table 5-1	Causes of Hematuria—contd	
Pathology	**Symptoms**	**Sonographic Findings**
AML (hamartoma)	Asymptomatic, with hemorrhage; flank pain, hematuria, hypertension	Well-defined, echogenic mass in cortex, increased posterior acoustic enhancement possible
RCC (or hypernephroma, adenocarcinoma)	Hematuria, palpable mass, flank pain, weight loss, fever, hypertension	Variable, solid, slightly hypoechoic, isoechoic with calcifications, complex mass arising in cortex
Nephroblastoma (Wilms' tumor)	Pain, malaise, weight loss, nausea, vomiting, hypertension, gross hematuria	Large, well-defined, slightly echogenic or complex mass; may cause obstruction or invade renal vein or IVC
TCC	Painless hematuria, pain with collecting system involvement	Bladder: bulky hypoechoic mass Kidney: separation of collecting system, dilation of collecting system
SCC	Painless gross hematuria, palpable mass	Bulky mass in renal pelvis; renal calculi may cause obstruction

AML, Angiomyolipoma; *IVC,* inferior vena cava; *RCC,* renal cell carcinoma; *SCC,* squamous cell carcinoma; *TCC,* transitional cell carcinoma.

CASE STUDIES FOR DISCUSSION

1. A 65-year-old patient with a history of abdominal pain and gas is seen for an abdominal and pelvic ultrasound. The laboratory results included hematuria. Ultrasound examination of the abdomen reveals a slightly enlarged spleen and a solid right renal upper pole mass (Fig. 5-16). No hydronephrosis is identified, and the right renal vein and IVC are patent. A CT scan is performed to further evaluate the right renal mass. What are the possible diagnoses?

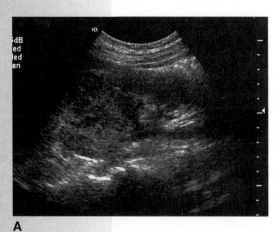

A

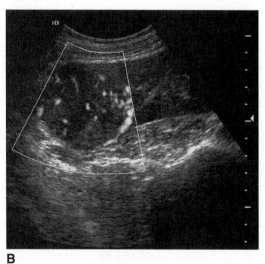

B

Fig. 5-16   A, Sagittal image of right kidney shows large, hypoechoic, well-defined mass. **B,** Sagittal image of right kidney upper pole documents blood flow to mass. (Courtesy Eileen Weinstein, Bellevue Medical Center, New York.)

2. A middle-aged woman with a history of microscopic hematuria is seen for an ultrasound of the kidneys. The renal fossae undergo bilateral sonographic imaging, and no kidneys are identified. The abdomen and pelvis are scanned to locate the kidneys. The kidneys are located in the pelvis posterior to the uterus (Fig. 5-17). No hydronephrosis, calculi, or perinephric fluid is seen. What are the most likely diagnoses consistent with the ultrasound findings?

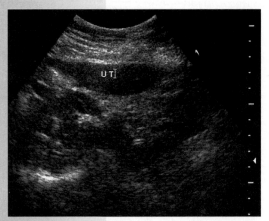

Fig. 5-17 Midline longitudinal view through pelvis, with mass posterior to uterus *(UT)*. (Courtesy Eileen Weinstein, Bellevue Medical Center, New York.)

3. A 46-year-old in-patient man with a clinical history of gross hematuria is seen for a urinary tract ultrasound. No prior imaging examinations of the urinary tract are available for comparison. The kidneys are identified in their normal location, no masses or hydronephrosis are seen, and the size and echotexture are consistent with normal kidneys. A Foley catheter is seen in the distended urinary bladder. A large, solid, irregular, marginated echogenic mass is identified adherent to the posterior bladder wall (Fig. 5-18). Echogenic debris is identified in the urinary bladder. Color Doppler does not definitely show vascularity. What is the most likely diagnosis?

4. An elderly man with abdominal pain and microscopic hematuria is seen for an abdominal ultrasound. The ultrasound shows a large echogenic mass extending superiorly from the right upper pole (Fig. 5-19). The left kidney appears grossly normal. What is the most likely diagnosis?

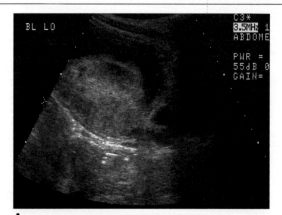

A

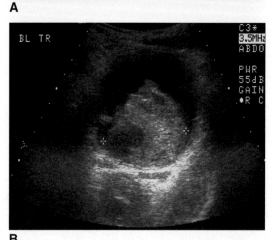

B

Fig. 5-18 Large bladder mass with hyperechoic and hypoechoic areas. **A,** Midline image of urinary bladder shows intraluminal mass. **B,** Transverse image of urinary bladder shows mass. (Courtesy Eileen Weinstein, Bellevue Medical Center, New York.)

5. An elderly male is seen by his physician for a routine examination. A routine laboratory workup is performed, and microscopic hematuria is found. A urinary tract ultrasound is requested to help find the cause of the hematuria. Two hypoechoic masses are imaged in the right kidney (Fig. 5-20). A complete abdominal ultrasound is performed, and no other pathology is noted. A CT scan is performed to aid in a diagnosis. What is the most likely diagnosis?

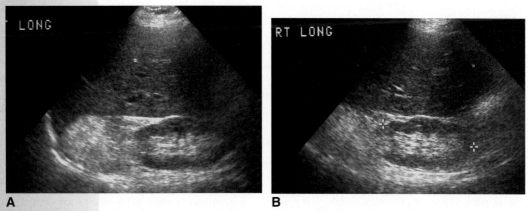

Fig. 5-19   **A,** Longitudinal view of right kidney with echogenic upper pole mass. **B,** Measurement of right kidney.

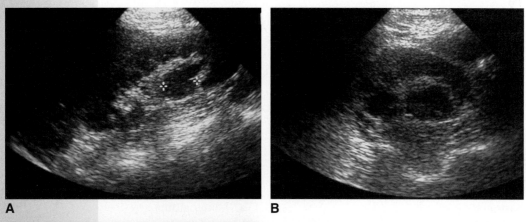

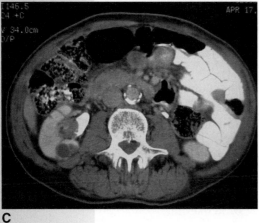

Fig. 5-20   **A,** Longitudinal image of right kidney with hypoechoic mass. **B,** Transverse view of right kidney with two central hypoechoic masses. **C,** Computed tomographic scan at level of kidneys. Two areas with decreased intensity.

STUDY QUESTIONS

1. A 40-year-old woman is seen for a renal ultrasound. Microscopic hematuria was found during her routine annual physical examination. A solid mass is identified in the renal cortex. The mass is more echogenic than the renal sinus, and the collecting system is not dilated. What is the most likely diagnosis?
   a. RCC
   b. renal calculi
   c. complex renal cyst
   d. AML
   e. hematoma

2. A 25-year-old patient with right flank pain, nausea, and vomiting is seen for a renal ultrasound. The ultrasound reveals large echogenic foci with posterior acoustic shadowing in the kidney. The calyces appear to be dilated. What is the most likely diagnosis?
   a. hematoma
   b. calculi
   c. TCC
   d. oncocytoma
   e. AML

3. A 2-year-old boy with a history of weight loss, vomiting, and hypertension and with dark pink urine is seen for an abdominal ultrasound. The sonographer identifies a large homogeneous echogenic mass distorting the kidney. What is the most likely diagnosis?
   a. nephroblastoma
   b. RCC
   c. congenital anomaly
   d. oncocytoma
   e. hematoma

4. A teenage boy is tackled roughly during a football game. After the game, he has abdominal pain. The pain becomes intense, and the next day he is seen at the emergency department. The laboratory values are abnormal, the hematocrit level is low, and microscopic hematuria is found. A renal ultrasound is ordered. The ultrasound of the left kidney is normal. The right kidney appears normal, but a sonolucent ring is seen surrounding the kidney. This is most consistent with:
   a. ruptured cyst
   b. lipoma
   c. perinephric hematoma
   d. AML
   e. hemangioma

5. A patient undergoing long-term dialysis with hypertension and flank pain is seen for a renal ultrasound. The ultrasound reveals a normal left kidney and a large complex lower pole mass of the right kidney. Low-level echoes are identified in the right renal vein. The most likely diagnosis of this mass is:
   a. hemangioma
   b. nephroblastoma
   c. TCC
   d. RCC
   e. AML

6. A 32-year-old patient with severe left flank pain and hematuria is seen for a renal ultrasound. The ultrasound reveals a dilated ureter, and no ureteral jet is seen on the left side. The right kidney appears normal, and the left renal collecting system is dilated. This is most consistent with:
   a. bladder hematoma
   b. ureteral stone
   c. kidney stone
   d. bladder stone
   e. hemangioma

7. A middle-aged patient with microscopic hematuria and no pain is seen for a renal ultrasound. The ultrasound reveals a small solid left renal mass that causes the renal cortex to bulge. No vascular flow is seen with color Doppler. This is most suggestive of:
   a. hemangioma
   b. oncocytoma
   c. TCC
   d. renal calculi
   e. adenoma

8. A patient with a history of tuberous sclerosis, recent onset of hematuria, and pain is seen for a renal ultrasound. The ultrasound reveals bilateral well-defined echogenic renal cortex masses with increased posterior acoustic enhancement. This finding is most consistent with:
   a. hemangioma
   b. hematoma
   c. AML
   d. RCC
   e. lipoma

9. A 42-year-old man who was recently told that he has hematuria is seen for an abdominal ultrasound. The ultrasound is unremarkable except for a 3-cm,

well-defined mass with a central scar in the left kidney. What is the most likely diagnosis?
a. hematoma
b. nephroblastoma
c. adenoma
d. oncocytoma
e. AML

10. An elderly patient with gross hematuria, pain, and a palpable abdominal mass is seen for an abdominal and pelvic ultrasound. The abdominal ultrasound reveals a hypoechoic mass in the renal sinus that is obstructing the renal collecting system and causing hydronephrosis of the left kidney. The left kidney does not lose its reniform shape. An irregularly shaped mass is identified in the urinary bladder. Color Doppler imaging of both masses does not show increased vascularity. This most likely represents which of the following?
a. TCC
b. nephroblastoma
c. adenoma
d. hematoma
e. SCC

REFERENCES

1. Patton T: *Anatomy & physiology*, ed 4, St Louis, 1999, Mosby.
2. Stec P: Intrarenal disorders. In Copstead L-EC, editor: *Perspectives on pathophysiology*, Philadelphia, 1995, WB Saunders.
3. Lee Y, Kim SH, Cho JY et al: Color and power Doppler twinkling artifacts from urinary stones, *Am J Roentgenol* 176:1441-1445, 2001.
4. Aytac SK, Ozcan H: Effects of Color Doppler system on the twinkling sign associated with urinary tract calculi, *J Clin Ultrasound* 27:433-439, 1999.
5. Bullock BL: Urinary excretion (unit 9). *Pathophysiology: adaptations and alterations in function*, ed 4, Philadelphia, 1996, Lippincott-Raven.
6. Hagen-Ansert SL: *Textbook of diagnostic ultrasonography*, vol 1, ed 5, St Louis, 2001, Mosby.
7. Gill K: *Abdominal ultrasound: a practitioner's guide*, Philadelphia, 2001, WB Saunders.
8. Joseph N, Neiman HL, Vogelzang RL: Renal masses, *Clin Diagn Ultrasound* 18:135-160, 1986.
9. Belville JS, Morgentaler A, Loughlin KR et al: Spontaneous perinephric and subcapsular hemorrhage: evaluation with CT, US and angiography, *Radiology* 172:733-738, 1989.
10. Kawamura DM: *Abdomen and superficial structures*, ed 2, Philadelphia, 1997, Lippincott.
11. De Carli P, Vidiri A, Lamanna L et al: Renal oncocytoma: image diagnosis and therapeutic aspects, *J Exp Clin Cancer Res*, 19:287-289, 2000.
12. Mittelstaedt CA: Kidney. In Mittelstaedt CA, editor: *General ultrasound*, New York, 1992, Churchill-Livingston.
13. Ruckle HC, Torres VE, Richardson RL et al: Renal tumors, *Curr Opin Nephrol Hypertens* 2:201-10, 1993.
14. Berkow R: *The Merick manual*, ed 16, Rahway, NJ, 1992, Merck Research Laboratories.
15. Rumack CM, Wilson SR, Charboneau JW: *Diagnostic ultrasound*, vol 1, ed 2, St Louis, 1998, Mosby.

BIBLIOGRAPHY

Little AF: Adrenal gland and renal sonography, *World J Surg* 24:171-182, 2000.
Yasumasu T, Koikawa Y, Uozumi J et al: Clinical study of asymptomatic microscopic haematuria, *Int Urol Nephrol* 26:1-6, 1994.
Hans B, Hans H, Sten H: The results of routine evaluation of adult patients with haematuria analysed according to referral form information with 2-year follow-up, *Scand J Urol Nephrol* 35:497-501, 2001.
Bichler K, Eipper E, Naber V: Urinary infection stones, *Int J Antimicrobial Agents* 19:488-498, 2002.
Lee HS, Hoh BH, Kim JW et al: Radiologic findings of renal hemangioma: report of three cases. *Korean J Radiol* 1:60-3, 2000.
McGahan JP, Goldberg BB: *Diagnostic ultrasound: a logical approach*, Philadelphia, 1997, Lippincott-Raven.

6

Rule Out Renal Failure

CHERYL A. VANCE

CLINICAL SCENARIO

■ A 64-year-old man with diabetes is seen in the ultrasound department for a renal ultrasound after routine laboratory test results were abnormal. The laboratory findings show an increase in blood urea nitrogen (BUN) level, an elevated creatinine level, and a decreased glomerular filtration rate (GFR). The patient has a recent diagnosis of hypertension. On inquiry, the patient revealed he is a "social" drinker and has a 40-year history of smoking 1.5 packs of cigarettes a day. In addition, he has had pain lately while walking.

The bilateral renal sonogram shows normal echogenicity of the renal parenchyma and sinus. No hydronephrosis, calculi, or evidence of obstruction is visualized during the sonogram. The right kidney measures 11.5 cm in length, and the left kidney measures 8.5 cm in length. Intrarenal Doppler examination of the right kidney (Fig. 6-1; see Color Plate 3) shows a steep systolic upstroke, a sharp systolic peak, and a second small peak in early systole. Intrarenal Doppler evaluation on the left kidney (Fig. 6-2; see Color Plate 4) shows a lengthened systolic rise time with a rounded systolic peak. What is the possible diagnosis for these sonographic findings?

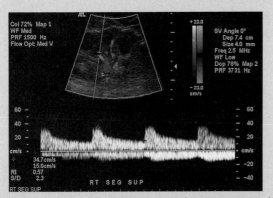

Fig. 6-1 Right kidney segmental artery Doppler. (Courtesy Cindy Rapp, Radiology Imaging Associates, Greenwood Village, Colorado.)

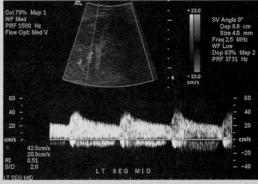

Fig. 6-2 Left kidney segmental artery Doppler. (Courtesy Cindy Rapp, Radiology Imaging Associates, Greenwood Village, Colorado.)

OBJECTIVES

■ Describe the typical causes and sonographic appearance of hydronephrosis.
■ List the common causes and characteristics of acute glomerulonephritis.
■ Describe the etiology and sonographic appearance of papillary necrosis.
■ Differentiate between acute and chronic renal failure sonographically.
■ Describe the Doppler characteristics typically found with renal artery stenosis.

■ Describe what may cause acute tubular necrosis.
■ Describe the sonographic appearance of pyonephrosis.
■ Differentiate between acute, chronic, emphysematous, and xanthogranulomatous pyelonephritis sonographically.
■ Describe possible causes and sonographic appearances of renal abscesses.
■ Describe the sonographic appearance of a typical fungal infection.

GLOSSARY OF TERMS

Anemia: a condition in which the number of red blood cells is less than normal

Anuria: no urine production

Azotemia: an excess of urea and other nitrogenous waste in the blood

Bacteriuria: the presence of bacteria in the urine

Blood urea nitrogen: value used to measure the concentration of nitrogen as urea in the blood

Cortex: the more peripheral segment of the kidney tissue that surrounds medulla and sinus

Creatinine: a laboratory value and byproduct of muscle metabolism

Diabetes mellitus: a metabolic disease in which carbohydrate use is reduced because of a deficiency of insulin

Dysuria: difficulty or pain in urination

Hematuria: the appearance of blood cells in the urine

Hyperkalemia: a greater than normal concentration of potassium ions in the circulating blood

Hypovolemia: a decreased amount of blood in the body

Ischemia: a local obstruction of the blood supply

Leukocytosis: an abnormally large number of leukocytes, as observed in acute infections

Neoplasm: any new growth or development, either malignant or benign, of an abnormal tissue

Oliguria: decreased urine output

Polyuria: increased urine output

Pharyngitis: inflammation of the mucous membrane and underlying parts of the pharynx

Proteinuria: increased presence of protein in the urine

Pyuria: presence of pus in the urine

Renal parenchyma: area from the renal sinus to the outer renal surface where the arcuate and interlobar vessels are found

Renal pyramids: the portion of the kidney that is composed of medullary substance consisting of a series of striated conical masses

Uremia: an excess of urea and other nitrogenous waste in the blood

A renal sonogram may be ordered for assessment of the kidneys when renal failure is suspected. Renal decline and failure is associated with significant morbidity and mortality. Renal failure results when the kidneys are no longer able to remove waste products from the bloodstream. Depending on the cause and the stage of the renal failure, a variety of patient symptoms exists. Initial symptoms may be understated, but the symptoms eventually progress to flank pain, nausea, vomiting, **anemia,** headaches, and increased **(polyuria),** decreased, or absent **(anuria)** urine production. Laboratory values may show **pyuria, hematuria,** white blood cells (WBCs) or bacteria in the urine (suggestive of inflammation or infection), and elevated blood urea nitrogen (BUN)/creatinine levels.

Renal failure may be caused by obstruction of urine flow, decreased renal blood flow, or renal parenchymal disease. Disease processes within the kidney that may be precursors to renal failure include hydronephrosis, acute glomerulonephritis, papillary necrosis, renal artery stenosis, acute tubular necrosis, and a variety of renal infections. Lower genitourinary tract diseases within the ureter, bladder, or urethra causing obstruction may lead to renal failure. In most cases, bilateral obstruction is necessary for renal insufficiency to develop.

Sonographic assessment for renal failure should include a thorough investigation of the genitourinary system with a search for signs of obstruction, tumors, anatomic abnormalities, calculi, infection, stenosis, and decreased renal vascular flow. The sonogram should be initiated with B-mode technology for assessment of the kidney's size and sonographic characteristics. Next, a Doppler evaluation (color and pulsed-wave) of the renal vascular system should be performed for determination of patency. Abnormal Doppler signals that suggest decreased vascular flow may include high systolic peak velocities, low or no diastolic flow, turbulence, and the tardus parvus effect (dampening of the waveform).[1]

HYDRONEPHROSIS

Hydronephrosis occurs when the renal collecting system of one or both kidneys becomes dilated from the obstruction of urine outflow. Hydronephrosis is caused by calculi, tumor, infection, previous obstruction, over-distended bladder, anatomic/congenital abnormalities, and pregnancy. Infection may occur with an extended period of urinary stasis. Prolonged hydronephrosis destroys the tubules in the **cortex,** resulting in renal parenchymal atrophy, scarring, or irreversible renal damage. This condition progressively leads to the loss of renal function. With long-standing hydronephrosis, the renal collecting system remains dilated after the obstruction is relieved. Patients with hydronephrosis may be asymptomatic, but this condition can also initiate with pain in the kidney region, infection, nausea, **dysuria,** fever, chills, vomiting, **uremia,** and microscopic hematuria.

Sonographic Findings

The distention of the renal pelvis and calyces found in patients with significant hydronephrosis causes overall renal enlargement. Sonographically, a hydronephrotic kidney will present with a group of anechoic, fluid-filled spaces within the renal sinus (Figs. 6-3 and 6-4). Acute obstruction may initially cause the kidney to

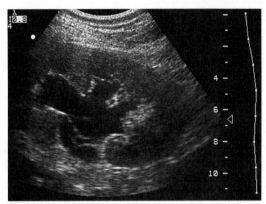

Fig. 6-3 Longitudinal image of right kidney shows hydronephrosis.

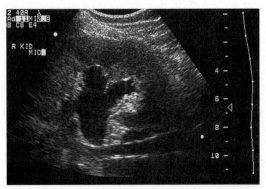

Fig. 6-4 Transverse image of right kidney shows hydronephrosis. (Courtesy Deborah A. Thomas, Wilford Hall Medical Center, Lackland Air Force Base, Texas.)

cease to excrete urine, which will delay the onset of any renal dilation. Echogenic calculi (with or without shadowing) may be located throughout the genitourinary system. Smaller stones blend into the echogenic renal sinus. Previous obstruction, pregnancy, megaureter, or an extremely full bladder also causes normal calyceal dilation. Chronic obstruction will cause atrophy of the renal parenchyma.

Hydronephrosis initiates with a slight distention of the collecting system displaying a small separation of the calyceal pattern (splaying).[2] As hydronephrosis progresses, the collecting system dilates with fluid extending into the major and minor calyceal systems (bear-claw effect).[2] Severe hydronephrosis presents with massive dilation including the renal pelvis. It is associated with cortical thinning/loss of the **renal parenchyma.** With assessment for hydronephrosis, parapelvic cysts should be ruled out. Generally, dilated calyces have a more echogenic margin than a parapelvic cyst. With assessment for hydronephrosis, one should search for an extra renal pelvis. The extra renal pelvis can be confused with hydronephrosis because of its large cystic appearance within the renal hilum.

Doppler evaluation is important in the evaluation for hydronephrosis. Doppler examination reveals prominent renal vasculature that may be confused with a dilated renal collecting system. Increased intrarenal pressure caused by urinary obstruction leads to a decline in renal blood flow and a thinning of the parenchyma. The resistance index on the affected side is increased when compared with the healthy kidney. In normal conditions, a relatively low renal vascular resistance is found. With partial obstruction, the resistive index may be unaffected. Ureteral jets (detectable with color Doppler examination) may be absent or decreased in frequency in acute obstruction.

ACUTE GLOMERULONEPHRITIS

Acute glomerulonephritis is an inflammation of the renal glomeruli that frequently occurs as a late complication of an infection, typically of the throat (**pharyngitis**).[3] Glomerulonephritis is characterized by bilateral inflammatory changes in the glomeruli that are not the result of infection of the kidneys. It is more common in males than in females and is more common in children than in adults.[4] Symptoms are variable and include smoky urine, history of recent fever, sore throat, joint pains, peripheral edema (e.g., face, ankles), nausea, **oliguria,** anemia, **azotemia,** and hypertension. Laboratory findings may include hematuria, proteinuria, decreased glomerular filtration rate (GFR), increased BUN value, and increased serum creatinine level.[5]

Inflammation and scarring of the glomeruli result in an inability to filter the blood properly to make urine.[6] The inflammation and scarring lead to poor kidney function and ultimately renal failure. Acute glomerulonephritis commonly leads to chronic glomerulonephritis. Chronic glomerulonephritis develops slowly and may not be detected until the kidneys fail, which could take 20 to 30 years.[3]

Chronic glomerulonephritis is characterized by irreversible and progressive glomerular fibrosis that leads to a reduction in the GFR and a retention of uremic toxins.[7] Chronic glomerulonephritis leads to chronic renal failure, end-stage renal disease, and eventually death. It requires long-term treatment with dialysis or transplantation.

Sonographic Findings

Acute glomerulonephritis may not present any differentiating sonographic features. An irregular cortical echopattern may be seen. When evident, the acute form of glomerulonephritis may cause an increase in the cortical echogenicity. The **renal pyramids** are well visualized. Bilateral renal enlargement is also a common sonographic finding. Chronic glomerulonephritis initially shows an increase in cortical echotexture without an increase in the medullary echotexture. It then progresses to increase both echodensities. Chronic glomerulonephritis shows small, smooth, echogenic kidneys.

PAPILLARY NECROSIS

The renal papillae are the rounded tips at the apex of each renal medullary pyramid. The renal papillae face toward the renal hilum and represent the confluence of the collecting ducts from each nephron within that pyramid. Necrosis of the renal papillae causes hydronephrosis from the sloughed papillae obstructing the calyces. Hydronephrosis is also caused by sloughed papillae obstructing the ureters. Any narrowed area can make a nesting spot for sloughed papilla, leading to obstruction. The sloughed papillae calcify, further increasing the potential for obstructive hydronephrosis. The actual sloughing of the renal papilla is the result of vascular **ischemia,** which leads to necrosis of the renal medullary pyramids.[8] Papillary necrosis is the result of medullary vasculature being compressed with inflammation.

Papillary necrosis is typically a bilateral process. Focal papillary necrosis involves only the tip of the papilla. Diffuse papillary necrosis involves the whole papilla and areas of the medulla. Papillary necrosis can affect a single papilla, or the entire kidney may be involved. Renal papillary necrosis is limited to the inner, more distal zone of the medulla and the papilla.

Patients with diabetes and women are more prone to papillary necrosis.[8] Patients have fever from infection, flank or abdominal pain, hypertension (from renal ischemia), dysuria, and hematuria. Laboratory results will typically show a positive urine culture (from passage of sloughed papillae), **proteinuria,** pyuria, **bacteriuria,** and low urine-specific gravity. Papillary necrosis can be a complication of severe pyelonephritis. Infection is also a complication of papillary necrosis because the necrotic papillae act as an origin for infection and the formation of stones. Papillary necrosis has the potential to lead to renal failure and ultimately death.

Sonographic Findings

Papillary necrosis is visualized sonographically as clubbing of the calyces as a result of obstruction caused by sloughed papillae.[5] Obstruction caused by sloughed papillae presents sonographically with signs of hydronephrosis. One should search sonographically for calculi or obstruction and look for stones large enough to produce a shadow and hydronephrosis resulting from papillary necrosis. Round or triangular cystic collections within the medullary pyramids may be visible. A sloughed papilla, when visualized, appears as an echogenic, nonshadowing structure within the renal collecting system. If the papillae calcify, acoustic shadowing would be shown. Severe papillary necrosis may cause the papillae to be replaced with urine-filled sacs.[9] Papillary necrosis would then appear as multiple cystic structures in the renal pyramid region that do not communicate with the renal pelvis.

RENAL FAILURE

Renal failure can be categorized as either acute or chronic. Acute symptoms are sudden and severe, whereas chronic symptoms are slow and irreversible. In both acute and chronic forms of renal failure, the excretory and regulatory functions of the kidneys are decreased. Obstructive causes of renal failure are treatable and therefore are an important diagnosis during patient evaluation. Renal disease is considered end stage once the kidneys are unable to fulfill more than 10% of their normal function.[3] At this point, dialysis may be necessary.

Acute Renal Failure

Acute renal failure is the generic term used to define an abrupt decrease in renal function resulting in retention of nitrogenous waste (BUN and creatinine). Acute renal failure may cause a decrease in renal blood flow and produce renal parenchymal insult or obstruction. Reduction of renal blood flow causes a decrease in the GFR, which leads to retention of water and salts. This causes oliguria, concentrated urine, and a progressive inability to excrete nitrogenous wastes. Decreased renal blood flow leads to ischemia and eventually to cell death. Recovery from acute renal failure is dependent on restoration of normal renal blood flow. Earlier blood flow normalization leads to a better prognosis for recovery of renal function. Patients with acute renal failure may have symptoms of **hypovolemia**, hypertension, edema, oliguria, and hematuria.[10] Laboratory results may include increased WBC counts, increased **creatinine** levels, and increased BUN values.

Acute renal failure may have different causes depending on the stage of the disease. Prerenal causes of acute renal failure are the result of hypoperfusion of the kidney. Renal causes result from parenchymal diseases, such as acute glomerulonephritis, renal vein thrombosis, and acute tubular necrosis.[10] Postrenal causes of acute renal failure are the result of obstruction.

Sonographic Findings. Acute renal failure may present sonographically with normal-sized or enlarged kidneys. The parenchymal echogenicity will be increased as compared with the liver.

Chronic Renal Failure

Chronic renal failure that necessitates dialysis or transplantation is referred to as end-stage renal disease. Failed kidneys are unable to regulate electrolyte, fluid, and acid-base balances.[11] In chronic renal failure, dialysis is necessary until a kidney transplant is performed. Chronic renal failure has many different causes that include infection, diabetes, hypertensive vascular disease, congenital and hereditary disorders, toxic nephropathy, and obstructive nephropathy.[11]

Renal failure produces no symptoms early in the course of the disease. The most common cause of chronic renal failure is **diabetes mellitus.**[5] Glomerulonephritis, interstitial nephritis, and chronic upper urinary tract infection are also causes of chronic renal failure. Patients with chronic renal failure may have malaise, increased concentration of urea in blood, fatigue, anorexia, nausea, hypotension, and **hyperkalemia.** Laboratory findings include decreased GFR, hyperkalemia, elevated BUN and serum creatinine levels, and anemia (from

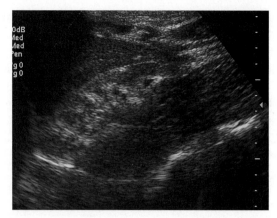

Fig. 6-5 Right kidney chronic renal failure; notice increased echogenicity of kidney as compared with liver and thin renal parenchyma. (Courtesy Deborah A. Thomas, Wilford Hall Medical Center, Lackland Air Force Base, Texas.)

loss of erythropoietin production).

Sonographic Findings. Initially, the kidneys are enlarged, but over time, patients with chronic renal disease encounter a progressive decrease in renal size bilaterally. With unilateral involvement, the affected kidney is almost impossible to visualize. Sonographically, patients with chronic renal disease have increased cortical echogenicity with poor corticomedullary differentiation (Fig. 6-5). With end-stage renal disease, the kidneys continue to become smaller and more echogenic. The renal parenchyma also becomes thinned.

RENAL ARTERY STENOSIS

Renal artery stenosis is a common cause of renovascular hypertension. Renal artery stenosis also causes chronic renal insufficiency and end-stage renal disease. Atherosclerosis is a common cause of renal artery stenosis in older patients. As the renal artery lumen progressively narrows, renal blood flow decreases and eventually compromises renal function and structure. In patients with renal artery stenosis, the chronic ischemia causes atrophy with decreased tubular cell size, patchy inflammation and fibrosis, and intrarenal arterial medial thickening.[12]

Renal artery stenosis causes a decrease in GFR once arterial luminal narrowing exceeds 50%.[12] Renal artery stenosis results in hypertension and a progressive loss of renal function. Bilateral renal artery stenosis causes renal failure. Renal artery stenosis is a common vascular complication of transplantation, and it affects the renal function.

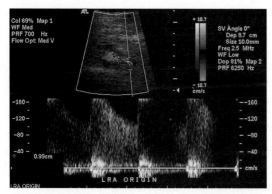

Fig. 6-6 Left main renal artery Doppler evaluation shows high velocities caused by renal artery stenosis. (Courtesy Cindy Rapp, Radiology Imaging Associates, Greenwood Village, Colorado.)

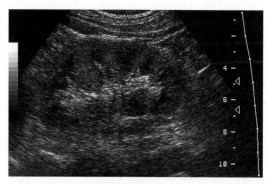

Fig. 6-7 Longitudinal image of left kidney; notice markedly increased echogenicity and enlarged renal pyramids. Diagnosis of acute tubular necrosis. (Courtesy Deborah A. Thomas, Wilford Hall Medical Center, Lackland Air Force Base, Texas.)

Sonographic Findings

Sonographically, a patient with renal artery stenosis shows significant asymmetry in kidney size. The affected kidney initially increases in size and then ultimately decreases significantly in size, although the renal structures appear normal. Early renal artery stenosis and severe long-standing renal artery stenosis do not show a reduced kidney size.

Doppler and color flow evaluations are helpful in showing reduced or no flow to the involved kidney or renal area. Duplex ultrasound combines B-mode sonography with pulsed Doppler to obtain flow velocity data. In healthy patients, a steep systolic upstroke will be seen with a second small peak in early systole and significant diastolic flow. Patients with renal artery stenosis have abnormal Doppler waveforms. Specifically, Doppler analysis in patients with renal artery stenosis shows high systolic peak velocities (Fig. 6-6; see Color Plate 5) with little or no diastolic flow at the site of stenosis. Flow disturbances occur up to 1 cm distal to the stenosis.[1] The stenotic area is typically at the junction of the renal artery and the aorta. The tardus parvus effect (seen distal to the stenosis) is apparent in the intrarenal vasculature of patients with renal artery stenosis. The tardus parvus effect is the dampening of the distal waveform–lengthened systolic rise time or slow systolic acceleration (tardus)/lowering and rounding of the systolic peak (parvus).[1]

ACUTE TUBULAR NECROSIS

Acute tubular necrosis results from the lack of blood being supplied to kidneys. This may be caused by trauma, surgery, or hypotension and leads to necrosis of the renal tubular epithelium. Acute tubular necrosis is a type of inherent renal failure that cannot be attributed to glomerular, vascular, or interstitial causes. Acute tubular necrosis is caused by the deposit of cellular debris within the renal collecting tubules. Both ischemic and toxic insults cause tubular damage. Acute tubular necrosis is a common cause of acute transplant failure. Acute tubular necrosis may have different causes: prerenal (normal kidney responding to hypoperfusion), renal (the pathology is within the kidney itself), or postrenal (caused by an urinary tract obstruction).

Patients with acute tubular necrosis may have hypertension, oliguria, edema, hypotension, intermittent flank pain (if caused by calculi), vomiting, hematuria, infection, sepsis, and muscle necrosis. Laboratory findings show an acute decrease in GFR to very low levels and a sudden increase in serum creatinine and BUN concentrations.

Sonographic Findings

Sonographically, acute tubular necrosis is a difficult diagnosis with ultrasound alone. The sonographic appearance of acute tubular necrosis depends on its cause. When hypotension is the cause, no sonographic abnormalities are apparent. Drugs, metal, and solvent exposure that results in acute tubular necrosis will cause enlarged echogenic kidneys. Severe cases of acute tubular necrosis also show bilateral renal enlargement. The increase is more apparent in the cross-sectional area than in the length. Less severe cases of acute tubular necrosis may not have any noticeable renal enlargement. The renal parenchymal pattern typically appears normal. Some patients may have an increase in the cortical echodensity with no increase in medullary echodensity. Enlarged renal pyramids may also be visualized (Fig. 6-7). In patients with acute tubular necrosis severe enough to cause renal failure, the Doppler patterns will show reduced diastolic flow.

RENAL INFECTION

Many renal diseases involve infection. The spectrum of severity varies depending on the type of renal infection. Renal infection can progress from pyelonephritis to focal nephritis to renal abscess. Most renal infections are contained in the kidney and may be resolved with antibiotics. Nephritis is a general term for any inflammation of the kidney. It may involve the glomeruli (glomerulonephritis), the spaces within the kidney (interstitial nephritis), or the main tissue of the kidney and pelvis (pyelonephritis). Nephritis may be acute (sudden onset) or chronic (slow onset).

Pyonephrosis

Pyonephrosis is distention of the renal collecting system with pus or infected urine. It usually occurs as a result of long-standing ureteral obstruction from calculus disease, stricture, or a congenital anomaly. Pyonephrosis may develop from a broad variety of conditions from an ascending urinary tract infection or the spread of a bacterial pathogen throughout the bloodstream. Upper urinary tract infection in combination with obstruction and hydronephrosis may lead to pyonephrosis. It may be caused by urinary obstruction in the presence of pyelonephritis. This would lead to a collection of WBCs, bacteria, and debris in the collecting system that would cause pyonephrosis. A hydronephrotic kidney filled with stagnant urine may become infected and filled with pus. This pus collects and eventually forms an abscess. Without early recognition, patients with pyonephrosis may have rapid deterioration and development of septic shock. Delayed diagnosis and treatment leads to irreversible kidney parenchymal damage and loss of renal function, ultimately requiring nephrectomy. Death results from excessively delayed diagnosis.

Pyonephrosis is relatively uncommon. It typically is associated with fever, chills, urinary tract infection, obstruction, hydronephrosis, and flank pain, although some patients are asymptomatic. Laboratory results may include **leukocytosis,** pyuria, and bacteriuria.

Sonographic Findings. Sonographic findings suggestive of pyonephrosis include the presence of hydronephrosis in conjunction with debris in the collecting system. The presence of debris and the layering of low-amplitude echoes in the hydronephrotic kidney are indicators of pyonephrosis. These low-level echoes in the collecting system are the most consistent finding in pyonephrosis. In some cases, echogenic pus can be seen filling the collecting system or layering in the dependent portion of the collecting system. Sometimes a kidney with pyonephrosis is indistinguishable from ordinary noninfected hydronephrosis.

Pyelonephritis

Pyelonephritis is an inflammation of the renal collecting system and renal parenchyma, particularly from local bacterial infection. It is categorized as acute or chronic. Pyelonephritis may localize and intensify to form a renal cortical abscess. It usually stems from the retrograde migration of bacteria up the ureter and into the kidney. Generally, pyelonephritis extends from the tip of the papilla to the periphery of the cortex, involving the kidney in a patchy manner. Differentiation between infected and normal parenchyma is usually noticeable.

Pyelonephritis is a common cause of flank pain (mild and dull). Fever, chills, nausea, dysuria, and vomiting are the most common symptoms. Leukocytosis, bacteriuria, and pyuria are typical findings in pyelonephritis.

Sonographic Findings. A renal ultrasound for identification of hydronephrosis may be helpful in some cases because pyelonephritis should not show any renal pelvic or ureteral dilation. If collecting system dilation is found, pyonephrosis should be suspected. Pyelonephritis shows isolated increases in the medullary echogenicity and renal enlargement. Focal pyelonephritis causes increased or decreased areas of echogenicity in the kidney that may bulge outside of the renal outline. Often there are no sonographic findings in cases of pyelonephritis.

Acute Pyelonephritis

Acute pyelonephritis is acute inflammation of the renal parenchyma and pelvis. It is characterized by small cortical abscesses in the medulla from pus in the collecting tubules and interstitial tissue. Acute pyelonephritis is usually the result of a bladder infection (cystitis) that has spread to the kidney.

Acute pyelonephritis is more common in females than in males.[4] Patients with acute pyelonephritis have sudden onset of pain in the lower back, fever with chills, nausea, dysuria, and frequent urination. Laboratory tests show WBCs, leukocytosis, pyuria, and bacteriuria.

Sonographic Findings. Sonographically, most cases of acute pyelonephritis appear normal. With unilateral involvement, renal enlargement with decreased cortical echogenicity may be apparent. The renal echogenicity varies from a normal appearance to generalized changes to focal decreases in the parenchyma. This decrease in corticomedullary echogenicity causes the renal sinus to appear more prominent. The renal sinus also appears compressed. A loss of corticomedullary differentiation and poorly marginated masses are also apparent in cases of pyelonephritis (Fig. 6-8). Severe cases of acute pyelonephritis show an enlarged kidney (both in length and cross-sectional area). Severe, prolonged, or multiple episodes of pyelonephritis cause calyceal clubbing and cortical scarring.[1]

Chronic Pyelonephritis

Chronic pyelonephritis is recurrent or persistent inflammation of the renal parenchyma and pelvis resulting from bacterial infection. It is characterized by calyceal deformities and large renal scars with patchy distribution. Chronic pyelonephritis is caused by destruction and scarring of the kidney tissue from untreated bacterial infections. It occurs mostly in patients with major anatomic anomalies, including urinary tract obstruction, calculi, renal dysplasia, or vesicoureteral reflux. Chronic pyelonephritis is associated with parenchymal narrowing and progressive renal scarring. If the condition is left untreated, renal failure occurs, requiring dialysis or transplantation.

Patients with chronic pyelonephritis, if symptomatic, have a high fever, lethargy, nausea, vomiting, intense flank pain, dysuria, and hypertension. Chronic pyelonephritis is more common in females than in males.[5] Laboratory findings may include pyuria, proteinuria,

bacteriuria, increased serum creatinine levels, and increased BUN values.

Sonographic Findings. Chronic pyelonephritis may have sonographic evidence of calculi. Renal changes are either unilateral or bilateral. Sonographically, a dilated blunt calyx may be visualized with an overlying cortical scar or atrophy. Chronic pyelonephritis shows an increase in cortical and medullary echodensity. Islands of normal tissue are visualized and are potentially confused with tumor formation. Patients with chronic pyelonephritis have clubbing of calyces, irregular renal outline, and thinning of the parenchymal tissue. The pelvis and calyces appear distorted, which causes difficult visualization of the renal boarders. A small, shrunken, misshapen kidney is a common sonographic finding of chronic pyelonephritis.

Emphysematous Pyelonephritis

Emphysematous pyelonephritis is an uncommon, life-threatening, severe infection that results in gas formation in the renal parenchyma. It is caused by vascular disease, high glucose levels, and necrotizing infection with a gas-forming organism.[9] Patients with emphysematous pyelonephritis usually need emergency nephrectomy. Generally, emphysematous pyelonephritis affects only one kidney. Emphysematous pyelitis is a less serious condition in which the gas forms in the collecting system (not in the renal parenchyma as in cases of emphysematous pyelonephritis).

Emphysematous pyelonephritis is more common in females than in males and is more common in patients with diabetes.[5] Patients are extremely ill with a fever of unknown origin, flank pain, dehydration, and electrolyte imbalance. Laboratory results include presence of *Escherichia coli* bacteria, hyperglycemia, and acidosis.[9]

Sonographic Findings. Emphysematous pyelonephritis rarely shows echogenic gas. Sonographically, intrarenal gas will appear as dirty shadows. Sonographic evaluation is made more difficult because of the gas producing echogenic foci with distal dirty shadows (Fig. 6-9). Bright reflectors with dirty shadows or ringdown artifacts are also demonstrated. Emphysematous pyelonephritis presents as a unilateral, enlarged, hypoechoic, inflamed kidney.

Xanthogranulomatous Pyelonephritis

Xanthogranulomatous pyelonephritis is a serious, long-term, debilitating illness characterized by an infectious renal inflammation. It is a chronic inflammatory disorder of the kidney characterized by a mass originating in the renal parenchyma. The xanthogranulomatous pyelo-

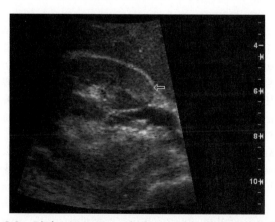

Fig. 6-8 Right transverse kidney with arrow pointing to area of altered cortical echogenicity in patient with acute pyelonephritis. (Courtesy Cindy Rapp, Radiology Imaging Associates, Greenwood Village, Colorado.)

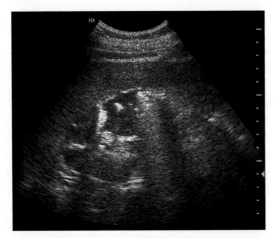

Fig. 6-9 Right kidney in patient with emphysematous pyelonephritis; note echogenic foci causing dirty shadows from intrarenal gas. (Courtesy Cindy Rapp, Radiology Imaging Associates, Greenwood Village, Colorado.)

nephritis kidney is usually nonfunctional and therefore typically requires nephrectomy. It is usually a unilateral disease. Xanthogranulomatous pyelonephritis results from long-term renal obstruction and infection. Frequently, xanthogranulomatous pyelonephritis presents with stones. Xanthogranulomatous pyelonephritis displays **neoplasm**-like properties, capable of local tissue invasion and destruction. Xanthogranulomatous pyelonephritis may be contained in the kidney, spread to the perinephric fat, or infiltrate the adjacent retroperitoneal structures. Xanthogranulomatous pyelonephritis has been known to fistulize (either in the renal parenchyma or gastrointestinal tract).

Patients with xanthogranulomatous pyelonephritis often are immunocompromised in some manner. Xanthogranulomatous pyelonephritis is more common in females than in males and is more common in patients with diabetes.[5] Patients with xanthogranulomatous pyelonephritis often appear chronically ill. Symptoms include anorexia, fever, weight loss, urinary tract infection, and a dull, persistent flank pain. Laboratory findings include leukocytosis, anemia, and bacteria in the urine.

Sonographic Findings. Sonographically, the patient with xanthogranulomatous pyelonephritis has a moderately enlarged kidney. Focal abscesses are also shown. Xanthogranulomatous pyelonephritis may be sonographically indistinguishable from renal cell carcinoma. Most patients have renal calculi, often in the form of a large, echogenic, shadowing staghorn calculus within the collecting system. A staghorn calculus is a calculus that takes the shape of the renal pelvis and sometimes the major calyces. These stones do not pass through the ureter and may require lithotripsy. A heterogeneous, inflammatory parenchymal mass and hydronephrosis may be apparent on the affected kidney. The mass will have through transmission and could appear to involve adjacent organs. Xanthogranulomatous pyelonephritis may show multiple areas of variable echogenicity. Multiple hypoechoic areas corresponding to dilated calyces are apparent. Xanthogranulomatous pyelonephritis causes a general decrease in echodensity with some areas of increased echogenicity. Perinephric fluid collections, inflammatory tissues, and dilated calyces are also seen.

Renal Abscess

An abscess is defined as a collection of pus. Renal abscesses tend to cause more intense pain than does pyelonephritis, possibly because the increased edema and inflammation stretching the renal capsule. Renal abscesses are corticomedullary or cortical. Cortico-medullary abscesses are derived from an ascending urinary infection and are associated with obstruction. Severe renal parenchymal involvement is observed with corticomedullary abscesses. Cortical abscesses develop from the spread of bacteria from elsewhere in the body through the vascular system. Renal abscesses result from acute focal bacterial nephritis, acute multifocal bacterial nephritis, emphysematous pyelonephritis, and xantho-granulomatous pyelonephritis. Acute pyelonephritis leads to parenchymal necrosis with abscess formation without adequate treatment.

Patients with renal abscesses may have intense flank or abdominal pain, palpable flank mass, fever, chills, dysuria, fatigue, nausea, vomiting, weight loss, and history of a recent urinary tract infection or renal calculi. Patients with diabetes are at an increased risk for renal abscesses. Laboratory findings include urinary infection, leukocytosis, positive urine and blood cultures, hematuria, increased WBC count, elevated BUN value, elevated creatinine level, bacteriuria, anemia, proteinuria, and pyuria.

Sonographic Findings. An intrarenal abscess presents sonographically as an ill-defined renal mass with low-amplitude internal echoes and disruption of the corticomedullary junction. Renal abscesses appear as thick-walled, hypoechoic, complex cystic masses. Internal mobile debris, gas with dirty shadowing, and septations are occasionally visualized within the abscess. Renal abscesses have irregular borders. Bowel loops filled with air and stool may mimic abscesses

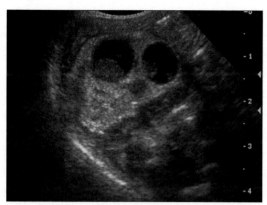

Fig. 6-10 Transverse lower pole of right kidney with *Candida albicans* (fungal balls). (Courtesy Carol Teal, Keesler Air Force Base, Mississippi.)

when the bowel is lying in close proximity to the kidney. Abscess formation generally appears as a complex fluid collection with varying degrees of internal echogenicity and a moderate increase in through transmission of sound. Renal abscesses tend to be solitary.

Fungal Infection

Fungal infections are diseases caused by the growth of fungi in or on the body. Fungal bezoars (fungal balls) are rare. When fungus balls are present, they can obstruct the renal pelvis or the ureters, resulting in pyonephrosis. Fungal infections diffusely involve the renal parenchyma. Multiple small focal parenchymal abscesses occur that may calcify over time. Fungal infections extend into the perinephric space. Fungal balls result from fungal infections invading the collecting system. Fungus balls are mobile and cause obstruction, leading to development of hydronephrosis. These fungal balls must be differentiated from other disorders such as blood clots, radiolucent stones, transitional cell tumors, and sloughed papilla.

Fungal infections of the urinary tract are more often found in diabetic and immunocompromised patients.[9] They are also found in patients with indwelling catheters, malignant diseases, hematopoietic disorders, and histories of long-term antibiotic or steroid therapy and intravenous drug abuse. Laboratory findings include hematuria, bacteriuria, and pyuria.

Sonographic Findings. A fungal infection appears sonographically as a medium echodensity, non-shadowing, mobile defect. Fungus balls are visualized as echogenic, nonshadowing, soft tissue masses within the renal collecting system (Fig. 6-10). Fungal infections also appear as small, hypoechoic parenchymal masses.

Tables 6-1 and 6-2 are summaries of the pathology, symptoms, and sonographic findings of renal failure and infections.

SUMMARY

Many precursors to renal failure must be considered in ruling out renal failure. Renal failure is caused by obstruction of urine flow, decreased renal blood flow, or renal parenchymal disease. Hydronephrosis is caused by a number of obstructive processes, including papillary necrosis, pyonephrosis, acute pyelonephritis, xanthogranulomatous pyelonephritis, and fungal infections. Any long-term obstructive process has the potential to lead to renal failure. In addition, any disease that reduces renal function has the ultimate risk of renal failure. Renal function may be ultimately reduced by any of the renal diseases discussed in this chapter. The cause and degree of renal function loss determines the medical path the patient will follow (e.g., percutaneous drainage, antibiotics, focal nephrectomy, nephrectomy, dialysis). Sonographically, a thorough B-mode assessment for hydronephrosis, masses, pyonephrosis, and calculi should be accomplished. Color evaluation should be used to distinguish between pathology and prominent vasculature and to determine patent renal blood flow. Finally, pulsed Doppler evaluation should be used in assessment of renal blood flow for stenosis or thrombosis.

CLINICAL SCENARIO—DIAGNOSIS

■ The advanced age of the patient, the history of diabetes, the abnormal laboratory values, and the hypertension all are clinical symptoms associated with processes that eventually lead to renal failure. The patient's excessive history of smoking and symptoms of painful walking are suggestive of atherosclerosis (plaque build-up narrowing the arteries). The decreased size of the left kidney and tardus parvus effect shown on intrarenal Doppler evaluation (see Fig. 6-1) lead to a renal artery stenosis diagnosis. The tardus parvus waveform suggests the stenosis is at a point proximal to the area of Doppler evaluation (possibly at some point between the renal hilum and aortic-renal junction). The stenotic area was presumably not visualized sonographically because of overlying bowel gas typically found around the renal arteries. The right kidney was normal sonographically in size, appearance, and Doppler assessment. Left renal artery stenosis is the only finding in this case study.

Table 6-1	Pathology Associated with Renal Failure	
Pathology	**Symptoms**	**Sonographic Findings**
Hydronephrosis	Asymptomatic, pain, infection, nausea, dysuria, fever, chills, vomiting, uremia, microscopic hematuria	Fluid-filled spaces that connect, increased resistance index; when severe, cortical thinning, renal enlargement
Acute glomerulonephritis	Smoky urine, recent fever, sore throat, joint pains, peripheral edema, nausea, oliguria, anemia, azotemia, hypertension	Irregular cortical echopattern, increased cortical echogenicity, prominent pyramids, bilateral renal enlargement; when chronic, small, smooth, echogenic kidneys
Papillary necrosis	Fever, hematuria hypertension, dysuria, pain	Hydronephrosis, clubbing of calyces, shadows from calculi, round or triangular anechoic collections in medullary pyramids; when severe, multiple anechoic noncommunicating structures in pyramid area
Acute renal failure	Hypovolemia, hypertension, edema, oliguria, hematuria	Normal or enlarged kidneys, increased parenchymal echogenicity
Chronic renal failure	Malaise, increased concentration of urea in blood, fatigue, anorexia, nausea, hypotension, hyperkalemia	Decreased renal size, increased cortical echogenicity, poor corticomedullary differentiation; when end-stage, small, echogenic kidney with thin parenchyma
Renal artery stenosis	Hypertension	Initially increased size progressing to decreased size, high systolic peak velocities, little or no diastolic flow at stenosis site, tardus parvus effect distal to stenosis
Acute tubular necrosis	Hypertension, oliguria, edema, hypotension, pain, vomiting, hematuria, infection, sepsis, muscle necrosis	Normal appearance, enlarged echogenic kidneys, increased cortical echogenicity, enlarged and hyperechoic pyramids; when severe, reduced diastolic flow

Table 6-2	Pathology Associated with Renal Infections	
Pathology	**Symptoms**	**Sonographic Findings**
Pyonephrosis	Asymptomatic, fever, hydronephrosis, urinary tract infection, pain, chills, obstruction	Hydronephrosis with layering of low-amplitude echoes
Acute pyelonephritis	Lower back pain, fever, chills, nausea, dysuria, frequent urination	Normal appearance, renal enlargement, decreased cortical echogenicity, focal decreased echogenicity in parenchyma, prominent renal sinus; when severe, cortical scarring, calyceal clubbing
Chronic pyelonephritis	Asymptomatic, high fever, lethargy, nausea, vomiting, intense flank pain, dysuria, hypertension	Shadowing from calculi, dilated blunt calyces, increased parenchymal echodensity, islands of normal tissue, irregular outline, thin parenchyma, decreased kidney size
Emphysematous pyelonephritis	Extreme illness, fever, flank pain, dehydration, electrolyte imbalance, artifacts, presence of *E. coli* bacteria	Rarely demonstrable, dirty shadows, echogenic foci with distal dirty shadows, ring-down unilateral enlarged and hypoechoic kidney

Table 6-2	*Pathology Associated with Renal Infections—cont'd*	
Pathology	Symptoms	Sonographic Findings
Xanthogranulomatous pyelonephritis	Chronic illness, anorexia, fever, weight loss, urinary tract infection, dull flank pain	Moderately enlarged kidney, focal abscesses, indistinguishable from renal cell carcinoma, large shadowing calculi, areas of variable echogenicity, hydronephrosis, dilated calyces, heterogeneous mass in parenchyma with through transmission, perinephric fluid
Renal abscess	Intense pain, palpable flank mass, fever, chills, dysuria, fatigue, nausea, vomiting, weight loss, recent urinary tract infection, renal calculi	Ill-defined renal mass with low-amplitude internal echoes, internal mobile debris, gas with dirty shadowing, septations, thick-walled, hypoechoic complex cystic mass, irregular borders, moderately increased through transmission
Fungal infection	Found in patients with diabetes, intravenous drug use, immune and hematopoietic disorders, indwelling catheters, malignant disease	Medium echodensity, nonshadowing, mobile defect within renal collecting system, small hypoechoic parenchymal masses

CASE STUDIES FOR DISCUSSION

1. A frail-appearing 55-year-old woman arrives at the ultrasound department for a renal sonogram. The patient has a long history of urinary tract obstruction. She has a fever, left flank pain, and recent unexplainable weight loss. Laboratory test results are positive for urinary infection. Sonographic examination reveals a normal right kidney. The left kidney is enlarged. It displays signs of hydronephrosis (Fig. 6-11) and also shows a large, echogenic, shadowing stone within the renal pelvis (not visualized in Fig. 6-11). Further analysis of the left upper pole of the kidney shows a heterogeneous parenchymal mass with varying echogenicities. What is the most likely diagnosis from this scenario?

2. A 45-year-old man with fatigue, pruritus, and nausea is sent from the emergency department for a renal ultrasound. He has a history of diabetes mellitus. The laboratory results show a decrease in the GFR, increased BUN level, elevated creatinine value of 5.1, and anemia. Sonographically, the kidneys are echogenic and decreased in size bilaterally in comparison with previous sonograms. The renal parenchyma appears thin (Fig. 6-12). What is a possible diagnosis of this study?

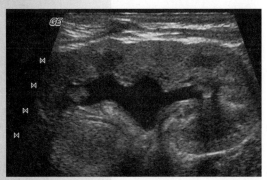

Fig. 6-11 Left longitudinal kidney. (Courtesy Cindy Rapp, Radiology Imaging Associates, Greenwood Village, Colorado.)

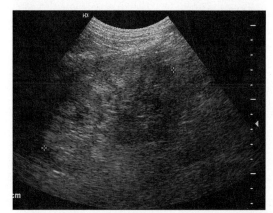

Fig. 6-12 Longitudinal left kidney. (Courtesy Deborah A. Thomas, Wilford Hall Medical Center, Lackland Air Force Base, Texas.)

CASE STUDIES FOR DISCUSSION—cont'd

3. A 33-year-old man, with a previous diagnosis of AIDS, is referred from the urology department for a renal sonogram. He has a 2-week history of flank pain, fever, and chills. Laboratory results show bacteriuria, leukocytosis, and pyuria. The renal sonogram shows a large, echogenic calculus (Fig. 6-13) with posterior shadowing in the right renal pelvis causing obstructive hydronephrosis (Fig. 6-14). Within the dilated, primarily anechoic calyces and pelvis are low-level echoes that show a layering effect within the collecting system. What are the most likely diagnoses?

4. A 12-year-old boy is sent to the ultrasound department for a renal sonogram. The patient has a recent fever, sore throat, foggy appearance to his urine, joint pains, and costovertebral tenderness. Laboratory test results show increased BUN and creatinine levels, hematuria, and proteinuria. Sonographically, the kidneys appear enlarged bilaterally. The left kidney shows irregular cortical echotexture (Fig. 6-15). What might be the diagnosis for this patient?

5. A 55-year old woman with diabetes is seen for a renal ultrasound and appears dehydrated and extremely ill. She has a fever and severe right flank pain. Laboratory results show the presence of *E. coli* bacteria. Sonographically, the left kidney appears normal. The right kidney (Fig. 6-16) displays dirty shadows intrarenally, making sonographic visualization difficult. The right kidney measures 14 cm in length and has a hypoechoic appearance. What is the diagnosis for this patient?

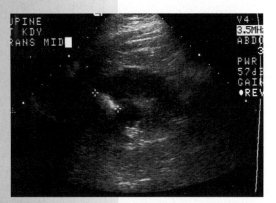

Fig. 6-13 Right kidney transverse. (Courtesy staff sonographers at John L. McClellen Memorial Veteran's Administration Medical Center, Little Rock, Arkansas.)

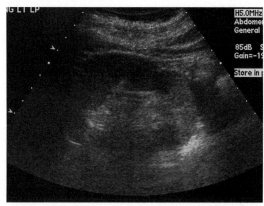

Fig. 6-15 Left kidney longitudinal. (Courtesy Cindy Rapp, Radiology Imaging Associates, Greenwood Village, Colorado.)

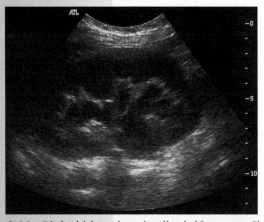

Fig. 6-14 Right kidney longitudinal. (Courtesy Cindy Rapp, Radiology Imaging Associates, Greenwood Village, Colorado.)

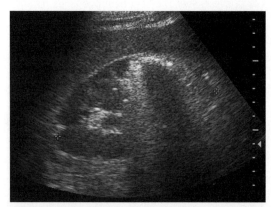

Fig. 6-16 Right kidney longitudinal. (Courtesy Cindy Rapp, Radiology Imaging Associates, Greenwood Village, Colorado.)

STUDY QUESTIONS

1. A 49-year-old woman is sent to the ultrasound department for sonographic evaluation of the kidneys. She has a history of long-term antibiotic usage for chronic renal infection. The laboratory test results show hematuria and bacteriuria. Sonographically, the left kidney is normal, whereas the right kidney shows a hypoechoic, dilated renal pelvis with medium echodensity and round, mobile, soft tissue masses throughout the collecting system. These masses do not shadow. This finding suggests which of the following?
   a. papillary necrosis
   b. renal abscess
   c. acute pyelonephritis
   d. chronic pyelonephritis
   e. fungal infection

2. An obese 61-year-old woman is seen for a renal sonogram. She has a history of hypertension, difficulty breathing, and lower back pain. The laboratory test results show a decrease in GFR. The kidneys have a normal sonographic appearance and measure within normal limits bilaterally. Doppler analysis of the left kidney appears normal. The right kidney show a lengthened systolic rise time, slow systolic acceleration, and rounding of the systolic peak on Doppler analysis. What is a possible diagnosis from these sonographic findings?
   a. pyonephrosis
   b. renal artery stenosis
   c. acute glomerulonephritis
   d. papillary necrosis
   e. hydronephrosis

3. A 59-year-old woman with diabetes is sent for a renal ultrasound. She has a history of recent fever, chills, abdominal pain, painful urination, and increased blood pressure. The laboratory test results reveal hematuria, pyuria, and bacteriuria. With ultrasound examination, large anechoic areas are revealed within left renal sinus. These anechoic areas appear to have a clubbing effect in relation to the adjacent calyx. The left renal parenchyma appears thin. Echogenic foci are causing shadowing within the collecting system. These findings are most suggestive of which of the following?
   a. chronic renal failure
   b. acute renal failure
   c. papillary necrosis

   d. acute tubular necrosis
   e. renal abscess

4. A 62-year-old woman with a history of diabetes is referred for a renal ultrasound from the emergency department. She is severely dehydrated and not coherent. Her temperature is 103° F. She has extreme pain along her left flank. The laboratory results of the urinary sample showed the presence of hematuria and E. coli bacteria. Sonographically, the right kidney appears normal. The left kidney has multiple echogenic foci throughout it. Visualization of the left kidney is difficult because of unusual shadowing throughout the left renal area. What is the most likely diagnosis?
   a. renal abscess
   b. xanthogranulomatous pyelonephritis
   c. pyonephrosis
   d. emphysematous pyelonephritis
   e. hydronephrosis

5. A 36-year-old firefighter is referred from the emergency department for a renal sonogram. His medical records indicate that he recently recovered from a bladder infection. He has intense left flank pain, palpable left flank mass, fever, painful urination, nausea, and vomiting. The laboratory test results reveal positive urine cultures, hematuria, increased WBC count, elevated BUN and creatinine levels, bacteriuria, and pyuria. Sonographically, the right kidney appears normal. The left kidney displays the presence of an ill-defined, complex fluid collection in the inferior renal pole. The complex fluid collection has septations, irregular, thick-walled borders, displays internal mobile debris, and shows dirty shadowing posterior to it. What is the most likely diagnosis from this sonographic examination?
   a. renal abscess
   b. emphysematous pyelonephritis
   c. fungal infection
   d. acute pyelonephritis
   e. acute glomerulonephritis

6. A 42-year-old man with a cocaine addiction is undergoing detoxification at a local facility and is seen for a renal sonogram. He has decreased urine output and hypertension. The laboratory test results reveal an acute decrease in the GFR to very low levels and a sudden increase in the serum creatinine and BUN concentrations. Sonographically, the

kidneys are enlarged bilaterally and have increased echogenicity when compared with the liver. The parenchymal echotexture appears normal in echogenicity, although the renal pyramids appear enlarged and hyperechoic. Doppler analysis reveals reduced diastolic flow. Which of the following is a possible diagnosis from the aforementioned clinical and sonographic findings?

a. chronic renal failure
b. acute pyelonephritis
c. chronic pyelonephritis
d. acute tubular necrosis
e. papillary necrosis

7. A 24-year-old woman with a 12-year history of recurring urinary tract infections arrives at the ultrasound department needing a renal sonogram. She has hypertension, a high fever, nausea, vomiting, and painful urination. The laboratory findings include bacteriuria, proteinuria, and increased BUN and creatinine levels. Sonographically, the right kidney appears normal, but the left renal parenchyma appears narrowed and has focal areas of increased echogenicity. In addition, the left kidney measures abnormally small and appears misshapen and its borders are difficult to visualize. What might be the cause of these sonographic findings?

a. acute pyelonephritis
b. chronic pyelonephritis
c. xanthogranulomatous pyelonephritis
d. emphysematous pyelonephritis
e. renal artery stenosis

8. A 37-year-old man with a history of smoking is sent for a renal ultrasound. The patient has a history of an upper urinary tract obstruction. He now has reduced urine output and hematuria. Laboratory results reveal increased creatinine levels, increased BUN values, and a decrease in the GFR. Sonographically, the kidneys are enlarged and show increased echogenicity when compared with the liver. What might be the cause of these findings?

a. emphysematous pyelonephritis
b. xanthogranulomatous pyelonephritis
c. fungal infection
d. acute renal failure
e. papillary necrosis

9. A 33-year-old male scuba diver presents with pharyngitis, edema, and decreased volume and frequency of urination. The laboratory results found

hematuria. The only sonographic findings were enlarged kidneys with increased echogenicity of the parenchymal cortex. Of the following, which diagnosis may result from these limited findings?

a. hydronephrosis
b. acute glomerulonephritis
c. pyonephrosis
d. fungal infection
e. renal abscess

10. A 49-year-old male construction worker with a history of an enlarged prostate is seen with right flank pain and painful urination. He claims to drink large amounts of milk every day. Laboratory findings include microscopic hematuria. An abdominal sonogram shows normal anatomy except for the right kidney. It displays a hypoechoic, dilated renal collecting system to include the ureter with no echogenic foci. This would be most consistent with which of the following?

a. hydronephrosis caused by the enlarged prostate obstructing flow
b. pyonephrosis caused by prolonged obstruction from staghorn calculi
c. pyelonephritis caused by infection spreading from the enlarged prostate
d. pyonephrosis caused by calcium deposits from excessive milk consumption
e. hydronephrosis caused by calcium deposits from excessive milk consumption

REFERENCES

1. McGahan J, Goldberg B et al: *Diagnostic ultrasound: a logical approach*, Philadelphia, 1998, Lippincott-Raven.
2. Hagen-Ansert SL: *Textbook of diagnostic ultrasonography*, vol 1, ed 5, St Louis, 2001, Mosby.
3. Cheers G: *Anatomica: the complete home medical reference*, Willoughby, 2000, Global Book Publishing Pty Ltd.
4. Hall R: *The ultrasound handbook: clinical, etiologic, pathologic, implications of sonographic findings*, ed 2, Philadelphia, 1993, JB Lippincott.
5. Rumack C, Wilson S, Charboneau J et al: *Diagnostic ultrasound*, vol 1, ed 2, St Louis, 1998, Mosby.
6. Parmar MS: Acute glomerulonephritis, http://www.emedicine.com/med/topic879.htm, retrieved July 9, 2003.
7. Salifu MO, Delano BG: Chronic glomerulonephritis, http://www.emedicine.com/med/topic880.htm, retrieved July 9, 2003.
8. Donohoe JM, Mydlo JH: Papillary necrosis, http://www.emedicine.com/med/topic2839.htm, retrieved July 9, 2003.

9. Kurtz A, Middleton W: *Ultrasound: the requisites*, St Louis, 1996, Mosby.
10. Acute renal failure, http://www.emedicine.com/med/topic1595.htm.
11. Verrelli M: Chronic renal failure, http://www.emedicine.com/med/topic374.htm, retrieved July 9, 2003.
12. Spinowitz BS, Rodriguez J: Renal artery stenosis, http://www.emedicine.com/med/topic2001.htm, retrieved July 9, 2003.

BIBLIOGRAPHY

Cheers G: *Anatomica: the complete home medical reference*, Willoughby, 2000, Global Book Publishing Pty Ltd.

Gray H: *Gray's anatomy: the classic collector's edition*, ed 15, New York, 1977, Crown Publishers.

Hagen-Ansert SL: *Textbook of diagnostic ultrasonography*, vol 1, ed 5, St Louis, 2001, Mosby.

Hall R: *The ultrasound handbook: clinical, etiologic, pathologic, implications of sonographic findings*, ed 2, Philadelphia, 1993, JB Lippincott.

Kurtz A, Middleton W: *Ultrasound: the requisites*, St Louis, 1996, Mosby.

McGahan J, Goldberg B et al: *Diagnostic ultrasound: a logical approach*, Philadelphia, 1998, Lippincott-Raven.

Rumack C, Wilson S, Charboneau J et al: *Diagnostic ultrasound*, vol 1, ed 2, St Louis, 1998, Mosby.

Sanders RC: *Clinical sonography: a practical guide*, vol 1, ed 3, Philadelphia, 1998, Lippincott-Raven.

Stedman T: *Stedman's medical dictionary*, ed 26, Baltimore, 1995, Williams & Wilkins.

Cystic Versus Solid Renal Mass

CHARLOTTE HENNINGSEN

CLINICAL SCENARIO

■ A 39-year-old echocardiographer with 15 years of experience has had sporadic back pain for about 5 years that she attributes to scanning. While scanning portables in the Cardiac Intensive Care Unit, she has a sharp pain on the right side. Curious as to whether she has gallstones, she places the 2.5-MHz transducer on her right upper quadrant. Somewhat familiar with the normal sonographic appearance of the liver, she identifies the homogeneous appearance of the liver parenchyma. Inferior to the liver, she sees multiple cystic structures. The next day she calls a friend who works in radiology ultrasound and describes her findings. The sonographer suggests that she seek a consultation with a nephrologist.

After an appointment with the nephrologist, a renal ultrasound is ordered and reveals the findings identified in Fig. 7-1. The left and right kidneys are similar in appearance. What is the most likely diagnosis?

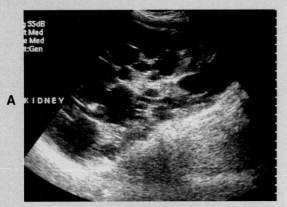
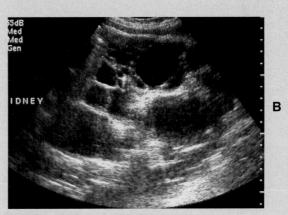

Fig. 7-1 Multiple cysts are identified on, **A**, right kidney and, **B**, left kidney.

OBJECTIVES

■ Describe cystic renal lesions that can be identified sonographically.

■ Differentiate the ultrasound findings of a variety of cystic renal lesions.

■ Describe the pattern of inheritance of specific hereditary cystic diseases.

■ List anomalies associated with cystic renal diseases.

■ Identify Doppler findings associated with cystic lesions.

■ List symptoms associated with specific renal cystic lesions.

GLOSSARY OF TERMS ▬

Autosomal recessive polycystic kidney disease: a hereditary disease characterized by varying degrees of dilation of the renal tubules and hepatic fibrosis; the most severe manifestations are considered inconsistent with life and are either diagnosed in utero or at birth

Caroli's disease: a hereditary disease of segmental or diffuse intrahepatic bile duct dilation; sonographically, saccular dilations that are contiguous with the ducts may be shown

Congenital familial anodontia: a congenital hereditary anomaly characterized by absence of some or all of the teeth

Dysuria: painful urination

Ehlers-Danlos syndrome: a hereditary syndrome characterized by hypermotility of the joints and skin laxity and fragility

Genotype: the identification of a disorder on the basis of a specific combination of genes or the location of the genes on a chromosome

Hematuria: blood in the urine

Hemihypertrophy: overgrowth of half of the body

Hippel-Lindau disease: an autosomal dominant disease characterized by development of a variety of cysts and neoplasms; renal cysts and renal cell carcinoma are prevalent in individuals with this disorder

Locus: relates to the specific location of a gene on a chromosome

Marfan syndrome: an autosomal dominant disorder characterized by elongated bones and abnormalities of the eyes and cardiovascular system

Multicystic dysplastic kidney: characterized by multiple, noncommunicating cysts of variable size in a nonfunctioning kidney; usually a unilateral process; may be a cause of an abdominal mass in a newborn; the cysts involute over time and may appear similar to a renal agenesis in an adult patient

Nephrocalcinosis: calcification within the renal parenchyma that may include the cortex or medulla

Tuberous sclerosis: an autosomal dominant or sporadic syndrome characterized by seizures, mental retardation, and cutaneous lesions; associated renal cysts and neoplasms are commonly identified in these patients as are lesions in the central nervous system, cardiovascular system, and pulmonary and skeletal systems

---

A renal ultrasound may be ordered to characterize the nature of a mass after other imaging procedures have been done. Then the task of the sonographer is to define whether the mass is of a cystic or solid nature. When the mass is cystic, it then must be further defined sonographically for determination of whether imaging or other diagnostic procedures are necessary. When cystic lesions are associated with decreasing renal function or other symptoms, such as hematuria or hypertension, a treatment plan must be explored to avoid other complications. Furthermore, the ultrasound examination may assist in defining whether or not the renal cysts are part of a genetic disease.

This chapter explores the numerous cystic lesions and cystic diseases of the kidneys. Sonography may also characterize a lesion as solid, and descriptions of a variety of renal neoplasms and the normal sonographic appearance of the kidneys are explored in Chapter 5.

RENAL CYSTS
Simple Cyst

Renal cysts are relatively common and have been identified in all ages, although they are seen with increasing frequency with increasing age. The exact origin of renal cysts is unknown, but they are thought to be acquired.[1] Cysts may be unilateral or bilateral, solitary or multiple. Simple cysts are usually asymptomatic, although pain or hematuria may be present. Depending on the size and location, cysts may be associated with hydronephrosis.

Sonographic Findings. The ultrasound appearance of a renal cyst should meet the criteria of a simple cyst. The cyst should be anechoic, thin walled, and round or oval and show acoustic enhancement posterior to the cyst (Fig. 7-2, *A* and *B*). Edge shadowing is frequently shown along the lateral margins of the cyst. Doppler of the cyst shows the absence of flow (Fig. 7-3).

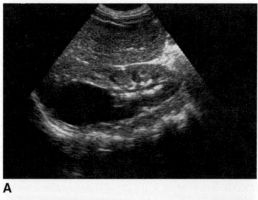

A

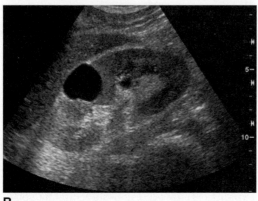

B

Fig. 7-2 Simple renal cysts are identified in **A** and **B**. (**B** Courtesy GE Medical Systems.)

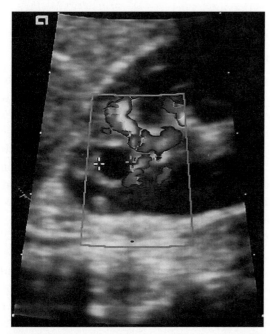

Fig. 7-3 Upper pole renal cyst with no blood flow to cyst. (Courtesy Shpetim Telegrafi, New York University.)

Atypical Cyst

When a cyst does not meet the criteria of a simple cyst, it may be classified as an atypical cyst. These cysts would include hemorrhagic cysts, infected cysts, multilocular or septated cysts, and calcified cysts (Fig. 7-4). The diagnosis may be made based on the patient's symptoms or may require additional imaging with computed tomography or needle aspiration and histologic examination.

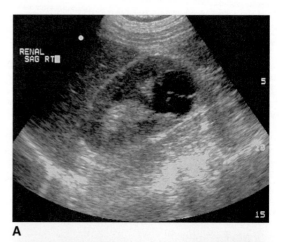

A

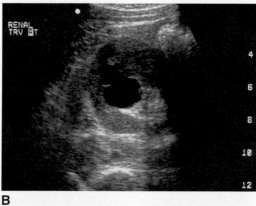

B

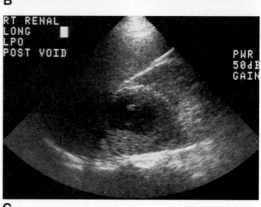

C

Fig. 7-4 Variable appearances of atypical cysts are shown in septate cyst identified in **A** and **B** and in infected cyst identified in **C**.

Hemorrhagic Cyst. Hemorrhage may occur in simple cysts or in cysts associated with cystic diseases. Patients may have flank pain and hematuria.

Sonographic findings. Blood has a variable appearance on ultrasound depending on whether the process is acute or chronic. The cyst may appear anechoic, contain low-level echoes, or have a complex appearance. A hemorrhagic cyst may or may not show acoustic enhancement. A retracted clot may have a similar appearance to a mass, and Doppler may assist in documenting the lack of flow in a hemorrhagic cyst.

Infected Cyst. When a cyst becomes infected, the patient may have flank pain, fever, hematuria, and white blood cells in the urine. Sonography can be useful in the diagnosis and treatment of these cysts through guided aspiration and drainage.

Sonographic findings. Infected cysts can have a variable appearance. Debris may appear as low-level echoes within the cyst and may show a layering effect that moves with a shift in the patient's position. In addition, the cyst wall may be thickened.

Multilocular Cyst. Cysts may contain loculations or septations and may be the result of resolved hemorrhage or infection. Thin septations typically are of no clinical significance, although aspiration may be used to exclude malignant disease.

Sonographic findings. A septated or multilocular cyst shows thin linear echoes within the cyst or an infolding of the cyst wall. If the septation is thick or shows papillary projections, it is suspicious for malignant disease.

Calcification in Cyst. Calcifications within a cyst wall may be identified in a cyst that has been previously infected or hemorrhagic. A small amount of calcification may be clinically insignificant; however, thick calcifications are worrisome for malignant disease and should be investigated further.

Sonographic findings. Calcifications appear echogenic and should display shadowing. If the calcification is significant in size, attenuation of the sound beam may prevent adequate visualization of the characteristics of the cyst.

Milk of Calcium Cyst

Milk of calcium cysts occur in patients with a calyceal diverticulum. Urine stasis in the cyst leads to formation of the milk of calcium, which is comprised primarily of calcium carbonate crystals. Milk of calcium cysts are usually asymptomatic and clinically insignificant. Few patients may have **hematuria**, flank pain, or infection.[2]

Sonographic Findings. Sonographically, a milk of calcium cyst shows a well-defined cystic lesion with echogenic milk of calcium that layers in the dependent portion of the cyst (Fig. 7-5) and shifts with changes in the patient's position.

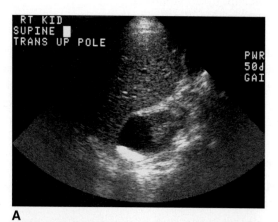

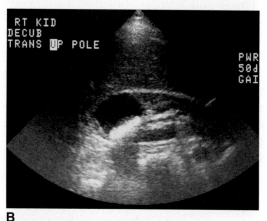

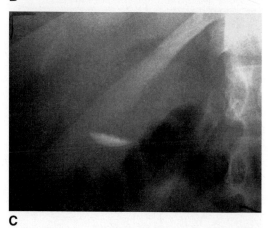

Fig. 7-5 Shift in position of milk of calcium is noted in cyst as patient is moved from, **A,** supine position to, **B,** decubitus position. **C,** Radiograph taken with patient standing also shows layering effect.

Parapelvic Cyst

Parapelvic cysts are located in the renal hilum and are thought to be of lymphatic origin.[1] These cysts do not communicate with the renal collecting system, although they may mimic hydronephrosis on ultrasound examination. Parapelvic cysts are usually asymptomatic. When present, clinical symptoms include hematuria, hypertension, and hydronephrosis.

Sonographic Findings. Sonographically, a parapelvic cyst appears as a cystic structure arising from the renal hilum. If multiple cysts exist, they may be confused with hydronephrosis. Sonographic differentiation may be made by demonstrating the lack of communication with the cyst or cysts and the collecting system (Fig. 7-6).

RENAL CYSTIC DISEASE
Autosomal Dominant Polycystic Kidney Disease

Autosomal dominant polycystic kidney disease (ADPKD) is a progressive disorder that leads to renal failure. ADPKD affects 1:1000 individuals, and three **genotypes** have been identified with a range of severity.[3] The most common type of ADPKD, *PKD1*, has been located on the short arm of chromosome 16. *PKD1* is also a more severe form of ADPKD that manifests at an earlier age, thus leading to end-stage renal disease (ESRD) approximately 20 years earlier than with *PKD2*. The *PKD2* **locus** has been identified on the long arm of chromosome 4. This milder form of the disease only affects approximately 10% of individuals with ADPKD, whereas *PKD1* affects approximately 85% of individuals with ADPKD.[4] A third type of ADPKD, *PKD3*, has been identified, but the genetic locus is unknown.[3,4]

Patients with ADPKD present clinically within the third to fourth decades of life.[5] Patients may have decreasing renal function and hypertension. ADPKD may also affect other organs, and cysts may be found in the liver, pancreas, and spleen. In addition, patients may also manifest with abnormalities of heart valves, colonic diverticula, and cerebral aneurysms. Patient symptoms may include flank pain and hematuria because cysts associated with ADPKD are prone to hemorrhage or become infected. Renal calculi may also be associated with ADPKD.

Sonographic Findings. Patients with ADPKD have multiple cysts of varying sizes noted bilaterally (Fig. 7-7). The identification of multiple cysts noted bilaterally aids in distinguishing this disease from

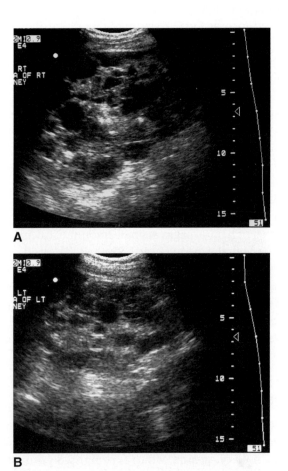

A

B

Fig. 7-7 Multiple cysts are identified in these enlarged kidneys (right **[A]** and left **[B]**) shown in a 65-year-old man with history of autosomal dominant polycystic kidney disease.

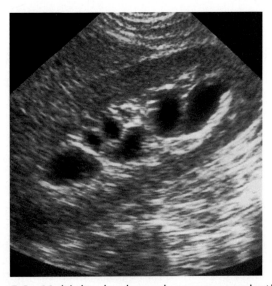

Fig. 7-6 Multiple, haphazard noncommunicating central cystic spaces represent parapelvic cysts.

multicystic dysplastic kidney (MCDK). As the disease progresses, the kidneys become markedly enlarged, and the presence of nephromegaly has been directly correlated with decreasing renal function.[3] The liver (Fig. 7-8), pancreas, and spleen should also be surveyed for the presence of cysts, although they generally appear later in the disease process. A polycystic liver rarely affects liver function, and the prevalence of liver cysts in females is debated in the literature.[3,4]

Sonography is a sensitive screening method for patients with a family history of ADPKD. DNA analysis is also available but is expensive and not as widely available as ultrasound screening. The sonographic criteria for diagnosis of the disease should be adjusted according to the patient's age. Findings suggestive of ADPKD include the identification of a total of two renal cysts, unilateral or bilateral in patients less than 30 years of age; two cysts in each kidney in patients 30 to 59 years of age; and four cysts in each kidney in patients 60 years of age or greater.[4,5]

Acquired Cystic Kidney Disease

Acquired cystic kidney disease (ACKD) is a progressive disorder that results in chronic renal failure from a noncystic renal disorder. It is characterized by the development of multiple cysts in the kidneys and is seen frequently in patients on long-term dialysis.[4,6]

ACKD is usually asymptomatic; however, clinical symptoms may present as the result of complications of ACKD, which include hemorrhage and the development of renal cell carcinoma.[4,6] When associated with renal cell carcinoma, the patient may have hematuria, flank pain, and fever.

Sonographic Findings. The diagnosis of ACKD can be made sonographically when three or more cysts are identified in each kidney (Figs. 7-9 and 7-10). The kidneys are usually decreased in size, but nephromegaly may also be identified.[4] Ultrasound may also be used in patients with known ACKD to monitor for the development of malignant neoplasm.

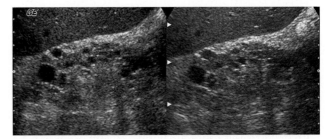

Fig. 7-9 Multiple cysts are identified in this patient consistent with acquired cystic kidney disease. (Courtesy GE Medical Systems.)

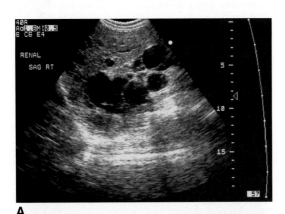

A

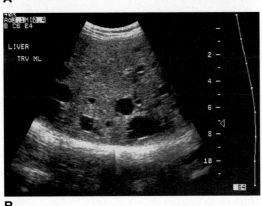

B

Fig. 7-8 A, Multiple cysts are identified in kidneys bilaterally in this 50-year-old woman in whom polycystic liver is also seen **(B).**

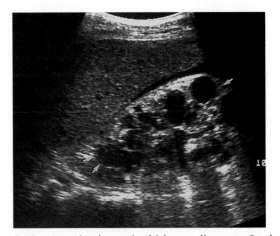

Fig. 7-10 Acquired cystic kidney disease. Sagittal sonogram shows echogenic kidney *(arrows)* with parenchymal loss and multiple cysts.

Medullary Sponge Kidney

Medullary sponge kidney is described as a cystic dilation of collecting tubules affecting the medullary and papillary portions of the collecting ducts.[7] It may present as a diffuse or focal disease but is usually a bilateral process. It is typically a congenital sporadic anomaly, although it rarely may be inherited in an autosomal dominant pattern or an autosomal recessive pattern (when associated with **Caroli's disease**).[7] Stone formation is not uncommon with medullary sponge kidney and may be the result of urinary stasis in the dilated collecting tubules or elevated urinary pH and hypercalciuria, which leads to stone formation.[4]

Patients with medullary sponge kidney are often asymptomatic but more commonly present in the third to fourth decades of life. When symptoms are seen, they are usually the result of infection from urinary stasis or from nephrolithiasis and may include flank pain, hematuria, **dysuria**, and fever. This condition has also been reported to be associated with other diseases and syndromes, including **hemihypertrophy, Ehlers-Danlos syndrome,** hypertrophic pyloric stenosis, hyperparathyroidism, Caroli's disease, polycystic kidney disease, **Marfan syndrome,** and **congenital familial anodontia.**[1,3] Additional symptoms may be present in patients with medullary sponge kidney related to the clinical features of the associated anomalies.

Sonographic Findings. Ultrasound examination of the kidneys may not show the tubular ectasia present with this disease, and radiographic examination may be necessary. When associated with **nephrocalcinosis,** sonographic findings of echogenic medullary pyramids (Fig. 7-11) with or without shadowing are identified. In addition, if the kidney is obstructed, hydronephrosis is shown.[1]

Table 7-1 is a summary of the pathology, symptoms, and sonographic findings of cystic lesions of the kidney.

SUMMARY

A variety of cysts and cystic diseases can be identified sonographically. Ultrasound imaging is an effective imaging method for identification of cysts, definition of their number and characteristics, and associated hydronephrosis when present.

Ultrasound imaging may also be used to identify hereditary disorders such as ADPKD. A thorough history, in addition to imaging, then plays an important role in the diagnosis. Renal cysts are also associated with uncommon and rare syndromes such as **tuberous**

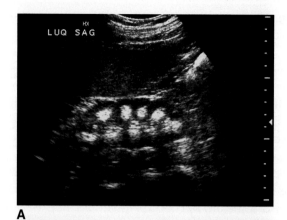

A

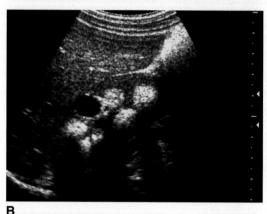

B

Fig. 7-11 Sonographic findings of nephrocalcinosis are identified in **A** and in **B**, which is also accompanied by simple renal cyst.

sclerosis and **Hippel-Lindau disease,** although they are not discussed in detail in this chapter. Some cystic renal diseases are seen more frequently in the pediatric patient, such as **autosomal recessive polycystic kidney disease** (ARPKD) and MCDK, and are discussed in detail in Chapter 9.

CLINICAL SCENARIO—DIAGNOSIS

■ The findings of multiple cysts bilaterally and increasing renal size are consistent with a diagnosis of ADPKD. The patient also discovered that she had hypertension, which is being controlled with medication. Because she grew up in an adopted family, this patient was unaware of any family history of renal cystic disease. She hopes to monitor her daughter as she grows older with ultrasound to determine whether she also will have this condition.

Table 7-1	*Cystic Lesions of Kidneys*	
Pathology	**Symptoms**	**Sonographic Findings**
Simple cyst	Usually asymptomatic	Round or oval, anechoic, thin-walled, posterior enhancement
Hemorrhagic cyst	Flank pain, hematuria	Anechoic, low-level echogenicity, or complex cystic lesion; with or without posterior enhancement
Infected cyst	Flank pain, fever, hematuria	Cyst with low-level echoes or fluid-debris level; cyst wall thickening
Milk of calcium cyst	Usually asymptomatic	Cystic lesion with layering of echogenic material in dependent portion
Parapelvic cyst	Usually asymptomatic	Cyst or cysts arising in renal hilum
Autosomal dominant polycystic kidney disease	Decreasing renal function, hypertension, flank pain, hematuria	Multiple cysts of variable size, bilateral, renal enlargement
Acquired cystic kidney disease	Usually asymptomatic	Three or more cysts in each kidney
Medullary sponge kidney	Asymptomatic, flank pain, hematuria, dysuria, fever	Echogenic medullary pyramids, with or without shadowing

CASE STUDIES FOR DISCUSSION

1. A 43-year-old man is seen with epigastric pain. An ultrasound is ordered to rule out gallbladder disease. The gallbladder is visualized and is contracted but otherwise unremarkable. A 1.5-cm cyst is also noted in the right lobe of the liver. The evaluation of the pancreas is suboptimal because of overlying bowel gas. The right kidney is enlarged, measuring 21 cm, and contains multiple cysts (Fig. 7-12). The sonographer also documents similar findings in the left kidney. What is the most likely diagnosis for this patient?

2. A 79-year-old man is seen with an "upset stomach" with vomiting. He has a history of a colon resection 1 year previously for a contained malignant neoplasm. Ultrasound examination results of the liver and gallbladder are un-

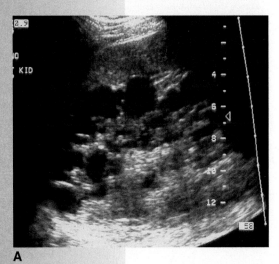

A

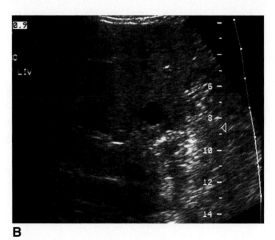

B

Fig. 7-12 **A,** Right kidney shows multiple cysts. **B,** Cyst is also noted in liver.

CASE STUDIES FOR DISCUSSION—cont'd ▬▬▬

remarkable. Imaging of the pancreas is limited. The right kidney contains a 5-cm anechoic lesion at the superior pole and a 2.5-cm anechoic lesion at the inferior pole as seen in Fig. 7-13, A. Imaging of the left kidney reveals a 2-cm anechoic lesion at the inferior pole (Fig. 7-13, B). What is the most likely diagnosis for this patient?

3. An 82-year-old man with a history of recurrent urinary tract infections (UTIs) is seen for intravenous pyelogram (IVP). The IVP reveals a right upper pole mass and left parapelvic mass. An ultrasound is ordered to characterize the nature of these radiolucent lesions. Ultrasound examination reveals a 6-cm anechoic lesion (Fig. 7-14, A) at the superior aspect of the right kidney and a 3.3-cm anechoic lesion arising in the renal sinus of the left kidney (Fig. 7-14, B). In addition, the images of the urinary bladder show an enlarged and irregular prostate indenting the base of the bladder. What is the diagnosis?

4. A 54-year-old man is seen with bilateral flank pain, which is greater on the left side. Ultrasound examination of the kidneys reveals bilaterally enlarged kidneys with multiple cysts too numerous to count (Fig. 7-15). Some cysts are complex in appearance, and multiple, small echogenic foci also are seen bilaterally. What is the most likely diagnosis?

5. A 74-year-old man with right-sided pain is referred to ultrasound to follow up on a finding of calcifications noted on a radiograph (Fig. 7-16, A). The ultrasound reveals a ring calcification (Fig. 7-16, B) at the superior aspect of the right kidney that shadows, preventing adequate visualization of the internal characteristics of this mass; however, it does appear to be anechoic. What is the most likely diagnosis and the significance of the finding?

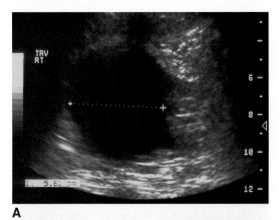

A

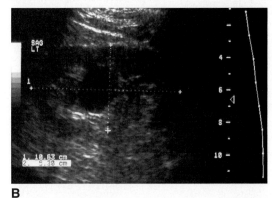

B

Fig. 7-14 A, Well-defined lesion is identified on right kidney. **B,** Smaller anechoic lesion is identified in left kidney.

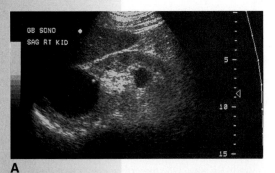

A

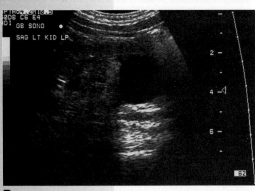

B

Fig. 7-13 A, Right kidney contains two anechoic lesions. **B,** Left kidney contains one anechoic lesion.

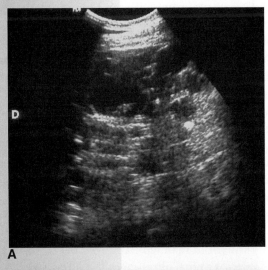

A

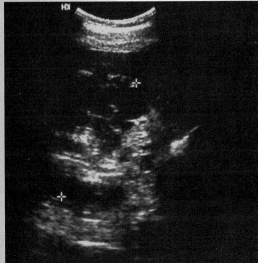

B

Fig. 7-15 **A,** Longitudinal image of right kidney and, **B,** transverse image of left kidney show multiple cysts bilaterally.

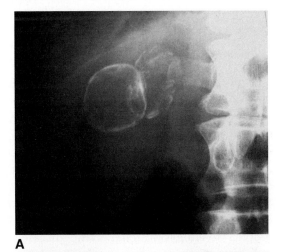

A

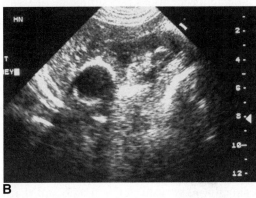

B

Fig. 7-16 **A,** Radiograph shows calcified lesion in region of right renal bed. **B,** Ultrasound examination shows ring calcification.

STUDY QUESTIONS

1. A 62-year-old man with a history of right flank pain is seen for a renal ultrasound. Sonographic examination of the right kidney reveals a 3-cm, round, anechoic lesion that is thin walled and has acoustic enhancement. This is most consistent with which of the following?
   a. acquired cystic kidney disease
   b. calcified cyst
   c. hemorrhagic cyst
   d. polycystic disease
   e. simple cyst

2. An asymptomatic, 26-year-old woman is seen with a family history of ADPKD. Because of the high cost of DNA testing, a screening renal ultrasound is ordered to rule out renal cystic disease. The sonographer identifies two simple cystic lesions in the right kidney and two simple cystic lesions in the left kidney. This is consistent with which of the following?
   a. acquired cystic kidney disease
   b. autosomal dominant polycystic kidney disease
   c. autosomal recessive polycystic kidney disease
   d. bilateral, simple cysts
   e. medullary sponge kidney

3. A 55-year-old man is seen with flank pain. Clinical evaluation reveals that he is febrile and that there are white blood cells in his urine. A renal ultrasound is ordered. Sonographic evaluation of the kidneys reveals a normal right kidney with a 1-cm simple cyst. The left kidney contains a 2.7-cm thick-walled cyst. This is most consistent with which of the following?
   a. right renal simple cyst, left renal simple cyst
   b. right renal infected cyst, left renal simple cyst
   c. right renal simple cyst, left renal infected cyst
   d. right renal simple cyst, left renal hemorrhagic cyst
   e. right renal simple cyst, left renal calcified cyst

4. A 47-year-old obese woman is seen for a right upper quadrant ultrasound to rule out gallstones. The right kidney contains a cyst with gravity-dependent echogenic matter that shifts in position as the patient rolls into a left lateral decubitus position. The patient has no renal symptoms. This finding is most consistent with which of the following?
   a. calcified cyst
   b. hemorrhagic cyst
   c. infected cyst

   d. milk of calcium cyst
   e. multilocular cyst

5. A 42-year-old woman is seen for a routine physical that reveals an elevated blood pressure. The patient had a first-degree relative who also had hypertension and died of a "kidney problem." A renal ultrasound is ordered and shows four cysts in the right kidney and five cysts in the left kidney. In addition, the kidneys are slightly increased in size. This is most consistent with which of the following?
   a. acquired cystic kidney disease
   b. autosomal dominant polycystic kidney disease
   c. autosomal recessive polycystic kidney disease
   d. bilateral, simple cysts
   e. multicystic dysplastic kidney

6. A 45-year-old man with a history of left flank pain is seen for a renal ultrasound. The ultrasound reveals a normal right kidney measuring 11.5 cm. The left kidney measures 12 cm and contains a round, anechoic lesion that has a thin, well-defined wall located at the superior aspect. No enhancement is identified. This would be characterized as which of the following?
   a. atypical cyst
   b. hemorrhagic cyst
   c. infected cyst
   d. multilocular cyst
   e. simple cyst

7. A 56-year-old woman with a history of a UTI is seen for a renal ultrasound. The ultrasound reveals mild hydronephrosis in the right kidney and a 2-cm cystic lesion within the renal hilum. This would be consistent with which of the following?
   a. hydronephrosis associated with a hemorrhagic cyst
   b. hydronephrosis associated with a milk of calcium cyst
   c. hydronephrosis associated with a parapelvic cyst
   d. hydronephrosis associated with an infected cyst
   e. hydronephrosis associated with a simple cyst

8. A 65-year-old man with diabetes and subsequent renal disease who has been on dialysis for 9 years is seen for a renal ultrasound. The ultrasound reveals kidneys that are decreased in size bilaterally with five small cysts on the left kidney and three small cysts on the right kidney. This would be most consistent with which of the following?

a. acquired cystic kidney disease
b. autosomal dominant polycystic kidney disease
c. autosomal recessive polycystic kidney disease
d. medullary sponge kidney
e. multiple, simple cysts

9. A 35-year-old man with a history of intermittent epigastric pain with meals is seen for a right upper quadrant ultrasound to rule out gallstones. The gallbladder, liver, and pancreas are unremarkable. The right kidney is normal in size, and the pyramids are highly echogenic. Examination of the left kidney reveals a similar appearance. This would be consistent with
a. acquired cystic kidney disease
b. calcified cystic disease
c. hydronephrosis
d. milk of calcium cyst
e. nephrocalcinosis

10. A 72-year-old man with intermittent flank pain is seen for a physical. Laboratory test results reveal abnormal renal function tests. A renal ultrasound is ordered and reveals bilateral, enlarged kidneys with multiple cysts too numerous to count. This would be consistent with which of the following?
a. acquired cystic kidney disease
b. ADPKD
c. ARPKD
d. medullary sponge kidney
e. MCDK

REFERENCES

1. Rumack CM, Wilson SR, Carboneau JW: *Diagnostic ultrasound*, ed 2, St Louis, 1998, Mosby.
2. Almeida A, Cavalcanti F, Medeiros A: Milk of calcium in a renal cyst, *Brazilian J Urol* 27:557-559, 2001.
3. Nicolau C et al: Abdominal sonographic study of autosomal dominant polycystic kidney disease, *J Clin Ultrasound* 22:277-282, 2000.
4. Levine E et al: Current concepts and controversies in imaging of renal cystic diseases, *Urol Clin North Am* 24:523-543, 1997.
5. Nicolau C et al: Autosomal dominant polycystic kidney disease types 1 and 2: assessment of US sensitivity for diagnosis, *Radiology* 213:273-276, 1999.
6. de Bruyn R, Gordon I: Imaging in cystic renal disease, *Arch Dis Child* 83:401-407, 2000.
7. Ghosh AK, Ghosh K: Medullary sponge kidney, http://www.emedicine.com/med/topic1413.htm, retrieved July 9, 2003.

BIBLIOGRAPHY

Anderson KN, Anderson LE, Glanze WD: *Mosby's medical, nursing, & allied health dictionary*, ed 5, St Louis, 1998, Mosby.
Baraitser M, Winter RM: *Color atlas of congenital malformation syndromes*, London, 1996, Mosby-Wolfe.
Hagen-Ansert SL: *Textbook of diagnostic ultrasonography*, vol 1, ed 5, St Louis, 2001, Mosby.
Kawamura DM: *Abdomen and superficial structures*, ed 2, Philadelphia, 1997, Lippincott.

8 Left Upper Quadrant Pain

CHARLOTTE HENNINGSEN

CLINICAL SCENARIO

■ A 68-year-old woman is seen for an upper gastrointestinal examination to rule out ulcer for persistent epigastric pain. The initial radiograph of the abdomen shows a large, calcified lesion in the left upper quadrant (Fig. 8-1, *A*). An abdominal ultrasound is ordered to clarify the finding on the radiograph.

The ultrasound reveals a small, echogenic lesion in the right lobe of the liver consistent with a hemangioma. A 7-cm mass in the left upper quadrant is identified and shows some enhancement and some shadowing (Fig. 8-1, *B*). The remainder of the ultrasound is unremarkable. What is the most likely diagnosis?

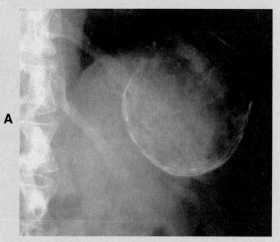

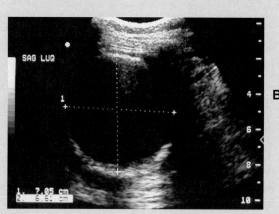

Fig. 8-1 **A,** Radiograph shows large calcified lesion. **B,** Ultrasound image of left upper quadrant confirms intrasplenic lesion.

OBJECTIVES

■ Describe the sonographic appearance of a normal spleen.

■ List the congenital variants of the spleen that may occur and describe the associated sonographic appearances.

■ List the causes of splenomegaly.

■ Describe the most common benign splenic neoplasms.

■ Identify risk factors associated with rupture of the spleen.

■ Identify the ultrasound findings associated with blunt trauma to the spleen.

■ Define the most common malignant splenic neoplasms.

■ Differentiate between the sonographic appearances of benign and malignant neoplasms.

■ List the causes of splenic infarct.

■ Identify Doppler findings associated with specific splenic anomalies.

GLOSSARY OF TERMS ▬▬▬

Anemia: decreased hemoglobin that may be from blood loss, an increase in destruction of red blood cells, or a decrease in production of red blood cells

Arsenic: a naturally occurring element that, in its inorganic form, is a known carcinogen

Computed tomography: a radiographic technique that allows detailed cross-sectional imaging

Cytomegalovirus: a group of herpes-type viruses that most greatly affects those who are immunocompromised and the fetus

Hematocrit: a measure of the amount of red blood cells

Hodgkin's disease: a malignant disease that involves lymphoid tissue

Infarction: an interruption in the blood supply to an area that may lead to necrosis of that area

Klippel-Trénaunay-Weber syndrome: a syndrome characterized by limb hypertrophy with associated large cutaneous hemangiomata

Leukocytosis: increased number of white blood cells that may be the result of infection or leukemia

Magnetic resonance imaging: a type of medical imaging that uses radiofrequencies and allows for excellent resolution and acquisition of data in multiple planes

Malaria: a serious infectious illness caused by a parasite and most commonly transmitted by the mosquito; seen most commonly in tropical areas

Mononucleosis: an acute infection caused by the Epstein-Barr virus that most commonly affects young persons; symptoms include fever, sore throat, enlarged lymph nodes, abnormal lymphocytes, and hepatosplenomegaly

Non-Hodgkin's lymphoma: a malignant disease of lymphoid tissue seen in increased frequency in individuals over 50 years of age

Situs: relates to the normal location of the organs in the body

Syncope: fainting

Thorium dioxide: a radiographic contrast agent previously used in angiography and myelography in the United States from approximately the early 1930s to the late 1950s; it has been associated with an increased risk of malignant diseases, including sarcomas of the liver and spleen

Thrombocytopenia: a decreased number of platelets

Vinyl chloride: a manufactured, flammable gas used in the plastics industry

---

An abdominal ultrasound ordered with a focus on the spleen is uncommon, but it may be used as a screening device because of the relatively low cost and portability. In the absence of a definitive diagnosis or when further clarification of pathology is needed, other imaging procedures, such as **computed tomography** (CT) and **magnetic resonance imaging** (MRI), may be used. The spleen is not often a site for primary disease, although it may be affected by pathologic processes such as hematologic and infectious disorders. This chapter explores a variety of congenital anomalies, neoplasms, and diseases that may affect the spleen in addition to the clinical significance and sonographic findings where indicated.

SPLEEN
Normal Sonographic Anatomy

The spleen is located in the left upper quadrant. Sonographically, the normal appearance of the spleen is that of a homogeneous, comma-shaped organ with an echogenicity similar to the liver and equal to or slightly hyperechoic to the kidney (Fig. 8-2; see Color Plate 6 for color version of Fig. 8-2, *C*). The normal size of the spleen is less than 13 cm in length.[1]

CONGENITAL VARIANTS
Accessory Spleen

Accessory spleen is the most common congenital anomaly, affecting the spleen in approximately 10% of the population.[2] This anomaly is most commonly located in the splenic hilum, although it may be located throughout the abdomen. The presence of an accessory spleen is usually insignificant, but accessory spleens rarely may undergo torsion or infarction and present with acute left upper quadrant pain.[3] Clinical symptoms should also be considered in differentiating between probable accessory spleens, neoplasms, and lymphadenopathy, which may have a similar sonographic appearance.

Sonographic Findings. Accessory spleens are usually round and have an echogenicity and homogeneity equal

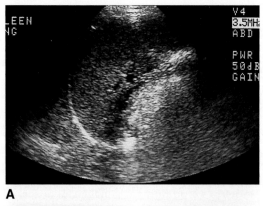

A

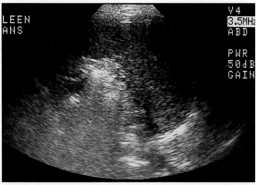

B

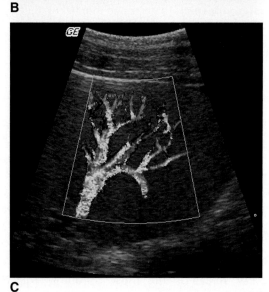

C

Fig. 8-2 **A** and **B**, Normal-appearing spleen. **C**, Normal splenic vasculature. (Courtesy GE Medical Systems.)

to that of the normal spleen (Fig. 8-3). Demonstration of the vascular connection from the accessory spleen to the normal spleen assists in confirmation of the diagnosis.

Ectopic Spleen

Ectopic spleen, a rare entity, may also be referred to as *splenia ectopia* or *wandering spleen*. It describes an anomaly in which the spleen migrates from its normal

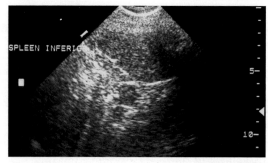

Fig. 8-3 Accessory spleen is identified in region of splenic hilum.

position because of congenital or acquired laxity of the suspensory ligaments. Because of the mobility of the spleen, it may also undergo torsion, resulting in acute abdominal pain and infarction.[4]

Sonographic Findings. The sonographic findings of an ectopic spleen include the absence of a normal spleen in the left upper quadrant. The ectopic spleen appears as a homogeneous structure consistent with the appearance of a spleen in the abdomen or pelvis. The use of power Doppler to show the presence or absence of flow may aid in the diagnosis of torsion and infarction.[4]

Polysplenia

Polysplenia is a rare congenital anomaly that is characterized by the development of multiple small spleens. Polysplenia is often associated with other anomalies that include congenital abnormalities of the heart and **situs** anomalies.[1,2]

Sonographic Findings. The diagnosis of polysplenia can be made when multiple small spleens are identified in the left upper quadrant.

SPLENOMEGALY

Enlargement of the spleen, or splenomegaly, is one of the most common anomalies of the spleen that sonographers encounter. Numerous causes of splenomegaly exist, with portal hypertension being the most common cause. Other causes include infection, hematologic disorders, immunologic disorders, trauma, neoplasia, vascular anomalies, and storage diseases.[2] In addition to clinical symptoms associated with the underlying disease, patients with splenomegaly may have left upper quadrant pain.

Sonographic Findings

The diagnosis of splenomegaly (Fig. 8-4) may be made when the length of the spleen is greater than or equal to

13 cm.[1] Splenomegaly may be noted subjectively when the inferior tip of the spleen covers the inferior pole of the left kidney.

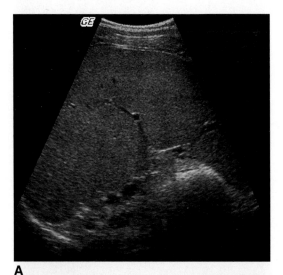

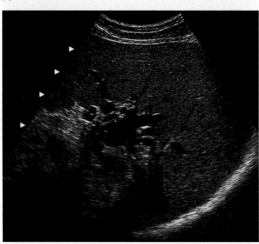

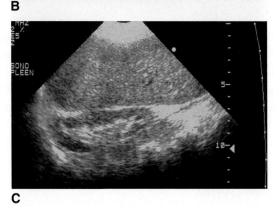

Fig. 8-4 Enlargement of spleen is shown in, **A,** longitudinal and, **B,** transverse images. Patient in **C** had cirrhosis and portal hypertension. (**A** and **B** Courtesy GE Medical Systems.)

CYSTS

With identification of a cyst in the left upper quadrant, ultrasound examination can also be useful in identification of the origin of cyst arising in the spleen or arising from adjacent organs such as the adrenal gland or gastrointestinal tract or a pancreatic pseudocyst extending into the spleen. Laboratory tests and patient history may also aid in the differentiation of cyst origin. Cysts arising in the spleen may be classified as primary when they have an epithelial or endothelial lining or secondary as the result of trauma, infection, or degeneration. Cysts in the spleen are uncommon and are usually benign.[5] Splenic cysts may be identified on ultrasound in asymptomatic patients as an incidental finding, although patients may have symptoms related to the cyst size or origin and may have left upper quadrant pain.

Sonographic Findings

A cyst should appear sonographically as a well-described, round or ovoid, thin-walled, anechoic lesion that shows acoustic enhancement (Fig. 8-5). Cysts affected by infection or trauma may show calcification of the cyst wall. Cysts may also show fluid-debris levels from purulent material or hemorrhage.[6]

ABSCESSES

Abscess formation in the spleen is considered rare and is associated with a variety of origins, including hematologic spread of infection, trauma, and malignant neoplasm. Abscesses may present as a solitary lesion or multiple masses. Patient symptoms may be silent or subtle, but patients may have left upper quadrant pain, fever, or referred pain to the chest or shoulder. Patients may also have splenomegaly, nausea and vomiting, and **leukocytosis.** Abscesses may rupture and are associated with a high mortality rate.[2] Ultrasound-guided aspiration may be used in combination with appropriate antibiotics to treat this disease; however, splenectomy may be necessary.[7]

Sonographic Findings

The sonographic appearance of splenic abscesses is variable (Fig. 8-6). Masses may appear round or ovoid with an irregular wall. Hypoechoic or anechoic lesions may be identified, and acoustic enhancement may also be noted. If gas is present, dirty shadowing may be seen.[2,7]

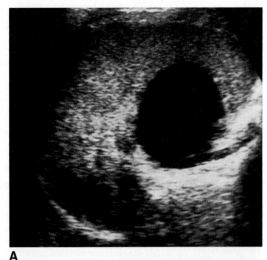

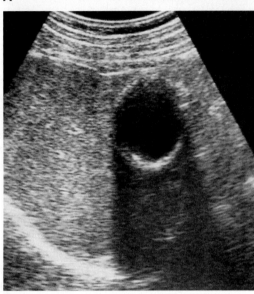

Fig. 8-5 **A,** Coronal scan of spleen shows 5-cm diameter cyst in hilar region of spleen adjacent to splenic vein. **B,** Calcified splenic cyst.

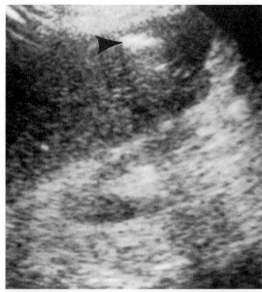

Fig. 8-6 Splenic abscess. Coronal scan shows gas collection with dirty shadowing.

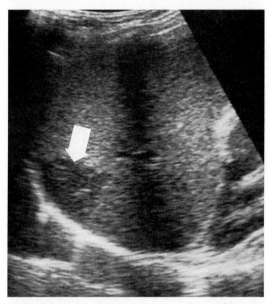

Fig. 8-7 Triangular echo-poor area *(arrow)* in superior aspect of spleen represents splenic infarct.

INFARCT

Splenic **infarction** may occur as the result of an embolic event, a hematologic disorder, vascular or pancreatic disease, congenital abnormalities, or neoplasm.[2] Infarction of the spleen, although uncommon, is one of the more common causes of focal splenic lesions and should be considered when patients have left upper quadrant pain.[2]

Sonographic Findings

The most specific ultrasound finding of a splenic infarct is that of a wedge-shaped, hypoechoic lesion (Fig. 8-7). Lesions may increase in echogenicity over time.[1,2,6] Lesions may appear round or be of variable echogenicity and shape and indistinguishable from other splenic lesions, including neoplasms, abscesses, and hematomas.

BENIGN NEOPLASMS
Hemangioma

Hemangiomas may be identified in the spleen and in the liver. Hemangioma is the most common benign tumor of the spleen, although benign neoplasms of the spleen are rare. They are usually isolated and

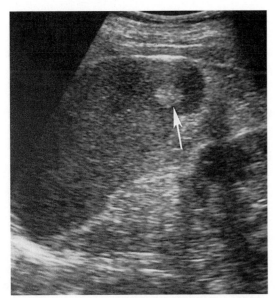

Fig. 8-8 Splenic hemangioma. Note small, well-defined, rounded, echogenic lesion *(arrow)* in spleen measuring 1.4 cm in diameter.

insignificant, but large lesions are at risk for rupture and hemorrhage, causing left upper quadrant pain. They may also occur in association with **Klippel-Trénaunay-Weber syndrome**.[6]

Sonographic Findings. The ultrasound appearance of a hemangioma may be similar to a hemangioma identified in the liver (Fig. 8-8): a well-defined, homogeneous, echogenic mass. Hemangiomas may also appear complex or contain calcifications.[2]

Hamartoma

Splenic hamartoma is a benign rare tumor that is usually asymptomatic. When clinical symptoms are present, they may include pancytopenia, **anemia**, and **thrombocytopenia**. This lesion can become greatly enlarged, compressing surrounding splenic tissues. Splenic hamartomas can also spontaneously rupture, causing acute pain.[8]

Sonographic Findings. The most common ultrasound appearance of a splenic hamartoma is a homogeneous, solid lesion of variable echogenicity. Hamartomas may also appear heterogeneous and complex and contain calcifications. This tumor may also show hypervascularity within the lesion with color Doppler, although this may not always be present.[8]

Lymphangioma

Splenic lymphangioma is a rare vascular tumor that occurs most commonly in childhood. The disease may be isolated to the spleen or involve multiple organs. Clinical symptoms are related to the developing splenomegaly and the subsequent compression of surrounding structures that occurs as the tumor grows.[9]

Sonographic Findings. Lymphangiomas present sonographically as a cystic lesion or multicystic lesions arising within the spleen with associated splenomegaly.[9]

Other Benign Neoplasms

Other benign neoplasms may arise in the spleen and are rarely identified. These splenic neoplasms that may be listed in the differential diagnosis include hemangioendothelioma, angiomyolipoma, littoral cell angioma, hemangiopericytoma, and lipoma.[2]

MALIGNANT NEOPLASMS
Lymphoma

The most common malignant disease that affects the spleen is lymphoma (**Hodgkin's disease** and **non-Hodgkin's lymphoma**), which presents as a primary splenic neoplasm or as a component of a disseminated disease process. Primary splenic lymphoma is more commonly identified in an older population.[2]

Sonographic Findings. Ultrasound examination of lymphoma of the spleen may reveal a diffuse, nodular spleen.[10] Hypoechoic lesions or diffuse inhomogeneity have been described.[1,2]

Angiosarcoma

Angiosarcoma is a primary neoplasm that usually arises in the spleen or liver and may also be termed hemangiosarcoma. Patients may have left upper quadrant pain, malaise, fever, and weight loss; however, splenic rupture may occur, causing acute abdominal pain and death.[11] Angiosarcoma has also been associated with exposure to **thorium dioxide**, **arsenic**, and **vinyl chloride**.[12] This is a highly aggressive tumor with a dismal prognosis.

Sonographic Findings. The sonographic appearance of angiosarcoma may be an inhomogeneous spleen with multiple hypoechoic lesions identified. Associated splenomegaly is also a typical finding. Doppler examination may reveal the vascular nature of this neoplasm.[12]

Metastasis

Metastasis to the spleen is uncommon and is usually a feature of widespread disease, originating more frequently from the breast, lung, stomach, prostate, ovary, and melanoma.[1,2,6]

Sonographic Findings. Most metastatic lesions in the spleen are hypoechoic, although hyperechoic and complex lesions have been identified (Fig. 8-9).

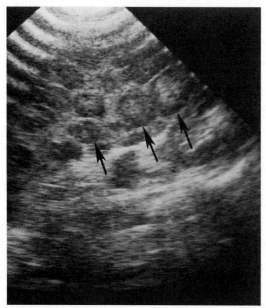

Fig. 8-9 Splenic metastases from malignant melanoma. Note multiple large lesions *(arrows)* in spleen.

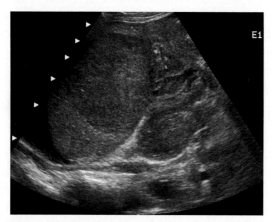

Fig. 8-10 Neoplasm is identified in spleen. Origin is unknown. Free fluid suggests malignant process. (Courtesy GE Medical Systems.)

Other Malignant Neoplasms

Other malignant neoplasms (Fig. 8-10) may arise in the spleen and are rarely identified. Depending on patient history and symptoms, malignant diseases that may be suggested in the differential diagnosis include Kaposi's sarcoma, leiomyosarcoma, fibrosarcoma, littoral cell angiosarcoma, malignant fibrous histiocytoma, cystadenocarcinoma, and teratoma.[2]

TRAUMA
Hematoma, Rupture

Blunt trauma to the left upper quadrant can cause a splenic hematoma or subcapsular hematoma with or

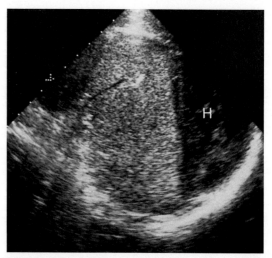

Fig. 8-11 Subcapsular hematoma of spleen. Transverse scan shows fluid-filled and debris-filled crescentic hematoma *(H)* in lateral aspect of spleen.

without rupture of the splenic capsule. Clinical symptoms may include severe left upper quadrant pain, falling **hematocrit, syncope,** and hypotension. Complications of nonsurgical management of blunt splenic injuries, although rare, include delayed splenic rupture, pseudocyst formation, and pseudoaneurysm formation.[13] Spontaneous splenic rupture has been identified in patients with infectious diseases, including **mononucleosis,** HIV, hepatitis A, **malaria,** and **cytomegalovirus.**[14] Ultrasound may be used as a prompt and cost-effective imaging method to diagnose the extent of trauma, to assist in determining the method of treatment, and to follow patients with a history of splenic injuries.

Sonographic Findings. The appearance of a hematoma is variable based on the age of the bleed. Blood may initially appear similar in echogenicity to the spleen becoming more anechoic over time. A subcapsular hematoma (Fig. 8-11) conforms to the shape of the spleen and, when isoechoic to splenic parenchyma, may mimic splenomegaly. Likewise, a hematoma within the spleen contains echoes initially but may appear inhomogeneous compared with the homogeneous splenic parenchyma. Rupture of the splenic capsule shows fluid within the peritoneal cavity.[6] Color Doppler of anechoic lesions should be used to rule out splenic pseudoaneuryms in patients with a splenic trauma.[15]

Table 8-1 is a summary of the pathology, symptoms, and sonographic findings for lesions of the spleen.

SUMMARY

The sonographer must understand and be able to differentiate pathology that may be identified in the

Table 8-1	*Lesions of Spleen*	
Pathology	**Symptoms**	**Sonographic Findings**
Simple cyst	Usually asymptomatic	Round or oval, anechoic, thin-walled, posterior enhancement
Abscess	Left upper quadrant pain, fever, nausea and vomiting	Round or oval lesion with irregular wall, hypoechoic or anechoic, with or without enhancement
Infarct	Left upper quadrant pain	Wedge-shaped hypoechoic lesion; may be round with variable echogenicity
Hemangioma	Usually asymptomatic	Well-defined, homogeneous, echogenic lesion
Hamartoma	Usually asymptomatic	Homogeneous, solid lesion of variable echogenicity; may appear inhomogeneous or complex
Lymphangioma	Left upper quadrant fullness or pain	Cystic or multicystic lesion
Angiosarcoma	Left upper quadrant pain, malaise, fever, weight loss	Inhomogeneous spleen with multiple, hypoechoic lesions and splenomegaly

spleen. Although the spleen is rarely the focus of an ultrasound examination, the sonographer may identify pathology as an incidental finding. Sonography may also be used in patients who cannot be transported or for follow-up of pathology previously identified with another imaging method. Knowledge of pathology, risk factors, symptoms, and the sonographic appearance of an anomaly ensures that the sonographer will provide the physician with the images necessary to make an accurate diagnosis.

CLINICAL SCENARIO—DIAGNOSIS

■ The radiologist recommended an MRI to further clarify the finding in the left upper quadrant. The MRI also showed and confirmed the ultrasound finding of a hemangioma in the right lobe of the liver. The mass in the left upper quadrant was identified as a cyst arising within the spleen with a partially calcified wall, suggesting a posttraumatic cyst.

CASE STUDIES FOR DISCUSSION

1. A 60-year-old woman is seen for a CT scan to rule out hypernephroma that revealed very small regions within the kidneys that were most likely cysts. The radiologist suggested an ultrasound for confirmation. The abdominal ultrasound reveals a normal gallbladder, pancreas, liver, and kidneys. The renal cysts are not identified on the ultrasound. In the left upper quadrant, medial to the splenic hilum, the homogeneous lesion shown in Fig. 8-12 is noted. What is a likely diagnosis?

2. A 17-year-old girl with a history of Gaucher's disease, a congenital disorder of lipid metabolism, is seen. An abdominal ultrasound is ordered for multiple organ involvement, although the primary symptom is hematuria. The right kidney measures 11 cm, and the left kidney measures 15.4 cm, with no focal abnormality or hydro-

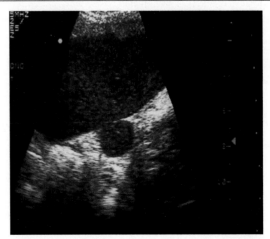

Fig. 8-12 Homogeneous lesion in splenic hilum is identified.

CASE STUDIES FOR DISCUSSION—cont'd

nephrosis identified. The spleen measures more than 20 cm in length (Fig. 8-13). This is consistent with what diagnosis?

3. A 70-year-old man is seen in the emergency department with pain in the left upper quadrant and weakness. His wife explains that he fell at home on the previous day. The emergency physician notes left-sided bruising, and laboratory tests reveal a falling hematocrit. The ultrasound identifies the finding in Fig. 8-14 and fluid in Morrison's pouch. What is the most likely diagnosis?

4. A 44-year-old man with a history of diarrhea and weight loss is seen for an abdominal ultrasound. Ultrasound reveals multiple hypoechoic lesions in the liver, kidneys, and spleen (Fig. 8-15, *A* and *B*). Lymphadenopathy is also noted. This would be most consistent with which diagnosis?

5. A 58-year-old man with a history of alcohol abuse and increasing abdominal girth is seen for an abdominal ultrasound. The liver appears small and nodular, with hepatofugal flow noted in the portal vein. The spleen measures more than 18 cm in length (Fig. 8-16). What is the most likely diagnosis?

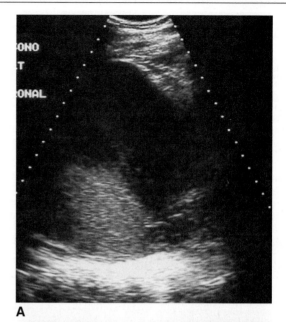

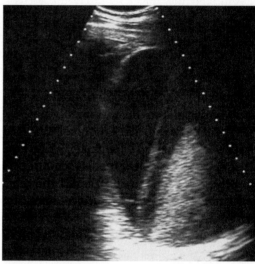

B

Fig. 8-14 **A,** Longitudinal and, **B,** transverse images of left upper quadrant.

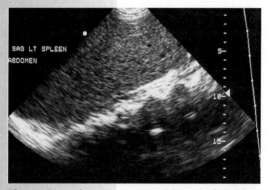

Fig. 8-13 Spleen measures 20 cm in length.

CASE STUDIES FOR DISCUSSION—cont'd

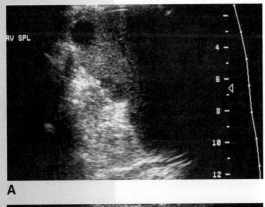

A

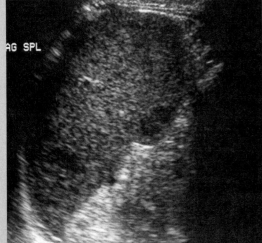

B

Fig. 8-15 Multiple hypoechoic lesions are identified in, **A,** transverse and, **B,** longitudinal images of spleen.

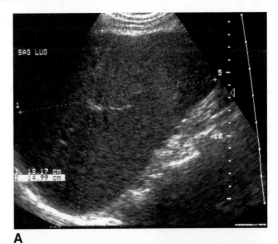

A

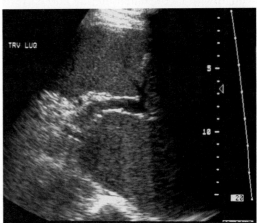

B

Fig. 8-16 Spleen is noted to be greater than 18 cm in length as shown in, **A,** longitudinal image of spleen; **B,** transverse image is also shown.

STUDY QUESTIONS

1. A 40-year-old man with left-sided pain is seen in the emergency department after a motorcycle accident. Clinical examination reveals left upper quadrant bruising and tenderness. Ultrasound examination reveals a comma-shaped, hypoechoic region surrounding the lateral aspect of the spleen. No free fluid is identified. This would be most consistent with which of the following?
   a. intrasplenic hematoma
   b. splenic neoplasm
   c. splenic rupture
   d. splenomegaly
   e. subcapsular hematoma

2. A renal ultrasound is ordered for a 30-year-old woman with a congenital uterine anomaly. Images of the left kidney reveal a well-defined, echogenic lesion in the spleen. This is most likely which of the following?
   a. angiomyolipoma
   b. hemangioma
   c. hemangiosarcoma
   d. lymphangioma
   e. metastasis

3. A patient is seen for an abdominal ultrasound for left upper quadrant pain. The ultrasound examination reveals a hypoechoic lesion that is triangular in shape. This would be most specific for which of the following?
   a. abscess
   b. hemangioma
   c. hematoma
   d. infarct
   e. metastasis

4. A 55-year-old man with epigastric pain is seen for abdominal ultrasound. The liver, kidney, gallbladder, and pancreas are unremarkable. The spleen is within normal limits and homogeneous. The splenic hilum contains a round 1.5-cm lesion that is homogeneous. Doppler examination shows a vessel connecting the spleen to the lesion. This would be consistent with which of the following?
   a. accessory spleen
   b. ectopic spleen
   c. lymphadenopathy
   d. nodularia splenia
   e. polysplenia

5. A 48-year-old woman with a history of cirrhosis and increasing abdominal girth is seen. Sonographic findings include abdominal ascites, hepatofugal flow in the portal vein consistent with portal hypertension, and a spleen measuring 17 cm in length. The finding in the spleen is consistent with:
   a. diffuse metastasis
   b. lymphoma
   c. splenic infarct
   d. splenic rupture
   e. splenomegaly

6. A 57-year-old man with a history of left flank pain is seen for renal ultrasound, which reveals a normal right kidney and a kidney stone in the left kidney. The sonographer incidentally notes a round, anechoic lesion in the spleen measuring 2 cm at its greatest diameter, with posterior acoustic enhancement. What is the most likely diagnosis?
   a. abscess
   b. cyst
   c. hematoma
   d. infarct
   e. lymphangioma

7. A 68-year-old man with a history of malaise, unexplained weight loss, and left upper quadrant pain is seen for an abdominal ultrasound. The patient recently retired from a wood treatment plant. The ultrasound examination reveals an enlarged spleen containing multiple hypoechoic lesions. Which of the following is the most likely diagnosis?
   a. angiosarcoma
   b. hemangioma
   c. lymphoma
   d. metastasis
   e. teratoma

8. A 28-year-old equestrian is seen in the emergency department after a fall from his horse at which time the horse stumbled and rolled over him. The patient has a pain response on palpation of the left upper quadrant, is having intermittent episodes of syncope, and has a falling hematocrit. The ultrasound reveals a hypoechoic splenic lesion that is increasing in size and fluid within the peritoneal cavity. What is the most likely diagnosis?
   a. lymphoma
   b. splenic abscess
   c. splenic infarct

d. splenic rupture

e. subcapsular hematoma

9. A 30-year-old woman with Hodgkin's disease and a history of left upper quadrant fullness is seen for an abdominal ultrasound. The ultrasound reveals an enlarged spleen that is diffusely heterogeneous. This would be consistent with which of the following?

a. fibrosarcoma

b. hemagioendothelioma

c. lymphangioma

d. metastasis

e. splenic lymphoma

10. A 56-year-old woman with a history of breast cancer and subsequent metastasis to the bones is seen for an abdominal ultrasound for abdominal pain. Ultrasound reveals hepatomegaly with multiple hypoechoic lesions throughout the liver. Splenomegaly is also noted with multiple hypo-echoic lesions within the spleen. This is consistent with which of the following?

a. angiosarcoma

b. multiple abscesses

c. metastasis to the liver and spleen

d. lymphoma

e. lymphangioma

REFERENCES

1. Hagen-Ansert SL: *Textbook of diagnostic ultrasonography*, vol 1, ed 5, St Louis, 2001, Mosby.

2. Robertson F, Leander P, Ekberg O: Radiology of the spleen, *Eur Radiol* 11:80-95, 2001.

3. Perez Fontan FJ, Soler R, Santos M et al: Accessory spleen torsion: US, CT and MR findings, *Eur Radiol* 11:509-512, 2001.

4. Danaci M et al: Power Doppler sonographic diagnosis of torsion in a wandering spleen, *J Clin Ultrasound* 28:246-248, 2000.

5. Lopes MAB, Ruano R, Bunduki V et al: Prenatal diagnosis and follow up of congenital splenic cyst: a case report, *Ultrasound Obstet Gynecol* 17:439-441, 2001.

6. Rumack CM, Wilson SR, Charboneau JW: *Diagnostic ultrasound*, vol 2, ed 2, St Louis, 1998, Mosby.

7. Chou Y-H et al: Ultrasound-guided interventional procedures in splenic abscesses, *Eur J Radiol* 28:167-170, 1998.

8. Tang S et al: Color Doppler sonographic findings in splenic hamartoma, *J Clin Ultrasound* 28:249-253, 2000.

9. Komatsuda T et al: Splenic lymphangioma: US and CT diagnosis and clinical manifestations, *Abdom Imaging* 24:414-417, 1999.

10. Konoshita LL, Yee J, Nash SR: Littoral cell angioma of the spleen: imaging features, *Am J Roentgenol AJR* 174:467-469, 2000.

11. Vrachliotis TG, Vaswani KK, Neimann TH et al: Primary angiosarcoma of the spleen—CT, MRI, and sonographic characteristics: report of two cases, *Abdom Imaging* 25:283-285, 2000.

12. Aytac S et al: Multimodality demonstration of primary splenic angiosarcoma, *J Clin Ultrasound* 27:92-95, 1999.

13. Emery KH, Babcock DS, Borgman AS et al: Splenic injury diagnosed with CT: US follow-up and healing rate in children and adolescents, *Radiology* 212:515-518, 1999.

14. Blaivas M, Quinn J: Diagnosis of spontaneous splenic rupture with emergency ultrasonography, *Ann Emerg Med* 32:627-630, 1998.

15. Fitoz S et al: Post-traumatic intrasplenic pseudo-aneurysms with delayed rupture: color Doppler sonographic and CT findings, *J Clin Ultrasound* 29:102-104, 2001.

9 Pediatric Mass

CHARLOTTE HENNINGSEN

CLINICAL SCENARIO

■ A 14-day-old girl is seen for renal ultrasound to follow an abdominal mass identified on an obstetric ultrasound examination. The ultrasound reveals a solid mass in the left suprarenal region (Fig. 9-1). Doppler interrogation shows blood flow within the mass. What is the most likely diagnosis?

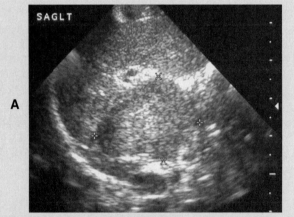

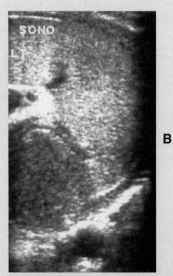

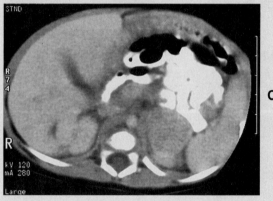

Fig. 9-1 Sonographic images show suprarenal lesion in, **A,** longitudinal and, **B,** transverse planes, which can also be seen with, **C,** computed tomographic scan.

OBJECTIVES

■ Describe the sonographic appearance of biliary tract anomalies that are common in the pediatric abdomen.

■ Differentiate abdominal neoplasms that occur in the pediatric patient.

■ Identify pertinent laboratory values associated with neoplasms in the pediatric abdomen.

■ Describe Doppler findings associated with pediatric neoplasms.

■ Differentiate the causes and sonographic findings of congenital hydronephrosis.

■ Describe the sonographic appearances of pediatric renal cystic diseases.

GLOSSARY OF TERMS ▰

Acholic: absence of bile

Anuria: absence of urinary output or production

Beckwith-Wiedemann syndrome: an autosomal recessive condition characterized by macroglossia, gigantism, hemihypertrophy, and exopthalmus; individuals may also manifest with organomegaly and are at increased risk for development of certain abdominal neoplasms

Catecholamines: a group of compounds that include epinephrine and norepinephrine

Familial adenomatous polyposis: a hereditary disease characterized by widespread development of polyps in the colon that begin to appear in late adolescence or early childhood and may lead to cancer of the colon

Hemihypertrophy: an asymmetric overgrowth of half of the body

Kasai operation: a surgical procedure to correct biliary atresia with establishment of a pathway for bile to flow from the ducts to the intestine; also known as *portoenterostomy*

Morbidity: a state of illness

Mortality: the state of having died

Neonate: an infant in the first 28 days of life

Oliguria: decreased urine output

Polysplenia syndrome: a syndrome characterized by abnormal development of the spleen, congenital heart defects, and situs anomalies

Precocious puberty: thelarche (breast development) and ovulatory activity before the age of 8 years

A sonographic examination of the abdomen in a pediatric patient may be based on the patient's symptoms, findings during a clinical examination of an enlarged girth or a palpable mass, or follow-up of an anomaly identified during an obstetric ultrasound. Symptoms may be nonspecific, and laboratory data, which may aid in the diagnosis, may be unavailable at the time of the sonogram.

A clinical finding of a palpable mass will precipitate a search for the origin of the mass, which may commonly arise from the kidney or adrenal gland or less commonly be associated with a liver, biliary, or gastrointestinal anomaly. A palpable mass may not directly relate to a specific neoplasm but may reflect the enlargement of an organ, as with renal cystic diseases or enlargement of the liver. This chapter focuses on abnormalities of the liver, biliary tract, genitourinary tract, and adrenal gland that more commonly occur in the pediatric patient and include neoplasms and diffuse disease processes. Anomalies of the gastrointestinal tract are discussed in Chapter 11.

BILIARY

Biliary Atresia

Biliary atresia is a serious progressive disease that is the result of narrowing or obliteration of the bile ducts. The different classifications of biliary atresia are dependent on which portion of the biliary tree is affected. Biliary atresia may affect intrahepatic or extrahepatic ducts and may or may not involve the gallbladder. The most common form of biliary atresia involves the extrahepatic portion of the biliary tree, including the gallbladder.[1] The cause of biliary atresia is unknown, although studies have suggested that biliary atresia may be the result of a congenital maldevelopment of the biliary tree or may be an acquired condition. The association of biliary atresia resulting from a viral infection has also been explored, and hereditary factors have been suggested.[2] Biliary atresia may also be associated with **polysplenia syndrome** (Fig. 9-2).

The clinical features of biliary atresia include persistent jaundice in the neonatal period, **acholic** stools, dark urine, and enlarged girth from hepatomegaly. Early diagnosis is important because surgical intervention is most effective when performed within the first 90 days of life.[3] The **Kasai operation** provides a pathway for biliary drainage of the liver through an anastomosis to the intestine. This may only delay biliary cirrhosis, or the surgery may fail and liver transplantation may be necessary. Left untreated, biliary atresia leads to cirrhosis, liver failure, and death.

Sonographic Findings. The most specific sonographic finding associated with biliary atresia is a small (<1.5 cm in length[3]) or absent gallbladder in a fasting infant. If a small gallbladder is identified, postprandial images should be taken and, in biliary atresia, the gallbladder will usually not contract. Another sonographic finding that has been identified is the triangular cord sign, which appears as an echogenic area superior to the portal vein bifurcation. The triangular cord sign represents the obliterated bile duct.[3]

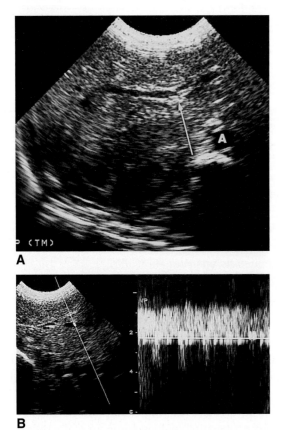

Fig. 9-2 **A,** Transverse liver sonogram in polysplenia syndrome in 3-month-old girl. Bifurcation of portal vein *(arrow)* is more anterior than usual. **B,** Right sagittal sonogram. Doppler cursor in portal vein shows normal hepatopetal flow. Inferior vena cava is missing on both views. Polysplenia is associated with biliary atresia.

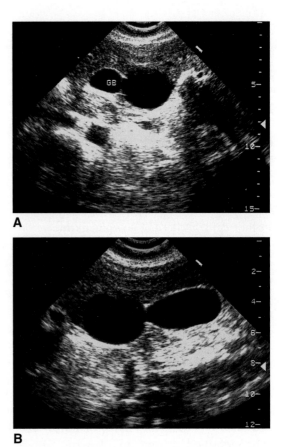

Fig. 9-3 Choledochal cyst may have appearance of cyst adjacent to gallbladder *(GB)* as shown in **A** and **B**.

Choledochal Cyst

Choledochal cyst is a cystic dilation of the biliary tree that most commonly affects the common bile duct (CBD). Five types of choledochal cysts are described by Todani.[4] Type I is characterized by a fusiform dilation of the CBD and is the most common. Type II presents as one or more diverticula of the CBD. Type III, known as a choledochocele, is a dilation of the intraduodenal portion of the CBD. Type IV consists of dilation of intrahepatic and extrahepatic ducts. And type V is classified as Caroli's disease and manifests with dilation of the intrahepatic ducts.[5]

The clinical presentation of choledochal cyst includes jaundice and pain. A palpable mass may also be present. Sonography is useful to differentiate choledochal cyst from other causes of jaundice in infancy, including biliary atresia and hepatitis. Surgical excision

of the choledochal cyst has a favorable outcome and early intervention is important, although when associated with concomitant biliary atresia, the long-term prognosis is considered poor.[6]

Sonographic Findings. Ultrasound investigation of a choledochal cyst most commonly shows the fusiform dilation of the CBD (Fig. 9-3), with associated intrahepatic ductal dilation. Depending on the type of choledochal cyst, multiple cysts in the area of the porta hepatis that are separate from the gallbladder may also be identified.

LIVER
Hemangioendothelioma

Infantile hepatic hemangioendothelioma is the most common vascular liver tumor of infancy that most commonly occurs within the first 6 months of life. A gender prevalence is seen, with most cases occurring in females.[7] This condition is a benign tumor, although it can be associated with serious complications.

The clinical presentation for infants with hemangioendothelioma includes hepatomegaly, which may

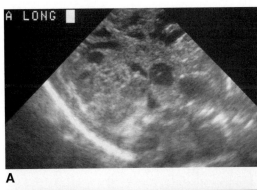

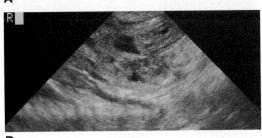

Fig. 9-4 One-day-old girl is seen with congestive heart failure and diffuse skin edema. **A,** Longitudinal and, **B,** transverse images of liver show diffuse irregular and complex appearance.

be accompanied by associated congestive heart failure (Fig. 9-4) and cutaneous hemangioma.[8] The serum α-fetoprotein level is usually within normal range but may be elevated. Hemangioendothelioma spontaneously regresses by 12 to 18 months of age, but complications may lead to significant **morbidity** and **mortality.** Medical treatment including steroids, chemotherapy, and radiation therapy may be used to shrink the tumor size, thus decreasing the vascularity.[7]

Sonographic Findings. The most common sonographic appearance of hemangioendothelioma is that of multiple hypoechoic lesions and hepatomegaly. The tumor may also be hyperechoic or isoechoic and contain cystic components (Fig. 9-5). Doppler (Fig. 9-6) may show the arteriovenous shunting that is frequently identified.[9]

Hepatoblastoma

Hepatoblastoma is the most common primary malignant disease of the liver and occurs most frequently in children who are less than 5 years of age.[5] Pathologically the hepatoblastoma is most commonly characterized as an epithelial tumor, but it may also be of mixed epithelial and mesenchymal cells.[10]

Hepatoblastoma has been associated with **Beckwith-Wiedemann syndrome, hemihypertrophy, familial adenomatous polyposis,** and **precocious puberty.** Clinical findings for hepatoblastoma include palpable abdominal mass and an elevated serum α-fetoprotein level. Patients may also have fever, pain, anorexia, and weight loss. The prognosis for this tumor depends on the resectability of the mass. Many patients are in the advanced stages at the time of diagnosis and so the prognosis is poor.

Sonographic Findings. The ultrasound appearance of hepatoblastoma (Fig. 9-7; see Color Plate 7) usually is a solitary mass, but it may also appear as a diffuse process with multiple lesions throughout the liver. Portal vein thrombosis may also be identified. Doppler evaluation of hepatoblastoma will reveal high-velocity, low-resistant flow pattern within the mass.

ADRENAL
Hemorrhage

Adrenal glands in fetuses and **neonates** are a risk for hemorrhage because of their large size and increased vascularity. Adrenal hemorrhage occurs in approximately 2:1000 live births and is usually diagnosed in the newborn but has also been detected in utero. Factors that increase the risk for adrenal hemorrhage include birth trauma, fetal hypoxia, maternal hypotension, sepsis, and other vascular factors.[11] Hemorrhage is also associated with large birth weight, prolonged labor, bleeding disorders, and renal vein thrombosis.[12] The right adrenal gland is more commonly affected, and adrenal hemorrhage is more common in males. Symptoms of adrenal hemorrhage include adrenal insufficiency, hyperbilirubinemia, anemia, and scrotal hematoma.

Sonographic Findings. Distinguishing adrenal hemorrhage from neuroblastoma is important because identification of a malignant neoplasm requires surgical intervention and adrenal hemorrhage (Fig. 9-8) usually spontaneously resolves. Adrenal hemorrhage initially appears echogenic and becomes hypoechoic over time. Follow-up sonograms (Fig. 9-9) show involution of the hemorrhage that may resolve to calcification or a residual cyst.

Neuroblastoma

Neuroblastoma is a tumor that arises in sympathetic neural crest tissues. Forty-five percent of neuroblastomas arise in the medulla of the adrenal gland, although tumors may also arise in the neck, mediastinum, retroperitoneum, and pelvis. The cause is unclear, but hereditary factors may be implicated and environmental factors during pregnancy may be associated, such as drug use, hair coloring, and exposure to electromagnetic fields.[13]

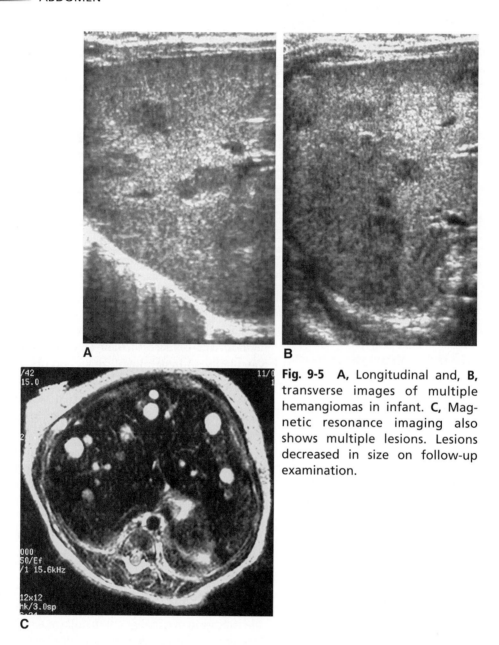

Fig. 9-5 **A,** Longitudinal and, **B,** transverse images of multiple hemangiomas in infant. **C,** Magnetic resonance imaging also shows multiple lesions. Lesions decreased in size on follow-up examination.

Diagnosis of neuroblastoma may occur during the perinatal period during obstetric ultrasound. Of those detected in utero, 90% arise in the adrenal gland.[13] The clinical presentation of neuroblastoma depends on the location of the tumor. Infants may have an abdominal mass, hypertension, diarrhea, and bone pain with metastasis. Most patients with neuroblastoma have increased **catecholamine** levels.

Sonographic Findings. The sonographic appearance (Fig. 9-10) of neuroblastoma is variable, with smaller tumors appearing more homogeneous and hyperechoic and larger tumors appearing more complex (Fig. 9-11). Tumors may contain calcifications or may also appear cystic.[14] Doppler evaluation may aid in differentiation of neuroblastoma from adrenal hemorrhage because

neuroblastoma reveals vascularity within the neoplasm whereas adrenal hemorrhage does not have flow patterns within the area of hemorrhage.

RENAL

Hydronephrosis

Hydronephrosis is characterized by dilation of the renal collecting system. The role of the ultrasound examination is to identify the severity of the dilation and the location of the obstruction. The most common cause of obstruction in the pediatric patient is the ureteropelvic junction obstruction (UPJ obstruction). UPJ obstruction may be the result of abnormal development of the muscle fibers of the UPJ, fibrosis

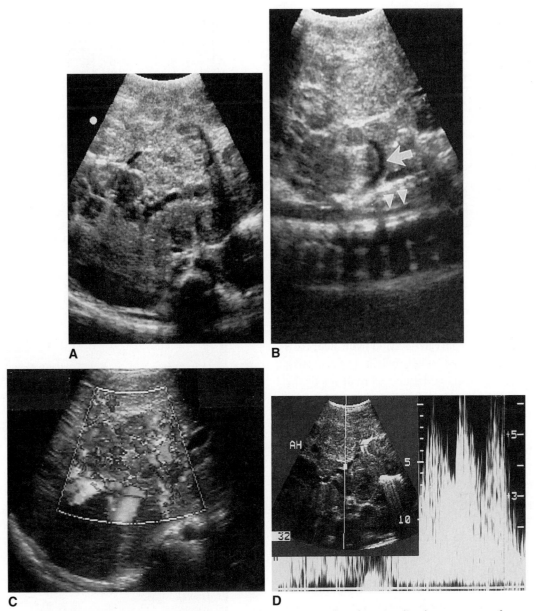

Fig. 9-6 Hemangioendothelioma. **A,** Transverse and, **B,** longitudinal sonogram of 4-month-old girl with greatly enlarged liver containing multiple nodules. Celiac axis is dilated *(arrow)*, and aorta distal to its origin is narrow *(arrowheads)*. **C,** Hepatic artery within liver is dilated. **D,** Low-resistance flow of great velocity is noted in hepatic artery, resembling malignant tumor flow. Cursor in hepatic artery.

and narrowing of the UPJ, compression of fetal vessels, an arrest in the normal development, or a failure of the recanalization of the proximal ureter. UPJ obstruction is usually unilateral, but associated contralateral renal anomalies may be present, including multicystic dysplastic kidney (MCDK), renal duplication, and agenesis.[15]

Hydronephrosis may also be the result of a ureterovesical junction obstruction (UVJ obstruction). UVJ obstruction is the result of an abnormal insertion of the ureter into the bladder wall.[16] This is usually part of a renal duplication anomaly, with the ureter arising from the upper pole of the kidney inserting into an ectopic ureterocele in the bladder.[15] UVJ obstruction is more commonly unilateral but may also be bilateral. Other causes of hydronephrosis include posterior urethral valves (PUVs) and megaureter, urethral atresia, prune-belly syndrome, and neoplasm. Clinical symptoms depend on the cause of the hydronephrosis and include follow-up of obstetric ultrasound, palpable abdominal mass, **oliguria,** or **anuria.**

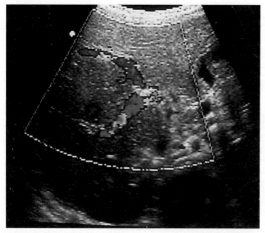

Fig. 9-7 Hepatoblastoma. Surrounding portal veins are displaced around mass.

Sonographic Findings. Hydronephrosis (Fig. 9-12) is identified when the renal pelvis is dilated with or without dilation of the renal calyces. Mild hydronephrosis is classified as a dilated renal pelvis (pyelectasis); moderate hydronephrosis is defined as dilation of the renal pelvis and calyces (pelvocaliectasis); and severe hydronephrosis is identified with significant pelvocaliectasis and thinning of the renal parenchyma.

Sonographic identification of the level of obstruction facilitates proper treatment and surgical management and predicts morbidity and mortality. UPJ obstruction can be diagnosed with obstruction of the kidney without dilation of the ureter or bladder (Fig. 9-13, *A* and *B*). UVJ obstruction is identified sonographically when the kidney is hydronephrotic and the ureter is dilated as well (Fig. 9-14, *A* and *B*). Ultrasound may also identify the ectopic ureterocele in the bladder that is associated with UVJ obstruction. PUV is evident when bilateral hydronephrosis and hydroureter are identified with an enlarged bladder (Fig. 9-15). A thickened bladder wall may also be identified with PUV in addition to the characteristic keyhole bladder (Fig. 9-15, *C*) that represents the dilated proximal urethra.

Renal Cystic Disease

Multiple types of cystic diseases of the kidney exist. This chapter focuses on those most commonly seen in the pediatric patient. Cystic diseases that more commonly affect the adult patient are discussed in Chapter 7.

Multicystic Dysplastic Kidney

Multicystic dysplastic kidney is an anomaly characterized by multiple cysts in a nonfunctioning kidney. It is considered to be a sporadic anomaly although, on

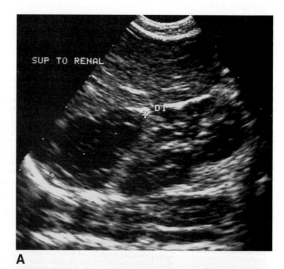

A

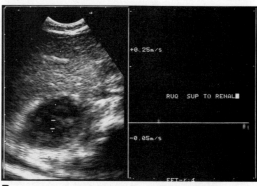

B

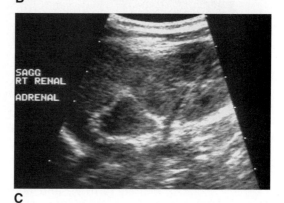

C

Fig. 9-8 **A,** Enlarged, complex adrenal gland is identified on, **B,** initial examination that is avascular. **C,** Follow-up examination shows decrease in size as hemorrhage regresses.

rare occasions, inheritance patterns have been described.[17] MCDK occurs in 1 in 4300 live births.[18] The cause is poorly understood, but it may be the result of an obstructive process in utero or a cessation of the embryologic development into the metanephros.[17] MCDK is usually unilateral but may be associated with a contralateral renal anomaly, the most common of

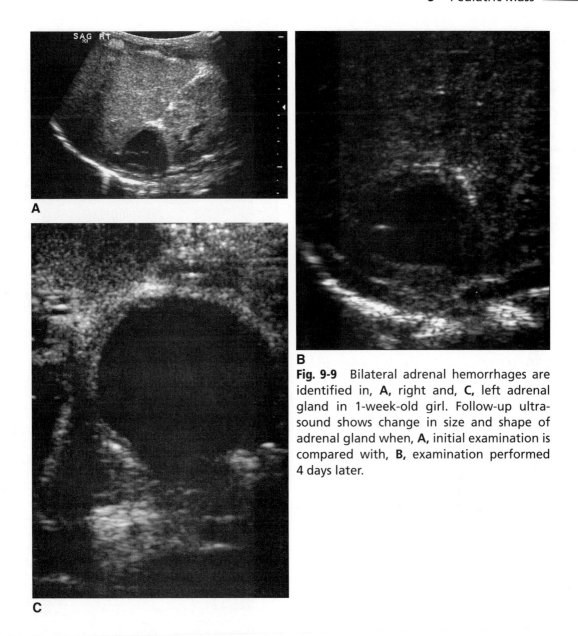

Fig. 9-9 Bilateral adrenal hemorrhages are identified in, **A,** right and, **C,** left adrenal gland in 1-week-old girl. Follow-up ultrasound shows change in size and shape of adrenal gland when, **A,** initial examination is compared with, **B,** examination performed 4 days later.

which is UPJ obstruction. MCDK may also be associated with genetic syndromes, such as Meckel syndrome and Patau syndrome.[15]

MCDK may present as a palpable abdominal mass, or a sonographic evaluation of an infant may follow an obstetric ultrasound finding. Infants with bilateral MCDK or a severe contralateral renal anomaly may have respiratory distress from the lack of amniotic fluid in utero. The prognosis for MCDK is poor when bilateral or associated with a syndrome. Patients with a unilateral MCDK are at increased risk for hypertension and the development of Wilms' tumors.

Sonographic Findings. Sonographic evaluation of the abdomen reveals multiple noncommunicating cysts in the renal bed (Fig. 9-16). Because this kidney is generally nonfunctioning, bilateral MCDK also present with an empty bladder (Fig. 9-17). The sonographic evaluation should include imaging of the contralateral kidney for associated anomalies such as UPJ obstruction, UVJ obstruction, and agenesis.

Autosomal Recessive Polycystic Kidney Disease

Autosomal recessive polycystic kidney disease (ARPKD) is a hereditary disorder that occurs in 1:10,000 live births. ARPKD, also known as *infantile polycystic kidney disease,* can manifest in various forms dependent on severity from perinatal (most severe), to neonatal, to infantile, to juvenile (least severe).[15] The perinatal form is the most common. ARPKD is characterized by varying

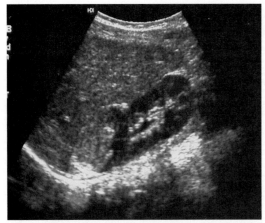

Fig. 9-10 Solid mass is identified at superior pole of kidney. Pathology results confirmed neuroblastoma.

degrees of renal tubular dilation and hepatic fibrosis. The degree of renal cystic disease, which can lead to renal failure, is more severe in the perinatal and neonatal forms, and the degree of hepatic fibrosis, which can lead to liver failure, is more prevalent in the infantile and juvenile forms of the disease.

The most severe forms of the disease present with renal failure. This may be identified in utero as large echogenic kidneys, oligohydramnios, and an absent bladder. The lack of amniotic fluid leads to pulmonary hypoplasia and a grave outcome for these infants when born live. In the less severe forms of the disease, portal hypertension and hypertension are more common clinical symptoms. Progression of the disease may result in the need for dialysis with subsequent renal transplantation and liver transplantation.

Sonographic Findings. The diagnostic criteria for ARPKD is the presence of bilateral enlarged kidneys with a loss of corticomedullary differentiation (Fig. 9-18). The bladder may appear empty or small in size. The less severe forms of the disease may present with portal hypertension, hepatomegaly, and splenomegaly, and the kidneys may appear normal, enlarged, and echogenic or may present with visible cysts.[19]

Nephroblastoma

Wilms' tumor, also known as *nephroblastoma,* is the most common renal tumor in children, with a peak age of 3 years old. This tumor is usually unilateral, but bilateral tumors (Fig. 9-19) may occur and may be associated with syndromes that include Beckwith-Wiedemann syndrome, hemihypertrophy, Drash syndrome, sporadic aniridia, and chromosomal anomalies.[20]

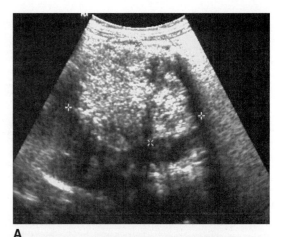

A

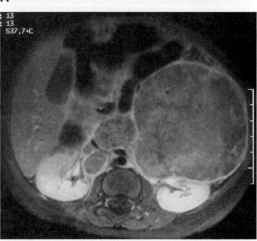

B

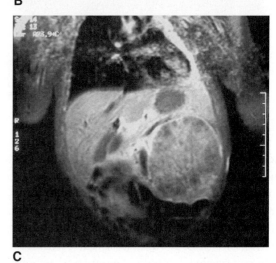

C

Fig. 9-11 **A,** Transverse image of suprarenal mass shows large, heterogeneous lesion, which is also shown on magnetic resonance imaging in, **B,** transverse and, **C,** coronal planes.

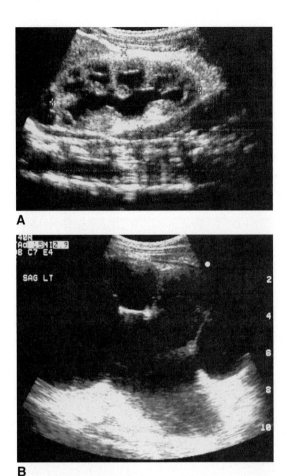

A

B

Fig. 9-12 A, Moderate hydronephrosis is identified. **B,** Severe hydronephrosis is seen with lack of identifiable renal parenchyma.

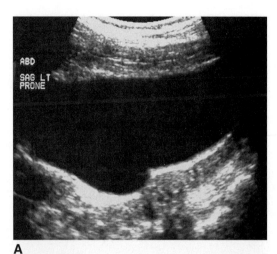

A

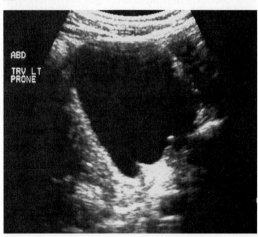

B

Fig. 9-13 A, Longitudinal and, **B,** transverse images of left kidney reveal severe dilation without evidence of dilated ureter consistent with ureteropelvic junction obstruction in 4-year-old girl with history of recurrent urinary tract infections.

The most common clinical presentation of a Wilms' tumor is that of a palpable abdominal mass. Other symptoms include pain, hematuria, hypertension, and malaise. Overall, Wilms' tumor is considered to have a favorable prognosis.

Sonographic Findings. The ultrasound appearance of Wilms' tumor is variable and may be a homogeneous or complex mass within the kidney. The mass usually is echogenic and may contain calcifications. The borders are usually well defined, and a hypoechoic or hyperechoic rim may outline the mass. The renal tissue may appear compressed and may be identified surrounding or partially surrounding the large mass. Depending on the size and location of the mass, hydronephrosis may also be identified. The sonographic examination should include imaging of the renal vein and inferior vena cava (IVC) for tumor thrombus (Fig. 9-20).

Mesoblastic Nephroma

Mesoblastic nephroma is the most common renal tumor in neonates. It is a rare benign tumor with a prevalence of 8:1,000,000.[21] Mesoblastic nephroma comprises connective tissue elements that can completely replace renal tissue.

These tumors may present in utero as a lateral abdominal mass with polyhydramnios. When associated with hydrops, the prognosis is grave. When identified in the neonatal period, the renal mass may grow through the renal capsule into the retroperitoneum; however, the prognosis is good because of the benign nature of this tumor.

Sonographic Findings. The most common sonographic appearance of a mesoblastic nephroma is that of a large, solid, homogeneous mass, but it may also contain cystic areas because of hemorrhage and necrosis. In utero, mesoblastic nephroma has been described as a solid or complex mass that may replace the kidney.[22,23]

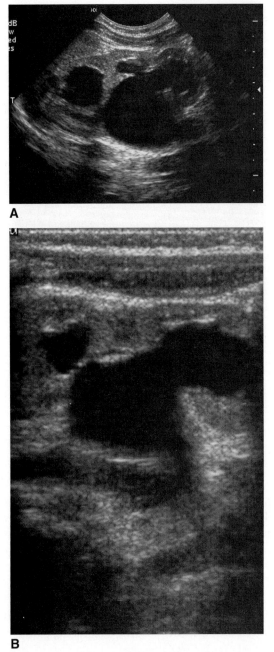

Fig. 9-14 Follow-up renal sonogram in neonate to confirm hydronephrosis identified in utero shows, **A,** moderate to severe hydronephrosis and, **B,** dilated ureter.

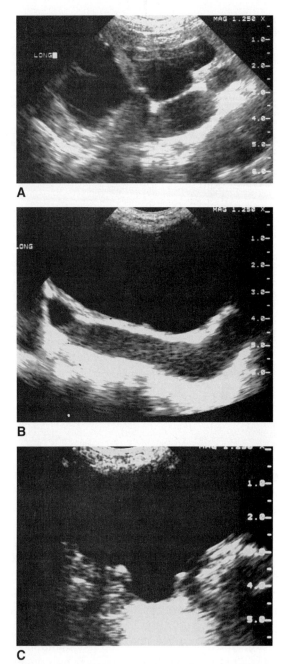

Fig. 9-15 **A,** Severe hydronephrosis is identified bilaterally in addition to, **B,** dilated ureters and, **C,** keyhole bladder in 8-month-old boy with abnormal urinalysis and fever.

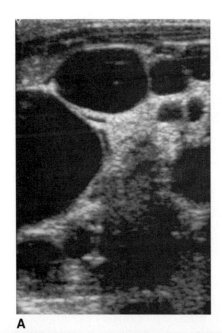

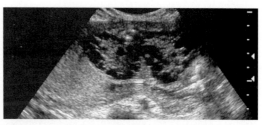

Fig. 9-17 Bilateral multicystic dysplastic kidney is shown in this fetus. No bladder was identified, and absence of amniotic fluid was also noted. Fetus died in utero.

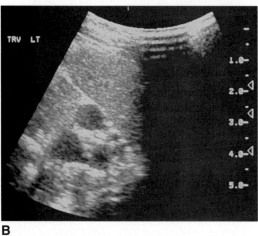

Fig. 9-16 **A** and **B**, Multicystic dysplastic kidney is shown in two different patients, both with normal contralateral kidneys.

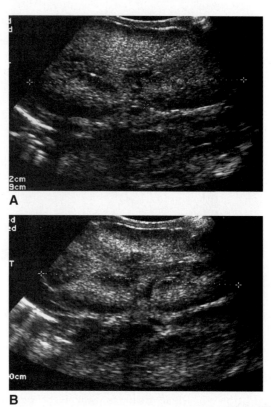

Fig. 9-18 Sonographic examination of kidneys in newborn confirmed bilateral enlarged kidneys measuring, **A**, 11.12 cm in length on right and, **B**, 10.40 cm in length on left, consistent with prenatal diagnosis of autosomal recessive polycystic kidney disease. Postnatal clinical findings include anuria and respiratory distress. Newborn died shortly after birth.

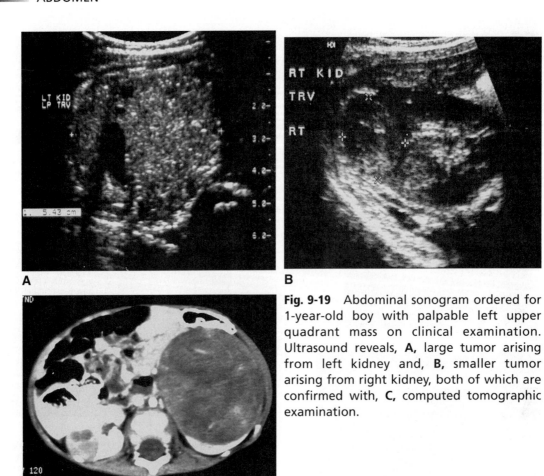

A

B

C

Fig. 9-19 Abdominal sonogram ordered for 1-year-old boy with palpable left upper quadrant mass on clinical examination. Ultrasound reveals, **A,** large tumor arising from left kidney and, **B,** smaller tumor arising from right kidney, both of which are confirmed with, **C,** computed tomographic examination.

Table 9-1 is a summary of the pathology, symptoms, and sonographic findings for pediatric neoplasms.

SUMMARY

In addition to those diseases that were described previously, sonographic examination of the pediatric patient with abdominal pain or a palpable mass may also aid in the diagnosis of a mesenteric cyst, duplication cyst, ovarian cyst, teratoma, cholecystitis, and other benign and malignant neoplasms that are more rarely seen in the pediatric patient. When an abdominal ultrasound fails to locate a mass in the liver, kidneys, or adrenal glands, the sonographer should also survey the lower quadrants of the abdomen to look for masses that may be associated with the retroperitoneum, gastrointestinal tract, and lower genitourinary systems.

CLINICAL SCENARIO—DIAGNOSIS

■ The infant underwent a follow-up ultrasound 4 days later that revealed no change and confirmed that this adrenal mass was most consistent with a neuroblastoma. Computed tomographic scan of the abdomen confirmed the ultrasound findings and also revealed absence of any metastatic disease. Surgery was preformed 6 days later, and the pathology report confirmed the classic histologic findings of a neuroblastoma without evidence of metastasis to the liver, lymph nodes, or bone marrow.

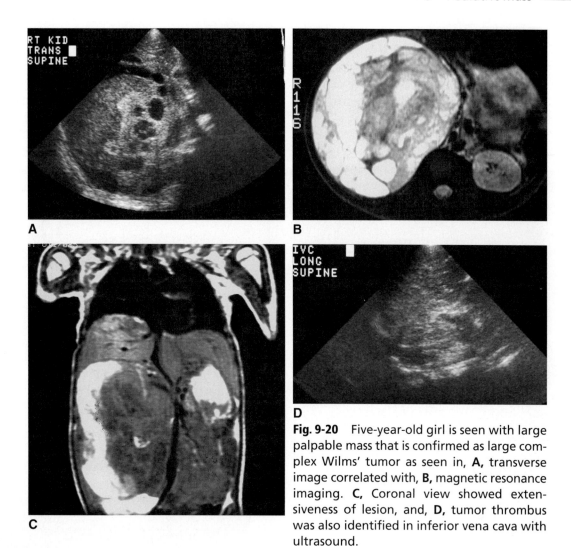

Fig. 9-20 Five-year-old girl is seen with large palpable mass that is confirmed as large complex Wilms' tumor as seen in, **A**, transverse image correlated with, **B**, magnetic resonance imaging. **C**, Coronal view showed extensiveness of lesion, and, **D**, tumor thrombus was also identified in inferior vena cava with ultrasound.

Table 9-1	*Pediatric Neoplasms*	
Pathology	**Symptoms**	**Sonographic Findings**
Hemangioendothelioma	Hepatomegaly, congestive heart failure	Multiple, hypoechoic lesions; hepatomegaly, arteriovenous shunting with Doppler
Hepatoblastoma	Palpable mass, fever, pain, anorexia, weight loss	Solitary mass or multiple lesions, increased vascularity with Doppler
Neuroblastoma	Abdominal mass, hypertension, diarrhea, bone pain	Homogeneous to complex, hyperechoic, calcifications, intratumoral flow with Doppler
Nephroblastoma	Palpable mass, hematuria, hypertension, malaise	Homogeneous or complex, hyperechoic, contains calcifications; associated hydronephrosis may be identified
Mesoblastic nephroma	Palpable mass	Large, solid, homogeneous mass, complex appearance with necrosis

CASE STUDIES FOR DISCUSSION

1. A 2-month old boy with a history of abdominal distension and tenderness is seen for an abdominal ultrasound. The ultrasound reveals a cystic dilation of the CBD as seen in Fig. 9-21. What is the most likely diagnosis?

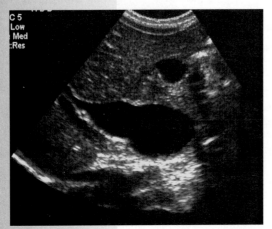

Fig. 9-21 Cystic dilation of common bile duct.

2. An abdominal ultrasound is requested for a 9-month-old boy with a left upper quadrant palpable mass on a well-baby examination. Ultrasound examination reveals an unremarkable liver, gallbladder, pancreas, and spleen. An approximately 7-cm complex mass is seen arising within the inferior pole of the left kidney (Fig. 9-22), and an approximately 2-cm echogenic mass is seen arising from within the middle of the right kidney. Doppler evaluation of the renal veins and IVC is within normal limits. What is the most likely diagnosis?

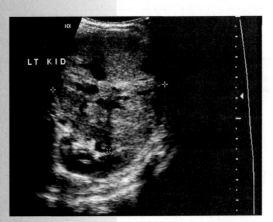

Fig. 9-22 Large complex mass is identified in left kidney.

3. A 15-day-old boy is seen for renal ultrasound to follow up an obstetric ultrasound that revealed unilateral renal agenesis. Ultrasound examination of the right kidney reveals dilation of the renal pelvis and calyces. The right ureter is not seen. The finding in the left renal bed is shown in Fig. 9-23, *A*, and the infant's bladder and pelvic region are also imaged as seen in Fig. 9-23, *B*. What is the probable diagnosis?

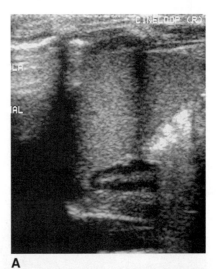

A

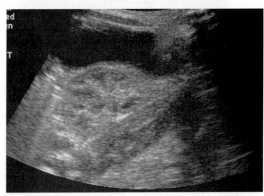

B

Fig. 9-23 Left renal bed is identified in **A**, and bladder and pelvic structures are identified in **B**.

4. A renal ultrasound was ordered for a 1-month-old girl to search congenital anomalies associated with a two-vessel umbilical cord that was identified at birth. Ultrasound examination of the right kidney was unremarkable. Survey of the left kidney revealed the hypoechoic mass at the superior aspect that measured 2 × 2 × 1 cm. Follow-up ultrasound 1 week later revealed a cystic mass measuring

CASE STUDIES FOR DISCUSSION—cont'd ▰▰▰

$3 \times 2 \times 2$ cm (Fig. 9-24). Another follow-up of this mass was performed 1 month later and revealed no abnormal finding in the left upper quadrant. What is the most likely diagnosis?

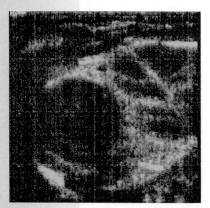

Fig. 9-24 Suprarenal lesion identified; follow-up sonogram shows complete resolution.

5. A 22-day-old boy is seen for renal ultrasound with a history of an obstetric ultrasound reporting a large cyst in the right renal bed and multiple cysts identified in the left kidney as seen in Fig. 9-25, *A* and *B*. The renal ultrasound identified the findings in the right renal bed as noted in Fig. 9-25, *C*, and the findings in the left renal bed as seen in Fig. 9-25, *D*. Normal adrenal glands and a normal bladder were also identified. What is the most likely diagnosis?

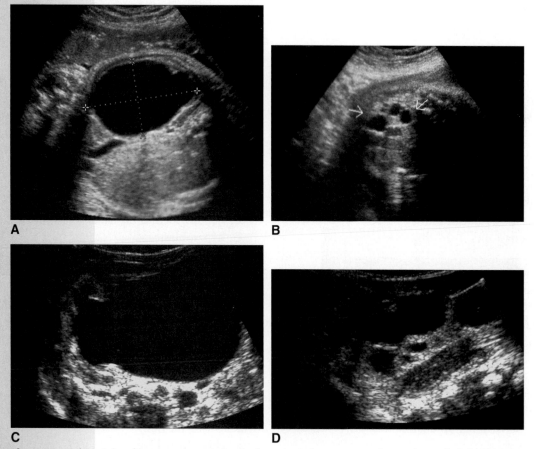

A
B
C
D

Fig. 9-25 Obstetric ultrasound reveals, **A**, large cystic structure in region of right kidney and, **B**, multiple noncommunicating cysts in region of left kidney. Postnatal ultrasound reveals findings in, **C**, right renal bed and, **D**, left renal bed.

STUDY QUESTIONS

1. A 2-year-old boy is seen with a palpable abdominal mass and malaise. Ultrasound examination of the abdomen reveals a 12-cm complex mass that appears to arise from the right kidney. This is most likely which of the following?
   a. hemangioendothelioma
   b. mesoblastic nephroma
   c. multicystic dysplastic kidney
   d. nephroblastoma
   e. neuroblastoma

2. A 1-month-old girl with a history of persistent jaundice, acholic stools, and increasing girth is seen for ultrasound. Ultrasound examination reveals an absent gallbladder and hepatomegaly. This is most consistent with which of the following?
   a. biliary atresia
   b. Caroli's disease
   c. cholecystitis
   d. choledochal cyst
   e. hepatoblastoma

3. A 2-week-old boy is seen with a palpable abdominal mass. Sonographic examination of the abdomen reveals a normal liver, gallbladder, pancreas, and right kidney. A discernible left kidney is not identified; however, a solid mass is identified in the left renal fossa. Obstetric ultrasound at 18 weeks' gestation confirmed two normally placed kidneys. This is most likely which of the following?
   a. adrenal hemorrhage
   b. autosomal polycystic kidney disease
   c. mesoblastic nephroma
   d. multicystic dysplastic kidney
   e. nephroblastoma

4. A newborn is seen for a renal ultrasound to follow up an obstetric ultrasound finding of hydronephrosis. Ultrasound reveals moderate hydronephrosis and ureterectasis of the right kidney. The left kidney is unremarkable. Evaluation of the bladder reveals a ureterocele. This is most consistent with which of the following congenital obstructive disorders?
   a. multicystic dysplastic kidney
   b. posterior urethral valve
   c. ureteropelvic junction obstruction
   d. urethral atresia
   e. ureterovesical junction obstruction

5. A sonographer is called to the neonatal intensive care unit to image a newborn in respiratory distress and anuria. The mother of the newborn was seen in the emergency department in labor without a history of prenatal care. Ultrasound examination reveals large, echogenic, reniform structures arising from the flanks. The bladder is empty. This is consistent with which of the following?
   a. autosomal recessive polycystic kidney disease
   b. multicystic dysplastic kidney
   c. mesoblastic nephroma
   d. posterior urethral valve
   e. renal agenesis

6. A 1-week-old girl with a history of unilateral severe hydronephrosis identified in utero is seen for renal ultrasound. The ultrasound reveals a normal left kidney and bladder. The right renal fossa is filled with multiple cysts that do not connect. This would be most consistent with which of the following?
   a. autosomal recessive polycystic kidney disease
   b. severe hydronephrosis
   c. mesoblastic nephroma
   d. multicystic dysplastic kidney
   e. ureteropelvic junction obstruction

7. A 6-week-old girl is seen with persistent jaundice. Ultrasound of the right upper quadrant shows a normal gallbladder with an adjacent cyst that appears to be contiguous with the common bile duct. This is most consistent with which of the following?
   a. biliary atresia
   b. choledochal cyst
   c. gallbladder duplication
   d. hemangioendothelioma
   e. hepatoblastoma

8. A 4-year-old girl is seen with fever and abdominal pain. On clinical examination, her pediatrician discovers a palpable mass in the right upper quadrant. Laboratory test results reveal an elevated serum alpha fetoprotein level. Ultrasound examination of the abdomen reveals a large mass in the liver. Doppler evaluation shows intratumoral vessels with a high-velocity, low-resistant flow pattern. This is most consistent with which of the following masses?
   a. choledochal cyst
   b. hemangioendothelioma

c. hepatoblastoma
d. hepatoma
e. neuroblastoma

9. A 9-month-old boy with leg pain is seen in the emergency department. A radiograph is ordered to rule out fracture and reveals bone metastasis. Clinical examination of the infant reveals a palpable mass in the left upper quadrant. Laboratory tests reveal increased catecholamine levels. The clinician orders an abdominal ultrasound to assess for which of the following masses?
a. adrenal hemorrhage
b. hemangioendothelioma
c. multicystic dysplastic kidney
d. nephroblastoma
e. neuroblastoma

10. An ultrasound is ordered on a newborn male with a history of an obstetric ultrasound that showed bilateral hydronephrosis, dilated tortuous ureters, and a "keyhole" bladder. The neonatal ultrasound will most likely confirm which of the following renal anomalies?
a. multicystic dysplastic kidney
b. posterior urethral valve
c. ureteropelvic junction obstruction
d. urethral atresia
e. ureterovesical junction obstruction

REFERENCES

1. Chardot C: *Biliary atresia,* http://www.pedihepa.org/BILIARYATRESIA.htm, retrieved July 9, 2003.
2. Ikeda S et al: Gallbladder contraction in biliary atresia: a pitfall of ultrasound diagnosis, *Pediatr Radiol* 28:451-453, 1998.
3. Kendrick A et al: Making the diagnosis of biliary atresia using the triangular cord sign and gallbladder length, *Pediatr Radiol* 30:69-73, 2000.
4. Lee HC et al: Dilation of the biliary tree in children: sonographic diagnosis and its clinical significance, *J Ultrasound Med* 19:177-182, 2000.
5. Rumack CM, Wilson SR, Charboneau JW: *Diagnostic ultrasound,* vol 2, ed 2, St Louis, 1998, Mosby.
6. Kim WS et al: Choledochal cyst with or without biliary atresia in neonates and young infants: US differentiation, *Radiology* 209:465-469, 1998.
7. Herman TE, Siegel MJ: Infantile hepatic hemangioendothelioma, *J Perinatol* 20:447-449, 2000.
8. Han SJ, Tsai CC, Tsai HM et al: Infantile hemangioendothelioma with a highly elevated serum alphafetoprotein level, *Hepto-Gastroenterology* 45:459-461, 1998.
9. Sato M et al: Liver tumors in children and young patients: sonographic and color Doppler findings, *Abdom Imaging* 25:596-601, 2000.
10. McCarville ME, Furman WL: Hepatoblastoma, http://www.emedicine.com/radio/topic331.htm, retrieved July 9, 2003.
11. Nadler EP, Barksdale EM Jr: Adrenal masses in the newborn, *Semin Pediatr Surg* 9:156-164, 2000.
12. Fang SB et al: Prenatal sonographic detection of adrenal hemorrhage confirmed by postnatal surgery, *J Clin Ultrasound* 27:206-209, 1999.
13. Lukens JN: Neuroblastoma in the neonate, *Semin Perinatol* 23:263-273, 1999.
14. Grando A et al: Prenatal sonographic diagnosis of adrenal neuroblastoma, *J Clin Ultrasound* 29:250-253, 2001.
15. Angtuaco TL, Collins HB, Quirk JG: The fetal genitourinary tract, *Semin Roentgenol* 34:13-28, 1999.
16. Zhou Q, Cardoza JD, Barth R: Prenatal sonography of congenital renal malformations, *Am J Roentgenol AJR* 173:1371-1376, 1999.
17. Srivastava T, Garola RE, Hellerstein S: Autosomal dominant inheritance of multicystic dysplastic kidney, *Pediatr Nephrol* 13:481-483, 1999.
18. Feldenberg LR, Siegel NJ: Clinical course and outcome for children with multicystic dysplastic kidneys, *Pediatr Nephrol* 14:1098-1101, 2000.
19. Lonergan GL, Rice RR, Suarez ES: Autosomal recessive polycystic kidney disease: radiologic-pathologic correlation, *RadioGraphics* 20:837-855, 2000.
20. Applegate KE, Ghei M, Perez-Atayde AR: Prenatal detection of a Wilms' tumor, *Pediatr Radiol* 1:65-67, 1999.
21. Schild RL, Plath H, Hofstaetter C et al: Diagnosis of a fetal mesoblastic nephroma by 3D-ultrasound, *Ultrasound Obstet Gynecol* 15:533-536, 2000.
22. Holley G, Labuski M, Kasales C: Congenital mesoblastic nephroma: antenatal and postnatal sonographic appearance with pathologic correlation, *J Diag Med Sonogr* 13:291-293, 1997.
23. Gernon CL, Alston B: Radiological case of the month, *Appl Radiol* Oct:41-42, 1999.

BIBLIOGRAPHY

Cushing B, Slovis TL: Sonography of the liver and biliary system in pediatric patients, *Appl Radiol* 14:71-77, 1985.
Kawamura DM: *Abdomen and superficial structures,* ed 2, Philadelphia, 1997, Lippincott.
Siegel MJ: *Pediatric sonography,* ed 2, New York, 1995, Raven Press.

Pulsatile Abdominal Mass

CHARLOTTE HENNINGSEN

CLINICAL SCENARIO

■ A 63-year-old obese woman with severe back pain is seen in the emergency department. The patient is hypotensive and goes into cardiac arrest, at which time her abdomen begins to swell. Ultrasound reveals the finding in Fig. 10-1 and free fluid in the abdomen. This is suggestive of what diagnosis?

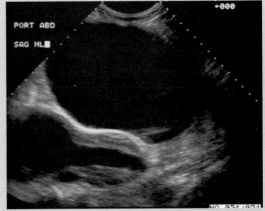

Fig. 10-1 Large cystic mass is identified anterior to aorta in longitudinal image.

OBJECTIVES

■ List the risk factors associated with aneurysm, dissection, and rupture.

■ Describe the technique for sonographic imaging of the aorta.

■ Identify the sonographic findings associated with aneurysm, dissection, and rupture.

■ Describe the symptoms associated with aneurysm, dissection, and rupture.

■ List the classifications used to characterize the various types of dissections.

The aorta is the largest artery and is responsible for supplying the body with blood through its many branches. The ascending aorta serves the head, neck, and upper extremities, and the descending aorta serves the abdomen, pelvis, and lower extremities by transporting gases, nutrients, and other substances to the tissues and transporting wastes to appropriate sites for excretion. The aorta is a tubular structure (as are other arteries) with a wall comprised of an inner layer, the tunica intima; a middle layer, the tunica media; and an outer layer, the tunica adventitia.

Sonographic examination of the abdominal aorta should include longitudinal and transverse images that show the proximal, middle, and distal segments and the iliac artery bifurcation. A normal aorta gradually tapers toward the distal segment (Fig. 10-2). The antero-posterior (AP) diameter should be measured in the longitudinal plane. The renal and iliac arteries should also be documented. The imaging limitation of overlying bowel gas can be diminished or alleviated with gentle transducer pressure and with patient preparation with an overnight fast. In addition, obese patients or patients with excessive bowel gas may benefit from the varying of imaging techniques, including patient placement in a left posterior oblique or decubitus position.

Because of the aorta's large size and the volume of blood transported through it, disruption of normal aortic flow can be catastrophic. One indicator of aortic disease is a palpable pulsatile mass that may be detected on clinical examination. The diagnosis of an aortic aneurysm should precipitate periodic follow-up of the mass to monitor for the potential life-threatening complications of rupture and dissection. This chapter explains the clinical symptoms and sonographic findings associated with aneurysm, rupture, and dissection.

ABDOMINAL AORTIC ANEURYSM

An abdominal aortic aneurysm (AAA) is a localized dilation of the aorta. AAAs have been identified in 2% to 4% of the general population who are over 50 years of age. AAAs develop as the tunica media, which is comprised largely of smooth muscle cells, collagen, and elastin, thins.[1] AAAs may be clinically silent, but the risk of rupture and the associated increased mortality rate show the importance of early detection and elective repair. Risk factors include a history of **atherosclerosis,** increased age, smoking, low serum high-density lipo-

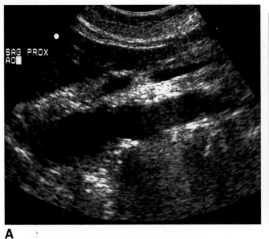 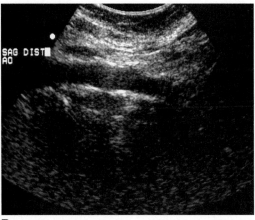

A **B**

Fig. 10-2 Longitudinal images of, **A,** proximal aorta and, **B,** distal aorta show tapering in healthy patient.

protein (HDL) cholesterol, and hypertension. The incidence of AAA is increased among men.[2]

An AAA may be suspected when clinical examination reveals a pulsatile abdominal mass located at the level of the umbilicus or slightly cephalic to the umbilicus, although a large girth may limit the sensitivity of clinical palpation. In addition, an AAA may be suspected when a tortuous calcified aorta is identified on a radiograph that may have been ordered for an unrelated condition or disease. Patients may have abdominal pain or back pain, which may indicate that the aneurysm is enlarging or, with severe symptoms, that rupture has occurred.

Sonographic Findings

Ultrasound imaging of the aorta for detection of aneurysm is the preferred test because of the high sensitivity and specificity of this examination, although results may be limited by obesity, prior abdominal surgery, and overlying bowel gas.[3] Ultrasound is more effective when the patient has had nothing by mouth (*nulla per os* [NPO]) 8 hours before the examination. Diagnosis of an aneurysm can be made when the AP diameter is 3 cm or greater in the longitudinal plane. Aortic aneurysms may be fusiform (uniform dilation) or saccular (asymmetric saclike dilation) in appearance, or the aorta may have a gradual widening referred to as *aortic ectasia*. Thrombus within the dilation may also be noted (Fig. 10-3) and most commonly appears as low-level echoes, although calcifications and liquefaction may also appear within thrombus, which may be clearly demonstrated with color Doppler. Also, an important part of the protocol is documentation of the location of the aneurysm relative to the renal arteries.

Ultrasound is also used in patient follow-up for assessment of the expansion of the aneurysm for planning of elective surgery. The current recommendation is yearly AAA scanning until the aneurysm reaches a diameter of 4 cm, then patient screening every 6 months until the aneurysm reaches a diameter of 5 cm, and then patient follow-up every 3 months until the aneurysm reaches a diameter of 5.5 cm, at which time elective repair (Fig. 10-4) can be scheduled.[3]

RUPTURED ANEURYSM

Rupture of AAA carries an 80% to 90% mortality rate and results in approximately 15,000 deaths each year in the United States.[3] The risk of rupture sharply increases with aneurysms of more than 6 cm in diameter, and high blood pressure and current smoking increase the growth rate of aneurysms and resultant rupture.[4] Patients

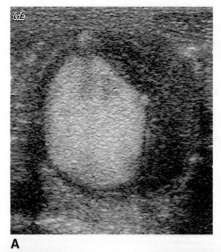

A

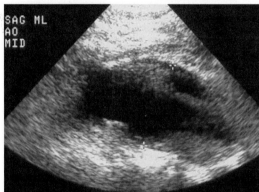

B

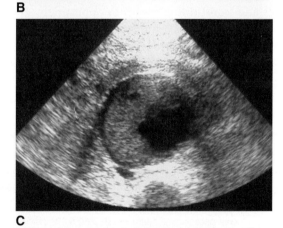

C

Fig. 10-3 A, Transverse image of aorta shows enlarged aorta with thrombus at periphery of vessel. **B,** Longitudinal and, **C,** transverse images of aneurysm in 68-year-old man with pulsatile abdominal mass. Thrombus within aneurysm measured 7 cm in AP diameter. (**A** Courtesy GE Medical Systems.)

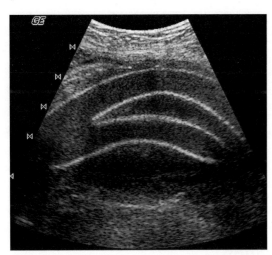

Fig. 10-4 Echogenic walls of aortic graft. (Courtesy GE Medical Systems.)

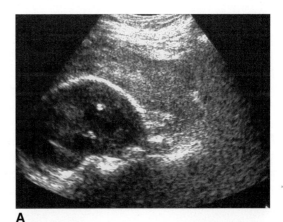

A

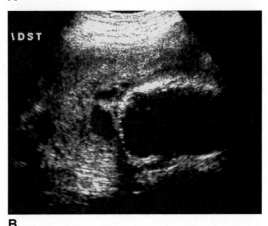

B

Fig. 10-5 Aortic aneurysm in elderly patient seen in unconscious state in emergency department. **A,** Longitudinal and, **B,** transverse images show dilated aorta, and transverse image shows large hematoma at left of umbilicus, which is worrisome for rupture.

with rapidly increasing aneurysms may be offered elective repair to decrease the mortality associated with rupture, and if the patient is a current smoker, smoking cessation should be encouraged. Blood pressure monitoring and control is also important in management for these patients.

The clinical presentation for aortic rupture includes **hypotension,** abdominal pain, and a palpable pulsatile mass. Pain may also radiate to the back, groin, or scrotum. Patients may present in **shock** and be unable to communicate, or they may not have a known history of AAA. A speedy diagnosis is imperative because of the rapid blood loss that can quickly lead to cardiovascular collapse and death.[1]

Sonographic Findings

Sonographic examination of the abdomen to rule out rupture (Fig. 10-5) should include a survey of the aorta to confirm the aneurysmal aorta, although the aorta may appear normal in size. The abdomen should also be explored for the presence of **hemoperitoneum.** Resolution of the disruption in the aortic wall may not be possible with ultrasound, but a periaortic hematoma may be identified, which would suggest rupture.[5] Fluid in the gutters or a perinephric hematoma may also be identified.

AORTIC DISSECTION

Aortic dissection occurs with the rupture of the intima of the aorta, which then separates from the media, with a column of blood between the two layers.[6] Causes of aortic dissection include hypertension, **Marfan syn-**drome, and less frequently, pregnancy and chest trauma. Dissection may result from the degenerative changes that occur in the aorta with atherosclerotic disease or may result from a congenital defect or an **iatrogenic** event.

Based on the extent and location of the dissection, characterization may be made with the Stanford or DeBakey classifications. The Stanford classification differentiates between dissections that involve the ascending aorta (type A) and dissections that do not involve the ascending aorta (type B). The DeBakey classification differentiates between dissections that involve the entire aorta (type I), dissections that involve only the ascending aorta (type II), and dissections that involve only the descending aorta (type III).[6,7] The classifications are used in the determination of treatment and prognosis. Dissection of the ascending aorta has a much higher mortality rate than that of the descending aorta, and type B dissections may be treated conservatively when life-threatening complications are not present, whereas type A dissections are generally treated surgically.

The clinical presentation of dissection is usually an acute onset of severe chest pain. Patients may also have neck or throat pain, pain in the abdomen or lower back, syncope, paresis, and dyspnea.[8] If the patient history includes hypertension, aortic aneurysm, or Marfan syndrome, dissection should be strongly considered. Clinical examination may also reveal absent pulses in the legs.

Sonographic Findings

The sonographic technique used in the diagnosis of dissection varies depending on the location of the dissection. Transesophageal echocardiography (TEE) is the most common method of imaging for dissections of the ascending aorta. Transabdominal ultrasound is used for imaging of the descending aorta, and computed tomography (CT) and magnetic resonance imaging (MRI) may also be used in evaluation of dissections of the ascending and descending aorta.

Dissection of the descending aorta may be diagnosed with identification of the intimal flap in the aorta (Fig. 10-6). Doppler can be used to document flow in the true lumen and, depending on whether the dissection is acute or chronic, flow may or may not be shown in the false lumen located between the tunica intima and tunica media. Because rupture is a complication of dissection, the sonographic findings of aorta rupture should also be evaluated.

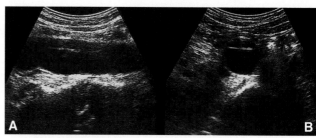

Fig. 10-6 Dissection of abdominal aorta. **A,** Sagittal and, **B,** transverse sonograms show intimal flap anteriorly separating true lumen from false lumen. (Courtesy Stephanie R. Wilson, MD, University of Toronto.)

SUMMARY

Aortic aneurysm may be identified in patients with a pulsatile mass or as an incidental finding. Patients with a history of aneurysm and severe symptoms should be considered at risk for dissection and rupture. Ultrasound findings plus correlation with patient symptoms and clinical examination can aid with a speedy diagnosis in potentially life-threatening situations. See Table 10-1 for a summary of the pathology, symptoms, and sonographic findings of the aorta.

CLINICAL SCENARIO—DIAGNOSIS

■ The aorta is dilated, and thrombus is seen in the aneurysm. The hypotensive state and the fluid in the abdomen suggest aortic rupture. This diagnosis was confirmed at surgery, and the condition was successfully repaired. Incidentally, the large cystic structure anterior to the aorta was not the bladder, although it did provide an excellent window for visualization of the aneurysm. After the aneurysm was repaired, this mass was removed and was confirmed to be an ovarian cystadenoma.

Table 10-1	*Pathology of Aorta*	
Pathology	**Symptoms**	**Sonographic Findings**
Aortic aneurysm	Pulsatile abdominal mass	Aortic AP diameter 3 cm, uniform or asymmetric dilation, with or without thrombus
Aortic rupture	Pulsatile abdominal mass, hypotension, abdominal pain, radiating pain	Aortic aneurysm, hemoperitoneum, periaortic hematoma
Aortic dissection	Severe chest pain, neck or throat pain, abdominal or back pain, syncope, paresis, dyspnea	Linear flap in aorta; flow may or may not be demonstrated on both sides of flap

CASE STUDIES FOR DISCUSSION

1. A 69-year-old man is seen for a right upper quadrant (RUQ) ultrasound for persistent RUQ pain. The ultrasound reveals cholelithiasis with pericholecystic fluid consistent with cholecystitis. Incidentally noted are the findings in the aorta (Fig. 10-7, *A* and *B*). The aorta measured 6.6 cm in the AP diameter. What is the most likely diagnosis of the finding in the aorta?

2. A 58-year-old man is seen for ultrasound of the aorta because of a pulsatile mass over the area of the umbilicus on physical examination. The distal aorta is shown in Fig. 10-8, *A* and *B*. What is the most likely diagnosis?

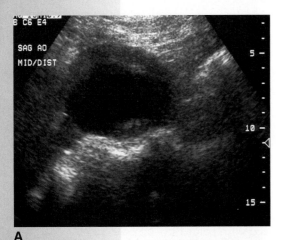

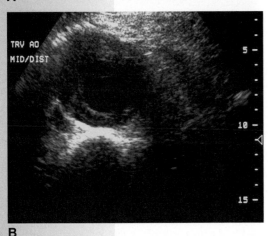

Fig. 10-7 **A,** Longitudinal and, **B,** transverse images of aorta with AP diameter of 6.6 cm.

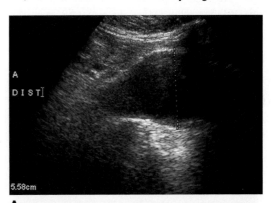

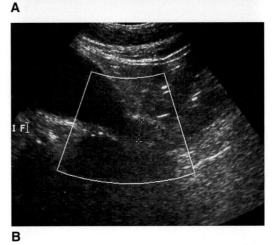

Fig. 10-8 **A** and **B,** Longitudinal images of distal aorta. **B,** Proximal left iliac artery is also identified.

CASE STUDIES FOR DISCUSSION—cont'd

3. An 82-year-old man arrives in the emergency department via ambulance from a nursing care facility. The patient is unconscious, and clinical examination reveals hypotension and an abdominal pulsatile mass. A portable ultrasound is requested immediately and reveals a dilated aorta that measures 8.5 cm in AP diameter (Fig. 10-9). The findings and clinical examination suggest what diagnosis?

4. A 79-year-old woman is seen for ultrasound of the aorta after multiple episodes of fainting. She has a history of poorly controlled hypertension and aneurysm and also has back pain. The ultrasound examination is technically limited because of obesity. The ultrasound findings confirm a dilated aorta that measures 7 cm in AP diameter (Fig. 10-10, A and B). A linear echo is also identified within the aorta, and color Doppler confirms flow on both sides of this flap. What is the most likely diagnosis?

5. An 82-year-old man is seen for follow-up of an AAA. The ultrasound reveals a dilated distal aorta that measures 3.9 cm in AP diameter. Mural thrombus is shown with color Doppler (Fig. 10-11). No increase in size is noted from the ultrasound performed 6 months prior. What is the appropriate follow-up for this patient at this time?

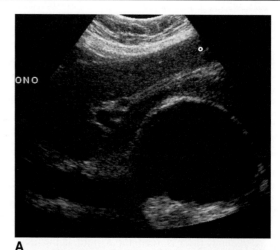

A

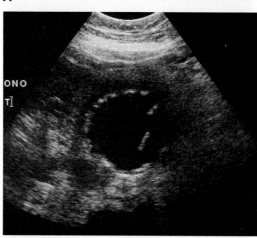

B

Fig. 10-10 **A,** Longitudinal and, **B,** transverse images of dilated aorta. Linear echo within vessel was documented with color flow on both sides.

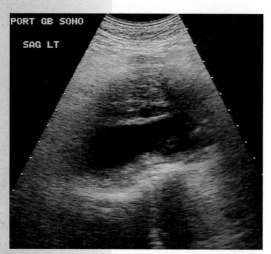

Fig. 10-9 Longitudinal image of aorta with measurement of 8.5 cm in AP diameter.

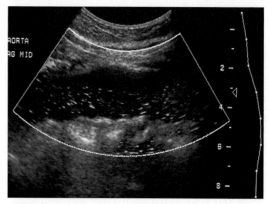

Fig. 10-11 Longitudinal image of aorta, with color Doppler outlining mural thrombus.

STUDY QUESTIONS

1. A 55-year-old man is seen for a routine physical examination. During the examination, the physician feels a pulsatile mass at the level of the umbilicus. An ultrasound is ordered for which of the following indications?
   a. to rule out abdominal aortic aneurysm
   b. to rule out atherosclerotic disease
   c. to rule out dissection
   d. to rule out neoplasm
   e. to rule out rupture

2. A 72-year-old woman is seen in an unconscious state in the emergency department. She is accompanied by her husband who states that she had an attack of severe abdominal pain and then passed out. Clinical evaluation reveals a hypotensive condition, and an abdominal ultrasound is ordered. The ultrasound reveals an aorta that measures 8 cm in diameter at the distal end and fluid in the peritoneal cavity. This would be consistent with which of the following?
   a. abdominal aortic aneurysm
   b. aortic dissection
   c. aortic rupture
   d. atherosclerotic disease
   e. Marfan syndrome

3. A 67-year-old man with vague abdominal pain is seen by his physician. A kidney-ureters-bladder radiograph (KUB) is ordered and is unremarkable except for calcifications noted along the aorta. An aortic ultrasound examination is ordered and reveals a distal aortic diameter of 4 cm. This would be consistent with which of the following?
   a. normal examination
   b. abdominal aortic aneurysm
   c. aortic dissection
   d. aortic rupture
   e. atherosclerotic disease

4. Based on the aortic dissection classification defined by Stanford, a dissection that involves the ascending and descending aorta would be given which of the following designations?
   a. type A
   b. type B
   c. type I
   d. type II
   e. type III

5. A 40-year-old man with a history of Marfan syndrome is seen with intense chest pain in the emergency department. Which of the following diagnoses should be the primary consideration?
   a. aortic aneurysm
   b. aortic dissection
   c. aortic rupture
   d. aortic thrombosis
   e. heart attack

6. All of the following are risk factors for abdominal aortic aneurysm except:
   a. advanced age
   b. atherosclerosis
   c. female gender
   d. hypertension
   e. smoking

7. A 72-year-old man has an abdominal aortic aneurysm that measures 4 cm in diameter. This patient should be followed with what frequency to monitor for expansion of the aneurysm?
   a. annually
   b. every 3 months
   c. every 6 months
   d. every 9 months
   e. no follow-up is needed

8. A 62-year-old woman is seen in the emergency department with chest pain and a fainting spell but is conscious and cognitive. Patient history includes a previously diagnosed abdominal aortic aneurysm. An ultrasound of the abdominal aorta and electrocardiography and echocardiography are ordered. The abdominal ultrasound reveals the aneurysm, which measures 4.8 cm. The sonographer also identifies a thin linear echo within the aorta and documents flow on both sides of this line with color Doppler examination. This would be consistent with which of the following diagnoses?
   a. aortic aneurysm
   b. aortic dissection
   c. aortic rupture
   d. aortic thrombosis
   e. heart attack

9. According to the DeBakey classification, an aortic dissection involving only the descending aorta would be classified as which of the following?

   a. type I
   b. type II
   c. type III
   d. type A
   e. type B

10. A 58-year-old woman with epigastric pain with eating is seen for an abdominal ultrasound to rule out gallstones. The sonographer identifies normal-appearing gallbladder, liver, pancreas, and spleen. The sonographer also documents a dilation of the aorta, which measures 6 cm at its greatest diameter. This would be consistent with which of the following?
   a. aortic aneurysm
   b. aortic dissection
   c. aortic rupture
   d. atherosclerotic disease
   e. hypertension

REFERENCES

1. Anderson LA: Abdominal aortic aneurysm, *J Cardiovasc Nurs* 15:1-14, 2001.
2. Singh K et al: Prevalence of and risk factors for abdominal aortic aneurysms in a population-based study, *Am J Epidemiol* 154:236-244, 2001.
3. Ebaugh JL, Garcia ND, Matsumura JS: Screening and surveillance for abdominal aortic aneurysms: who needs it and when, *Semin Vasc Surg* 14:193-199, 2001.
4. Powell JT, Brown LC: The natural history of abdominal aortic aneurysms and their risk of rupture, *Acta Chir Belg* 101:11-16, 2001.
5. Ballard RB, Rozycki GS, Knudson MM et al: The surgeon's use of ultrasound in the acute setting, *Surg Clin North Am* 78:337-364, 1998.
6. Flachskampf FA, Daniel WG: Aortic dissection, *Cardiol Clin* 18:807-817, 2000.
7. Erbel R et al: Diagnosis and management of aortic dissection, *Eur Heart J* 22:1642-1681, 2001.
8. Stöllberger C et al: Headache as the initial manifestation of acute aortic dissection type A, *Cephalalgia* 18:583-584, 1998.

11 Gastrointestinal Imaging

KIMBERLY EISEN

CLINICAL SCENARIO

■ A mother brought her 1-month-old twin baby girl to the emergency department because the baby had had projectile vomiting after every meal for the past 24 hours. The baby was also unusually irritable and would not stop fussing. During the pediatrician's initial examination, he felt a small 3-cm mass in the infant's right upper quadrant, close to midline. The baby did not show signs of jaundice but was somewhat lethargic. The baby was immediately given intravenous fluids for dehydration, and an ultrasound of the abdomen was ordered. The abdominal sonogram was performed focusing on the area of the pylorus (Figs. 11-1 to 11-3). What is the most likely diagnosis of this infant's illness?

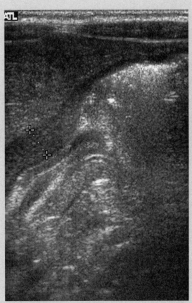

Fig. 11-2 Anteroposterior pyloric wall thickness of 6.1 mm.

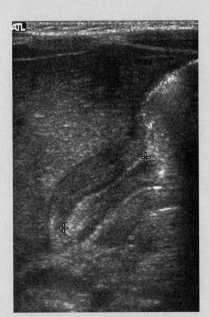

Fig. 11-1 One-month-old infant with pyloric canal length of 2.17 cm.

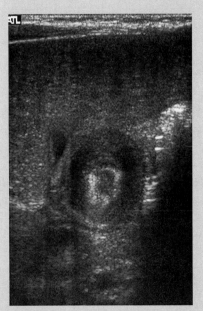

Fig. 11-3 Transverse view of inflamed pyloric canal.

OBJECTIVES

■ Describe the epidemiology, anatomy and pathophysiology, and causes of appendicitis.

■ Describe the clinical presentation and sonographic findings of appendicitis, including the best method of imaging the appendix with ultrasound.

■ Describe the epidemiology and anatomy and pathophysiology of infantile hypertrophic pyloric stenosis.

■ Describe the clinical presentation, sonographic findings, and treatment of infantile hypertrophic pyloric stenosis.

■ Describe the epidemiology and anatomy and pathophysiology of intussusception.

■ Describe the clinical presentation, sonographic findings, and treatment of intussusception.

GLOSSARY OF TERMS

Abscess: a localized collection of pus surrounded by inflamed tissue that is formed as a result of tissue disintegration from an infection

Appendicolith: a fecalith or calcification located in the appendix

Ascites: free fluid in the abdomen

Barium enema: a radiographic procedure in which barium is introduced into the rectum in a retrograde fashion for visualization of the bowel lining with fluoroscopy

Cervix sign: sometimes used to describe a stenotic pyloric channel; the sonographic appearance of pyloric stenosis resembles the appearance of the cervix in pregnancy and thus is nicknamed the "cervix" sign

Computed tomography: a radiographic technique that uses a narrowly collimated beam of radiographs that rotates in a continuous 360-degree motion around the patient to image the body in cross section

Diverticulum: a pouchlike herniation through the muscular wall of a tubular organ that occurs in the stomach, the small intestine, or most commonly, the colon

Fecalith: a hard, impacted mass of feces in the colon

Hydrostatic enema: a retrograde water enema used as a first attempt at reducing an intussusception

Icteric: a term used to describe a condition of jaundice

Intraperitoneal: inside the peritoneum

Jaundice: a yellow discoloration of the skin, mucous membranes, and sclerae of the eyes caused by greater than normal amounts of bilirubin in the blood

Mandibular frenulum: a normal midline craniofacial structure extending from the vestibular mucosa of the lower lip to the gingival mucosa of the lower jaw

McBurney's sign: pain in the right lower quadrant with rebound tenderness in cases of appendicitis

Meckel's diverticulum: an anomalous sac of embryologic origin that protrudes from the wall of the ileum usually between 30 and 90 cm from the ileocecal sphincter

Meconium ileus: obstruction of the small intestine in the newborn caused by impaction of thick, dry, tenacious meconium, usually at or near the ileocecal valve

Metabolic alkalosis: an abnormal condition characterized by the significant loss of acid in the body or by increased levels of base bicarbonate

Necrosis: localized tissue death that occurs in groups of cells in response to disease or injury

Nuclear medicine: a medical discipline in which radioactive isotopes are used in the diagnosis and treatment of disease; major fields of nuclear medicine are physiologic function studies, radionuclide imaging, and therapeutic techniques

Peritoneum: an extensive serous membrane that covers the entire abdominal wall of the body and is reflected over the contained viscera

Peritonitis: an inflammation of the peritoneum produced by bacteria or irritating substances introduced into the abdominal cavity by a penetrating wound or perforation of an organ in the gastrointestinal or reproductive tract

Polyp: a small tumorlike growth that projects from a mucous membrane surface

Pyloric canal (channel): muscle that connects the stomach to the proximal duodenum

Pyloromyotomy, or Fredet-Ramstedt operation: a surgical procedure that involves the cutting of the muscle fibers of the gastric outlet to widen the opening; used as a treatment for pyloric stenosis

Upper gastrointestinal: fluoroscopic radiographic imaging of the upper gastrointestinal tract after the ingestion of barium

Ultrasound is an appropriate imaging method for the diagnosis of several types of gastrointestinal (GI) diseases, the most common of which is appendicitis. Patients of all ages with right lower quadrant pain or nausea and vomiting must be considered at risk for appendicitis. Clinical symptoms such as vomiting and pain can also be indicative of other GI illnesses, including infantile hypertrophic pyloric stenosis (IHPS) and intussusception. Clinicians must presume the most likely cause of the symptoms and follow-up with diagnostic studies, such as sonography, to confirm or exclude the initial diagnosis.

APPENDICITIS

Acute appendicitis is one of the most common diseases that necessitates emergency surgery[1] and is the most common atraumatic surgical abdominal disorder in children 2 years of age and older.[2] Males and females have a lifetime appendicitis risk of 8.6% and 6.7%, respectively, yet the mortality rate in nonperforated appendicitis is less than 1%.[2] Early diagnosis of appendicitis in patients is essential in prevention of perforation, **abscess** formation, and postoperative complications.[3] A delay in diagnosis often occurs with young, pregnant, or elderly patients, increasing the risk of perforation. The mortality rate can be as high as 5% in these patients.[2] During the past 10 years, ultrasonography, along with **nuclear medicine** and **computed tomography** (CT), has been used in the diagnosis of appendicitis. Despite technologic advances, the diagnosis of appendicitis is still based primarily on patient history and physical examination.[2]

Epidemiology

Appendicitis usually results from an obstructing object or obstructive disorder within the appendix. The risk for an obstruction can be linked to diet or genetic predisposition. Generally, unhealthy diets, including decreased dietary fiber along with increased refined carbohydrates (e.g., pure sugars and starches), can increase the incidence rate of appendicitis.[3] Genetically, a history of appendicitis in a first-degree relative is associated with a 3.5% to 10% relative risk for the disorder. The strongest familial associations occur in children between birth and 6 years of age.[3]

Anatomy and Pathophysiology

The appendix is a long, thin **diverticulum** that arises from the inferior tip of the cecum (Fig. 11-4). Although the average length of the appendix is 3 inches, it may measure as long as 9 inches.[4] The appendix usually has an anterior **intraperitoneal** location that, when inflamed, may come in contact with the anterior parietal peritoneum and cause right lower quadrant pain. As much as 30% of the time, the appendix may be "hidden" from the anterior peritoneum when in a pelvic, retroileal, or retrocecal position (Fig. 11-5).[2] The differing locations of the appendix can make sonographic imaging a challenge. The shape of the appendix also differs depending on age. At birth, the appendix is funnel-shaped, which limits the chance for obstruction to occur (Fig. 11-6). By age 2 years, the appendix assumes a more normal conic shape, which increases the chance for luminal obstruction (Figs. 11-7 and 11-8).[3] Although the appendix itself is not necessary for survival, the lining of the appendix, composed of

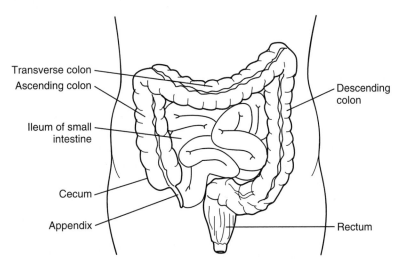

Fig. 11-4 Diagram of normal location of appendix. Appendix lies at junction of terminal ileum of small intestine and proximal ascending colon.

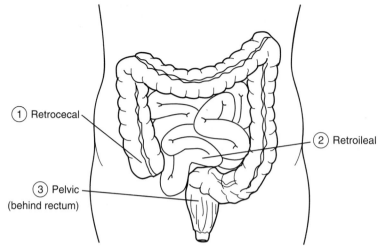

Fig. 11-5 Appendix is sometimes in atypical location as shown in diagram. *1,* Retrocecal location (behind cecum); *2,* retroileal location (behind ileum of small intestine); and *3,* pelvic location (hidden behind uterus, rectum, or ovaries).

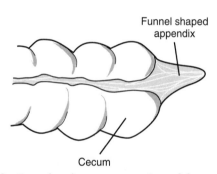

Fig. 11-6 Drawing is representative of funnel-shaped appendix, which is shape of normal appendix in infants up to 2 years of age.

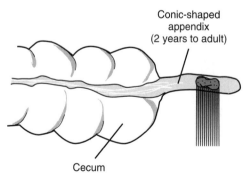

Fig. 11-7 By age 2 years, appendix assumes more adultlike conic shape, increasing chance for proximal luminal obstruction.

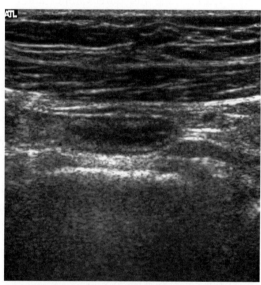

Fig. 11-8 Longitudinal sonographic image of normal conic-shaped appendix in 9-year-old girl.

lymphatic tissue, is thought to play a specialized role in the immune system.

Obstruction of the appendiceal lumen usually precludes appendicitis. This obstruction can be caused by several different diseases, including lymphoid follicle hyperplasia, **fecalith** (a hard, impacted mass of feces), foreign bodies, seeds, or parasites. An obstruction to the proximal lumen of the appendix inhibits the drainage of mucous secretions from the walls of the appendix, which eventually causes distension in the distal appendiceal lumen. This distension allows for bacterial invasion and edema to the wall of the appendix and finally results in inflammation and pain.

Some cases of appendicitis can occur without obstruction. These cases begin with direct mucosal ulceration caused by a buildup of mucus within the appendix, sometimes called a *mucocele*,[5] which then leads to bacterial invasion and resultant appendicitis.[3] Regardless of the cause of appendicitis, the patient must seek immediate medical attention. If the patient does not have symptoms, chooses to ignore the symptoms, or cannot communicate their symptoms (e.g., infants and young children), failure to receive medical attention within 36 hours will likely result in rupture of the appendix.

A ruptured appendix places the patient at much greater risk for postsurgical complications. Rupture causes the bacteria-filled mucus to spill into the **peritoneum** and can lead to diffuse **peritonitis** or abscess formation.[3] When the appendix has ruptured, sonographic visualization is much more difficult because the lumen is no longer distended and the anatomy is distorted by surrounding inflammation and adjacent abscess.[5]

Clinical Presentation

The first classic symptom of appendicitis is periumbilical pain, followed by nausea, right lower quadrant pain, and subsequent vomiting with fever.[3] Fifty percent of adult cases have all of these symptoms.[3] Other adult cases, and many pediatric cases, may have more inconspicuous symptoms, such as irritability, lethargy, abdominal pain, anorexia, fever, or diarrhea, which make diagnosis more of a challenge. The most important clinical finding is right lower quadrant pain with palpation. Physicians also use the quick release method to rule out appendicitis. The quick release is performed by applying pressure with the fingertips directly over the area of the appendix and then quickly letting go. With appendicitis, the patient will usually have rebound tenderness (**McBurney's sign**) associated with peritoneal irritation.[2] Although an elevated white blood cell (WBC) count ($>10,000/mm^3$) can be an indicator for appendicitis, the accuracy of this test alone is limited.[3] Some painful gynecologic conditions, such as ovarian cyst, can mimic appendicitis, so a pelvic examination or ultrasound in women with suspicious right lower quadrant pain is common.[2] A pregnancy test for all women of childbearing age is also common to rule out ectopic pregnancy.

Sonographic Findings

Graded-compression sonography is useful in diagnosis with equivocal clinical findings. Graded-compression sonography is a rapid, noninvasive, and inexpensive means of imaging the normal or inflamed appendix.

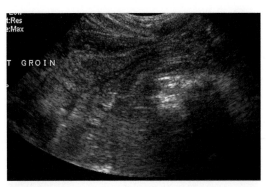

Fig. 11-9 Sonographic image of ascending colon in 4-year-old boy.

The technique requires no patient preparation, and scanning can be performed at the most tender site, which enables correlation of imaging findings with patient symptoms.[6] A high-frequency linear array probe ranging from 7 to 12 MHz is most commonly used. Before scanning, the patient is asked to point with one finger to the point of maximal pain. This technique also helps in identification of the location of an abnormally positioned appendix.[1] Graded compression uses gradual pressure, with the transducer moving in a cephalad to caudad fashion to displace the normal gas-containing bowel loops for visualization of the inflamed appendix. When inflamed, the appendix will not compress.

If the patient is unable to point to a specific area of pain, the sonographer must seek the appendix. Real-time scanning is initiated in the transverse plane and directed toward the cecal tip and the origin of the appendix.[6] Scanning begins laterally in the iliac fossa at the level of the umbilicus. Gradual pressure is applied with the transducer to compress bowel loops and express all gas and fluid contents. The ascending colon is first identified as a gas-filled peristaltic structure with the sonographic appearance of bowel (i.e., an inner echogenic ring surrounded by five concentric bowel wall layers; Fig. 11-9). The ascending colon is scanned caudally to its termination at the cecum. With the transducer in the transverse plane, the cecum is scanned inferiorly to its tip. The normal cecum and terminal ileum are easily compressible with moderate pressure. The terminal ileum is identified as a compressible peristaltic bowel segment adjacent to the cecum. The examination is continued inferiorly with identification of the psoas and iliacus muscles and the external iliac artery and vein.

The examination is considered diagnostic when the psoas muscle and external iliac vessels are identified and

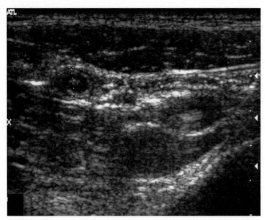

Fig. 11-10 Transverse image of normal appendix in 9-year-old boy. Anteroposterior (AP) diameter is 4.1 mm (normal AP measurement, <7 mm).

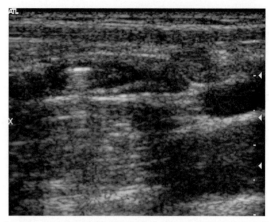

Fig. 11-12 Longitudinal view of normal appendix in same 9-year-old male patient.

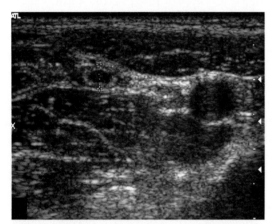

Fig. 11-11 Normal transverse anteroposterior (AP) measurement in same 9-year-old patient shows compression. With compression, AP diameter is 3.5 mm. Note that compression of appendix is not achievable in positive cases of appendicitis.

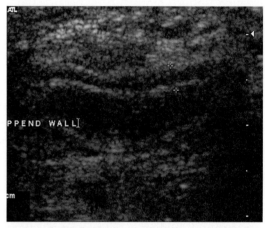

Fig. 11-13 Longitudinal sonographic image of inflamed appendix wall in 18-year-old female patient. Anteroposterior (AP) measurement, 2.7 mm (normal, <2 mm).

when the cecum and terminal ileum can be adequately compressed with the transducer for evaluation of the retrocecal region. Identification of the appendix is not always possible. The appendix originates from the cecal tip but can vary in position. It is most commonly directed medially or caudally but may be retrocecal or lateral to the cecum.[1] The normal appendix, when identified, will appear as a tubular structure with a blind end that measures 6 mm or less in anterior-posterior (AP) dimension from outer wall to outer wall (Figs. 11-10 to 11-12).[1,6] A normal appendix must be identified to rule out appendicitis.

Ultrasound findings in nonperforated appendicitis include a muscular wall thickness greater than 2 mm (Fig. 11-13), an appendiceal diameter (outer wall to

outer wall) greater than 7 mm that does not compress (Fig. 11-14), a "target" sign (bull's-eye appearance) of abnormally thickened bowel wall layers when viewed in the short axis, and sometimes distension or obstruction of the appendiceal lumen accompanied by increased echogenicity (edema) surrounding the appendix. Findings may also include an echogenic shadowing **appendicolith** (Figs. 11-15 to 11-17), pericecal or perivesical free fluid (Fig. 11-18), or increased color Doppler in the wall of the appendix, indicating increased appendiceal perfusion.

Ultrasound findings with a perforated or ruptured appendix may include the target sign with inhomogeneous or missing layers in the wall and with inhomogeneous pericecal or perivesical mass without

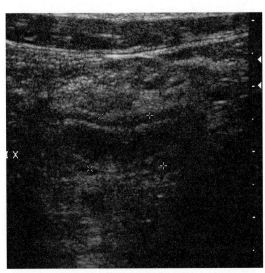

Fig. 11-14 Longitudinal anteroposterior (AP) diameter in same 18-year-old female patient with appendicitis. AP diameter measurement, 8.2 mm (normal, <7 mm).

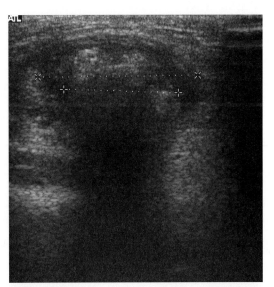

Fig. 11-16 Transverse view of inflamed appendix with 1.7-cm appendicolith.

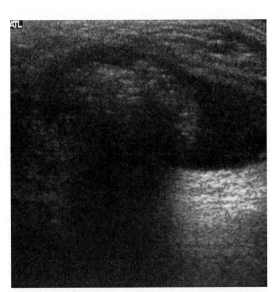

Fig. 11-15 Longitudinal view of inflamed appendix with appendicolith in 4-year-old male patient.

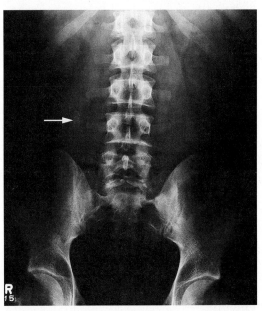

Fig. 11-17 Radiograph of abdomen including kidneys, ureters, and bladder in 20-year-old male patient with appendicitis. Note calcified appendicolith visible in right lower quadrant *(arrow)*.

peristalsis or free fluid in the abdomen.[3] Gangrenous appendicitis may be suggested when sonographic imaging shows a loss of the echogenic submucosal layer and absent color Doppler flow in that segment of the appendix.[6] Periappendiceal abscesses may be found in cases of rupture either before or after appendectomy and generally appear as vague hypoechoic or complex masses (Fig. 11-19). Abscesses are usually successfully drained after appendectomy with a transrectal biopsy guide on an endocavitary transducer. Insertion of the transducer into the rectum allows for adequate visuali-

zation and drainage of the abscess with ultrasound guidance.

A false-negative ultrasound diagnosis is common when nonvisualization of the appendix occurs. Reasons for nonvisualization may include superimposed air or feces, obesity, abdominal wall rigidity or pain, scanning of an uncooperative child, or atypical appendiceal location.[3] In these cases, a CT scan of the appendix may be ordered to confirm the diagnosis before surgery.

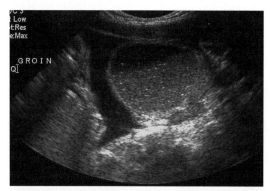

Fig. 11-18 Free fluid (ascites) surrounded by loops of bowel in 4-year-old male patient with appendicitis.

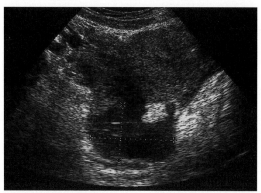

Fig. 11-19 Postappendectomy abscess found in right lower quadrant (adjacent to uterus) of 22-year-old patient with ruptured appendix.

Graded-compression sonography has proven to be of considerable value in the diagnosis of acute appendicitis. A positive finding on sonographic examination speeds diagnosis and therapy in clinically doubtful cases and at the same time reduces the number of negative laparotomy cases.[1]

PYLORIC STENOSIS

Hypertrophic pyloric stenosis is a GI tract disorder common in infancy that can also occur in adults as the result of ulcer or fibrosis at the gastric outlet. The disorder causes projectile vomiting, weight loss, and fluid and electrolyte abnormalities. The problem can usually be diagnosed with clinical symptoms along with manual detection of an enlarged pylorus, described as an olive-sized lump to the right of the stomach. When diagnosis cannot be confirmed with clinical examination, imaging studies, including sonography and fluoroscopy, are appropriate.[7]

Epidemiology

Infantile hypertrophic pyloric stenosis has a rate of occurrence of 3 per 1000 infants[9] and is four times more likely to occur in male infants than in female infants.[7] The symptoms usually begin within 1 to 10 weeks after birth[8]; however, IHPS can occur in infants up to 6 months of age.[5] The etiology of IHPS is unknown, although familial predisposition has shown in 10% of males born after an affected child and 2% of females born after an affected child. To date, no physical markers exist for identification of infants at risk for IHPS, but one study recently linked a hypoplastic or absent **mandibular frenulum** (a normal midline craniofacial structure extending from the lower lip to the lower jaw) in 92% of 25 patients with IHPS.[9]

Anatomy and Pathophysiology

Hypertrophic pyloric stenosis is the result of hypertrophy of the circular musculature that surrounds the pylorus, which causes constriction and obstruction of the gastric outlet.[7] The pylorus is a tubular structure located on the right side of the stomach. It is the sphincter that connects the stomach with the duodenum of the small intestine. The most common position of the pylorus is about 3 cm to the right of the sagittal axis at the level of the first lumbar vertebra (Fig. 11-20).

Clinical Presentation

Pyloric stenosis classically is seen with nonbilious projectile vomiting and, if prolonged, could result in dehydration and **metabolic alkalosis**. Nonprojectile vomiting and **jaundice** may also occur.[7,10] The hypertrophic pylorus can usually be palpated after a feeding and is described as an olive-shaped mass, about 2 cm in diameter, in the right side of the epigastrium, representing the constricted pyloric muscle. If this mass is felt, the diagnosis is confirmed; however, in many cases, the olive-shaped mass cannot be felt, so diagnostic sonography of the pylorus or fluoroscopic **upper gastrointestinal** (UGI) examination is needed to rule out stenosis.

Sonographic Findings

Ultrasonography is the imaging method of choice for pyloric stenosis because it is highly accurate and lacks the ionizing radiation associated with radiologic fluoroscopic procedures, such as UGI.[7] With evaluation for pyloric stenosis, the role of any imaging method is to first identify the pyloric muscle, measure its length and AP wall thickness, and document passage of fluid from the stomach through the pylorus.[7] Plain film

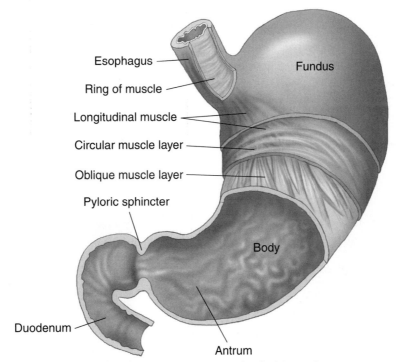

Fig. 11-20 Diagram of pylorus. Pylorus muscle (sphincter) connects antrum of stomach with duodenum of small intestine.

Labels: Esophagus, Ring of muscle, Longitudinal muscle, Circular muscle layer, Oblique muscle layer, Pyloric sphincter, Duodenum, Fundus, Body, Antrum

radiographs or UGI contrast studies can be used; however, ultrasonography is superior in direct visualization of the muscle hypertrophy and the **pyloric channel length**.

Pyloric stenosis can be viewed with real-time imaging of the pylorus muscle preferably 2 to 3 hours after the last meal. A high-frequency linear array probe ranging from 7 to 12 MHz is most commonly used, but in older patients, a 3-MHz to 7-MHz curvilinear probe may be necessary. Patients should undergo scanning in the right posterior oblique (RPO) position if possible. The RPO position helps with visualization of the pylorus with use of the fluid-filled stomach as a scanning window. The location of the pylorus can be identified with scanning in a transverse plain along the lesser curvature of the stomach through the left lobe of the liver just to the right of midline. The pylorus lies inferior and to the right of the antrum of the stomach.[5] If the pylorus is not well visualized, the patient may drink some water for display of the gastric lumen.[5] Gastric peristalsis can be seen in real time after the ingestion of approximately 10 ml of an electrolyte replacement fluid or water. The sonographer should remember to keep a towel handy because the infant is prone to vomiting after ingestion of the fluids. Absent peristalsis and lack of movement of fluid through the pylorus, along with a thickened AP muscle wall and

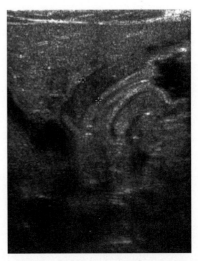

Fig. 11-21 Longitudinal image of stenotic pylorus in 5-week-old male infant. Anteroposterior (AP) wall thickness, 5.1 mm (normal wall thickness, <3.5 mm).

increased pylorus channel length indicate stenosis. Measurements should be taken to document the size of the muscle. An AP muscle wall thickness of 3.5 mm or more (Figs. 11-21 and 11-22) along with a pylorus length of 17 mm or more indicates stenosis. A stenotic pyloric channel resembles the appearance of the cervix in pregnancy and thus is nicknamed the **"cervix sign"** (Figs. 11-23 to 11-25) .

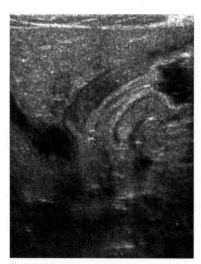

Fig. 11-22 Longitudinal image of pyloric stenosis in same 5-week-old male infant. Pyloric canal length is at upper limits of normal at 1.7 cm (normal, <1.7 cm).

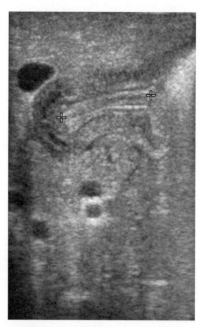

Fig. 11-24 Longitudinal view of pyloric stenosis in 1-month-old male patient. Canal length measured abnormally at 1.9 cm (normal, <1.7 cm).

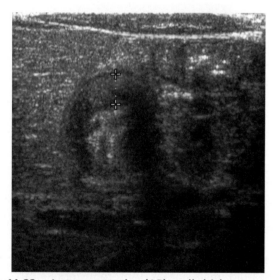

Fig. 11-23 Anteroposterior (AP) wall thickness can be measured in either longitudinal or transverse image of pylorus. Here AP wall thickness is abnormal at 4.3 mm (normal, <3.5 mm).

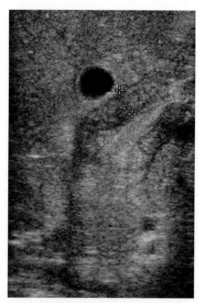

Fig. 11-25 Thickened anteroposterior (AP) wall is shown in same 1-month-old male patient with measurement of 5.3 mm (normal, <3.5 mm).

Pyloric stenosis can be dangerous if not diagnosed within several days of the onset of symptoms. Severe dehydration and biochemical disturbances, such as hypokalemic metabolic alkalosis, occur when the condition is untreated. Patients in whom the hypertrophied pylorus can be reliably palpated by an experienced clinician may not need ultrasound evaluation. The use of ultrasound imaging is best reserved for those cases in which the clinical examination results are negative.[11]

Treatment

Once diagnosis is made, the usual treatment for hypertrophic pyloric stenosis involves fluid replacement therapy followed by the **Fredet-Ramstedt operation**, or

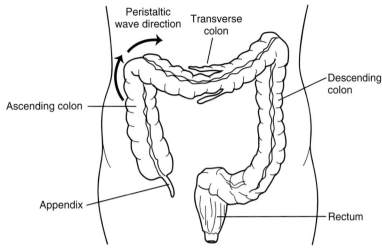

Fig. 11-26 Diagram of colocolic intussusception. Proximal transverse colon is undergoing peristalsis into distal transverse colon.

pyloromyotomy.[7] This surgical procedure is performed with mild anesthesia and involves cutting of the muscle fibers of the gastric outlet to widen the opening. Most patients successfully recover from this procedure without recurrence of the stenosis.

INTUSSUSCEPTION

Intussusception is the telescoping or invagination of a proximal portion of the intestine into a more distal portion, resulting in vascular compromise and subsequent bowel **necrosis** (Fig. 11-26).[8] It is an emergent condition and most commonly affects infants between 5 and 9 months of age but can occur in all age groups.[12] Intussusception is also common in patients with cystic fibrosis, a disease that causes the exocrine glands to produce abnormally thick secretions of mucus that result in chronic cough, frequent foul-smelling stools, and persistent upper respiratory infections.[8]

   Barium enema (BE) is the gold standard for diagnosis of all types of intestinal obstructive processes. This examination involves a rectal infusion of barium sulfate, a radiopaque contrast medium, for diagnosis of obstruction, tumors, or other abnormalities. In children, the procedure is used therapeutically to reduce nonstrangulated intussusception. Recently, however, diagnostic ultrasound is more frequently used as an accurate low-risk screening tool for intussusception when performed by an experienced sonographer and pediatric radiologist.[12]

Epidemiology

The incidence rate of intussusception is 2 to 4 cases per 1000 births, with a 3:2 male predominance ratio.[8] In the United States, the mortality rate is less than 1%, but morbidity increases with delays in diagnosis.[12] Although intussusception is most common in infants 5 to 9 months of age, children with cystic fibrosis may also have intussusception because of **meconium ileus,** an obstruction of the small bowel by viscid stool in the terminal ileum.[8] A seasonal incidence has also been noted, with peaks in the spring, summer, and middle of winter. These periods correspond to peaks in the occurrence of seasonal gastroenteritis and upper respiratory tract infection.[8]

Anatomy and Pathophysiology

Intussusception may involve segments of the small intestine, colon, or terminal ileum and is described as a prolapse of one segment of bowel into the lumen of another segment. It can be ileoileal, colocolic, ileoileocolic, or, most commonly, ileocolic (Fig. 11-27). A specific lead point, which draws the proximal intestine and its mesentery inward, propagating it distally through peristalsis, is identified in only 5% of cases and is most commonly seen in ileoileal intussusception. Lead points are more commonly found in older children and nearly always in adults.[8] A lead point is any intestinal disorder that can cause an intussusception. **Meckel's diverticulum** (an anomalous sac of embryologic origin protruding from the wall of the ileum usually between 30 and 90 cm from the ileocecal sphincter) is the most common lead point, followed by **polyps** and then tumors such as lymphoma.[5,8] The cause of intussusception in patients without a lead point is mostly unknown; however, infantile cases are more common in fat and healthy infants than in thin, undernourished infants.[8]

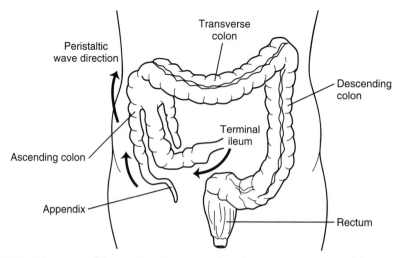

Fig. 11-27 Diagram of ileocolic intussusception (most common type) in ascending colon. Distal ileum of small intestine is being drawn by peristalsis into proximal ascending colon

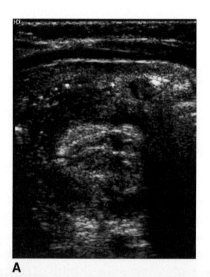

A

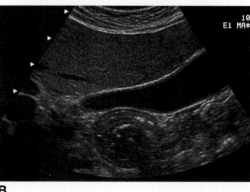

B

Fig. 11-28 **A,** Transverse view (doughnut sign) of ileocolic intussusception in 12-year-old male patient. **B,** Target sign is clearly shown in this patient. (Courtesy GE Medical Systems.)

Clinical Presentation

The most common triad of clinical symptoms in patients with intussusception includes crampy abdominal pain, vomiting, and bloody stools.[12] Patients may also have lethargy, fever, diarrhea, abdominal distension, irritability, or right upper quadrant mass. A rectal examination, with testing for occult blood or mucus, is an important part of the evaluation and frequently has positive results.[12] Laboratory testing may also reveal dehydration, anemia, or leukocytosis.[8] The peristaltic nature of the intestine may cause the abdominal pain to occur in spasms. Careful palpation during physical examination will reveal an ill-defined or sausage-shaped mass in the right upper quadrant in 85% of patients.[8]

Sonographic Findings

The patient should undergo scanning in the supine position. A complete survey of the upper abdomen should always be performed, followed by an examination of the lower abdomen, with focus on the bowel with a 5-MHz to 7-MHz linear or curved array transducer.[4] The classic sonographic appearance of intussusception includes the "doughnut," or target, sign and the "pseudokidney," or "sandwich," sign.[13] A doughnut sign, a hypoechoic rim of homogenous thickness and contour with a central hyperechoic core, is seen in a transverse view of intussusception (Fig. 11-28, *A* and *B*). A hyperechoic tubular center is seen longitudinally covered by a hypoechoic ring 3 to 5 cm in diameter, resembling a pseudokidney (Fig. 11-29).[12] Free peritoneal fluid or **ascites** is not an uncommon finding with uncomplicated intussusception.[4] Color flow Doppler

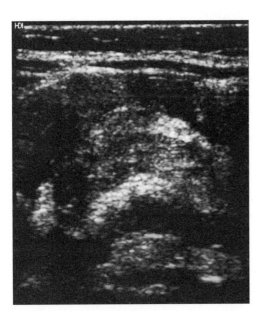

Fig. 11-29 Sagittal view of ileocolic intussusception (resembles pseudokidney).

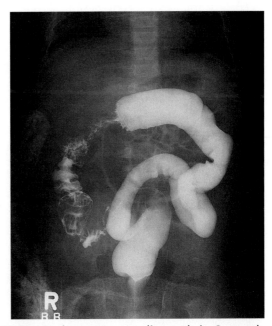

Fig. 11-30 Barium enema radiograph in 8-month-old male shows ileocolic intussusception that would not reduce on three attempts. Patient was sent for surgical reduction.

can be used to help determine whether the involved bowel should be reduced (cured with retrograde fluid pressure) or surgically resected. Absent blood flow in the bowel walls means that the bowel has probably necrosed and will need surgical resection. If adequate color flow is seen to all areas of the telescoping bowel, the chances are better for a reduction.[4]

Diagnostic fluoroscopic enema studies have remained the imaging method of choice for intussusception for both diagnosis and therapy in patients with stable conditions.[8] However, in recent years, increasing numbers of radiologists are relying on sonography for diagnosis or exclusion of intussusception. The quality of the study and its interpretation are operator dependent, although sonographic diagnosis in positive cases has shown an accuracy rate of 100%.[8] Sonography is best used as a diagnostic tool of exclusion in patients with a lower suspicion of intussusception.

Treatment

The diagnostic BE is therapeutic in approximately 80% of cases because of the retrograde flow of barium through the large intestine. As the barium fills and expands the colon, the pressure can spontaneously reduce the intussusception (Figs. 11-30 to 11-32). In instances in which the enema fails to reduce the intussusception, the reduction may be attempted a second or third time with air or **hydrostatic enema**, or if the patient's condition is unstable, surgery can provide a mode for manual reduction.[8] Patients in whom a lead point is suspected or diagnosed are not candidates for radiologic enema

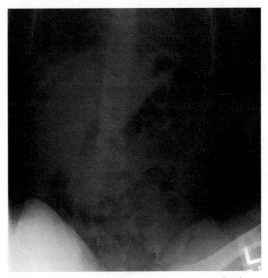

Fig. 11-31 Preliminary barium enema (BE) scout radiograph on 2-year-old female patient. Mass effect is seen outlined by air in right side of abdomen. Mass was found to be intussusception at hepatic flexure, which was successfully reduced during BE examination (see Fig. 11-32).

reduction and would directly undergo surgery.[12] The overall mortality rate of intussusception is less than 1%. Recurrence after nonoperative reduction is 5% to 10% and after surgical reduction is 1% to 4%. The risk of postoperative adhesive small bowel obstruction after nonoperative reduction is 0% and after operative reduction is up to 7%.[8] Without treatment, the patient may have complications, such as bowel obstruction, perforation, peritonitis, and vascular compromise, which could lead to edema or gangrene of the bowel.[5]

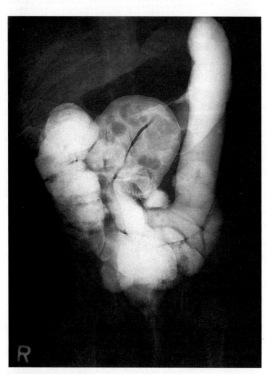

Fig. 11-32 Postreduction radiograph on same 2-year-old female patient.

SUMMARY

The confirmation of GI disease such as appendicitis, pyloric stenosis, and intussusception by sonography requires skill on the part of the sonographer and radiologist. These skills can easily be acquired through education and experience. Sonography does have limitations in imaging of the GI tract, and other methods such as fluoroscopic radiography or CT scan may be needed to follow up nondiagnostic or questionable ultrasound findings. Table 11-1 summarizes the symptoms and sonographic findings in positive cases of GI disease.

CLINICAL SCENARIO—DIAGNOSIS

◼ The abdominal sonogram was performed by the sonographer while the pediatric surgeon and pediatric radiologist observed. Although the infant had eaten 4 hours previously, the stomach was still full of fluid. No additional fluid was needed for the diagnosis. The radiology report indicated that the pyloric muscle was thickened. Single-wall thickness was measured at 6 mm, with a channel length of 2.1 cm. These findings were compatible with IHPS. Surgery was scheduled and performed the same afternoon.

Table 11-1	*Pathology of Gastrointestinal System*	
Pathology	**Symptoms**	**Sonographic Findings**
Appendicitis	Right lower quadrant pain, nausea and vomiting, fever	Muscle wall, >2 mm; AP thickness of appendix (outer to outer), >7 mm
Pyloric stenosis	Projectile vomiting, weight loss, dehydration, right upper quadrant mass	AP muscle wall, >3.5 mm; pyloric channel length, >17 mm
Intussusception	Abdominal pain, vomiting, bloody stool, lethargy, fever, diarrhea, abdomen distension, right upper quadrant mass	Doughnut or target sign (transverse); pseudokidney or sandwich sign ascites

CASE STUDIES FOR DISCUSSION

1. A 22-year-old woman presents to the emergency department (ED) with right lower quadrant pain and fever. The results of a urine pregnancy test are positive. The ED physician orders an appendix and pregnancy ultrasound examination. The endovaginal ultrasound reveals a viable 10-week and 2-day intrauterine pregnancy and a moderate amount of fluid in the cul-de-sac. The ultrasound of the appendix reveals an inflamed appendix with a corresponding AP muscle wall thickness of 4.2 mm. The patient undergoes surgery for immediate appendectomy. The surgeon's notes indicate a ruptured appendix. Three days later, the patient returns to the ED with vaginal bleeding and cramping. The ultrasound notes a 10-week and 6-day gestation with a heart rate of 152 beats per minute and a **complex mass** and free fluid in the right adnexa. Nine days later the patient returns to the operating room (OR) for a dilation and curettage (D&C) for missed abortion. The surgeon requested ultrasound assistance in the OR. Transabdominal scanning revealed a missed abortion, and a D&C was performed (Figs. 11-33 to 11-35). The endocavitary probe with needle guide was then used to guide drainage of the right adnexal complex mass (Fig. 11-36). What is the most likely origin of the complex mass?

2. A 3300-g male infant is born after a full-term uneventful pregnancy. His parents are healthy and have no history of **icteric** episodes. The infant is bottle fed, and jaundice does not develop during the first 10 days. At 4 weeks old, the infant is admitted to the hospital for projectile vomiting. He then weighs 3950 g and is mildly icteric. Serum bilirubin is 165 μmol/L and is entirely unconjugated. An

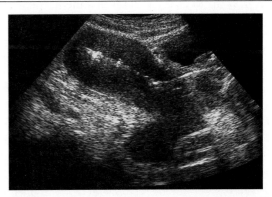

Fig. 11-34 Image of sagittal uterus during surgical dilation and curettage. Note echogenic reflection of surgeon's tool in endometrium.

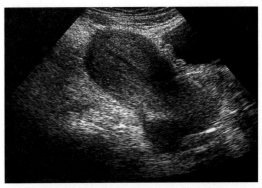

Fig. 11-35 Image of normal endometrium after dilation and curettage.

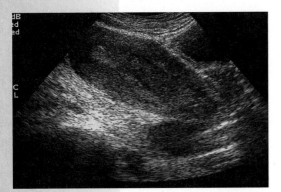

Fig. 11-33 Missed abortion with right adnexal complex mass. Note thickened complex endometrium that shows remaining products of conception.

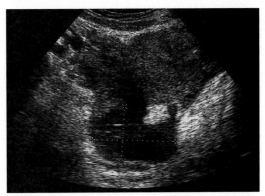

Fig. 11-36 With insertion of endocavitary probe with biopsy guide into rectum, surgeon successfully drained the complex mass.

CASE STUDIES FOR DISCUSSION—*cont'd*

abdominal ultrasound is ordered and reveals the finding in Fig. 11-37. What is the most likely diagnosis?

3. An 8-month-old male infant is brought to the office for a well-child visit. The infant's mother incidentally notes that he had several episodes of vomiting since the previous night, without fever or diarrhea. On physician examination, the infant is observed to be listless, with a temperature of 100.4° F, otitis media on the right side, and moderate dehydration. Findings on abdominal examination are unremarkable. A rectal examination is not performed. The infant is sent to the ED where he is aggressively rehydrated and observed. Results of laboratory tests are not specific. After several hours of rehydration, the child's condition is unchanged and he passes a large, grossly bloody stool. An abdominal radiograph is ordered but is unremarkable. A barium enema is ordered for diagnosis

and therapeutic purposes (Fig. 11-38). What is the most likely diagnosis?

4. A 7-year-old girl is seen in the ED with 2 days of vomiting, right lower quadrant pain, and fever. The white blood cell count is elevated. The physician notes rebound tenderness (McBurney's sign) on the right side. What is the most likely diagnosis?

5. A 5-week-old male infant is seen by the pediatrician with symptoms that include 3 days of nausea, vomiting, and lethargy. The baby's abdomen is taunt and slightly distended, and a small amount of blood is present in the stool. What is the most likely reason for this baby's condition?

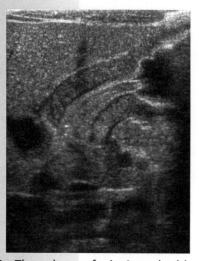

Fig. 11-37 The pylorus of a in 4-week-old male.

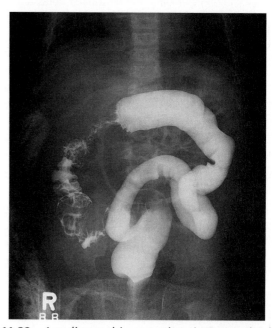

Fig. 11-38 A radiographic procedure in 8-month-old male.

STUDY QUESTIONS

1. A 7-week-old male infant is seen with projectile vomiting for 3 days. He is dehydrated and, on physical examination, has an olive-shaped mass in the right upper quadrant. What is the most likely diagnosis?
   a. appendicitis
   b. intussusception
   c. pyloric stenosis
   d. the flu

2. A 6-month-old, chubby female infant is seen with lethargy, fever, and diarrhea. A small amount of blood is found in the stool. What is the most likely diagnosis?
   a. pyloric stenosis
   b. intussusception
   c. appendicitis
   d. cystic fibrosis

3. A 31-year-old woman is seen with right lower quadrant pain, fever, and an elevated WBC count. What is the most likely diagnosis?
   a. gallstones
   b. ovarian cyst
   c. ectopic pregnancy
   d. appendicitis

4. A 50-year-old man with a history of stomach ulcers is seen with weight loss and projectile vomiting. What is the most likely diagnosis?
   a. gallstones
   b. pyloric stenosis
   c. appendicitis
   d. intussusception

5. A 5-year-old boy is seen with periumbilical pain, nausea, and fever. Both of his parents had surgical appendectomies as children. What is the most likely diagnosis?
   a. intussusception
   b. hepatitis
   c. meningitis
   d. appendicitis

6. A 10-year-old girl with cystic fibrosis is seen with abdominal pain, vomiting, and lethargy. A sausage-shaped mass is palpated in the right upper quadrant. What is the most likely diagnosis?
   a. appendicitis
   b. pyloric stenosis
   c. intussusception
   d. hepatitis

7. A 3-week-old male infant with an absent mandibular frenulum is seen with projectile vomiting. What is the most likely diagnosis?
   a. pyloric stenosis
   b. intussusception
   c. appendicitis
   d. the flu

8. A pregnant 23-year-old patient is seen with right lower quadrant pain and vomiting. The WBC count is elevated. What is the most likely diagnosis?
   a. ectopic pregnancy
   b. appendicitis
   c. right ovarian cyst
   d. pyloric stenosis

9. A 63-year-old man with a history of diverticulitis is seen with abdominal pain and bloody stools. He is lethargic with fever and diarrhea. What is the most likely diagnosis?
   a. appendicitis
   b. gallstones
   c. intussusception
   d. pyloric stenosis

10. A 45-year-old woman with a history of fibrosis and stomach ulcers is seen with vomiting, weight loss, and electrolyte imbalance. What is the most likely diagnosis?
    a. pyloric stenosis
    b. intussusception
    c. gallstones
    d. appendicitis

REFERENCES

1. Hagen-Ansert S: Textbook of diagnostic ultrasonography, St Louis, 2001, Mosby.
2. Yacoe ME, Jeffrey RB Jr: Sonography of appendicitis and diverticulitis, Radiol Clin North Am 32:899-912, 1994.
3. Hardin DM Jr: Acute appendicitis: review and update, Am Fam Physician 60:2027-2034, 1999.
4. Kawamura DM: Diagnostic medical sonography: abdomen, Philadelphia, 1992, JB Lippincott.
5. McAlister WH: Intussusception: even Hippocrates did not standardize his technique of enema reduction, Radiology 206:595-598, 1998.

6. Rothrock SG, Pagane J: Acute appendicitis in children: emergency department diagnosis and management, *Ann Emerg Med* 36:39-51, 2001.

7. Irish MS et al: The approach to common abdominal diagnosis in infants and children, *Pediatr Clin North Am* 45:729-772, 1988.

8. De Felice C et al: Hypoplastic or absent mandibular frenulum: a new predictive sign of infantile hypertrophic pyloric stenosis, *J Pediatr* 136:408-410, 2000.

9. Birnbaum BA, Jeffrey RB Jr: CT and sonographic evaluation of acute right lower quadrant abdominal pain, *AJR Am J Roentgenol* 170:361-371, 1998.

10. Deluca SA: Hypertrophic pyloric stenosis, *Am Fam Physician* 47:1771-1773, 1993.

11. Trioche P et al: Jaundice with hypertrophic pyloric stenosis as an early manifestation of Gilbert syndrome, *Arch Dis Child* 81:301-303, 1999.

12. Godbole P, Sprigg A, Dickson JA et al: Ultrasound compared with clinical examination in infantile hypertrophic pyloric stenosis, *Arch Dis Child* 75:335-337, 1996.

13. Winslow BT, Westfall JM, Nicholas RA: Intussusception, *Am Fam Physician* 54:213-217, 1996.

Retroperitoneum

CHARLOTTE HENNINGSEN

CLINICAL SCENARIO

■ A 66-year-old man with lung cancer is seen for a renal ultrasound for increased blood urea nitrogen and creatinine values. The kidneys measure within normal limits without evidence of hydronephrosis or neoplasm. Superior to both kidneys are large adrenal masses (Fig. 12-1) that are confirmed with computed tomography (CT). Pleural fluid is also noted. An increase in the size of the adrenal glands is noted when compared with a CT performed 3 months previously. What is the most likely diagnosis?

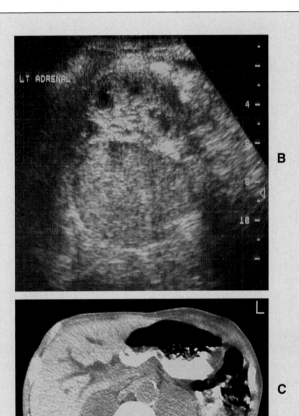

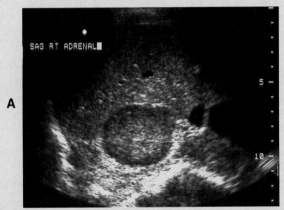

Fig. 12-1 A, Right and, **B,** left adrenal glands are identified. **C,** Enlargement of glands is confirmed.

OBJECTIVES

■ Define the application of ultrasound in the imaging of the anatomy and pathology of the retroperitoneum.

■ Describe the ultrasound appearance of abdominal lymphadenopathy.

■ List malignant and benign tumors of the adrenal gland.

■ Identify risk factors and symptoms associated with adrenal gland neoplasms.

■ Describe the ultrasound findings associated with retroperitoneal fibrosis.

Except for ultrasound imaging of the kidneys, imaging of the retroperitoneum is often accomplished with other imaging methods, such as computed tomography (CT) or magnetic resonance imaging (MRI). Adequate sonographic evaluation of the retroperitoneum is difficult because of the significant amount of gastrointestinal tract and the subsequent bowel gas that creates excessive artifact in that region. Sonographers may identify lymphadenopathy, adrenal masses, and other retroperitoneal lesions incidentally, or they may be asked to follow a process that has already been diagnosed with another method. Therefore, an understanding of the anatomy and associated pathologies that may be encountered is important.

LYMPHADENOPATHY

The abdominal lymph node chain follows the course of the aorta and iliac arteries. These retroperitoneal lymph nodes are typically less than 1 cm and are not visualized with ultrasound.[1] Lymph nodes may enlarge in the presence of infection or malignant disease, with **lymphoma** the most common disease process associated with retroperitoneal **adenopathy**. Ultrasound may be used in the detection of lymphadenopathy and may also be used to guide biopsy for the determination of the etiology of the enlarged nodes for implementation of appropriate treatment.

Sonographic Findings

Abnormal lymph nodes (Fig. 12-2) are round or oval, measure greater than 1 cm, and have low-amplitude echogenicity.[2] Transducer pressure may be used to displace bowel gas. A mantle of lymph nodes in the paraspinal region may anteriorly displace the aorta, referred to as a "floating" aorta, or multiple enlarged nodes may surround and "sandwich" the aorta and inferior vena cava (IVC).

ADRENAL MASS

Ultrasound imaging is infrequently used as the primary diagnostic imaging method of the adrenal gland, except in pediatric patients (see Chapter 9). Sonography may be used to follow an adrenal mass, or an adrenal mass may be an incidental finding and generically referred to as an *incidentaloma*. The most common adrenal tumors include adrenal adenoma, pheochromocytoma, adrenocortical carcinoma, and adrenal metastasis. Lesions of the adrenal gland less commonly include hydatid cyst, endothelial cyst, hemangioma, ganglioneuroma, angiosarcoma, and myelolipoma.[3]

Adrenal Cyst

Adrenal cysts are rare asymptomatic lesions that may be unilateral or bilateral. An adrenal cyst may be of endothelial or epithelial origin or may be characterized as a pseudocyst as a result of infection or hemorrhage.

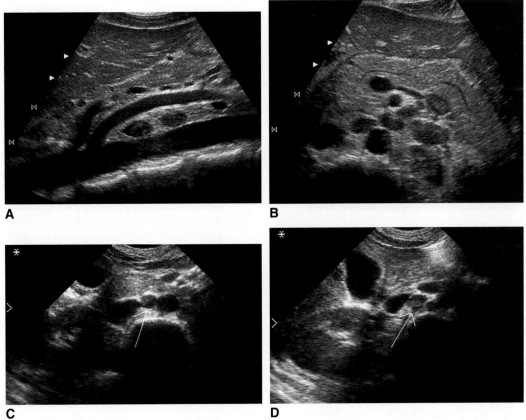

Fig. 12-2 Multiple enlarged abdominal lymph nodes are identified in, **A,** longitudinal and, **B,** transverse images. **C** and **D,** A few enlarged lymph nodes are identified in patient. (**A** and **B** Courtesy GE Medical Systems.)

The infectious adrenal cyst may be parasitic, occurring most commonly in patients infected with *Echinococcus granulosus*.[2]

Clinical signs, when evident, include palpable mass or pain, which may relate to the compression of surrounding organs.[4] In addition, cysts may become infected, link with an endocrinologic dysfunction, or rupture, leading to anemia and shock. Symptoms may be specific to the cyst origin and cause nausea and vomiting or back pain.

Sonographic Findings. Simple adrenal cysts (Fig. 12-3) appear anechoic and thin walled, with acoustic enhancement. Pseudocysts and hemorrhagic cysts may have thick walls that contain calcifications, septations, or low-level echoes. Cysts that do not meet the sonographic criteria of a simple cyst should be followed with other imaging methods or with interventional or surgical correlation.[5]

Pheochromocytoma

Pheochromocytoma is a rare catecholamine-secreting tumor that occurs in approximately 1:1000 patients

with hypertension.[6] Pheochromocytoma arises from the medullary region of the adrenal gland. It is usually a benign lesion, although approximately 10% have been reported to be malignant.[7] When the condition is symptomatic, hypertension is the most common symptom. Patients may also have sweating, palpitations, and headache. Laboratory screening tests for pheochromocytoma include a 24-hour urinary **metanephrine, vanillylmandelic acid,** or **catecholamine** assessment.[8]

Sonographic Findings. Pheochromocytomas are usually solitary solid tumors that occur most frequently in the right adrenal gland. These tumors are fairly easy to detect with ultrasound because of their large size. The tumors are usually homogeneous masses (Fig. 12-4), although they may appear heterogeneous and complex and contain calcifications.[2]

Adrenal Cortical Disease

Benign adrenal **neoplasms** that arise from the adrenal cortex include adrenal adenomas and myelolipomas. Adrenal adenomas (Fig. 12-5) may be functioning tumors and associated with **Cushing's syndrome** or

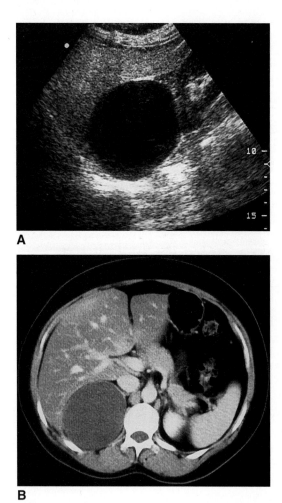

A

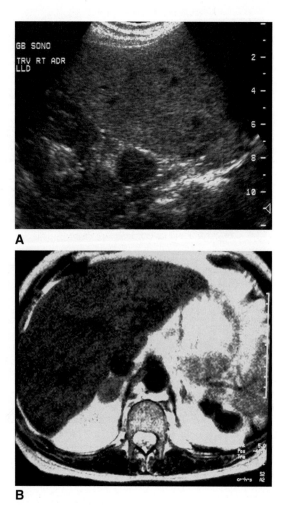

A

B

Fig. 12-3 Adrenal cyst. **A,** Sagittal sonogram shows large, well-defined anechoic cyst with through transmission. **B,** Computed tomography shows low attenuation lesion in right adrenal gland.

B

Fig. 12-5 **A,** Ultrasound and, **B,** magnetic resonance imaging show adrenal mass consistent with adrenal adenoma.

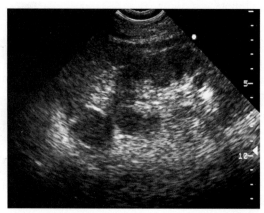

Fig. 12-4 Left adrenal mass in 44-year-old woman with hypertension. Ultrasound findings are consistent with pheochromocytoma.

Conn's syndrome, or they may be nonfunctioning and discovered incidentally or at autopsy. An adrenal adenoma is found sonographically to be a round, small, solid mass (Fig. 12-6), although differentiation of adrenal neoplasm from adrenal **hyperplasia** may be difficult. On follow-up examination, the lack of an increase in size of a neoplasm or the lack of a change in echogenicity suggests a benign condition.[9] Ultrasound or CT may be used in the follow-up of these lesions.

Adrenal myelolipomas are rare benign neoplasms that are composed of fat and elements of bone marrow. These neoplasms are usually asymptomatic nonfunctioning tumors that are discovered incidentally, although symptoms may occur with large tumors from pressure, hemorrhage, and necrosis. Because of the fatty nature of this mass, the sonographic finding associated with myelolipoma (Fig. 12-7) is that of an echogenic lesion.[10]

Adrenocortical carcinoma is a rare primary malignant disease of the adrenal gland that may be functioning or

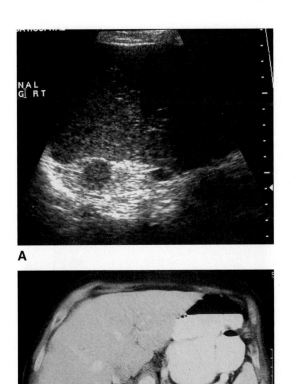

A

B

Fig 12-6 **A,** Homogeneous adrenal mass, identified in 84-year-old woman, was also shown on computed tomography **(B)** and was consistent with benign adenoma.

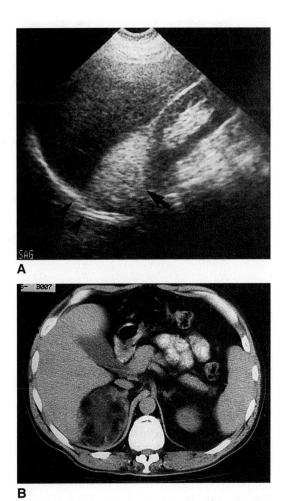

A

B

Fig 12-7 Myelolipoma. **A,** Sagittal sonogram shows large echogenic adrenal mass *(arrows)* with apparent diaphragmatic disruption *(arrowheads)* as result of propagation speed artifact. **B,** Confirmatory computed tomography shows presence of fat within right adrenal mass.

nonfunctioning. Symptoms are related to the functional status of the tumor and may include Cushing's syndrome, **virilization**/feminization, **precocious puberty,** and Conn's syndrome.[2] Patients who are seen at a late stage may also have pain and a palpable mass at the time of diagnosis. The sonographic findings depend on the size of the mass. Smaller neoplasms appear homogeneous, and larger lesions may show mixed echogenicity (Fig. 12-8) because of hemorrhage and necrosis. Masses may also contain calcifications. The size of the lesion also relates to the risk of malignant disease, with adrenal masses greater than 6 cm at increased risk for malignant disease.[8]

Metastatic disease to the adrenal glands occurs in patients with a primary malignant disease. Lung, breast, melanoma, kidney, thyroid, and colon cancers are the most common primary malignant diseases to metastasize to the adrenal gland. The adrenal lesions may be unilateral or bilateral and may be clinically silent. The sonographic findings (Fig. 12-9) are consistent with a solid mass of variable size, with mixed echogenicity when hemorrhage or necrosis is present.[2]

RETROPERITONEAL FIBROSIS

Retroperitoneal fibrosis is a disease that is characterized by a bulky mass of fibrous tissue. It is usually idiopathic, although it has also been associated with malignant disease, aneurysm, and **methysergide** usage.[1,2] Retroperitoneal fibrosis may envelop the aorta, IVC, and ureters, with resultant hydronephrosis. Symptoms include flank and back pain, weight loss, nausea and vomiting, and **malaise.**

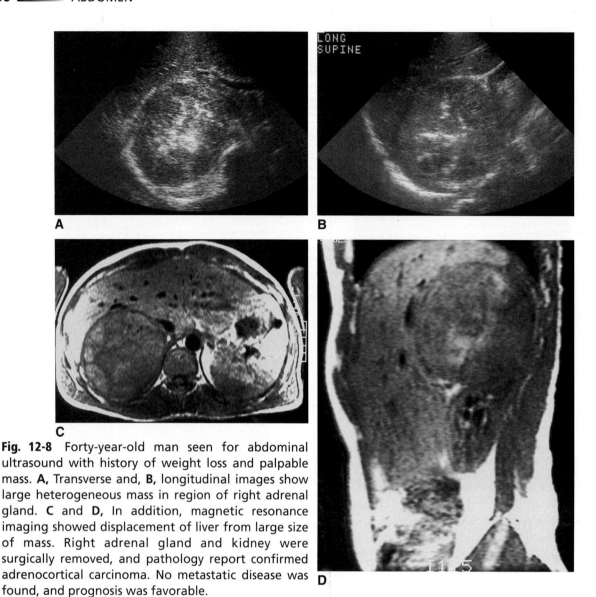

Fig. 12-8 Forty-year-old man seen for abdominal ultrasound with history of weight loss and palpable mass. **A,** Transverse and, **B,** longitudinal images show large heterogeneous mass in region of right adrenal gland. **C** and **D,** In addition, magnetic resonance imaging showed displacement of liver from large size of mass. Right adrenal gland and kidney were surgically removed, and pathology report confirmed adrenocortical carcinoma. No metastatic disease was found, and prognosis was favorable.

Sonographic Findings

Ultrasound examination may show a fibrous mass surrounding the aorta and IVC (Fig. 12-10). Associated hydronephrosis may also be identified. If retroperitoneal fibrosis is suspected, CT is the imaging method of choice.[2]

Table 12-1 is a summary of the pathology, symptoms, and sonographic findings of lesions of the adrenal gland.

SUMMARY

Sonographic imaging of the retroperitoneum is limited; however, ultrasound may be used to follow pathology or may provide an incidental finding. In addition to the pathology discussed in this chapter, a variety of benign and malignant primary tumors of the retroperitoneum, although rare, exists and includes lipoma, leiomyosarcoma, fibrosarcoma, mesothelioma, and teratoma. The sonographic appearances are often nonspecific, and other diagnostic procedures may be used to ascertain the specific diagnosis so that an appropriate treatment plan can be formulated.

CLINICAL SCENARIO—DIAGNOSIS

■ The history of lung cancer plus the increasing size of the adrenal masses suggest metastatic disease. Lymphadenopathy is also identified in the most current imaging study.

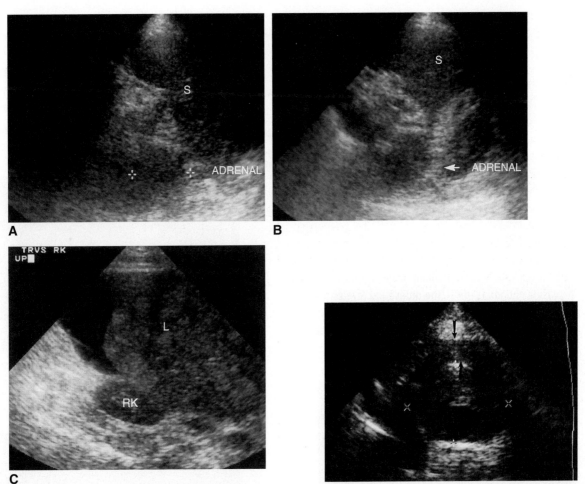

Fig. 12-9 A and **B,** Ill-defined mass demonstrated in area of adrenal gland identified in patient with **(C),** metastatic liver disease. *L,* Liver, *RK,* right kidney; *S,* spleen.

Fig. 12-10 Retroperitoneal fibrosis. Transverse scan shows aneurysm with thin layer *(arrows)* of fibrous tissue, anterior and adjacent to aortic wall.

Table 12-1	*Lesions of Adrenal Gland*	
Pathology	**Symptoms**	**Sonographic Findings**
Adrenal cyst	Usually asymptomatic	Anechoic, round, thin-walled, posterior enhancement
Pheochromocytoma	Asymptomatic, hypertension, sweating, palpitations, headache	Solid, homogeneous
Adrenal adenoma	Asymptomatic, Conn's syndrome or Cushing's syndrome	Solid, round, small
Adrenal myelolipoma	Usually asymptomatic	Solid, echogenic
Adrenocortical carcinoma	Pain, palpable mass, Cushing's syndrome, virilization, feminization, precocious puberty, Conn's syndrome	Small lesions: homogeneous; large lesions: mixed echogenicity

CASE STUDIES FOR DISCUSSION

1. A 42-year-old woman is seen for a right upper quadrant (RUQ) ultrasound for RUQ pain. The ultrasound results are unremarkable except for the finding in Fig. 12-11. What is the most likely diagnosis?

2. A 26-year-old woman with a 2-year history of intermittent hypertension is seen for a renal ultrasound. A 24-hour urine collection also reveals increased catecholamine values. The mass identified in Fig. 12-12 measures 4.4 × 4.3 × 3.8 cm. What is the most likely diagnosis?

3. An 18-month-old female is seen with the phenotypic appearance of Cushing's syndrome and increased facial hair. A right upper quadrant ultrasound examination is ordered to rule out abdominal mass because of the increasing abdominal girth. The ultrasound reveals a small homogeneous mass that measures less than 2 cm in greatest diameter superior to the right kidney, as seen in Fig. 12-13. What is the most likely diagnosis?

4. An 89-year-old woman with a history of unexplained weight loss is seen for an abdominal ultrasound. The ultrasound reveals the multiple ovoid lesions identified in Fig. 12-14. What is the most likely diagnosis?

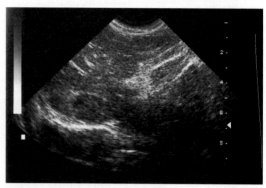

Fig. 12-13 Homogeneous mass is identified superior to right kidney.

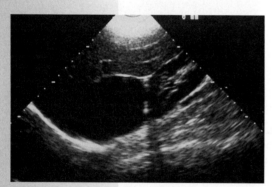

Fig. 12-11 Anechoic lesion is identified superior to right kidney.

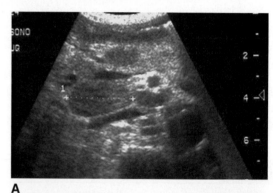

A

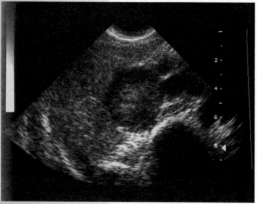

Fig. 12-12 Solid mass is identified in area of adrenal gland.

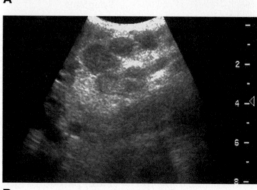

B

Fig. 12-14 Multiple oval and round lesions are identified in, **A**, transverse and, **B**, longitudinal planes.

---

5. A 74-year-old woman is seen for a renal ultrasound because of renal failure. Lung cancer and metastatic disease to the ribs were diagnosed 6 months previously. The renal ultrasound reveals a normal right kidney and a left kidney that is decreased in size. A pleural effusion is also noted on the right side. An approximately 2-cm hypoechoic mass is shown superior to the left kidney, as seen in Fig. 12-15. This is suggestive of what diagnosis?

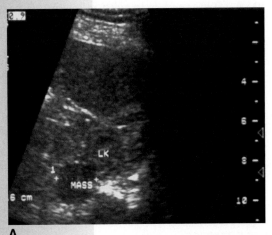 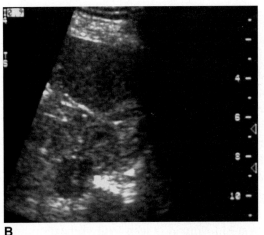

A   **B**

Fig. 12-15 Mass is identified superior and medial to left kidney with **(A)** and without **(B)** calipers.

STUDY QUESTIONS

1. A patient is seen with a persistent headache. Physical examination reveals hypertension, and laboratory tests reveal increased catecholamine values. This is most suggestive of which of the following?
   a. adrenal adenoma
   b. adrenal carcinoma
   c. adrenal cyst
   d. adrenal myelolipoma
   e. pheochromocytoma

2. A patient with a history of pancreatic cancer with liver metastasis is seen for a follow-up ultrasound examination. The ultrasound reveals progression of the liver involvement. In addition, multiple ovoid hypoechoic lesions are identified around the aorta and IVC. These additional findings are consistent with which of the following?
   a. incidentaloma
   b. lymphadenopathy
   c. lymphoma
   d. pseudocysts
   e. retroperitoneal fibrosis

3. A 58-year-old woman is seen with flank pain and loss of appetite. An ultrasound of the abdomen reveals bilateral hydronephrosis and an echogenic mass surrounding the aorta and IVC. This would be most consistent with which of the following?
   a. lymphadenopathy
   b. lymphoma
   c. myelolipoma
   d. pheochromocytoma
   e. retroperitoneal fibrosis

4. A 32-year-old woman is seen for an RUQ ultrasound to rule out gallstones. The sonographer notes a 2-cm, thin-walled, round anechoic lesion at the superior aspect of the right kidney. This is most likely which of the following?
   a. adrenal adenoma
   b. adrenal cyst
   c. adrenocortical carcinoma
   d. lymphadenopathy
   e. pseudocyst

5. A 66-year-old woman is seen with back pain and a history of aneurysm. An ultrasound of the aorta

reveals a dilated aorta enveloped by an echogenic mass. Hydronephrosis is also noted incidentally. The most likely diagnosis is:
a. aortic aneurysm
b. lymphadenopathy
c. metastasis
d. retroperitoneal fibrosis
e. retroperitoneal lipoma

6. A 70-year-old man with a history of carcinoma of the lung is seen for ultrasound. The patient has malaise and weight loss. An abdominal ultrasound is ordered and identifies mild ascites. In addition, bilateral solid masses are noted superior to the kidneys. This is suggestive of which of the following?
a. adrenal adenomas
b. adrenal hyperplasia
c. adrenal metastasis
d. lymphadenopathy
e. pheochromocytomas

7. A 42-year-old woman is seen with virilization and abdominal pain. Ultrasound examination of the abdomen reveals a 7.5-cm adrenal mass that is complex, with areas of calcification and necrosis. This would be most consistent with which of the following?
a. adrenal adenoma
b. adrenal hyperplasia
c. adrenal metastasis
d. adrenocortical carcinoma
e. pheochromocytoma

8. A 50-year-old man is seen by his clinician with palpitations and headaches. Clinical evaluation reveals hypertension and increased vanillylmandelic acid values on 24-hour urine collection. Ultrasound examination reveals an enlarged homogeneous right adrenal gland. This is most consistent with which of the following?
a. adrenal adenoma
b. adrenal carcinoma
c. adrenal hyperplasia
d. adrenal myelolipoma
e. pheochromocytoma

9. A 67-year-old man is seen with a history of lymphoma. Ultrasound reveals multiple oval hypoechoic

lesions surrounding the abdominal aorta. This would be consistent with which of the following?
a. incidentaloma
b. lymphadenopathy
c. pseudocyst formation
d. retroperitoneal fibrosis
e. retroperitoneal fibroma

10. A 60-year-old man with a history of vague flank or back pain is seen for renal ultrasound. The ultrasound reveals a large renal cyst causing mild hydronephrosis on the right kidney. Incidentally noted are bilateral round lesions superior to both kidneys that are anechoic and thin walled. This is consistent with which of the following?
a. adrenal adenomas
b. adrenal cysts
c. adrenal pseudocysts
d. adrenocortical carcinoma
e. hemorrhagic cysts

REFERENCES

1. Hagen-Ansert S: *Textbook of diagnostic ultrasound*, ed 5, St Louis, 2001, Mosby.
2. Rumack CM, Wilson SR, Charboneau JW: *Diagnostic ultrasound*, vol 2, ed 2, St Louis, 1998, Mosby.
3. Otal P et al: Imaging features of uncommon adrenal masses with histopathologic correlation, *Radiographics* 19:569-581, 1999.
4. Bellantone R et al: Adrenal cystic lesions: report of 12 surgically treated cases and review of the literature, *J Endocrinol* 21:109-112, 1998.
5. Udelsman R, Fishman EK: Radiology of the adrenal, *Endocrinol Metab Clin North Am* 29:27-42, 2000.
6. Huddle KR, Nagar A: Phaeochromocytoma in pregnancy, *Aust N Z Obstet Gynaecol* 39:203-206, 1999.
7. Yeh CN, Jeng LB, Chen MF, Hung CF: Nonfunctioning malignant pheochromocytoma associated with dermatomyositis: case report and literature review, *World J Urol* 19:148-150, 2001.
8. Higgins JC, Fitzgerald JM: Evaluation of incidental renal and adrenal masses, *Am Fam Physician* 63:288-294, 2001.
9. Fontana D et al: What is the role of ultrasonography in the follow-up of adrenal incidentalomas? *Urology* 54:612-616, 1999.
10. Tanaka D, Oyama T, Niwatsuino H et al: A case of asymptomatic giant myelolipoma of the adrenal gland, *Radiat Med* 16:213-216, 1998.

II   GYNECOLOGY

13

Abnormal Uterine Bleeding

D. ASHLEY HILL

CLINICAL SCENARIO

■ A 32-year-old nulligravid woman is seen by her physician with increasingly heavy menses. Her menses used to occur every 28 days and last 5 days. For the past year, menses still occurs every 28 days but now is preceded by 2 to 5 days of brown spotting followed by 6 to 7 days of heavy bleeding. Occasional painless coital spotting still occurs. The patient takes two iron pills a day for mild anemia from heavy menses and has no significant medical or surgical history and specifically no bleeding disorders. She is married and monogamous and is a registered nurse in the neonatal intensive care unit. Physical examination findings are unremarkable and include a normal-sized nontender uterus. What are the possible diagnoses? What are the appropriate diagnostic imaging options?

OBJECTIVES

■ Describe the common clinical presentation of nonpregnant patients with abnormal uterine bleeding.

■ Differentiate the sonographic appearances of the more common causes of abnormal uterine bleeding.

■ List the appropriate imaging studies available for evaluation of abnormal uterine bleeding.

■ Describe the differences in sonographic appearance between endometrial polyps and submucosal leiomyomas (fibroids).

■ List treatment options for the most common causes of abnormal uterine bleeding.

GLOSSARY OF TERMS

Abnormal uterine bleeding: a general term that describes a change in menstrual bleeding pattern, including infrequent, irregular, heavy, or intermenstrual bleeding, from either organic causes or endocrine abnormalities; organic causes include either systemic illnesses that cause uterine bleeding or true lesions of the uterus or endometrium; endocrine dysfunction is more appropriately termed "dysfunctional uterine bleeding"

Adenomyosis: a common benign condition in which endometrial tissue invades the uterine muscular layer (myometrium)

Dysfunctional uterine bleeding: prolonged uterine bleeding without an anatomic (organic) cause; the term implies abnormal uterine bleeding from a hormonal abnormality

Endometrial carcinoma: a uterine malignant disease that originates from the endometrium

Endometrial hyperplasia: abnormal proliferation (growth) of the endometrium; different designations of endometrial hyperplasia include simple, complex, and atypical

Endometrial polyp: a focal growth of endometrial tissue that projects into the endometrial cavity

Endometrium: the inner lining of the uterus that responds to hormonal stimulation and produces both menstrual and abnormal uterine bleeding

Hematometra: a uterus distended with blood from obstruction of the cervix or vagina

Hysterosalpingography: a radiologic technique in which dye is infused into the uterus and fallopian tubes for identification of endometrial lesions or tubal blockage

Hysteroscopy: a procedure in which a flexible or rigid hysteroscope is inserted into the uterus for direct visualization of the endometrial cavity; this allows the gynecologic surgeon to diagnose and treat many intrauterine abnormalities

Intermenstrual bleeding: bleeding or spotting between regular menstrual periods

Leiomyoma, or myoma, or fibroid: a benign smooth muscle tumor that usually occurs in the uterus

Menometrorrhagia: prolonged or excessive bleeding at irregular intervals

Menorrhagia: prolonged or excessive uterine bleeding at regular intervals that lasts more than 7 days or with greater than 80 ml of blood

Sensitivity: ability to accurately determine the presence of a disease

Sonohysterography, or saline-infusion ultrasound, or saline-infusion sonography: a technique in which sterile saline solution is infused into the endometrial cavity during vaginal ultrasound for better visualization of endometrial abnormalities

Specificity: ability to accurately determine the absence of a disease

Abnormal uterine bleeding (AUB) is a common problem that leads to pelvic sonography. Patients may be seen by their healthcare provider with infrequent menses, prolonged menses (**menorrhagia**), intermenstrual spotting or bleeding, postcoital spotting, or irregular and heavy menses (**menometrorrhagia**). Accordingly, a number of possible diagnoses are considered in the evaluation of AUB. AUB may arise from organic causes, a lesion within the uterus or **endometrium,** or from a reproductive tract or systemic illness that affects the uterus. AUB that is not caused by an organic problem is usually from an endocrinologic source such as hormonal dysfunction and is called "**dysfunctional uterine bleeding.**"

Although the study of female reproductive hormones is fascinating, it is beyond the scope of this chapter. Sonographers most often will evaluate suspected anatomic lesions, such as **endometrial polyps**, fibroids,

adenomyosis, or **endometrial hyperplasia** or **carcinoma** (Box 13-1). Some other causes of AUB, some of which are discussed in this text, do not arise from anatomic lesions within the uterus or endometrium and include reproductive tract diseases, systemic illnesses, and endocrinologic causes (see Box 13-1). Although sonographers most often will see patients with suspected anatomic causes of AUB, one should be versed in the many possible causes of AUB for a thoughtful evaluation.

Pelvic sonography is a useful adjunct to the pelvic physical examination. For example, with clinician palpation of an enlarged uterus or with patient body habitus, anxiety, or tenderness that makes the examination difficult, the clinician may order or perform a sonogram for better assessment of uterine and adnexal anatomy. Many authors have studied whether pelvic sonography correlates with bimanual pelvic examination. Despite use of transabdominal transducers, which are less sensitive

BOX 13-1

Causes of Abnormal Uterine Bleeding

REPRODUCTIVE

Cervicitis (cervical infection)
Cervical carcinoma
Cervical polyp
Endometrial infection
Foreign objects (i.e., lost intrauterine device)
Hydatidiform molar pregnancy
Iatrogenic (i.e., contraceptives, hormone replacement
    medications, some psychotropic medications)
Ovarian or fallopian tube malignancy (uncommon)
Pelvic inflammatory disease
Trauma (iatrogenic, sexual intercourse, sexual assault)

SYSTEMIC ILLNESSES

Cirrhosis
Hypothyroidism
Uremia
Thrombocytopenia
Leukemia
von Willebrand's disease

ENDOCRINOLOGIC

Anorexia
Anovulation
Hyperprolactenemia
Hypothyroidism
Polycystic ovary syndrome
Prolongation of the corpus luteum cyst (controversial)
Significant stress (may cause anovulation)

than endovaginal transducers for pelvic sonography, one group found that ultrasound had a similar **specificity** compared with physical examination.[1] However, the **sensitivity** of ultrasound exceeded that of the pelvic examination. Another study evaluated cases both with physical examination and with endovaginal sonography within 48 hours of gynecologic surgery. The authors found that endovaginal sonography was very useful.[2] Some authors advocate consideration of office endovaginal sonography as a helpful part of the gynecologic physical examination.[3]

NORMAL UTERINE ANATOMY

Because anatomic lesions within the body of the uterus or involving the endometrial lining can cause AUB,

sonographers must have an understanding of normal uterine anatomy. The normal uterus is a pear-shaped organ located in the mid pelvis, adjacent to the bladder (anteriorly) and rectum (posteriorly; Fig. 13-1). The uterus is a muscular organ with an inner hollow endometrial cavity (Fig. 13-2) that responds to hormonal stimulation and can cause AUB.

The uterus is composed of three layers: the serosa (outer), the myometrium (middle), and the endometrium (inner). Each of the three uterine layers can have anatomic abnormalities that may cause AUB. Fibroids can develop within any of the three uterine layers, as discussed subsequently (Fig. 13-3). Adenomyosis is a common condition in which endometrial tissue invades the myometrium, sometimes causing pain or heavy bleeding. Many lesions can involve the endometrium, including hyperplasia, cancer, polyps, fibroids, and infection.

Uterine size varies throughout a woman's life, depending on hormonal stimulation, pregnancy, and anatomic disorders. After menarche but before childbirth, the uterus generally measures approximately 8 cm long, 5 cm wide, and 2.5 cm thick and weighs about 40 g.[4] Ultrasound measurements closely correlate with hysterectomy specimen measurements.[5]

Pelvic sonography for AUB should focus on the uterus and endometrium. The examination should begin with a view of the uterus in the sagittal plane (Fig. 13-4). The myometrium should have a homogeneous echo texture (Fig. 13-5). The uterine veins within the myometrium commonly will be visualized and appear hypoechoic or anechoic (see Fig. 13-4). The uterus should be measured in the sagittal (anterior/posterior) plane (Fig. 13-6). The uterus should be completely surveyed, with a search for hypoechoic or hyperechoic areas, which, as discussed subsequently, may represent fibroids or adenomyosis. Thinking of the uterus in three dimensions during the scan is helpful. The transducer is adjusted for a view of the uterus in the coronal (transverse) plane, in which the uterus is measured again (Fig. 13-7). Sonographers should take care to avoid a falsely increased transverse uterine measurement as the result of lateral fibroid, prominent ovarian veins, adnexal mass, or prominent bowel surrounding the uterus (Fig. 13-8).

UTERINE PHYSIOLOGY

The endometrium changes appearance on the basis of hormonal stimulation. During the first half of the menstrual cycle, the proliferative (follicular) phase, the endometrium appears as three hyperechoic lines separated by two hypoechoic areas (Figs. 13-9 and

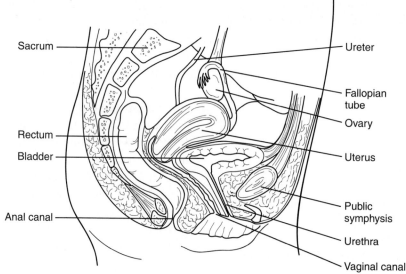

Fig. 13-1 Normal pelvic anatomy. Note close relationship between uterus and surrounding organs such as bladder and intestines.

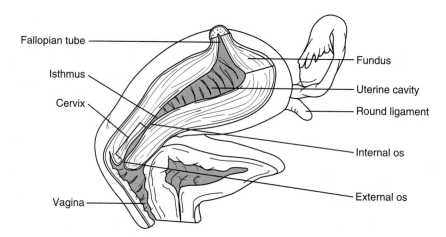

Fig. 13-2 Normal uterine anatomy. Thick, muscular uterine walls normally compress endometrial cavity.

13-10). The inner hyperechoic line represents the endometrial cavity, and the outer hyperechoic lines denote the junction of the myometrium and endometrium. Usually ovulation occurs at mid cycle, on about day 14 of the menstrual cycle. After ovulation, the endometrium progresses through the secretory, or luteal, phase. During this latter half of the menstrual cycle, the three hyperechoic lines are absent. Instead the endometrium appears thicker and entirely hyperechoic (Fig. 13-11). As discussed subsequently, sonographers may see irregularities of the endometrium, such as polyps, fibroids, and endometrial hyperplasia or cancer,

in evaluation of patients with AUB. The endometrium should be measured with placement of the calipers at the outer endometrium of one side and measurement to the outer endometrium of the opposing side (see Figs. 13-10 and 13-11).

LEIOMYOMA

Leiomyomas, usually called *uterine fibroids,* are benign smooth muscle tumors that develop from the myometrium but may involve any of the uterine layers (Fig. 13-12; see also Fig. 13-3). Fibroids less commonly can

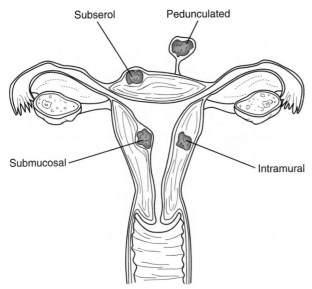

Fig. 13-3 Illustration of cut uterus. Uterine fibroids can develop in any of three uterine layers. Note subserosal, intramural, and submucosal fibroids.

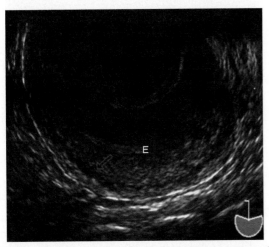

Fig. 13-4 Sagittal view of uterus shows hypoechoic uterine vessels in posterior myometrium (*arrow*). *E,* Endometrium.

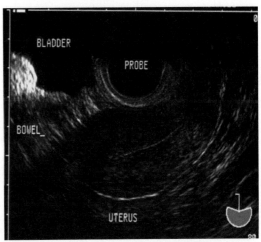

Fig. 13-5 Sagittal plane of normal uterus shows close approximation of surrounding organs.

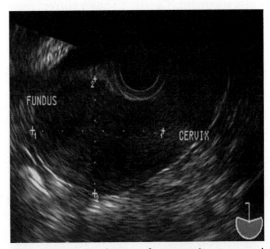

Fig. 13-6 Sagittal plane of normal uterus shows anterior/posterior (caliper 2) and fundus to cervix (caliper 1) measurements.

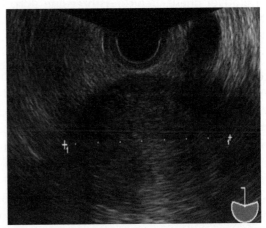

Fig. 13-7 Transverse (coronal) plane of normal uterus. Calipers show correct technique for measurement of transverse plane.

develop within the vagina, cervix, broad ligament, or fallopian tubes or on the omentum (so-called parasitic fibroids). Fibroids are the most common pelvic tumors and are a leading cause of hysterectomy. They are more common in black women than in other ethnic groups.[6] Fibroids can have a tremendous variation in size, ranging from a millimeter to more than 20 cm. Some women have multiple fibroids, usually with a wide variation in size. Generally only submucosal or large intramural fibroids cause AUB. Pedunculated fibroids are remote from the endometrium and myometrium and typically

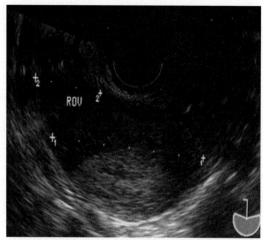

Fig. 13-8 Transverse uterine plane. Figure shows right ovary adjacent to uterus, which could give falsely elevated measurement if ovary is included in transverse measurement. Caliper 1 shows correct measurement of transverse plane.

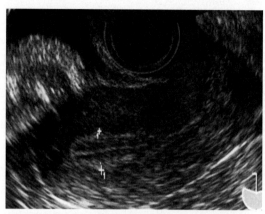

Fig. 13-10 Sagittal view of uterus shows hyperechoic follicular endometrium. Calipers show correct location for measurement of endometrial anterior/posterior endometrial thickness. Endometrial thickness is normal (12 mm) for 26-year-old woman during follicular phase.

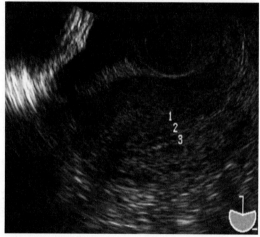

Fig. 13-9 Sagittal view of uterus during follicular (proliferative) phase, depicting three-line sign. Note hyperechoic endometrium found during follicular phase (1).

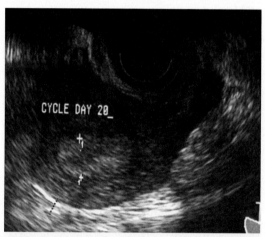

Fig. 13-11 Sagittal view of normal hyperechoic luteal phase endometrium. Measurement of 13 mm is normal for endometrium of menstruating woman on cycle day 20.

do not cause menorrhagia. Although fibroids might be presumed to cause AUB because of mechanical compression or irritation of the endometrium, researchers have not elucidated the exact mechanism of fibroid-induced bleeding. Current theory suggests that fibroids alter the uterine vascular system, which causes abnormal bleeding.[7]

Clinicians may suspect uterine fibroids from patient history or physical examination and may order a sonogram for assessment of the location and size of the fibroids for help in development of a treatment plan. Some gynecologists obtain a sonogram before surgery

to help determine the best surgical procedure plan for the patient. For example, patients who undergo removal of fibroids (myomectomy) may need a combined approach in which the gynecologist removes large subserosal fibroids via an abdominal incision and also removes submucosal fibroids with placement of an operative hysteroscope through the cervix and into the endometrial cavity. Fibroids do not necessarily necessitate treatment because many women with uterine fibroids have asymptomatic conditions. Clinicians base treatment plans on the size and location of the fibroid, patient symptoms, and patient wishes on whether or not to

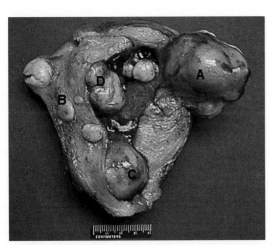

Fig. 13-12 Cut pathology specimen shows subserosal *(A)*, intramural *(B)*, and submucosal *(C)* uterine fibroids. Compare with Fig. 13-3. (Courtesy Michael Radi, MD, Department of Pathology, Florida Hospital Orlando).

undergo surgery. Examples of possible medical therapy for uterine fibroids include nonnarcotic analgesics for symptoms such as pressure and painful intercourse and gonadotropin-releasing hormone (GnRH) agonists to temporarily decrease uterine size before surgery. Surgical treatment methods include outpatient hysteroscopic removal of submucosal myomas for patients with abnormal bleeding, or perhaps recurrent miscarriages, and surgical removal via abdominal or laparoscopic approaches for intramural, subserosal, or pedunculated fibroids. A more recent treatment for uterine fibroids is uterine artery embolization in which invasive radiologists use vascular catheters to embolize the fibroid's vascular supply for patients unable or unwilling to undergo surgery. Clinicians find pelvic sonography useful for development of a coherent treatment plan.

Sonographic Findings

Fibroids visualized with sonography may cause obvious distortion of the uterine contour, generalized enlargement of the uterus, an altered echo texture (hypoechogenicity or hyperechogenicity), or calcifications with shadowing. Gross, Silver, and Jaffe[8] analyzed 41 patients with proven uterine fibroids to determine which sonographic features predicted uterine myomas. The three most common abnormalities that predicted uterine myomas were uterine contour irregularity (76%), altered echo texture (68%), and generalized uterine enlargement (66%). Most fibroid uteri had two or more abnormalities visible sonographically. Documentation should include

the size, location, and appearance of each fibroid. Submucosal fibroids may focally distort the endometrium, appearing as an area of increased echogenicity, although they may be difficult to differentiate from intramural fibroids or endometrial polyps. Fedele and colleagues[9] performed endovaginal sonography and hysteroscopy to compare these two methods for diagnosis of submucosal fibroids. Both methods had similar sensitivities and specificities, but vaginal sonography could not distinguish between a polyp and a submucosal fibroid. As discussed subsequently in this chapter, the infusion of contrast into the uterus will clarify the location of submucosal fibroids and help differentiate fibroids from polyps. Intramural fibroids may impinge on and distort the endometrium (Fig. 13-13). Fibroids are relatively easy to visualize when they are single, hypoechoic, and well encapsulated within the myometrium (Figs. 13-14 and 13-15). However, visualization of multiple fibroids can be challenging (Fig. 13-16). This is particularly true with large fibroids that distort the myometrium. Also, visualization of calcified fibroids may be difficult as they can cast large shadows because of their attenuating hyperechoic appearance (Fig. 13-17). Subserosal fibroids can be quite large and may extend laterally, mimicking an adnexal mass or a bicornuate uterus.[10] Pedunculated fibroids also may be difficult to visualize because of their size and location and, in some cases, may necessitate imaging with both endovaginal and transabdominal probes if the fibroid extends out of the pelvis.

A number of situations may make visualization of uterine fibroids difficult. Baltarowich et al[10] studied 44 cases with proven fibroids in which so-nography initially pointed to other disorders. The most common misdiagnosis noted was with a pedunculated or lateral fibroid misdiagnosed as an adnexal mass (19/44 cases). In addition, fibroids may undergo degeneration in which the central portion of the fibroid loses its blood supply and becomes necrotic (Fig. 13-18). Clinically, patients with degenerating fibroids may have abdominal pain. (Pregnant patients with a degenerating fibroid present a difficult diagnostic challenge because placental abruption and preterm labor can both be seen with abdominal pain). Degenerating fibroids may appear as hypoechoic masses and, if situated laterally, can mimic cystic adnexal masses.[10] Although endovaginal sonography generally is preferred in visualization of uterine fibroids, use of the transabdominal probe in addition to the vaginal probe may be necessary when the entire dimensions of large or pedunculated fibroids cannot see be seen with endovaginal sonography alone. In a large study of 405 women, Fedele et al[11] could not

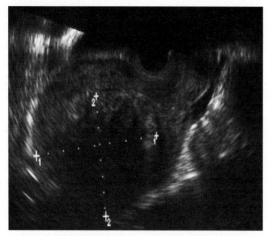

Fig. 13-13 Large posterior intramural fibroid measuring 8 × 7.7 cm is distorting endometrium.

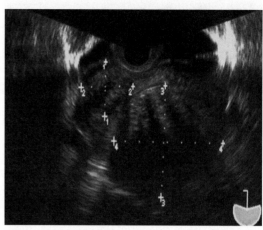

Fig. 13-16 Large myomatous uterus with 8-cm posterior fibroid (caliper 3) and smaller adjacent fibroid (caliper 2). Full evaluation is difficult because of size of fibroids.

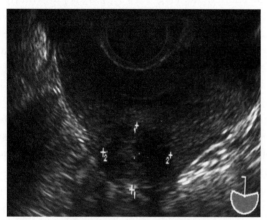

Fig. 13-14 Transverse uterine plane. Note well-encapsulated posterior subserosal fibroid.

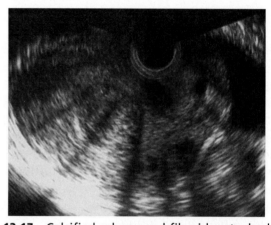

Fig. 13-17 Calcified submucosal fibroid casts shadows posteriorly. Note smaller subserosal fibroid in posterior wall that also casts shadows.

fully visualize the uterus in 6% of patients because of marked uterine enlargement.

ADENOMYOSIS

Adenomyosis is a common gynecologic condition in which endometrial glands and stroma penetrate into the myometrium, causing distortion of the myometrium from smooth muscle hyperplasia. The exact incidence rate is unknown, with reports in the medical literature ranging from 5% to 70%.[12] The most definitive method for diagnosis of adenomyosis is a pathologic specimen of the myometrium, usually obtained at hysterectomy. The wide variation noted previously may be a consequence of the disparity between pathologists in microscopic evaluation of a specimen for the presence

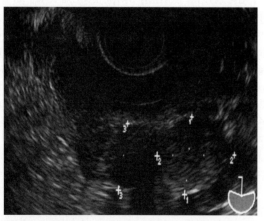

Fig. 13-15 Sagittal uterine plane shows two well-encapsulated posterior fibroids.

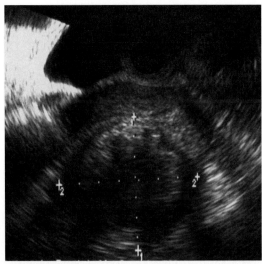

Fig. 13-18 Large necrotic fibroid seen in sagittal plane. Patient underwent abdominal uterine myomectomy. Pathologic evaluation revealed necrotic fibroid.

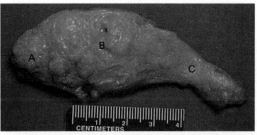

Fig. 13-19 Cut pathology specimen of uterus shows fundal adenomyoma *(A)* and extensive adenomyosis within myometrium *(B)*. *C,* Cervix. (Courtesy Michael Radi, MD, Department of Pathology, Florida Hospital Orlando).

of adenomyosis. For example, one team examined 200 consecutive hysterectomy specimens and found that the incidence rate of adenomyosis rose from 31% to 61% when only six extra tissue specimens were examined microscopically.[13]

Adenomyosis is a problematic condition for clinicians because the most common symptoms, painful menstruation (dysmenorrhea), AUB, and pelvic pain, can be caused by a number of other common gynecologic conditions. The mechanism with which adenomyosis causes or contributes to AUB is unknown. Adenomyosis is not an uncommon pathologic diagnosis in patients who are asymptomatic. Even when adenomyosis is found in a hysterectomy specimen (Fig. 13-19), attribution of the patient's symptoms to only adenomyosis may be difficult. This is particularly true because adenomyosis, fibroids, and other gynecologic conditions may coexist. Further, adenomyosis is notoriously difficult to diagnose clinically. One group found that adenomyosis was suspected before surgery in only 10% of cases.[14] Clinicians may suspect adenomyosis when a patient has a globally enlarged "boggy" uterus on bimanual examination. Treatment options other than hysterectomy are limited and include GnRH agonist therapy,[15] endometrial ablation or resection,[16] nonnarcotic analgesics, and uterine artery embolization.[17]

Sonographic Findings

Gynecologists and pathologists have noted that adenomyosis may be diffuse or localized into circumscribed foci called *adenomyomas*. Diffuse adenomyosis, in which endometrial glands and stroma are diffusely incorporated into the myometrium, is more common. Adenomyomas can appear sonographically similar to uterine fibroids. Many authors have studied diffuse adenomyosis with transabdominal or endovaginal sonography. There are several sonographic criteria for adenomyosis. A number of authors,[18-22] some with transabdominal probes and others with endovaginal probes, report that ill-defined myometrial heterogenicity (Fig. 13-20) is suggestive of adenomyosis. Two smaller studies noted uterine enlargement as a marker for adenomyosis.[19,23] Walsh, Taylor, and Rosenfield[20] studied four patients with adenomyosis and reported that transabdominal sonography revealed irregular cystic spaces from 5 to 7 mm in size that produced a honeycomb pattern to the myometrium. One group found that somewhat similar cystic areas could be used presumptively in the diagnosis of adenomyosis.[24] A study of 119 patients revealed that the most common sonographic appearances of adenomyosis were poorly defined hypoechoic and heterogenous areas within the myometrium (Figs. 13-21 and 13-22).[22] No patients with proven adenomyosis had increased echogenicity. The exact mechanism of myometrial disruption in patients with adenomyosis is unknown, although smooth muscle hypertrophy and ectopic foci of endometrial tissue with cystic spaces may contribute to the altered myometrial heterogenicity. Sonographic imaging of diffuse adenomyosis may be difficult, particularly if the uterus is markedly enlarged, calcified fibroids cast acoustic shadows, or multiple fibroids or adenomyomas distort the myometrium.

ADENOMYOMAS

Adenomyomas are focal areas of adenomyosis that may resemble uterine fibroids sonographically (Figs. 13-23 to 13-25).

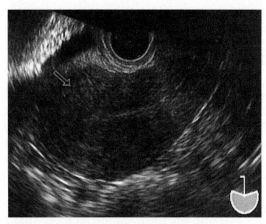

Fig. 13-20 Sagittal plane of uterus. Arrow points to ill-defined myometrial hypergenicity at fundus. This 34-year-old multigravid patient underwent vaginal hysterectomy. Pathology specimen revealed extensive adenomyosis.

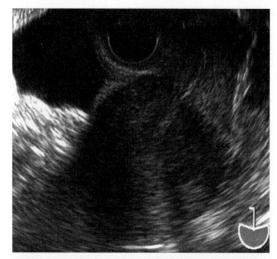

Fig. 13-21 Sagittal view of uterus. Note oval-shaped hypoechoic area just posterior to myometrium that casts shadows *(arrows)*. Evaluation of hysterectomy specimen revealed adenomyosis.

Sonographic Findings

The largest sonographic evaluation of adenomyomas to date studied 405 women and found that sonography had a high success rate for diagnosis of adenomyomas.[11] The authors used a 6.5-MHz endovaginal probe before surgery, with a inhomogeneous circumscribed area in the endometrium containing anechoic lacunae, for diagnosis of adenomyomas. Marked uterine enlargement prevented full sonographic evaluation in 24 patients (6%). The authors note that endovaginal sonography had a 74% positive predictive value, so that in 25% of patients the diagnosis of an adenomyoma was made when the patient actually had one or more uterine fibroids. This finding may have important clinical implications for gynecologists planning surgery because fibroids generally are easier to remove than adenomyomas as the former usually is well encapsulated and the latter is diffusely involved with the surrounding myometrium.

As stated, endovaginal sonography has reasonable ability in the diagnosis of adenomyosis, but the subtle findings necessary for a presumptive diagnosis of adenomyosis require real-time sonography and operator experience. Some authors have advocated magnetic resonance imaging (MRI) as a more accurate diagnostic test for adenomyosis. In one series of 20 patients, Ascher and coworkers[26] found MRI to be significantly more accurate than endovaginal sonography. However, in a larger series of 119 patients, one group reported that endovaginal sonography and MRI were similar in the ability to diagnose adenomyosis. But the authors

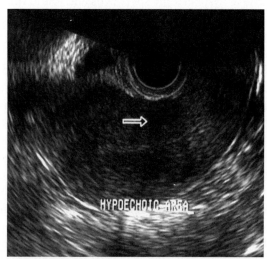

Fig. 13-22 Sagittal view of uterus. Arrow points to hypoechoic area above endometrium at mid uterus consistent with adenomyosis.

correctly noted that ultrasound evaluation of suspected adenomyosis is highly operator dependent, necessitates real-time images, and may not be reproducible from one examiner (or examination) to another.[22] Further, researchers studied 106 women before hysterectomy to compare endovaginal ultrasound with MRI and found that although MRI and endovaginal sonography were equally good at diagnosis of adenomyosis, neither was accurate with larger uteri with volumes of more than 400 ml.[27] However, other authors have found MRI accurate for diagnosis of adenomyosis in the presence of a large palpable uterus.[28] If further studies suggest

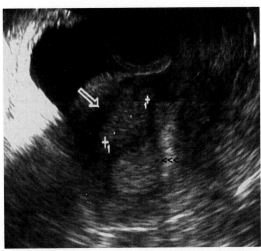

Fig. 13-23 Sagittal view of uterus. Open arrow points to focal hyperechoic area in anterior uterine wall. Patient underwent myomectomy, but focal area was not well encapsulated as expected of fibroid. Pathology evaluation revealed adenomyoma. Closed arrows point to endometrium.

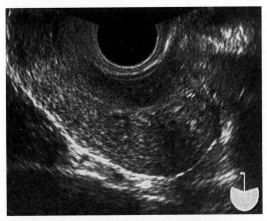

Fig. 13-24 Sagittal view of uterus with fundus to right. Hyperechoic ill-defined area extends from endometrium toward fundus. Pathologic evaluation revealed oblong-shaped adenomyoma. See also Fig. 13-25.

that MRI is more accurate than endovaginal sonography in the presence of very large uteri, MRI might be preferable in this subset of patients. However, the current expense of MRI precludes its use for most patients with suspected adenomyosis.

ENDOMETRIAL HYPERPLASIA AND CARCINOMA

Clinicians who care for women with AUB must always consider the possibility of endometrial hyperplasia or endometrial carcinoma as the possible etiology. Endo-

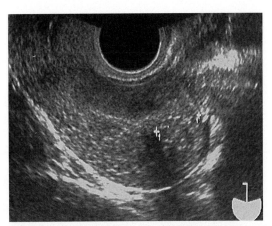

Fig. 13-25 Same patient as depicted in Fig. 13-24. Calipers mark extent of adenomyoma.

metrial adenocarcinoma is the most common gynecologic cancer, affecting almost one in every 50 women. Most cases are diagnosed in women between the ages of 50 and 65 years, although about 5% of cases are diagnosed in women of less than age 40 years. The risk factors for endometrial carcinoma include obesity, nulliparity, early menarche, menopause after age 52 years,[29] diabetes, tamoxifen therapy for breast cancer, white race, chronic anovulation, and unopposed estrogen stimulation. Clinically, endometrial hyperplasia and cancer usually present with AUB. (Bleeding in menopausal women is termed postmenopausal bleeding). Clinicians may order or perform vaginal sonography when patients have AUB, particularly heavy or frequent bleeding (menorrhagia or menometrorrhagia), or postmenopausal bleeding. Some patients will have an enlarged uterus, but most patients will have normal physical examination findings. Although the most accurate method for diagnosis of endometrial cancer is an endometrial biopsy or a hysterectomy specimen (Figs. 13-26 and 13-27), many patients with AUB undergo pelvic sonography before a biopsy or as part of a triage system to determine the need for a biopsy.

Familiarity of the normal menstrual cycle and its effect on endometrial anatomy is imperative for an effective pelvic sonogram. Unopposed estrogen stimulation is the most important to the sonographer because this is visible sonographically as a thickened or abnormal-appearing endometrium. As discussed previously, the endometrium responds to hormonal stimuli from the ovarian hormones estrogen and progesterone. During the early phase of the menstrual cycle, the follicular phase, estrogen stimulates endometrial growth. At about mid cycle, or day 14 of a 28-day cycle, ovulation occurs. After the egg is released from the ovary, a corpus luteum cyst develops on the ovary and produces pro-

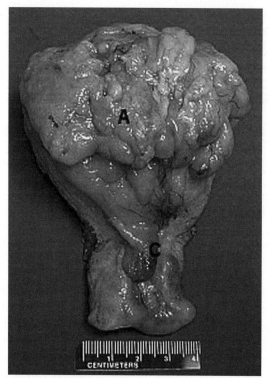

Fig. 13-26 Cut hysterectomy specimen shows endometrial hyperplasia at fundal portion of specimen *(A)*. *C,* Cervix. (Courtesy Michael Radi, MD, Department of Pathology, Florida Hospital Orlando).

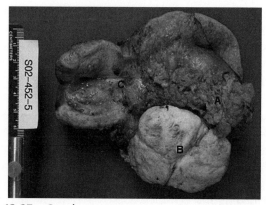

Fig. 13-27 Cut hysterectomy specimen shows endometrial carcinoma *(A)* and associated leiomyoma *(B)*. Distinguishing hyperplasia from carcinoma with visualization is often difficult. *C,* Cervix. (Courtesy Michael Radi, MD, Department of Pathology, Florida Hospital Orlando).

gesterone. Progesterone levels peak about a week after ovulation and then decline (unless pregnancy occurs). If pregnancy does not occur, estrogen and progesterone levels decrease and the loss of hormonal stimulus leads to menses. When the endometrium is exposed to

estrogen, the endometrial layer closest to the endometrial cavity, the stratum functionale, increases in size. Bakos and colleagues[30] used endovaginal sonography to evaluate the endometrium of 16 women throughout a normal ovulatory cycle. The follicular endometrium measured about 4 mm, the ovulatory endometrium about 13 mm, and the luteal endometrium about 12 mm. Fleischer, Kalemeris, and Entman[31] also measured the endometrium during the menstrual cycle. They reported follicular measurements of 4 to 8 mm (see Figs. 13-9 and 13-10), ovulatory measurements of 6 to 10 mm, and luteal measurements of 10 to 12 mm (see Fig. 13-11). (Note that the Fleisher group reported half-thickness measurements of "one side" of the endometrium, which have been doubled here). In addition, they reported that the endometrium during menstruation measured about 1 mm (Fig. 13-28). Table 13-1 summarizes the findings of these two studies, which reveal that the endometrium increases in size throughout the proliferative phase until ovulation and then stabilizes through the luteal phase until menstruation occurs. After menstruation, the endometrium begins growing in response to increasing estrogen levels.

Endometrial thickness measurements can be confusing. Many studies report normal and abnormal values for endometrial thickness in postmenopausal patients, including those undergoing hormone replacement therapy or with postmenopausal bleeding. The endometrial thickness ranges discussed previously (4 to 13 mm) are for normally menstruating women. In contrast, many authors have reported that an endometrial thickness of less than or equal to 4 to 5 mm almost always excludes endometrial abnormalities in postmenopausal women.[32-35] This finding is discussed later in this chapter. Therefore, clinicians, radiologists, and sonographers should be aware that, for example, a 10-mm endometrial thickness is probably normal in a menstruating woman, whereas a 10-mm endometrium may be abnormal in a postmenopausal woman.

Endometrial hyperplasia is an abnormal proliferation (growth) of the endometrium in response to excess or unopposed estrogen. Patients taking estrogen-only hormone replacement medications or women with chronic anovulation are at risk for endometrial hyperplasia or endometrial carcinoma. An anovulatory patient does not always produce a corpus luteum cyst, so the endometrium does not receive adequate progesterone stimulation. The unopposed estrogen continues to "fertilize" the endometrium, potentially leading to abnormal growth. Pathologists and gynecologists use specific terminology to categorize endometrial hyper-

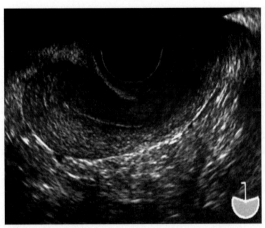

Fig. 13-28 Sagittal view of uterus shows normal menstrual endometrium of 21-year-old woman. Thin hyperechoic endometrial stripe measures only 1 mm.

Table 13-1	*Endometrial Thickness (mm) during Normal Menstrual Cycle*		
Reference	Follicular Phase	Ovulation	Luteal Phase
Bakos et al[30]	4	13	12
Fleischer, Kalemeris, and Entman[31]	4 to 8	6 to 10	10 to 12

plasia, depending on the appearance of the endometrial glands and whether or not cellular abnormalities (atypia) are visible microscopically. Ultrasound cannot be used to distinguish between the different classifications of endometrial hyperplasia. However, clinically this information is important because the potential for endometrial hyperplasia to progress to cancer increases as cellular atypia increases. Kurman, Kaminski, and Norris[36] reported that progression to endometrial cancer occurred in only 1 of 93 patients (1%) with simple hyperplasia, about 1 of 29 patients (3%) with complex hyperplasia, and 8% of patients with simple atypical hyperplasia. However, 29% of patients with complex atypical hyperplasia had carcinoma develop.[36] The treatment of endometrial hyperplasia depends on the degree of atypia and the age and health of the patient particularly because simple hyperplasia without atypia uncommonly progresses to cancer. In some cases, hormonal therapy with progestin is effective for treatment of endometrial hyperplasia, and hysterectomy may be indicated for older patients finished with childbearing or those with significant

atypia. The treatment for endometrial cancer depends on the age and health of the patient, the histologic characteristics of the tumor, and the degree of spread. Cancers limited to the endometrium or inner uterus without metastases have cure rates in the 90% range. In general, endometrial carcinoma limited to the uterus may be treatable with hysterectomy. Carcinoma that has spread to adjacent or distant organs may necessitate hysterectomy, chemotherapy, or radiation therapy.

Sonographic Findings

Only a biopsy can be used to differentiate between endometrial hyperplasia and carcinoma, but useful information may be obtained from a sonographic examination that may point to or help exclude either of these diagnoses. Chambers and Unis[37] studied a small number of patients and reported that sonographic signs suggestive of endometrial carcinoma were present in 67% of patients. Blood distending the endometrial cavity is called **hematometra** (Fig. 13-29), which can be caused by obstruction of the endocervical os from prior endometrial surgery or a large submucosal fibroid or from endometrial carcinoma or previous pelvic radiation therapy.[38] Other authors have examined uterine size and endometrial carcinoma. One group studied 21 patients with endometrial adenocarcinoma and reported that about 70% of the patients had an enlarged uterus (>8 cm sagittal and 3 cm anterior-posterior).[39] Further, the group reported that those patients with early stage endometrial cancer had a normal-sized uterus and a normal endometrial echo pattern but that patients with advanced disease (stages III to IV) had a lobular or enlarged uterus and a mixed endometrial echo pattern. Unfortunately, increased uterine size is a nonspecific finding that can occur with many gynecologic conditions, such as fibroids and adenomyosis. Evaluation of the endometrium is more specific for determination of the potential for or the exclusion of the likelihood of endometrial carcinoma.

Many authors have studied the endometrium sonographically to determine whether characteristics exist that are suggestive of endometrial hyperplasia or carcinoma. Some groups have evaluated vaginal sonography as a screening tool in asymptomatic postmenopausal women.[40-43] Transvaginal ultrasound currently is not used as a screening study to rule out endometrial hyperplasia or malignant disease in asymptomatic women because of its poor positive predictive value for detection of endometrial abnormalities.[44] Further, endometrial cancer is relatively uncommon, occurring in 1 of 50 women, and most women with endometrial cancer have

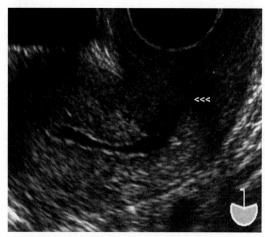

Fig. 13-29 Sagittal view of uterus shows hematometra. Endometrial canal is distended by blood, which appears hypoechoic. This 56-year-old patient had cervical stenosis at level of internal os *(arrows)*.

Table 13-2	*Average Endometrial Thickness (mm) of Various Endometrial Anomalies in Postmenopausal Women*		
Normal Biopsy	**Polyps**	**Hyperplasia**	**Carcinoma**
4	10	14	20

Data from Smith-Bindman et al.[45]

vaginal bleeding. Smith-Bindman and colleagues[45] performed a metaanalysis of 35 prospective studies in which authors used endovaginal sonography to evaluate the endometrium before tissue biopsy. The metaanalysis included 5892 women and found that 94% of patients were seen with vaginal bleeding at a mean age of 61 years. The prevalence of endometrial hyperplasia or polyps was 40% and of endometrial cancer was 13%. The authors reported that patients with normal biopsy results had an average endometrial thickness of only 4 mm but that patients with endometrial cancer had an average thickness of 20 mm (Table 13-2). Other authors have reported similar findings with retrospective data.[46] The metaanalysis data also revealed that with a 5-mm cutoff to define abnormal endometrial thickness, vaginal ultrasound identified 95% of endometrial disease among women not using hormone replacement therapy and 91% of endometrial disease among women using hormone replacement medications. (The sensitivity of vaginal sonography for detection of endometrial pathology is less for women taking hormone replacement therapy because these medications can cause endometrial proliferation). The authors conclude that with a 5-mm threshold, endovaginal sonography is similar to endometrial biopsy for exclusion of serious endometrial disease. These data are important because clinicians typically perform an office endometrial biopsy, uterine curettage, or hysteroscopically directed biopsy when postmenopausal patients are seen with vaginal bleeding. Some patients cannot tolerate the biopsy procedure because of age, cervical stenosis, or pain. Further, office biopsy devices may miss focal abnormalities such as polyps or focal carcinoma.[47-50] Postmenopausal patients with an endometrial thickness of less than or equal to 4 to 5 mm have a very low risk for endometrial carcinoma or other serious endometrial disease. Several authors advocate endovaginal ultrasound as a triage method for such patients to determine whether office or operative biopsy is necessary.[45,50-52]

Figs. 13-30, 13-31, and 13-32 show the endovaginal ultrasound findings and give a discussion of the clinical scenario for perimenopausal and postmenopausal patients with abnormal vaginal bleeding and with subsequent diagnosis of either endometrial hyperplasia or carcinoma. Note that for all patients the physician or sonographer used full-thickness caliper measurements of the endometrium. See Fig. 13-26 for a hysterectomy specimen from a patient with endometrial hyperplasia, and see Fig. 13-27 for a hysterectomy specimen from a patient with endometrial carcinoma.

ENDOMETRIAL POLYPS

Endometrial polyps are focal overgrowths of the endometrial glands and stroma. Their size is variable. Some are as small as 1 mm, and others fill the entire endometrial cavity and can prolapse from the cervix. Endometrial polyps are soft, fleshy, tan or red growths that can be attached to the endometrium by a long pedunculated stalk or a broad base. Pedunculated polyps can prolapse from the cervix and are difficult to remove with endometrial curettage (D&C) because they tend to move away from the curette. Polyps are most common in women between the ages of 40 and 49 years,[53] although they may be incidental findings in reproductive-aged women. Most polyps are asymptomatic. Polyps can cause coital spotting, **intermenstrual bleeding,** menorrhagia, menometrorrhagia, and prolonged staining after normal menstruation.

Endometrial polyps contain blood vessels, stroma, and endometrial glands and can respond to hormonal

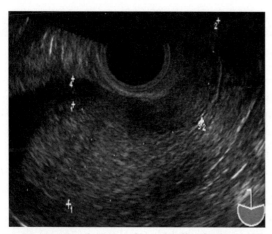

Fig. 13-30 Sagittal view of markedly thickened endometrium, measuring 22 mm, of postmenopausal woman. Endometrium has regular contour. Hysteroscopically directed biopsy with uterine curettage revealed simple endometrial hyperplasia without atypia. Patient received oral progesterone therapy and had normal endometrial biopsy results 6 months later.

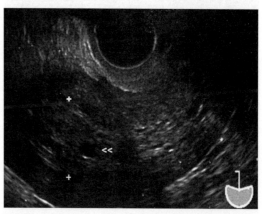

Fig. 13-32 Sagittal view of uterus of 60-year-old woman with new-onset heavy vaginal bleeding. Note thickened endometrium (between calipers) and cystic space within endometrial tissue *(arrows)*. Biopsy revealed grade I, well-differentiated endometrial carcinoma that was successfully treated with abdominal hysterectomy.

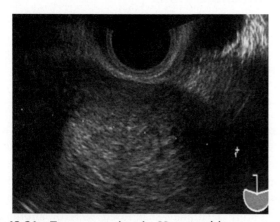

Fig. 13-31 Transverse view in 62-year-old woman with new-onset vaginal bleeding. Endometrium is thickened at 18 mm but has regular contour. Biopsy revealed simple hyperplasia with atypia. Patient also had uterine prolapse and underwent uncomplicated vaginal hysterectomy.

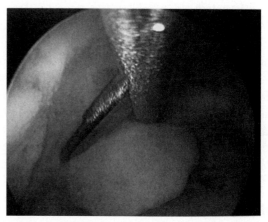

Fig. 13-33 Gynecologist removing endometrial polyp during hysteroscopy.

stimuli. In addition, endometrial polyps may harbor foci of endometrial hyperplasia or carcinoma. Fortunately, the risk of endometrial carcinoma in a polyp is low.[54] Gynecologists treat endometrial polyps with hysteroscopic endometrial polypectomy[55] because uterine curettage can miss endometrial polyps,[56] leading to inadequate treatment. With **hysteroscopy,** gynecologists can directly visualize the polyp, its base, and the entire endometrial cavity. Direct visualization allows the surgeon to remove the polyp (Fig. 13-33; see Color Plate 8). Pathologists can examine the excised

polyps histologically to document the absence of hyperplasia or malignant disease.

Sonographic Findings

Polyps appear sonographically as hyperechoic endometrial foci (Fig. 13-34). The hyperechoic area can be a well-defined, as in the case of a larger or broad-based polyp, or an ill-defined global thickening of the endometrium, as in the case of a pedunculated polyp with a long stalk. In one series of 68 postmenopausal women with previously discovered thickened endometria, Hulka and coworkers[57] found that cystic spaces within the endometrium were predictive of polyps. Indman[58] found that endovaginal sonography was used to

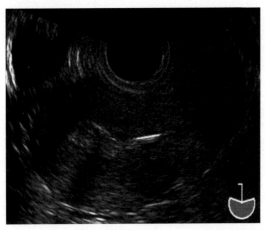

Fig. 13-34 Sagittal view of uterus shows circular hyperechoic area at fundus. *White line* in endometrial canal is sonohysterography catheter before saline infusion. Benign polyp was removed during hysteroscopy.

accurately diagnose 89% of endometrial polyps. However, endovaginal sonography may miss focal endometrial polyps because the walls of the endometrial cavity compress the polyps, making discrimination of a polyp from a globally thickened endometrium difficult (see Fig. 13-34). For intrauterine contrast to better visualize endometrial cavity lesions, clinicians began using saline-infusion sonography, often called **sonohysterography**. Sonohysterography has become a valuable method for diagnosis of endometrial polyps and other endometrial lesions.

SONOHYSTEROGRAPHY

Sonohysterography is simply endovaginal sonography enhanced with infusion of sterile saline solution into the endometrial cavity with a small catheter. Like **hysterosalpingography** (HSG), it allows visualization of the endometrial cavity. But instead of having a static image, it allows the operator to image the endometrium, uterus, and adnexa in real time. Box 13-2 lists current indications and relative contraindications, which have not been well studied, for sonohysterography. Researchers have compared sonohysterography with several other procedures to determine the accuracy of this technique for correct diagnosis of endometrial cavity abnormalities. Authors have compared sonohysterography with endovaginal sonography, HSG, hysteroscopy, and hysterectomy specimens.

Sonohysterography is an accurate technique for diagnosis of endometrial polyps and submucosal fibroids, particularly compared with traditional endovaginal

---

BOX 13-2

Indications and Contraindications for Sonohysterography

INDICATIONS

Evaluation of abnormal uterine bleeding (59, 60, 61)
Evaluation of perimenopausal bleeding (62, 63, 64)
Evaluation of postmenopausal bleeding (65, 66)
Detection of endometrial polyps (67, 68)
Detection of submucosal fibroids (68, 69)
Diagnosis of intrauterine adhesions (70, 71)
Preoperative evaluation prior to surgery (72)
Diagnosis of residual placental tissue (73, 74)
Evaluation of patients with recurrent pregnancy loss (75)
Evaluation of infertility patients (71, 76, 77, 78)
Evaluation of patients taking tamoxifen (79, 80, 81)
Localization of intrauterine foreign objects (82, 83)

CONTRAINDICATIONS

Known or suspected intrauterine pregnancy.
Unstable uterine hemorrhage.
Acute salpingitis (pelvic inflammatory disease).
Possibly: known endometrial carcinoma

---

sonography. For example, in a study of 62 patients with infertility, Alatas and colleagues[76] found that traditional endovaginal sonography was able to diagnose 36% of cavity defects and HSG was able to diagnose 73% of abnormalities but that saline-infusion endovaginal sonography accurately diagnosed 90% of anomalies. Another group studied 105 patients and found a 96% agreement between sonohysterography and hysteroscopy but also found that conventional endovaginal ultrasound missed half of endometrial polyps.[66] Conventional endovaginal sonography fails to resolve endometrial polyps because the anterior and posterior uterine walls compress the endometrium so that polyps cannot be seen easily. Infusion of saline solution removes the compression and allows visualization of the polyps. Sonohysterography also compares well with other methods of visualization of the endometrium. Widrich and coworkers[84] evaluated 130 patients to compare sonohysterography with hysteroscopy and found no significant difference between the two procedures. Further, Parsons, Hill, and Spicer[85] performed sonohysterography before hysterectomy in 53 patients and found that the procedure had a 95% sensitivity and a 100% specificity for diagnosis of polyps, submucosal

Equipment Used for Sonohysterography

Vaginal ultrasound
Appropriate intrauterine catheter
Speculum (open-sided if possible)
Sterile saline with 20- to 30-ml syringe
Absorbent under-buttocks pad
Ring forceps
Have available: Single-tooth tenaculum or cervical
    stabilizer, cervical dilators

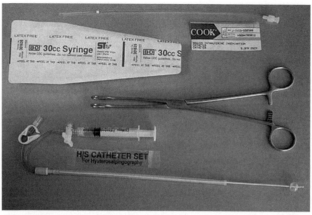

Fig. 13-35 Supplies necessary for sonohysterography (5.3F Soules intrauterine insemination catheter *[top]*, ring forceps, 30-ml syringe, and Ackrad H/S balloon catheter).

fibroids, a small number of endometrial carcinomas, and normal cavities, as verified by pathologic specimens.

Sonohysterography is clearly an accurate technique for detection of endometrial abnormalities and is also simple to learn. Box 13-3 lists the equipment necessary for sonohysterography. A urine or serum pregnancy test should be considered for those patients for sonohysterography in the luteal phase who are not using contraceptives and are not postmenopausal. The room is prepared before the examination with the collection of instruments, catheters, and the saline solution–filled syringe. The syringe is filled with prefilled bottles of sterile saline solution or saline solution from a 500- or 1000-ml intravenous bag with sterile technique and an 18-gauge needle. The needle is discarded. The patient is positioned in the lithotomy position in stirrups on an absorbent under-buttocks pad to absorb spilled saline solution. After traditional endovaginal sonography is performed, the probe is removed, an open-sided speculum is placed, and the cervix is swabbed with a disinfectant, such as Betadine. The following two catheter types are preferred: a 5.3F Soules intrauterine insemination catheter (Cook Urological, Inc., Spencer, Indiana) or a 5F HSG catheter with a 2-ml balloon (H/S catheter, Ackrad Laboratories, Cranford, New Jersey; Fig. 13-35). The latter is useful for women with a large cervical os that causes the smaller Soules catheter to fall out or saline solution to flush back out of the cervix into the vagina. A potential drawback to the balloon catheter is that if the balloon is inflated at the internal cervical os, it may obscure small polyps located at the internal os. In practice, this is probably an uncommon situation. The Goldstein sonohysterography catheter (Cook Urological, Inc) is a 1.8 mm–diameter modified version of the Soules catheter that uses a small acorn to help reduce saline solution outflow from the cervix. The acorn

inserts into the external os, allowing full visualization of the internal os and endometrial cavity. The choice of catheter reflects operator preference. Dessole and colleagues[86] compared six sonohysterography catheters during 610 sonohysterography procedures. They evaluated the catheters for ease of use, time for insertion, volume of contrast media used, reliability, cost, and patient tolerability. They found no statistically significant differences between the various catheters, although patients best tolerated the Goldstein catheter.

The sonographer should flush saline solution through the catheter to remove all air bubbles, which cause artifact during the procedure. Then the sonographer will assist the physician in the following procedure. The catheter is grasped about 2 to 3 cm from the tip with a ring forceps and then gently fed through the external os into the uterus. It is useful to let the physician know whether the uterus is anteverted or retroverted. The insemination or sonohysterography catheter, or the H/S balloon catheter, should be placed at the level of the internal os. If the balloon catheter is used, 1 ml (instead of 2 ml) of saline solution should be used to expand the balloon to prevent cramping, and the balloon may be placed in the cervix, and not the endometrial cavity, to prevent obscuring polyps adjacent to the internal os. The acorn on the Goldstein catheter should abut the external os, although nulliparous or postmenopausal patients may not need the acorn, which can be removed. Catheter insertion is usually easy, although patients with cervical stenosis uncommonly may need a tenaculum or cervical stabilizer on the anterior cervix and care should be taken not to apply the tenaculum to the bladder base. In addition, the tenaculum may cause pain or point bleeding, which may necessitate application of silver nitrate or rarely, a suture. Stenotic cervices may need cervical dilation, although this is uncommon. The author has required the use of cervical dilators for fewer than 0.5% of sonohysterography procedures. After the catheter is placed, the speculum is gently removed without dislodging the catheter. An open-sided Graves speculum makes the catheter less likely to pull out during speculum removal. The endovaginal probe is reinserted, and saline solution is slowly infused through the catheter. Rapidly infusion of the saline solution can be painful.

The sonographer should scan the uterus in both sagittal and transverse planes to appreciate the three-dimensional nature of the endometrial cavity. Note that missing smaller polyps is easy if the entire uterus is not scanned from cervix to fundus (sagittal plane) and cornu to cornu (transverse plane). Appreciate the enhanced ability to visualize the endometrium with saline-infusion sonography compared with traditional sonography. If saline solution flushes out of the cervix, slow steady pressure may be applied to the syringe to keep the endometrial cavity partially distended. (Full distention is not necessary and may produce pain). Endometrial measurements should be taken (Fig. 13-36), and documentation of any endometrial abnormalities identified.

Figs. 13-37 to 13-41 show the ability of sonohysterography to identify endometrial abnormalities. When possible, traditional endovaginal sonography is compared with sonohysterography for the same patient.

Sonohysterography is a well-tolerated procedure. Most patients have minimal, if any, discomfort. The author has had to stop the procedure one time (for patient anxiety) but has not had to abandon the procedure for pain. The procedure adds only a few minutes to a traditional endovaginal sonogram, is inexpensive, and replaces more invasive, painful, and expensive procedures such as HSG or hysteroscopy for diagnosis of endometrial cavity abnormalities.

Table 13-3 provides a summary of pathology, symptoms, and sonographic findings of the anatomic causes of abnormal uterine bleeding.

SUMMARY

Abnormal uterine bleeding is a common gynecologic problem that often leads to pelvic sonography. Sonographers are able to provide clinicians with valuable information that directly affects treatment plans. In the case of postmenopausal bleeding, pelvic sonogram results may prevent the patient from undergoing unnecessary invasive surgery.

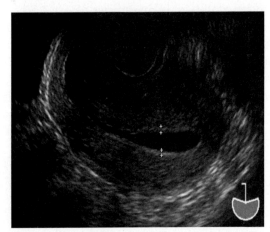

Fig. 13-36 Sagittal view of normal sonohysterography study. Only 12 ml of saline solution was used to distend endometrium for this study. Calipers show correct technique for measurement of endometrial thickness of both anterior and posterior endometrium. Total (anterior and posterior combined) endometrial thickness should be reported.

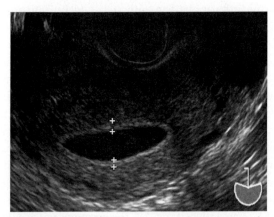

Fig. 13-37 Transverse uterine view shows normal sonohysterography study. Calipers show correct technique for measurement of anterior and posterior endometrial thickness.

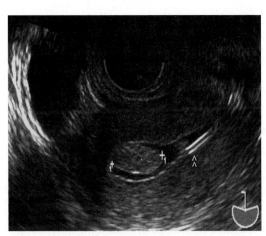

Fig. 13-38 Sagittal view of uterus during sonohysterography reveals 1.7-cm submucosal fibroid. Fibroid has smooth continuous border. Soules infusion catheter is seen as it rests just past internal cervical os. Fibroid was causing heavy and regular vaginal bleeding (menorrhagia) and was removed with operative hysteroscopy (see Fig. 13-42).

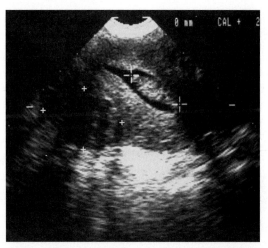

Fig. 13-40 Sagittal view of uterus during sonohysterography of 26-year-old woman with coital spotting and intermenstrual vaginal bleeding. Long polyp arises from broad base on anterior uterine wall. Also note hypoechoic fibroid in posterior uterine wall (smaller calipers).

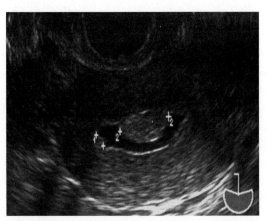

Fig. 13-39 Transverse view of uterus during sonohysterography of same patient in Fig. 13-38. Note small adjacent polyp.

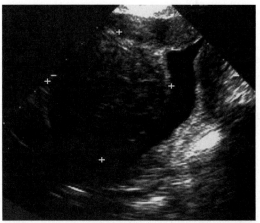

Fig. 13-41 Sonohysterogram of large submucosal fibroid. Patient was seen in emergency department with anemia requiring blood transfusion. Patient received intramuscular GnRH therapy and later underwent successful hysteroscopic myomectomy. More pressure and saline solution than normal may be required to distend uterus during sonohysterography when patient has large submucosal fibroid.

CLINICAL SCENARIO—DIAGNOSIS

■ The 32-year-old patient has menorrhagia. She initially undergoes a pelvic sonogram during an emergency department visit that reveals a normal-sized uterus and adnexa, no free fluid, and an irregular, 10.2-mm endometrial lining. Her gynecologist orders a sonohysterogram. The sonographer notes a 9-mm by 6-mm fundal endometrial polyp that the gynecologist removes a week later with outpatient hysteroscopy (see Fig. 13-33). The patient reports complete resolution of symptoms during the past three menstrual cycles.

Table 13-3	*Anatomic Causes of Abnormal Uterine Bleeding*	
Pathology	**Symptoms**	**Sonographic Findings**
Adenomyosis	May be asymptomatic; painful menses, heavy but regular bleeding, pelvic pain	1-3 mm anechoic lakes, ill-defined myometrial heterogenicity, diffuse uterine enlargement, thickened posterior uterine wall, irregular 5-7 mm cystic spaces with honeycomb pattern
Endometrial polyps	Often asymptomatic; spotting; heavy and regular menses, or bleeding with intercourse	Hyperechoic endometrial foci, cystic spaces within the endometrium
Endometrial hyperplasia	Abnormal uterine bleeding, postmenopausal bleeding	Abnormally thickened endometrium, prominent echogenicity of the endometrial cavity
Endometrial carcinoma	Abnormal uterine bleeding, postmenopausal bleeding	Distended uterine cavity, enlarged or lobular uterus, fluid-filled endometrial cavity, prominent echogenicity of the endometrial cavity
Leiomyomas (fibroids)	May be asymptommatic; pain, heavy bleeding, painful menses, rectal pressure, back pain	Uterine contour irregularity, altered echo texture (hypo- or hyperechogenicity), generalized uterine enlargement, calcifications with shadowing

CASE STUDIES FOR DISCUSSION

1. A 38-year-old multiparous woman is seen with pelvic pain and regular but heavy menstrual bleeding for the past 7 months. Her physician orders a pelvic sonogram. The sonographer notes an enlarged uterus with a smooth 4-mm endometrium and multiple areas with a heterogenous appearance within the myometrium. The adnexa are normal in appearance. What is the most likely diagnosis?

2. A 58-year-old multiparous woman is seen with new-onset postmenopausal bleeding over the past 3 days. She undergoes a pelvic sonogram that reveals an irregular thickened (9-mm) endometrium with a focal area measuring 11 mm. What is the next diagnostic procedure?

3. A 54-year-old woman is seen with 5 days of post-menopausal bleeding. The sonogram reveals a smooth 16-mm endometrium. What is the next diagnostic procedure?

4. A 28-year-old nulliparous patient has pelvic pressure and painful intercourse. Her body habitus precludes a satisfactory pelvic examination, so the physician orders pelvic sonography. Vaginal sonography reveals a 12-cm subserosal fibroid. What are the treatment options?

5. A 30-year-old nulliparous patient with a history of three miscarriages has intermittent brown spotting and 7-day

menses. A pelvic sonogram reveals focal endometrial thickening. Her physician refers her for a sonohysterogram, which reveals a 1.4-cm well-defined lesion within the endometrium. Her gynecologist removes the lesion hysteroscopically (Fig. 13-42; see Color Plate 8). What is the most likely diagnosis?

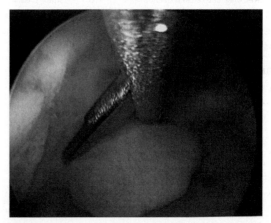

Fig. 13-42 Photo taken during hysteroscopic removal of lesion. Gynecologist used electrocautery wire to shave lesion off of anterior uterine wall.

STUDY QUESTIONS

1. A 32-year-old woman is seen with pelvic pain and intermittently painful intercourse. The pelvic sonogram reveals a hypoechoic area at the fundus of the uterus measuring 6 cm by 6 cm. What is the most likely diagnosis?
   a. adenomyosis
   b. submucosal fibroid
   c. endometrial polyp
   d. intramural fibroid
   e. endometrial hyperplasia

2. A 46-year-old woman has heavy regular vaginal bleeding. The sonogram reveals a 14-mm endometrium that is globally thickened. What is the most likely cause of the bleeding?
   a. endometrial hyperplasia
   b. submucosal fibroid
   c. endometrial carcinoma
   d. adenomyosis
   e. endometrial polyp

3. A 42-year-old is seen with brown spotting 4 days before normal menses and undergoes a pelvic sonogram. The gynecologist performs a saline-infusion vaginal ultrasound. The gynecologist most likely sees which one of the following?
   a. endometrial carcinoma
   b. endometrial hyperplasia
   c. an endometrial polyp
   d. a 4-cm subserosal fibroid
   e. adenomyosis

4. A 56-year-old woman undergoing estrogen replacement therapy is seen with new-onset vaginal bleeding. The pelvic sonogram reveals a 23-mm endometrium with irregular borders and a focal anechoic area consistent with an endometrial fluid collection. This patient most likely has what condition?
   a. endometrial hyperplasia
   b. adenomyosis
   c. a submucosal fibroid
   d. endometrial carcinoma
   e. nothing; this is a normal sonogram report

5. A 40-year-old woman is seen with worsening pelvic pressure and pain. The vaginal sonogram reveals an enlarged uterus with a 6-mm regular endometrium. A heterogenous-appearing myometrium is seen with focal areas of small anechoic lakes and enlargement of the posterior uterine wall in the sagittal plane. What condition does this patient most likely have?
   a. endometrial carcinoma
   b. multiple small intramural fibroids
   c. this is a normal pelvic sonogram report
   d. endometrial hyperplasia
   e. adenomyosis

6. A 32-year-old black woman is seen by her gynecologist for a routine pelvic examination. Her physician palpates an enlarged uterus and orders a pelvic sonogram. The sonographic examination reveals a 2-cm hypoechoic lesion within the uterine myometrium. This is most likely which of the following?
   a. adenomyoma
   b. leiomyoma
   c. a normal finding
   d. uterine carcinoma
   e. uterine fibrosis

7. A 70-year-old woman is seen by her family physician with a history of prolonged uterine bleeding. She reports that she has not undergone a pelvic examination since the birth of her last child at the age of 42 years. A sonographic evaluation of her pelvis is ordered and reveals an echogenic heterogeneous endometrium that measures 12 mm in thickness. What is the most likely diagnosis?
   a. endometrial carcinoma
   b. endometrial hyperplasia
   c. endometrial hypoplasia
   d. submucosal leiomyoma
   e. uterine polyp

8. A 35-year-old woman is seen for a pelvic ultrasound examination for a right adnexal mass palpated on clinical evaluation. The ultrasound reveals normal right and left ovaries. A hypoechoic well-defined lesion is identified in the right adnexal region connected by a stalk to the uterus. What is the most likely diagnosis?
   a. interligamentous fibroid
   b. parasitic fibroid
   c. pedunculated fibroid
   d. submucosal fibroid
   e. subserosal fibroid

9. A 40-year-old woman is seen with painful periods and a tender enlarged uterus on clinical examination.

A pelvic sonogram reveals an enlarged inhomogeneous uterus. What is the most likely diagnosis?

a. adenomyoma
b. adenomyosis
c. endometrial hyperplasia
d. leiomyoma
e. myometrial hypertrophy

10. A 47-year-old woman is seen by her physician because she can no longer button her favorite pair of jeans despite her weight loss efforts. Physical examination results reveal that her uterine fundus extends to her umbilicus. A pelvic ultrasound shows an enlarged inhomogeneous uterus containing multiple calcifications with shadowing. What is the most likely diagnosis?

a. adenomyosis
b. leiomyomata
c. myometrial hypertrophy
d. uterine cancer
e. uterine polyposis

REFERENCES

1. Andolf E, Jorgensen C: A prospective comparison of clinical ultrasound and operative examination of the female pelvis, *Ultrasound Med* 7:617-620, 1988.
2. Frederick JL, Paulson RJ, Sauer MV: Routine use of vaginal ultrasonography in the preoperative evaluation of gynecologic patients: an adjunct to resident education, *J Reprod Med* 36:779-782, 1991.
3. Goldstein SR: Incorporating endovaginal ultrasonography into the overall gynecologic examination, *Am J Obstet Gynecol* 162:625-632, 1990.
4. Langlois PL: The size of the normal uterus, *J Reprod Med* 4:220-228, 1970.
5. Platt JF, Bree RL, Davidson D: Ultrasound of the normal nongravid uterus: correlation with gross and histopathology, *J Clin Ultrasound* 18:15-19, 1990.
6. Faerstein E, Szklo M, Rosenshein N: Risk factors for uterine leiomyoma: a practice-based case-control study. I. African-American heritage, reproductive history, body size, and smoking, *Am J Epidemiol* 153:1-10, 2001.
7. Stewart EA, Nowak RA: Leiomyoma-related bleeding: a classic hypothesis updated for the molecular era, *Hum Reprod Update* 2:295-306, 1996.
8. Gross BH, Silver TM, Jaffe MH: Sonographic features of uterine leiomyomas: analysis of 41 proven cases, *J Ultrasound Med* 2:401-406, 1983.
9. Fedele L, Bianchi S, Dorta M et al: Transvaginal ultrasonography versus hysteroscopy in the diagnosis of uterine submucous myomas, *Obstet Gynecol* 77:745-748, 1991.
10. Baltarowich OH, Kurtz AB, Pennell RG et al: Pitfalls in the sonographic diagnosis of uterine fibroids, *AJR Am J Roentgenol* 151:725-728, 1988.
11. Fedele L, Bianchi S, Dorta M et al: Transvaginal ultrasonography in the differential diagnosis of adenomyoma versus leiomyoma, *Am J Obstet Gynecol* 167:603-606, 1992.
12. Azziz R: Adenomyosis: current perspectives, *Obstet Gynecol Clin North Am* 16:221-235, 1989.
13. Bird CC, McElin TS, Manalo-Eastrella P: The elusive adenomyosis of the uterus, *Am J Obstet Gynecol* 112:583-593, 1972.
14. Owolabi OT, Strickler RC: Adenomyosis: a neglected diagnosis, *Obstet Gynecol* 50:424-427, 1977.
15. Wang PH, Yang TS, Lee WL et al: Treatment of infertile women with adenomyosis with a conservative microsurgical technique and a gonadotropin-releasing hormone agonist, *Fertil Steril* 73:1061-1062, 2000.
16. Wood C, Maher P, Hill D: Biopsy diagnosis and conservative surgical treatment of adenomyosis, *J Am Assoc Gynecol Laparosc* 1(4 Pt 1):313-316, 1994.
17. Siskin GP, Tublin ME, Stainken BF et al: Uterine artery embolization for the treatment of adenomyosis: clinical response and evaluation with MR imaging, *AJR Am J Roentgenol* 177:297-302, 2001.
18. Fedele L, Bianchi S, Dorta M et al: Transvaginal ultrasonography in the diagnosis of diffuse adenomyosis, *Fertil Steril* 58:94-97, 1992.
19. Bohlman ME, Ensor RE, Sanders RC: Sonographic findings in adenomyosis of the uterus, *AJR Am J Roentgenol* 148:765-766, 1987.
20. Walsh JW, Taylor KJ, Rosenfield AT: Gray scale ultrasonography in the diagnosis of endometriosis and adenomyosis, *AJR Am J Roentgenol* 132:87-90, 1979.
21. Brosens J, De Souza NM, Barker FG et al: Endovaginal ultrasonography in the diagnosis of adenomyosis uteri: identifying the predictive characteristics, *Am J Obstet Gynecol* 102:471-474, 1995.
22. Reinhold C, McCarthy S, Bret PM et al: Diffuse adenomyosis: comparison of endovaginal US and MR imaging with histiopathic correlation, *Radiology* 199:151-158, 1996.
23. Seidler D, Laing FC, Jeffrey RB et al: Uterine adenomyosis: a difficult sonographic diagnosis, *J Ultrasound Med* 6:345-349, 1987.
24. Reinhold C, Atri M, Mehio A et al: Diffuse uterine adenomyosis: morphologic criteria and diagnostic accuracy of endovaginal sonography, *Radiology* 197:609-614, 1995.
25. Chiang CH, Chang MY, Hsu JJ et al: Tumor vascular pattern and blood flow impedance in the differential diagnosis of leiomyoma and adenomyosis by color Doppler sonography, *J Assist Reprod Genet* 16:268-275, 1999.

26. Ascher SM, Arnold LL, Patt RH et al: Adenomyosis: prospective comparison of MR imaging and trans-vaginal sonography, *Radiology* 190:803-806, 1994.

27. Dueholm M, Lundorf E, Hansen ES et al: Magnetic resonance imaging and transvaginal ultrasonography for the diagnosis of adenomyosis, *Fertil Steril* 76:588-594, 2001.

28. Togashi K, Ozasa I, Konishi I et al: Enlarged uterus: differentiation between adenomyosis and leiomyoma with MRI, *Radiology* 171:531-534, 1989.

29. Elwood JM, Cole P, Rothman KJ et al: Epidemiology of endometrial cancer, *J Natl Cancer Inst* 59:1055-1060, 1977.

30. Bakos O, Lundkvist O, Wide L et al: Ultrasono-graphical and hormonal description of the normal ovulatory menstrual cycle, *Acta Obstet Gynecol Scand* 73:790-796, 1994.

31. Fleischer AC, Kalemeris GC, Entman SS: Sonographic depiction of the endometrium during normal cycles, *Ultrasound Med Biol* 2:271-277, 1986.

32. Nasri MN, Coast GJ: Correlation of ultrasound findings and endometrial histopathology in postmenopausal women, *Br J Obstet Gynaecol* 96:1333-1338, 1989.

33. Osmers R, Volksen M, Schnauer A: Vaginosonography for early detection of endometrial carcinoma? *Lancet* 335:1569-1571, 1990.

34. Goldstein SR, Nachtigall M, Snyder JR et al: Endometrial assessment by vaginal ultrasonography before endometrial sampling in patients with post menopausal bleeding, *Am J Obstet Gynecol* 163:119-123, 1990.

35. Granberg S, Wikland M, Karlsson B et al: Endometrial thickness as measured by endovaginal ultrasonography for identifying endometrial abnormality, *Am J Obstet Gynecol* 164:47-52, 1991.

36. Kurman RJ, Kaminski PF, Norris HJ: The behavior of endometrial hyperplasia. A long-term study of "untreated" hyperplasia in 170 patients, *Cancer* 56:403-412, 1985.

37. Chambers CB, Unis JS: Ultrasonographic evidence of uterine malignancy in the postmenopausal uterus, *Am J Obstet Gynecol* 154:1194-1199, 1986.

38. Scott WW Jr, Rosenshein NB, Siegelman SS et al: The obstructed uterus, *Radiology* 141:767-770, 1981.

39. Requard CK, Wicks JD, Mettler FA: Ultrasonography in the staging of endometrial adenocarcinoma, *Radiology* 140:781-785, 1981.

40. Archer DF, McIntyre-Seltman K, Wilborn WW et al: Endometrial morphology in asymptomatic post-menopausal women, *Am J Obstet Gynecol* 165:317-322, 1991.

41. Zacchi V, Zini R, Canino A: Transvaginal sonography as a screening method for the identification of patients at risk of postmenopausal endometrial pathology, *Minerva Gynecol* 45:339-342, 1993.

42. Castelo-Branco C, Puerto B, Duran M et al: Trans-vaginal sonography of the endometrium in post-menopausal women: monitoring the effect of hormone replacement therapy, *Maturitas* 19:59-65, 1994.

43. Shipley CR, Simmons CL, Nelson GH: Comparison of transvaginal sonography with endometrial biopsy in asymptomatic postmenopausal women, *J Ultrasound Med* 13:99-104, 1994.

44. Langer RD, Pierce JJ, O'Hanlan KA et al: Transvaginal ultrasonography compared with endometrial biopsy for the detection of endometrial disease. Post-menopausal Estrogen/Progestin Interventions Trial, *N Engl J Med* 337:1792-1798, 1997.

45. Smith-Bindman R, Kerlikowske K, Feldstein VA et al: Endovaginal ultrasound to exclude endometrial cancer and other endometrial abnormalities, *JAMA* 280:1510-1517, 1998.

46. Malpani A, Singer J, Wolverson MK et al: Endometrial hyperplasia: value of endometrial thickness in ultrasonographic diagnosis and clinical significance, *J Clin Ultrasound* 18:173-177, 1990.

47. Dubinsky TJ, Pravey HR, Gormaz G et al: Transvaginal hysterosonography: comparison with biopsy in the evaluation of postmenopausal bleeding, *J Ultrasound Med* 14:887-893, 1995.

48. Dubinsky TJ, Parvey HR, Gormaz G et al: Transvaginal hysterosonography in the evaluation of small endo-luminal masses, *J Ultrasound Med* 14:1-6, 1995.

49. Guido RS, Kanbour A, Ruhn M et al: Pipelle endometrial sampling sensitivity in the detection of endometrial cancer, *J Reprod Med* 40:553-555, 1995.

50. Goldstein SR, Zeltser I, Horan CK et al: Ultrasonography-based triage for perimenopausal patients with abnormal uterine bleeding, *Am J Obstet Gynecol* 177:102-108, 1977.

51. Karlsson B, Granberg S, Wikland M et al: Transvaginal ultrasonography of the endometrium in women with postmenopausal bleeding: a Nordic multicenter study, *Am J Obstet Gynecol* 172:1488-1494, 1995.

52. Gull B, Carlsson S, Karlsson B et al: Transvaginal ultrasonography of the endometrium in women with postmenopausal bleeding: is it always necessary to perform an endometrial biopsy? *Am J Obstet Gynecol* 182:509-515, 2000.

53. Novak ER, Woodruff JD, editors: *Novak's gynecology and obstetric pathology with clinical and endocrine relations*, ed 8, Philadelphia, 1979, WB Saunders.

54. Pettersson B, Adami HO, Lindgren A et al: Endometrial polyps and hyperplasia as risk factors for endometrial carcinoma: a case-control study of curettage specimens, *Acta Obstet Gynecol Scand* 64:653-659, 1985.

55. Tjarks M, Van Voorhis BJ: Treatment of endometrial polyps, *Obstet Gynecol* 96:886-889, 2000.

56. Gebauer G, Hafner A, Siebzehnrubl E et al: Role of hysteroscopy in detection and extraction of endometrial polyps: results of a prospective study, *Am J Obstet Gynecol* 184:59-603, 2001.

57. Hulka CA, Hall DA, McCarthy K et al: Endometrial polyps, hyperplasia, and carcinoma in the postmenopausal women: differentiation with endovaginal sonography, *Radiology* 191:755-758, 1994.

58. Indman PD: Abnormal uterine bleeding: accuracy of vaginal probe ultrasound in predicting abnormal hysteroscopic findings, *J Reprod Med* 40:545-548, 1995.

59. Lev-Toaff AS, Toaff ME, Liu JB et al: Value of sonohysterography in the diagnosis and management of abnormal uterine bleeding, *Radiology* 201:179-184, 1996.

60. Laughead MK, Stones LM: Clinical utility of saline solution infusion sonohysterography in a primary care obstetric-gynecologic practice, *Am J Obstet Gynecol* 176:1313-1316, 1997.

61. Chittacharoen A, Theppisai U, Linasmita V et al: Sonohysterography in the diagnosis of abnormal uterine bleeding, *J Obstet Gynaecol Res* 26:277-281, 2000.

62. Goldstein SR: Use of ultrasonohysterography for triage of perimenopausal patients with unexplained uterine bleeding, *Am J Obstet Gynecol* 170:565-566, 1994.

63. Wolman I, Jaffa AJ, Hartoov J et al: Sensitivity and specificity of sonohysterography for the evaluation of the uterine cavity in perimenopausal patients, *J Ultrasound Med* 15:285-288, 1996.

64. Bernard JP, Lecuru F, Darles C et al: Saline contrast sonohysterography as first-line investigation for women with uterine bleeding, *Ultrasound Obstet Gynecol* 10:121-125, 1997.

65. O'Connell LP, Fries MH, Zeringue E et al: Triage of abnormal postmenopausal bleeding: a comparison of endometrial biopsy and transvaginal sonohysterography versus fractional curettage with hysteroscopy, *Am J Obstet Gynecol* 178:956-961, 1998.

66. Epstein E, Ramirez A, Skoog L et al: Transvaginal sonography, saline contrast sonohysterography and hysteroscopy for the investigation of women with postmenopausal bleeding and endometrium > 5 mm, *Ultrasound Obstet Gynecol* 18:157-162, 2001.

67. Syrop CH, Sahakian V: Transvaginal sonographic detection of endometrial polyps with fluid contrast augmentation, *Obstet Gynecol* 79:1041-1043, 1992.

68. Turner RT, Berman AM, Topel HC: Improved demonstration of endometrial polyps and submucous myomas using saline-enhanced vaginal sonohysterography, *J Am Assoc Gynecol Laparosc* 2:421-425, 1995.

69. Cicinelli E, Romano F, Anastasio PS et al: Transabdominal sonohysterography, transvaginal sonography, and hysteroscopy in the evaluation of submucous myomas, *Obstet Gynecol* 85:42-47, 1995.

70. Salle B, Gaucherand P, de Saint Hilaire P et al: Transvaginal sonohysterographic evaluation of intrauterine adhesions, *J Clin Ultrasound* 27:131-134, 1999.

71. Soares SR, Barbosa dos Reis MM, Camargos AF: Diagnostic accuracy of sonohysterography, transvaginal sonography, and hysterosalpingography in patients with uterine cavity diseases, *Fertil Steril* 73:406-411, 2000.

72. Bernard JP, Rizk E, Camatte S et al: Saline contrast sonohysterography in the preoperative assessment of benign intrauterine disorders, *Ultrasound Obstet Gynecol* 17:145-149, 2001.

73. Wolman I, Jaffa AJ, Pauzner D et al: Transvaginal sonohysterography: a new aid in the diagnosis of residual trophoblastic tissue, *J Clin Ultrasound* 24:257-261, 1996.

74. Zalel Y, Cohen SB, Oren M et al: Sonohysterography for the diagnosis of residual trophoblastic tissue, *J Ultrasound Med* 20:877-881, 2001.

75. Keltz MD, Olive DL, Kim AH et al: Sonohysterography for screening in recurrent pregnancy loss, *Fertil Steril* 67:670-674, 1997.

76. Alatas C, Aksoy E, Akarsu C et al: Evaluation of intrauterine abnormalities in infertile patients by sonohysterography, *Hum Reprod* 12:487-490, 1997.

77. Kim AH, McKay H, Keltz MD et al: Sonohysterographic screening before in vitro fertilization, *Fertil Steril* 69:841-844, 1998.

78. Alatas C, Urman B, Aksoy S et al: Evaluation of uterine cavity by sonohysterography in women scheduled for intracytoplasmic sperm injection, *Hum Reprod* 13:2461-2462, 1998.

79. Tepper R, Beyth Y, Altaras MM et al: Value of sonohysterography in asymptomatic postmenopausal tamoxifen-treated patients, *Gynecol Oncol* 64:386-391, 1997.

80. Elhelw B, Ghorab MN, Farrag SH: Saline sonohysterography for monitoring asymptomatic postmenopausal breast cancer patients taking tamoxifen, *Int J Gynaecol Obstet* 67:81-86, 1999.

81. Hann LE, Gretz EM, Bach AM et al: Sonohysterography for evaluation of the endometrium in women treated with tamoxifen, *AJR Am J Roentgenol* 177:337-342, 2001.

82. van Roessel J, Wamsteker K, Exalto N: Sonographic investigation of the uterus during artificial uterine cavity distention, *J Clin Ultrasound* 15:439-450, 1987.

83. Bussey LA, Laing FC: Sonohysterography for detection of a retained laminaria fragment, *J Ultrasound Med* 15:249-251, 1996.

84. Widrich T, Bradley LD, Mitchinson AR et al: Comparison of saline infusion sonography with office hysteroscopy for the evaluation of the endometrium, *Am J Obstet Gynecol* 174:1327-1334, 1996.

85. Parsons A, Hill DA, Spicer D: Sonohysterographic imaging of the endometrial cavity, *Front Biosci* 1:f1-5, 1996, http://www.bioscience.org/1996/v1/f/parsons/res.htm, retrieved September 9, 2002.

86. Dessole S, Farina M, Capobianco G et al: Determining the best catheter for sonohysterography, *Fertil Steril* 76:605-609, 2001.

14 Lost Intrauterine Device

JOHN W. VAN WERT and CHARLOTTE HENNINGSEN

CLINICAL SCENARIO

■ A 27-year-old woman is seen for a pelvic ultrasound. The patient had a Copper T intrauterine device inserted 9 months ago and is having persistent **menometrorrhagia.** Her gynecologist attempted to remove the device, but the strings broke with attempted removal and are no longer visible.

A transvaginal ultrasound reveals a homogeneous uterus. Both ovaries appear normal. An echogenic object (Fig. 14-1, *A* and *B*) appears in the endometrial cavity. What are the possibilities for the location and the removal of the device?

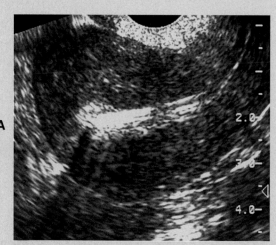 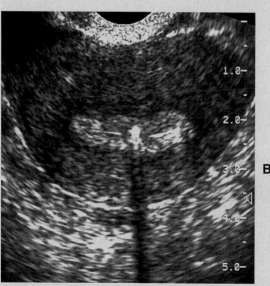

Fig. 14-1   **A,** Longitudinal and, **B,** transverse images of uterus. Note shadowing extending from echogenic structure.

OBJECTIVES

■ Describe the sonographic appearance of properly positioned intrauterine devices.
■ Describe the sonographic appearance of abnormally positioned intrauterine devices.
■ Differentiate the sonographic characteristics of intrauterine devices in association with complicating factors, including infection, perforation, pregnancy, and ectopic pregnancy.
■ Identify gynecologic symptoms associated with intrauterine device use.
■ List the factors associated with lost intrauterine devices.

GLOSSARY OF TERMS ■

Ectopic pregnancy: any pregnancy positioned outside of the normal intrauterine location

Endometrium: the glandular mucous membrane that lines the inside of the uterus

Endomyometritis: infection of the endometrium and inner myometrium of the uterus characterized by pelvic pain, fever, uterine tenderness, and vaginal discharge

Forceps: an instrument that resembles a pair of tongs that is used for grasping or extracting

Hysteroscopy: a surgical technique of direct visualization of the endometrial cavity through a scope placed through the cervical canal

Infertility: the inability to conceive a child, usually over a 1-year time frame

Intrauterine device: a foreign body placed in the endometrial cavity of the uterus to prevent conception

Menometrorrhagia: irregular or excessive bleeding during menstruation and between menstrual periods

Myometrium: the smooth muscle body of the uterus

Pelvic inflammatory disease: inflammation of the female genital tract, especially of the fallopian tubes, caused by any of several microorganisms, characterized by severe abdominal pain, high fever, foul-smelling vaginal discharge, and in some cases, destruction of tissue that can result in sterility

Retroverted uterus: a uterus that is turned posteriorly

Spontaneous abortion: the premature expulsion of a nonviable pregnancy from the uterus

During the past few years, new designs and manufacturing techniques have caused increased interest in the use of **intrauterine devices** (IUDs) as a contraceptive option in the United States. The IUD is the most common form of reversible contraception used worldwide and is the most cost-effective method of birth control if used for more than 2 years.[1,2] IUD use had declined in the United States since the 1960s after the rate of pelvic inflammatory disease was found to increase in users of one IUD, the Dalkon Shield (AH Robins, St. Davids, Pennsylvania). The type of string that was attached to the base allowed bacteria to travel to the upper genital tract. This type of string tail is no longer in use.[1,2] Since the days of the ill-fated Dalkon Shield, other IUDs have been designed and approved, such as the Copper T (ParaGard T380A Intrauterine Copper Contraceptive, Ortho-McNeil Pharmaceutical, Raritan, New Jersey). This IUD consists of copper wire wound around the arms and stem of the T.[3] Studies suggest that the release of copper ions changes the chemical composition of the fluid in the **endometrium.** The presence of a foreign body in the endometrial canal induces morphologic changes, and the alteration in the endometrial fluid milieu causes an inflammatory reaction that is spermicidal and prevents fertilization.[2] The Copper T IUD is approved for 10 years of continuous use before removal is necessary.

Recently, progesterone-releasing or progestin-releasing IUDs have become a popular option. These IUDs also induce a foreign-body reaction but to a lesser degree than the copper-containing devices. The release of progestational hormone causes the endometrial glands to shrink and atrophy, reducing sperm survival and inhibiting embryo implantation. The cervical mucous is also thickened with progesterone, diminishing sperm motility.[1,2] The thinning of the endometrium with the progestational hormones has the benefit of reducing the amount of menstrual flow, which adds to the appeal of the IUD as a contraceptive option. The progestin-releasing IUD requires removal every 5 years, whereas the progesterone-releasing IUD must be changed every year.

SONOGRAPHIC APPEARANCE OF AN INTRAUTERINE DEVICE

When the IUD has been properly inserted, the device expands from its temporarily constricted state (used for insertion through the endocervical canal) and lies in the plane of the endometrial cavity. All of the IUDs currently approved by the U.S. Food and Drug Administration (FDA) are created from an echogenic plastic, with or without copper, in a T configuration (Fig. 14-2, A). The top bars of the T unfold after insertion to lie across the fundal portion of the endometrial cavity, and the stem lies vertically. Occasionally, other IUD shapes (Fig. 14-2, B and C) may be identified sonographically if a patient has not had regular gynecologic care and has not had an older IUD removed. Some of the varying configurations include serpentine- and 7-shaped devices. IUDs appear highly echogenic (Fig. 14-2, D), may exhibit entrance-exit reflections (Fig. 14-2, E), and may cast a shadow.

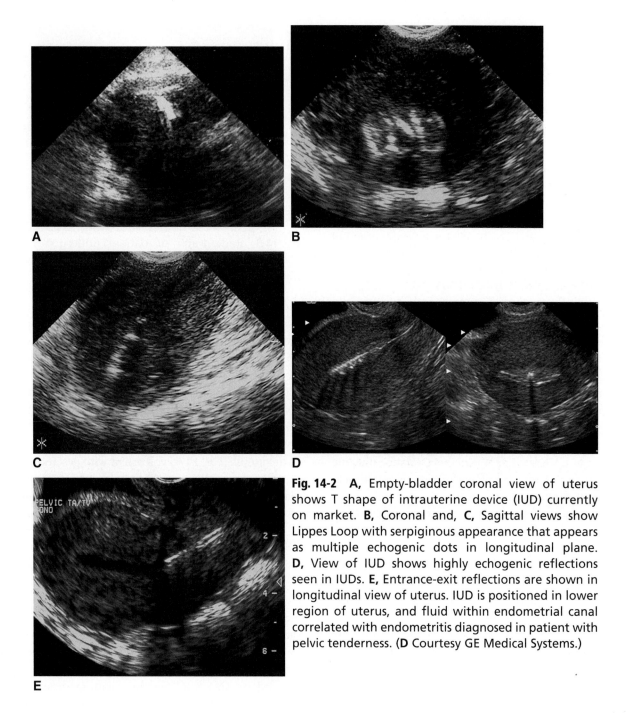

Fig. 14-2 A, Empty-bladder coronal view of uterus shows T shape of intrauterine device (IUD) currently on market. **B,** Coronal and, **C,** Sagittal views show Lippes Loop with serpiginous appearance that appears as multiple echogenic dots in longitudinal plane. **D,** View of IUD shows highly echogenic reflections seen in IUDs. **E,** Entrance-exit reflections are shown in longitudinal view of uterus. IUD is positioned in lower region of uterus, and fluid within endometrial canal correlated with endometritis diagnosed in patient with pelvic tenderness. (**D** Courtesy GE Medical Systems.)

The IUD strings (usually two) are attached to the bottom of the stem and pass through the endocervical canal and into the upper portion of the vagina, where they typically coil asymptomatically. The strings are the consistency of fine fishing line and are not usually visualized with ultrasound. Patient with an IUD needs to palpate the IUD strings to ensure that the IUD is still in place because expulsion may occur and go unrecognized by the patient. Missing strings may also be the result of breakage or detachment of the strings, strings migrating into the cervix, or IUD perforation into or through the uterus. When a patient or the clinician cannot locate the strings, an ultrasound may be ordered to locate the lost IUD.

INTRAUTERINE DEVICE COMPLICATIONS

Infection

One of the most concerning aspects of placement of a foreign object into the body is the introduction of bacteria into a sterile locale. The design improvements and the use of sterile technique with insertion have minimized IUD-associated infection, but occasional cases of **endomyometritis, pelvic inflammatory disease,** and even tuboovarian abscesses can be seen with IUDs.

Sonographic Findings. A thickened irregular endometrial cavity with possible echogenic debris or fluid (see Fig. 14-2, *E*) may be seen in advanced endomyometritis. Dilated cylindric or serpiginous fallopian tubes, tuboovarian complexes appearing as complex or inhomogeneous adnexal masses, and excess cul-de-sac fluid are commonly noted with pelvic inflammatory disease (see Chapter 15). The IUD is typically noted in its usual endometrial location.

Perforation or Ectopic Location

Perforation occurs in approximately one per 1000 insertions[4] and is associated with improper insertion procedure, the level of experience and skill of the inserter, and an extremely **retroverted** or **posterior uterus.**[5,6] Perforation may also occur in patients with congenital uterine anomalies. Perforation is expected whenever the strings are not palpable or visible from the cervical os. If the device is no longer in the uterus, other radiographic techniques may be necessary to localize the IUD, such as magnetic resonance imaging or flat plate radiography. If perforation is confirmed, not only is there no contraceptive efficacy, but immediate removal is necessary to prevent other complications, such as perforation of the bowel or bladder.[1]

Sonographic Findings. The endometrial cavity can be clearly delineated separately from the location of the IUD. The IUD may be visible in the **myometrium,** the cervix, or the pelvic or abdominal cavity. It is possible that no IUD is seen whatsoever, suggesting expulsion or an extrapelvic location. A radiograph will show the presence of the IUD (Fig. 14-3) if it has perforated the uterus because IUDs are radiopaque.

Pregnancy

Although IUDs have an exceptionally low failure rate compared with other forms of contraception, the failure rate of two to three per 100 woman-years leads to 300,000 or more pregnancies with IUDs in situ worldwide each year.[7,8] A relatively high risk of complications in pregnancy with IUDs in situ exists, including **spontaneous abortion,** premature rupture of membranes, preterm labor, septic abortion, and maternal death.[8-14] Appropriate care is removal of the IUD from the pregnant uterus if the strings are visible at the cervix.[8,10-15] During the past several years, ultrasound has been

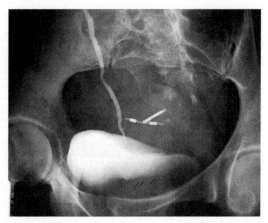

Fig. 14-3 Radiograph of patient undergoing intravenous pyelography for flank pain shows radiopaque nature of Copper T intrauterine device.

successfully used to aid in the removal of IUDs with strings that are not visible with excellent fetal and maternal results.[7] Laparoscopy is the procedure of choice for removal of ectopic abdominally located IUDs, even in pregnancy. The importance of ultrasound in **infertility** evaluations has also been confirmed with several reports of "forgotten" IUDs sonographically revealed in patients referred to infertility clinics.[16]

Sonographic Findings. The pregnancy is visualized in the uterus (Fig. 14-4) consistent with gestational age. The echogenic IUD is commonly found apparently displaced to the inner surface of the myometrium, outside of the amniotic sac, and may be in any orientation.

Ectopic Pregnancy

Women who conceive with an IUD in place have an increased risk of **ectopic pregnancy** (30% of conceptions).[17] Infection, one of the risks of IUD use, may increase the incidence of ectopic pregnancies by causing tubal damage and scarring. Patients who desire to keep properly placed IUDs may opt for traditional surgical management of the ectopic pregnancy and also can undergo successful treatment with medical therapy, such as methotrexate, leaving the IUD in situ and functional.[17]

Sonographic Findings. Ultrasound can determine the location of the IUD and also its relationship to the presence of an ectopic gestation (Fig. 14-5). Care is taken to note whether the highly echogenic IUD is in its normal intrauterine location, has migrated away, or has perforated through the myometrium. The ectopic gestation most commonly is identified in the adnexal region because most ectopic pregnancies are located in the fallopian tubes (see Chapter 21). Sonographic findings may also include cul-de-sac fluid and the

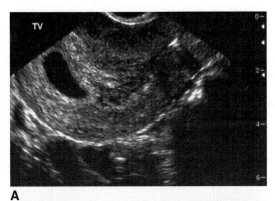

A

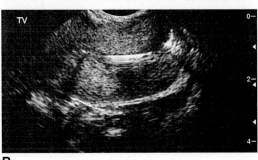

B

Fig. 14-4 This 23-year-old patient was seen with history of skipped period and positive pregnancy test. Ultrasound shows, **A,** gestational sac identified in longitudinal image, yolk sac, and, **B,** intrauterine device positioned in cervical region. Mean sac diameter corresponded to 5.5-week gestation. (Courtesy Lori Davis and Natalie Cauffman, Florida Hospital Deland.)

absence of an intrauterine gestation. The presence or absence of an intrauterine pregnancy should be carefully correlated with beta human chorionic gonadotropin levels.

Table 14-1 is a summary of the symptoms and pathologic findings of the complications of IUDs.

SUMMARY

The choice of an IUD for contraception is prevalent, so ultrasound is commonly used for determination of proper placement, location, and orientation of the device. Ultrasound will help evaluate the nature of concurrent complications, such as infection, perforation, ectopic location (lost IUD), and contraceptive failures, including both intrauterine and ectopic pregnancies.

The future of evaluation of IUD placement and complications lies with three-dimensional ultrasound (Fig. 14-6). This technique enables imaging of both the arms and the shaft of the entire IUD simultaneously, allowing for faster and more accurate localization.[18]

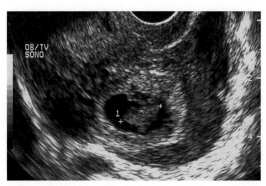

Fig. 14-5 Viable ectopic pregnancy was identified in adnexal region of 30-year-old woman with positive pregnancy test and intrauterine device that was identified within uterus.

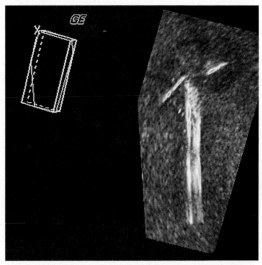

Fig. 14-6 Three-dimensional ultrasound of intrauterine device (IUD) shows IUD within endometrial canal. (Courtesy GE Medical Systems.)

CLINICAL SCENARIO—DIAGNOSIS

■ The fact that the IUD strings were initially visible suggests that the IUD is in the uterus and not abdominally located. The IUD strings may break from the age of the IUD (unlikely in this case because of the fairly recent insertion); from a severely retroverted uterine location, making the string tension vector at right angles to the axis of the IUD; or more commonly, from an IUD embedded in the myometrium. Options for removal include gynecologic tools, such as an IUD hook, ultrasound-guided **forceps** removal, and **hysteroscopic** removal with direct visualization.

Table 14-1	Complications Associated with Intrauterine Devices	
Complication	**Symptoms**	**Sonographic Findings**
Infection	Pelvic pain, fever, purulent discharge	Thick endometrial cavity and intrauterine device (IUD), dilated fallopian tubes, tuboovarian abscesses, cul-de-sac fluid
IUD expulsion	None; pregnancy	Normal-appearing uterus; no IUD visible
IUD perforation	None; pregnancy, abdominal pain	IUD not visible within endometrial cavity, may be seen in myometrium or cervix or may not be identified; radiograph can confirm intraabdominal location
Pregnancy	Positive pregnancy test, may lead to pregnancy complications	Gestational sac; IUD at inner surface of myometrium
Ectopic pregnancy	Positive pregnancy test, pain, bleeding	IUD in endometrium, ectopic location of gestational sac, cul-de-sac fluid

CASE STUDIES FOR DISCUSSION

1. A 22-year-old woman is seen for an ultrasound with a last menstrual period of approximately 10 weeks prior and an IUD insertion 6 months ago. The ultrasound reveals the findings in Fig. 14-7, *A* and *B*. What is the most likely diagnosis?
2. A 25-year-old woman with pelvic pain is seen for pelvic ultrasound. The ultrasound reveals the highly echogenic structure noted in Fig. 14-8 and confirms the presence of an IUD. What is the likely diagnosis for this patient?
3. A 42-year-old woman is seen with lower quadrant abdominal pain. She has a history of IUD usage but has been unable to palpate the string. An ultrasound reveals a normal-appearing uterus with a minimal amount of cul-de-sac fluid. A radiograph is ordered and shows the findings in Fig. 14-9. What is the most likely diagnosis?
4. A 32-year-old woman is seen with bleeding and a positive pregnancy test. The ultrasound shows the finding in Fig. 14-10. What is the most likely diagnosis?

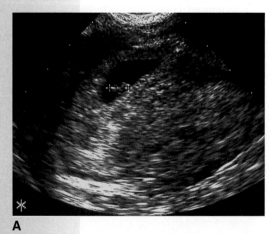
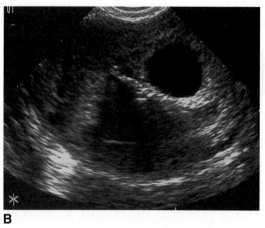

A   **B**

Fig. 14-7 **A,** Longitudinal image of uterus shows crown-rump length corresponding to 6.5-week gestation. No evidence is found of heartbeat. **B,** Transverse image shows echogenic structure that shadows lateral to gestational sac.

5. A 40-year-old woman is seen for a pelvic ultrasound for missing strings. The patient has had an IUD in place for the past 3 years. The ultrasound reveals the finding in Fig. 14-11. What is the most likely diagnosis?

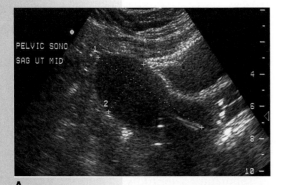

A

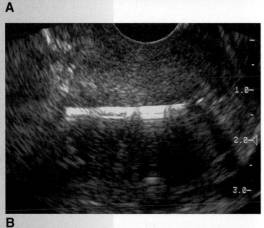

B

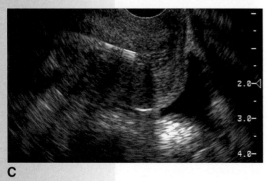

C

Fig. 14-8 A, Transabdominal ultrasound of longitudinal uterus correlates with endovaginal cervical findings in **B** and **C.**

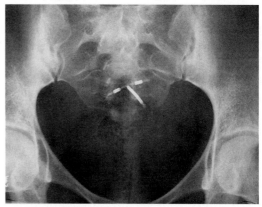

Fig. 14-9 Radiograph of pelvis shows T-shaped intrauterine device.

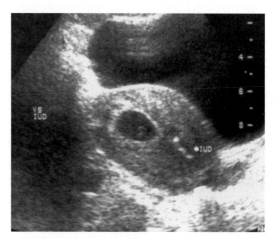

Fig. 14-10 Longitudinal image of uterus.

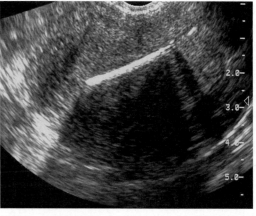

Fig. 14-11 Endovaginal ultrasound of longitudinal view of uterus.

STUDY QUESTIONS

1. A 42-year-old woman is seen with severe pelvic pain. The patient has a history of IUD insertion after her most recent pregnancy. The IUD is not identified on endovaginal ultrasound of the uterus. A radiograph shows the IUD in the pelvis. What is the most likely diagnosis?
   a. ectopic pregnancy
   b. IUD perforation
   c. pelvic inflammatory disease
   d. IUD string detachment
   e. tuboovarian abscess

2. The sonographic appearance of an IUD includes which of the following?
   a. highly echogenic, entrance-exit reflections, shadowing
   b. hypoechoic, entrance-exit reflections, enhancement
   c. anechoic with shadowing
   d. highly echogenic, entrance-exit reverberation, enhancement
   e. hypoechoic, entrance-exit reflections, enhancement

3. A young women with severe pelvic pain and IUD usage is seen for ultrasound. Ultrasound reveals the T-shaped IUD within the endometrium. Bilateral enlarged tubular structures are identified in the adnexae. This patient should be treated for which of the following?
   a. cul-de-sac fluid
   b. ectopic pregnancy
   c. ectopic IUD
   d. IUD perforation
   e. pelvic inflammatory disease

4. Currently, the IUDs on the market have which of the following shapes?
   a. circle
   b. T
   c. 7
   d. serpiginous
   e. triangle

5. A patient is seen with a positive pregnancy test and IUD usage. An ultrasound reveals a 7-week, live gestation within the uterus. The IUD is identified at the lower uterine segment, and the strings are visible to the obstetrician as they protrude through the external cervical os. What is most likely course of treatment for this patient?
   a. expectant management
   b. laparoscopic surgery to remove the IUD
   c. laparoscopic concurrent IUD removal and abortion
   d. IUD removal through the cervix
   e. medical abortion

6. A patient with a positive serum pregnancy test and IUD usage is seen for sonographic examination. The ultrasound reveals the IUD with no evidence of an intrauterine gestation. Cul-de-sac fluid is also noted. The patient's last menstrual period is 7.5 weeks prior. What is the most likely diagnosis for this patient?
   a. ectopic pregnancy
   b. false-positive pregnancy test
   c. intrauterine pregnancy
   d. pelvic inflammatory disease
   e. spontaneous abortion

7. A 27-year-old woman is seen with pelvic pain and IUD usage of 1-year duration. The pelvic ultrasound reveals a normal-appearing uterus without evidence of an IUD. The patient denies IUD expulsion, but a radiograph also fails to reveal an IUD. What is the most likely explanation regarding the IUD?
   a. unrecognized IUD expulsion
   b. perforation of the IUD into the abdomen
   c. a normally placed IUD unrecognized with ultrasound
   d. pelvic inflammatory disease preventing recognition of the IUD

8. A 35-year-old woman is seen for a pelvic ultrasound for pelvic pain. She has had an IUD for the past 3 years without complication. The ultrasound reveals a normal-appearing uterus with a T-shaped IUD located in the endometrium with the T arms positioned toward the fundus. This is consistent with which of the following?
   a. a normally positioned IUD
   b. ectopic pregnancy
   c. IUD perforation
   d. pelvic inflammatory disease

9. A 37-year-old woman with a history of heavy bleeding with pregnancy is seen for ultrasound. Her last menstrual period was 8 weeks prior. The ultrasound reveals a slightly enlarged uterus without evidence of an intrauterine pregnancy. The sonographer also identifies a highly echogenic serpiginous structure within the uterus that

shadows. No evidence is found of cul-de-sac fluid or adnexal masses. This would be most consistent with which of the following?

a. ectopic pregnancy

b. endometritis

c. forgotten IUD with a spontaneous abortion

d. IUD perforation

e. pelvic inflammatory disease

10. A 28-year-old woman is seen for pelvic ultrasound for missing strings from her IUD. The ultrasound reveals a T-shaped, highly echogenic structure arising within the endometrium. This would be consistent with which of the following?

a. a normally positioned IUD

b. endometritis

c. IUD expulsion

d. IUD perforation

REFERENCES

1. Kent MG: Sonographic evaluation of an abnormal location of an intrauterine device, *J Diagn Med Sonogr* 15:203-205, 1999.

2. Mishell DR: Intrauterine devices: mechanisms of action, safety and efficacy, *Contraception* 58(suppl):45S-53S, 1998.

3. Stewart GK: Intrauterine devices. In Trussell J, Stewart F, Cates W et al, editors: *Contraceptive technology,* ed 17, New York, 1998, Ardent Media.

4. Bjornerem A, Tollan A: Uterine device: primary and secondary perforation of the urinary bladder, *Acta Obstet Gynecol Scand* 76:383-385, 1997.

5. *Intrauterine devices: technical and managerial guidelines for services,* Geneva, 1997, World Health Organization.

6. Speroff L, Darney P: Intrauterine contraception. The IUD. In Speroff L, Darney P, editors: *A clinical guide for contraception,* ed 2, Baltimore, 1996, Williams & Wilkins.

7. Stubblefield PG, Fuller AF, Foster SC: Ultrasound guided intrauterine removal of intrauterine contraceptive devices in pregnancy, *Obstet Gynecol* 72:961-964, 1988.

8. Fallon JH: Pregnancy with IUD in situ, *Kans Med* 86:322-324, 1985.

9. Lewit S: Outcome of pregnancy with intrauterine devices, *Contraception* 2:47-57, 1970.

10. Christian CD: Maternal deaths associated with an intrauterine device, *Am J Obstet Gynecol* 119:441-444, 1974.

11. Wiles PJ, Zeiderman AM: Pregnancy complicated by intrauterine contraceptive devices, *Obstet Gynecol* 44:484-490, 1974.

12. Tatum HJ, Schmidt FH, Jain AK: Management and outcome of pregnancies associated with the Copper T intrauterine contraceptive device, *Am J Obstet Gynecol* 126:869-877, 1976.

13. Eisinger SH: Second trimester spontaneous abortion, the IUD and infection, *Am J Obstet Gynecol* 124:393-397, 1976.

14. Koetsawang S, Rachawat D, Piya-Anant M. Outcome of pregnancy in the presence of intrauterine device, *Acta Obstet Gynecol Scand* 56:479-482, 1977.

15. American College of Obstetricians and Gynecologists: *The intrauterine device, ACOG technical bulletin 104,* Washington, DC, 1987, The American College of Obstetricians and Gynecologists.

16. Ron-el R, Weinraub Z, Langer R et al: The importance of ultrasonography in infertile women with "forgotten" intrauterine contraceptive devices, *Am J Obstet Gynecol* 161:211-212, 1989.

17. Sites CK: Treatment of ectopic pregnancy with single-dose methotrexate in a patient with an intrauterine device; a case report, *J Reprod Med* 40:800-802, 1995.

18. Lee A, Eppel W, Sam C et al: Intrauterine device localization by three-dimensional transvaginal sonography, *Ultrasound Obstet Gynecol* 10:289-292, 1997.

Pelvic Inflammatory Disease

REGINA SWEARENGIN

CLINICAL SCENARIO

■ A 21-year-old college student is seen in the emergency department with lower abdominal pain and fever. The patient states that the abdominal pain has become increasingly severe since her period finished 3 days ago. She has been using an over-the-counter treatment for what she thought was a vaginal infection that somewhat improved her symptoms of itching and burning. Physical examination reveals abdominal guarding and rebound tenderness. Manual pelvic examination elicits such severe pain that a thorough examination of the pelvic organs cannot be completed. Laboratory test results show elevated white blood cell counts and a negative human chorionic gonadotropin level. The patient also denies pregnancy.

A sonogram of the pelvis is ordered. Transabdominal scanning shows bilateral complex masses, fluid in the cul-de-sac, and ovarian enlargement (Fig. 15-1). Thickening of the endometrium is also noted. Endovaginal scanning is attempted, although only a limited amount of information is gained because of the patient's pain during the procedure. What is the possible diagnosis?

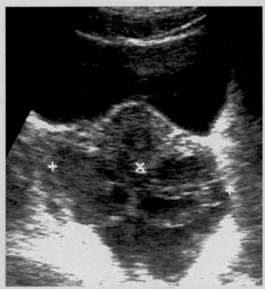

Fig. 15-1 Transverse scan of uterus shows bilateral adnexal masses, pyosalpinx, and thickened endometrium.

OBJECTIVES

■ List and describe the etiology and risk factors associated with pelvic inflammatory disease.
■ Describe the progression of pelvic inflammatory disease, and identify the specific sequela of pelvic inflammatory disease.
■ Describe the sonographic appearances of pelvic inflammatory disease, including salpingitis,

pyosalpinx, hydrosalpinx, and tuboovarian abscess.
■ Identify Doppler findings associated with pelvic inflammatory disease.
■ Identify pertinent laboratory values and related diagnostic studies associated with pelvic inflammatory disease.

GLOSSARY OF TERMS

Dyspareunia: painful or difficult intercourse

Endotoxemia: presence of bacterial toxins in the blood

Erythrocyte sedimentation rate: nonspecific indicator of inflammation

Fitz-Hugh–Curtis syndrome: right upper quadrant pain that occurs with tuboovarian abscess; perihepatitis

Gonorrhea: inflammation of the genital mucous membrane caused by *Neisseria gonorrhoeae*

Leukocytosis: increased numbers of white blood cells; seen with infection

Rebound tenderness: pain that can be produced or intensified with release of pressure

Salpingitis: inflammation of the fallopian tubes

Sexually transmitted disease: disease acquired as a result of intercourse with an infected individual

Tuboovarian abscess: abscess formed when purulent material escapes the fallopian tube and forms a pocket of abscess near the ovary

Pelvic inflammatory disease (PID) is a type of **sexually transmitted disease** (STD), although this bilateral infection may be associated with the use of an intrauterine contraceptive device (IUCD). Less commonly, unilateral PID may result from direct extension of primary lower abdominal/pelvic abscesses or postabortion or postchildbirth complications. The diagnosis of PID is usually made clinically through the assessment of patient history and symptoms, pelvic examination, urine test, and culture of vaginal secretions.[1] Early and vigorous antibiotic treatment is needed to stop the progression of the disease and prevent the development of infertility.

Chlamydia is more common than gonorrhea as a source of infection, but numerous aerobic and anaerobic organisms may also be present. In many cases, the symptoms of chlamydia and gonorrhea are mild or nonexistent in both females and males; however, males are more likely to seek treatment when symptoms are present. Eighty-five percent of females and 40% of males with chlamydia infection are asymptomatic, but 75% to 80% of men do not know that **gonorrhea** and chlamydia can be asymptomatic and can have serious consequences.[2]

Risk factors for PID include female gender under the age of 35 years, sexual activity (two or more partners), and the use of IUCD. The risk of recurrent infection is high, and the consequences of PID include chronic pelvic pain from adhesions, peritonitis, ectopic pregnancy, maternal death from ectopic pregnancy, and infertility (increased risk with each occurrence). Early and appropriate treatment is usually with two antibiotics to cover the possibility of multiple organisms; the patient's partners must also be treated. Symptoms may abate without the infection being cured, which can lead to the patient not completing the course of medication.

Because PID is readily diagnosed with assessment of the patient's symptoms and signs, sonography of the pelvis may not provide additional diagnostic information because the anatomy many times will appear normal. However, pelvic sonography is frequently performed because of physical findings such as fever, severe pain with manipulation of the cervix or adnexal areas, presence of purulent vaginal discharge, abdominal/rebound tenderness, and possible elevated white blood cell (WBC) count and **erythrocyte sedimentation rate** (ESR). Sonography is useful in showing the presence and extent of endometritis, **salpingitis**, pyosalpinx, hydrosalpinx, and **tuboovarian abscess** (TOA). Occasionally, the only sonographic feature of PID will be a loss of definition of the posterior uterine border.[3,4]

Both transabdominal (TA) and endovaginal (EV) scanning techniques are recommended for evaluation of the presence and extent of PID. TA scanning allows for the overall evaluation of the entire pelvis and delineation of large structures/masses. EV scanning allows for the high-resolution evaluation of the uterus/endometrial cavity, fallopian tubes, ovaries, cul-de-sac, and adnexal areas.[3] However, the patient's condition (i.e., pelvic pain) may make full distention of the urinary bladder or insertion and manipulation of the EV transducer impossible. The sonographer must be aware of these possibilities and should tailor the examination to decrease pain for the patient and increase information gained. Gentle and slow scanning motions are imperative, and a thorough explanation of the procedure may help to increase patient compliance.

The symptoms of acute PID include: fever (low or high), shaking chills, abdominal pain (mild/moderate/severe), nausea, vomiting, vaginal discharge, and irregular vaginal bleeding. Signs of acute PID include abdominal guarding, rebound tenderness, increased pain with cervical or adnexal manipulation, dyspareunia, **leukocytosis**, elevated ESR, paralytic ileus, and shock from peritonitis.

Symptoms of chronic PID are persistent pelvic/lower abdominal pain, irregular menses, and possibly infertility. Signs of chronic PID may include presence of an adnexal masses without fever.[1]

Related diagnostic studies include: urine test, cultures of vaginal secretions/discharge, culdocentesis, laparoscopy, and computed tomographic (CT) and magnetic resonance imaging (MRI) imaging.

SONOGRAPHIC FINDINGS

Fallopian Tubes

The fallopian tubes are contained within the broad ligament and are not appreciated with sonography unless surrounded by ascites or involved in a disease process, such as salpingitis, pyosalpinx, or hydrosalpinx. Fallopian tubes are best shown with radiographic salpingography, which involves pressure injection of radiopaque contrast through the tubes.

Salpingitis

Salpingitis is an infection of the fallopian tubes that may be acute, subacute, or chronic.[5] The sonographic appearance of acute salpingitis includes nodular thickening of the walls of the fallopian tubes with diverticula. Hyperemia is also present and can be shown color Doppler imaging. Anechoic or echogenic (pus-containing) fluid may be seen in the posterior cul-de-sac (pouch of Douglas) as may uterine enlargement with endometrial fluid or thickening (endometritis). Subacute salpingitis indicates that infectious changes have taken place without significant clinical signs and symptoms.

Chronic salpingitis is related to recurrent bouts of PID and may result in significant tubal scarring and the presence of hydrosalpinx (Fig. 15-2). The patient may have pain during intercourse or bowel movements (from adhesions involving the bowel and peritoneal surface) and during menses.[1] Tubal scarring may be seen sonographically as several cystic structures extending from the uterus to the adnexa; this is sometimes referred to as the "chain of lakes" or "string of pearls" sonographic appearance. Infertility and ectopic pregnancy may result from the tubal scarring.

Pyosalpinx

Pyosalpinx is a progression of PID in which the fallopian tubes become swollen with purulent exudates

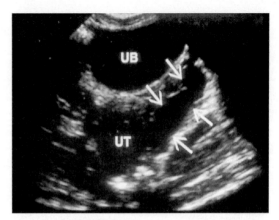

Fig. 15-2 Hydrosalpinx.

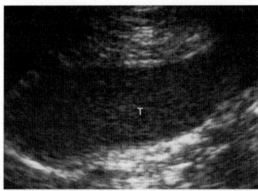

Fig. 15-3 Pyosalpinx. Endovaginal image of fallopian tube filled with pus.

(Fig. 15-3). The sonographic appearance of pyosalpinx is consistent with visualization of thick-walled tubular or serpiginous structures surrounding the ovaries. The interstitial portion of the tube is tapered at the cornu of the uterus. The tube may also be described as sausage shaped. Echogenic material or debris related to the presence of pus may be seen within the fallopian tubes. In addition, blurring of the normal tissue planes in the pelvis can occur, making delineation of the organs and structures difficult.

Endovaginal scanning can differentiate pyosalpinx from other pelvic masses by showing the tubular nature of the tube. Pyosalpinx can also be differentiated from fluid-filled bowel with visualization of peristalsis in the bowel. Color Doppler imaging will show increased flow in the pelvic structures.

Hydrosalpinx

Hydrosalpinx is a consequence of PID in which the fallopian tube or tubes become closed at the fimbriae and the pus within a pyosalpinx gradually liquefies, leaving serous fluid. In addition, the walls of the tubes

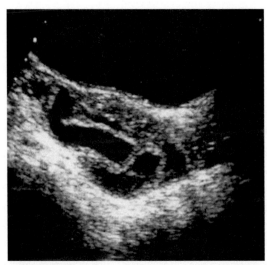

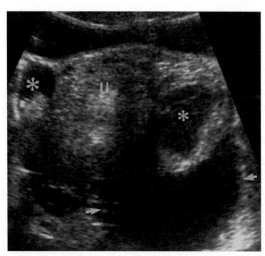

Fig. 15-4 Hydrosalpinx. Long left image of fallopian tube dilated with serous fluid.

Fig. 15-6 Transverse scan of uterus *(U)* shows bilateral adnexal masses *(*)* with fluid in cul-de-sac.

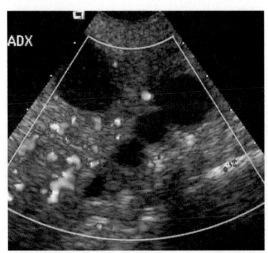

Fig. 15-5 Hydrosalpinx. No flow in anechoic tubular structure; blood flow seen in vessels around structure.

become thinner and the tubes may dilate to twice the normal diameter. The patient may be asymptomatic or may have colicky pain. Hydrosalpinx may be present for a significant length of time before diagnosis of infertility from blockage of the fallopian tubes.

Sonographically, the fallopian tubes appear as anechoic thin-walled structures with a multicystic or fusiform mass effect (Fig. 15-4). Color Doppler is useful to differentiate hydrosalpinx from bowel or prominent pelvic veins (Fig. 15-5). The sonographer should carefully show the pathway of the tube and the ovary.[5]

Tuboovarian Abscess

Tuboovarian abscess results from pus leaking from an infected fallopian tube (pyosalpinx) and may occur

from communication with the ovary. TOA is a result of serious pelvic infection and is generally seen in the later stages of PID. Small abscesses develop but still respond to the antibiotic treatment. Large abscesses may necessitate surgical removal/drainage. A surgical emergency can occur with massive perforation by a pelvic abscess during which the patient has a rapid progression of severe abdominal pain, nausea, vomiting, peritonitis, shock from peritonitis, and **endotoxemia**.[6]

Sonographically, TOA appears as a thick-walled, complex hypoechoic mass with fluid in the cul-de-sac and adnexa (Fig. 15-6). TOA may be bilateral or unilateral and can be found in the adnexa or in the posterior cul-de-sac. Additional sonographic appearances include a mass with septations, irregular margins, and fluid-debris levels. Serial ultrasound examinations can follow the response of the TOA to antibiotic therapy or can provide guidance during a drainage procedure. If untreated, TOA may progress to peritonitis. The presence of air/gas within the abscess may make sonographic detection and delineation of the disease process difficult unless the examination correlates with clinical findings.

In pelvic abscess with peritonitis, the patient has a high fever and a significantly elevated WBC count associated with the severe lower abdominal pain, nausea, and vomiting.[6] Diffuse spread of purulent fluid into the surrounding pelvic cavity is seen. Ten percent of patients may have **Fitz-Hugh–Curtis syndrome** develop in which the patient has right upper quadrant (RUQ) pain.[4] Sonographically, free fluid may be noted in the cul-de-sac and the hepatorenal space (Morison's pouch), with an indistinct appearance of the pelvic organs due from tissue edema and abscesses.

Endometritis

Fifty percent to 80% of patients with endometritis, inflammation of the endometrium, are asymptomatic. The most common symptoms are vaginal discharge, urethral burning, pelvic pain, and elevated WBC and ESR. Endometritis may result from cesarean section birth, IUCD perforation, retained products of conception (POC), or contamination with gonorrhea or chlamydia. Endometritis therefore is not always related to PID but may be the first presentation of PID.[4]

Sonographic appearances of endometritis include: normal uterus in approximately 75% of cases, uterine enlargement, widened or thickened echogenic endometrium, air in the endometrium (from gas-forming infection), fluid in endometrial cavity, or hypoechoic halo around the endometrium (Fig. 15-7).[4] The ovaries

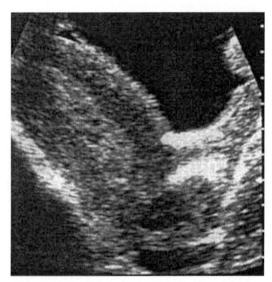

Fig. 15-7 Prominent endometrium with fluid in cul-de-sac.

may be enlarged and indistinct because of inflammation. Endometritis may progress to myometritis, parametritis, pelvic abscess, or peritonitis.

Table 15-1 is a summary of the pathology, symptoms, and sonographic findings of PID.

SUMMARY

Sonographic examination of the female pelvis is useful in determination of the extent of PID and in demonstration of the sequela of the disease process. Sonography can follow the course of PID, thus enabling the physician to treat the disease successfully. Guidance for drainage procedures in the case of TOA or pelvic abscess can be provided with ultrasound imaging. Because of the severe pain often experienced with PID, the pelvic sonogram can be a challenging examination to perform. Sonographic appearances must be correlated with clinical and laboratory findings to provide a definitive sonographic diagnosis.

CLINICAL SCENARIO—DIAGNOSIS

■ Although the sonogram was limited in quality because of the inability of the patient to cooperate fully for the examination, a diagnosis of PID with bilateral TOA was made. The patient was treated with antibiotics, and follow-up sonograms revealed resolution of the PID and bilateral TOA. Additional follow-up was recommended to determine whether the PID affected her fertility status.

Table 15-1	*Pelvic Inflammatory Disease*	
Pathology	**Symptoms**	**Sonographic Findings**
Endometritis	Often asymptomatic; vaginal discharge, urethral burning, pelvic pain; patient history of cesarean section, IUCD perforation, retained POC; STD	Normal uterus; uterine enlargement, thickened endometrium; air or fluid in endometrial cavity; hypoechoic halo around endometrium; ovarian enlargement with indistinct borders
Salpingitis	Subacute: no clinical symptoms Acute: fever, chills, abdominal pain, nausea, vomiting, vaginal discharge, irregular vaginal bleeding, abdominal guarding, rebound tenderness, pain with manipulation of cervix Chronic: dyspareunia, painful bowel movements, infertility, ectopic pregnancy	Subacute/acute: nodular thickening of fallopian tube walls with diverticula; hyperemia; anechoic or echogenic fluid in cul-de-sac; uterine enlargement, endometrial fluid or thickening Chronic: hydrosalpinx, cystic structures extending from uterus to adnexa, ectopic pregnancy
Pyosalpinx	Fever, chills, abdominal pain, nausea, vomiting, vaginal discharge, irregular vaginal bleeding, abdominal guarding, rebound tenderness, pain with manipulation of cervix	Swollen, thick-walled fallopian tubes; echogenic debris within tubes; blurring of normal tissue planes
Hydrosalpinx	Asymptomatic or colicky pain	Dilated, thin-walled tubes filled with fluid
TOA	High fever, elevated WBC count, severe lower abdominal pain, nausea and vomiting; RUQ pain; peritonitis	Variable appearance; unilateral or bilateral thick-walled, complex hypoechoic mass in adnexa or cul-de-sac; mass with septations, irregular margins, fluid-debris levels; air within mass; free fluid in cul-de-sac and Morison's pouch; blurring of normal tissue planes

IUCD, Intrauterine contraceptive device; *POC,* products of conception; *RUQ,* right upper quadrant; *STD,* sexually transmitted disease; *WBC,* white blood cell.

CASE STUDIES FOR DISCUSSION

1. A 15-year-old girl is seen in the emergency department with a high fever and some abdominal pain. Her mother is afraid that she has appendicitis. During the physical examination, the patient was reluctant to discuss her symptoms and sexual history with her mother present. When the mother left the examination room, the physician was able to elicit from the patient that she had had sex just once for the first time the previous week with a boy from school. The patient also revealed that she had not noticed any vaginal discharge and thought she just had cramps because her period was about to start. Laboratory work revealed negative pregnancy test results and leukocytosis. A pelvic sonogram was ordered and showed a complex mass posterior and to the left of the uterus (Fig. 15-8). An endovaginal scan was attempted but was discontinued by the mother because of the patient's pain. What is the differential diagnosis?

2. A 23-year-old unmarried woman sees her physician for the second time in 2 weeks. Ten days ago, the physician diagnosed PID based on the patient symptoms and physical examination. Vaginal cultures were sent for laboratory analysis, but the patient was started on a course of oral antibiotics at the time of the first office visit. The patient now has severe abdominal pain and a fever. Once again, the physician performs a pelvic examination, only now the patient has exquisite pain as the cervix and adnexal areas are manipulated. With suspicion that the PID has not responded to the medication so that the infection has possibly progressed to abscess, the physician sends the patient to the hospital for a pelvic sonogram. The sonogram (Fig. 15-9) reveals complex mass and free fluid in the cul-de-sac. Color Doppler reveals increased flow consistent with hyperemia. The patient is admitted to the hospital for intravenous antibiotics and close monitoring of her condition. What is the most likely diagnosis?

3. A 25-year-old woman who is a recent immigrant from Europe is seen in the emergency department with stomach symptoms. The patient's use of the English language is limited, so she is unable to answer many of the physician's questions during the work-up and physical examination. The patient denies pregnancy. The physical examination is limited by the patient's pain and inability to communicate. The physician orders abdominal and pelvic ultrasounds to locate the source of the pain. The upper abdominal sonogram is unremarkable, but the pelvic sonogram reveals the presence of an IUCD in the uterus. The sonographer is unable to perform an endovaginal scan because of the patient's refusal. The transabdominal images show some uterine enlargement, with the IUCD centrally located in the uterus (Fig. 15-10). Bilateral ovarian volumes are increased when compared with the normal range. What is the diagnosis?

4. A patient is seen for a pelvic ultrasound. She is G4P2022, and her last menstrual period was 2 weeks ago. The patient's symptoms consist of moderate pelvic pain and a sensation of fullness. She relates that her physician told her "there might be something going on" in her pelvis, which

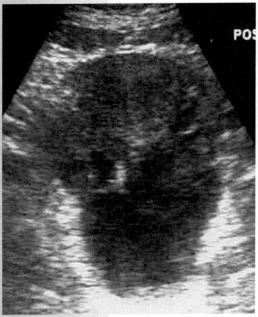

Fig. 15-8 Large complex mass posterior to uterus.

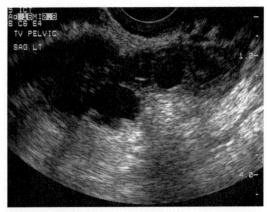

Fig. 15-9 Uterus is seen posterior to bladder and is bordered by complex lesions.

CASE STUDIES FOR DISCUSSION—cont'd

is why she needs the ultrasound. She denies vaginal discharge or dyspareunia. The sonogram reveals bilateral enlarged ovaries and a prominent endometrium with a hypoechoic halo (Fig. 15-11). What is the most likely diagnosis?

5. A 50-year-old postmenopausal woman in the emergency department relates a history of recent divorce and resumption of an active sexual life (multiple partners). She also reveals that because of her menstrual status, she did not use any contraceptive protection. Her symptoms are "fever, pain, and a smelly vaginal discharge." She has had the symptoms for a few days and sought treatment when the pain became severe. Physical examination reveals significant pelvic tenderness and a purulent vaginal discharge. A pelvic sonogram reveals bilateral tubular structures that are thick walled (Fig. 15-12). Although the condition was painful, the patient was able to tolerate an endovaginal scan, which confirmed the presence of large tubular structures, the ovaries, and free fluid in the cul-de-sac. What is the most likely diagnosis?

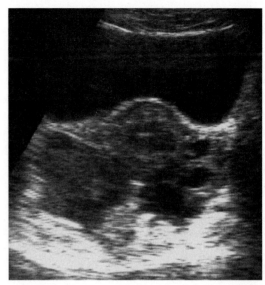

Fig. 15-11 Transverse scan of uterus shows bilateral ovarian enlargement and prominent endometrium.

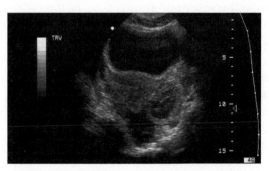

Fig. 15-12 Left fallopian tube is representative of finding also identified in right adnexa.

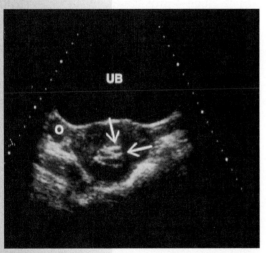

Fig. 15-10 Intrauterine contraceptive device *(arrows)*.

STUDY QUESTIONS

1. A sexually active 18-year-old woman is seen with symptoms of pelvic pain, vaginal discharge, dyspareunia, and pain during bowel movements. She relates a history of treatment for vaginal infection twice in the past year. Laboratory values reveal some leukocytosis. Ultrasound of the pelvis is unremarkable except for pain experienced by the patient during the EV scan and lack of movement of the uterus and ovaries with slight pressure by the EV transducer. What is the most likely diagnosis?
   a. acute pelvic inflammatory disease with tubo-ovarian abscess
   b. endometriosis
   c. chronic pelvic inflammatory disease; possible adhesions
   d. hydrosalpinx

2. A 24-year-old college student is seen for a pelvic ultrasound for vague symptoms of pelvic discomfort. The sonogram reveals fluid in the cul-de-sac, slightly enlarged ovaries, an indistinct posterior uterine border, and increased blood flow in all pelvic structures. These findings are most likely related to which of the following?
   a. ectopic pregnancy
   b. acute pelvic inflammatory disease
   c. chronic pelvic inflammatory disease
   d. pyosalpinx

3. During a pelvic sonogram, the sonographer visualizes prominent anechoic tubular structures in both adnexa. The patient has symptoms of pelvic pain but denies history of PID. What should the sonographer do to further evaluate the tubular structures?
   a. use color Doppler to check for blood flow in the structures
   b. require that the patient increase her fluid intake to further distend the urinary bladder
   c. have another sonographer complete the examination
   d. nothing; the sonographer has done all that is needed to make the diagnosis

4. A friend brings a 30-year-old woman who has recently undergone an elective abortion to the emergency department. The patient has severe abdominal pain and a high fever. The friend states that the patient began feeling sick the day before, 3 days after the elective abortion. The patient displays abdominal guarding and a purulent vaginal discharge. A pelvic sonogram reveals large complex masses in both adnexae and enlargement of the uterus with air in the endometrium. The ovaries are not well seen because of the presence of the adnexal masses. A sonogram of the upper abdomen reveals some fluid in the hepatorenal space. These sonographic findings are most suggestive of which of the following?
   a. chronic pelvic inflammatory disease with hydrosalpinx and adhesions
   b. ruptured ectopic pregnancy
   c. pelvic inflammatory disease with pyosalpinx
   d. endometritis, tuboovarian abscess, and Fitz-Hugh–Curtis syndrome

5. During a pelvic sonogram for workup of infertility in a 30-year-old woman, the sonographer sees several cystic structures that extend bilaterally from the uterus to the region of the ovaries. This finding can be described as which of the following?
   a. Fitz-Hugh–Curtis syndrome
   b. chain-of-lakes appearance
   c. sausage-shaped fallopian tubes
   d. dilated pelvic veins

6. A 38-year-old woman undergoes a pelvic ultrasound because her physician felt some fullness in both adnexal regions during her last check-up. The patient denies history of venereal disease or use of an IUCD. The ultrasound examination reveals bilateral fluid-filled structures. With EV scanning, these structures are determined to be tubular. Which of the following is a possible diagnosis?
   a. pyosalpinx
   b. ascites
   c. tuboovarian abscess
   d. hydrosalpinx

7. A follow-up pelvic sonogram for a patient with diagnosis of TOA is performed. The ultrasound reveals little or no change in the appearance of the pelvic abscesses since the first sonogram 1 week ago. What may be the next step in the treatment of this case of PID?
   a. surgical removal of the uterus and ovaries
   b. ultrasound-guided drainage of the abscesses
   c. serial sonograms and continued oral antibiotics

d. continued antibiotic therapy with no further need for ultrasound

8. A patient with suspected acute PID is sent for a pelvic ultrasound examination. The sonogram reveals normal-appearing uterus, ovaries, and adnexal regions. Why is this possible?

a. inappropriate techniques used by the sonographer have created a false-negative sonogram

b. the sonographer did not get a complete patient history and therefore missed the pelvic inflammatory disease

c. the patient had a complete resolution of the pelvic inflammatory disease before the sonogram was performed

d. the sonographic appearance of normal pelvic structures is seen in approximately 75% of acute pelvic inflammatory disease cases

9. A patient with a known diagnosis of Crohn's disease is seen with left lower quadrant pain and fever. The pelvic sonogram reveals the presence of an echogenic, sausage-shaped mass in the left adnexa. This most likely is related to which of the following?

a. unilateral pyosalpinx

b. bilateral pyosalpinx

c. bilateral tuboovarian abscess

d. unilateral hydrosalpinx

10. A patient with long-standing pelvic pain is seen for a pelvic sonogram. The ultrasound examination reveals bilateral extraovarian adnexal masses that contain low-level echoes. The differential diagnosis for this sonographic appearance includes all of the following except:

a. endometriosis

b. pelvic inflammatory disease/tuboovarian abscess

c. pelvic abscess

d. ovarian torsion

REFERENCES

1. Berkow R, Beers M: *The Merck manual of diagnosis and therapy*, ed 17, Rahway, NJ, 1999, Merck & Co.
2. Yates B: *Low level of STD knowledge is serious*, http://www.docguide.com/dgc.nsf/news/html, retrieved June 16, 2000.
3. Rumack CM, Wilson SR, Charboneau JW: *Diagnostic ultrasound*, vol 1, ed 2, St Louis, 1998, Mosby.
4. Hall R: *The ultrasound handbook*, ed 3, Philadelphia, 1999, Lippincott.
5. Hagen-Ansert SL: *Textbook of diagnostic ultrasonography*, vol 2, ed 5, St Louis, 2001, Mosby.
6. National Institutes of Health/National Institute of Allergy and Infectious Diseases: *Sexually transmitted diseases statistics, fact sheet, 1998*, http://www.niaid.nih.gov/factsheets/stdstats.html, retrieved June 16, 2000.

BIBLIOGRAPHY

Sanders RC: *Clinical sonography*, ed 3, Philadelphia, 1998, Lippincott.

Henningsen C: *National certification examination review, obstetrics and gynecology*, ed 3, Dallas, 2001, Society of Diagnostic Medical Sonography.

Johnson PT, Kurtz AB: *Case review obstetric and gynecologic ultrasound*, ed 1, St Louis, 2001, Mosby.

Bisset RA, Khan AN: *Differential diagnosis in abdominal ultrasound*, ed 2, Philadelphia, 2002, WB Saunders.

Callen PW: *Ultrasonography in obstetrics and gynecology*, ed 4, Philadelphia, 2000, WB Saunders.

McGahan JP, Goldberg BB: *Diagnostic ultrasound a logical approach*, Philadelphia, 1998, Lippincott.

16

Infertility

PAMELA A. KUNAU SZCZESNIAK

CLINICAL SCENARIO

◼ An 18-year-old woman is seen for a pelvic ultrasound with 1 week of severe pelvic pain and spotting. She is nauseated but not vomiting. A pregnancy test is ordered and is positive. The ultrasound examination reveals the findings in Figs. 16-1 and 16-2. What is the most likely diagnosis for this patient?

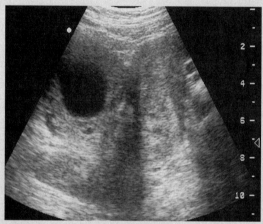

Fig. 16-2 Two horns are identified. The horn on the right demonstrates a gestational sac.

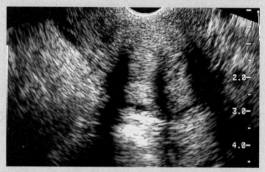

Fig. 16-1 Transverse image demonstrating two cervices.

OBJECTIVES

◼ List and describe the ovarian factors that can lead to infertility.

◼ Differentiate the sonographic appearances of ovarian causes of infertility.

◼ Describe the normal embryologic development of the uterus.

◼ Define a variety of congenital uterine anomalies.

◼ Describe the sonographic features that differentiate the types of congenital uterine anomalies.

GLOSSARY OF TERMS

Amenorrhea: lack of menstruation

Anovulation: absence of ovulation

Dysmenorrhea: pain that corresponds with menstruation

Ectopia: an abnormal location of an organ

Hematocolpos: menstrual blood within the vagina

Hematometracolpos: menstrual blood within the vagina and uterus

Hirsutism: abnormal excess growth of hair

Hysterosalpingography: radiographic procedure with injection of contrast medium into the uterus and fallopian tubes for evaluation

Hysteroscopy: use of an endoscope for evaluation of the uterus

Menorrhagia: extreme bleeding during a menstrual period

Oligomenorrhea: very little or irregular menstrual flow

Stein-Leventhal syndrome: endocrine disorder linked with anovulation; symptoms include infertility, hirsutism, and oligomenorrhea

Pelvic ultrasound may be used in the identification of various causes of infertility. Many of the abnormalities may be found incidentally because the patient is asymptomatic. Clinical examinations and correlative imaging procedures may assist in a definitive diagnosis so that treatment, surgery, or pregnancy options can be explored.

This chapter is limited to a discussion of factors linked with infertility that may be identified with ultrasound. The most common ovarian factors linked with infertility are explored, and differentiations of congenital uterine anomalies are discussed. Tubal factors associated with infertility are discussed in Chapter 15.

ENDOMETRIOSIS

Endometriosis is the result of functioning endometrial tissue being located outside the uterus. The condition is hormonally stimulated during the reproductive years and can affect up to 25% to 35% of infertile women.[1] Symptoms of endometriosis besides infertility include pain, **menorrhagia**, and **dysmenorrhea**, although patients may be asymptomatic.[2] Endometriosis can be localized or diffuse. The ovaries are the most common

place for endometriosis to occur, although endometrial implants may be located anywhere in the body.[3] Endometriosis can be treated medically, with hormones or hormone-suppression therapy, or surgically, depending on the extent of disease and the desired outcome. The purpose of treatment may be to decrease or alleviate symptoms of pain associated with endometriosis or to improve the chances of pregnancy with removal of endometrial implants that may be impeding ovulation or obstructing fallopian tubes. Surgery is the better option if the endometriosis is moderate to severe,[4] although recurrence of the disease is possible. The rate of pregnancy after laparoscopy or laparotomy is 42.8% and 46.6%, respectively.[5] Patients who no longer desire fertility may elect hysterectomy and bilateral salpingoooophorectomy to decrease symptoms of the disease.

Sonographic Findings

The localized form of endometriosis, endometrioma, presents as a mass involving the ovary and is also known as a *chocolate cyst*. The classic ultrasound appearance is a well-defined, thin-walled mass containing low-level, internal echoes with through transmission. Endometriomas can be unilocular or multilocular and are frequently multiple in number.[3] Other sonographic appearances include masses with thick walls, internal septations, or fluid-debris levels in the dependent portion of the lesion (Figs. 16-3 to 16-8).[2,3] Endometriomas are most easily characterized with endovaginal ultrasound with better definition of the degree of internal echoes when compared with transabdominal ultrasound.[6]

The diffuse form of endometriosis is more difficult to evaluate because the implants of diffuse endometriosis are usually too small to be seen. Endometriosis may be suggested when the tissue planes between the pelvic structures blend indistinctly from adhesions. When the focal form is not visualized, sonographic examination will usually be nondiagnostic.[2,3]

POLYCYSTIC OVARIAN DISEASE

Polycystic ovarian disease (PCOD) is an endocrine disorder that produces **anovulation** and results in infertility. Patients with PCOD have an imbalance of luteinizing hormone (LH) and follicle-stimulating hormone (FSH).[3] The LH level may be elevated or the ratio of LH to FSH may be elevated. Testosterone levels are increased, and estrogen levels are also abnormal.

PCOD is a cause for infertility in approximately 6% of women of reproductive age.[7] Clinical symptoms include infertility, early pregnancy loss, hirsutism,

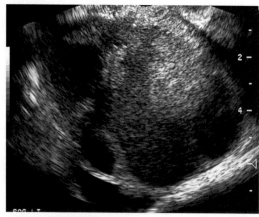

Fig. 16-3 Endovaginal scan of sagittal view of a complex endometrioma.

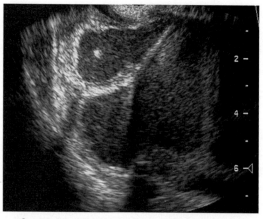

Fig. 16-4 Ultrasound of endometrioma.

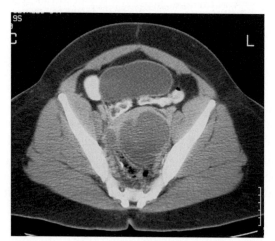

Fig. 16-5 Computed tomographic scan of endometrioma.

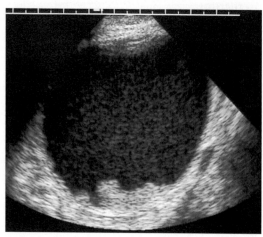

Fig. 16-6 Endovaginal ultrasound of left ovarian endometrioma with internal debris.

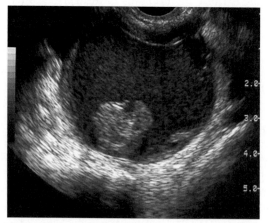

Fig. 16-7 Complex endometrioma shown with ultrasound.

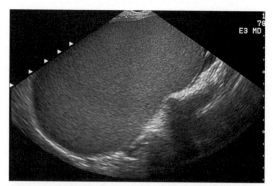

Fig. 16-8 Endometrioma completely filled with internal echoes. (Courtesy GE Medical Systems.)

Stein-Leventhal syndrome, and amenorrhea; although some patients with PCOD have no symptoms. The diagnosis is generally made with evaluation of the clinical presentation and hormone levels, but ultrasound is also used to look for the positive findings of PCOD. In addition, patients with PCOD may incur the risks associated with unopposed estrogen and may be monitored for endometrial carcinoma and breast cancer.[3]

Sonographic Findings

Sonographic examination of PCOD may reveal bilateral ovaries that contain multiple small follicles. The follicles are usually located in the periphery of the ovary and are 0.5 to 0.8 cm in size.[3] This produces a sonographic appearance of a "string of pearls" (Figs. 16-9 and 16-10). The ovaries also have an increase in stromal echogenicity (Fig. 16-11). The size of the ovaries may be normal or enlarged.[2]

CONGENITAL UTERINE ANOMALY

Congenital uterine anomalies can be a contributing factor in infertility. The uterus and fallopian tubes develop from paired müllerian ducts that fuse, and then the uterine septum formed from the fusion is reabsorbed. The development of the uterus occurs between 7 and 12 weeks of gestation. Anomalies that occur may be caused by failure of development of one or both of the müllerian ducts (uterine agenesis, unicornuate uterus), failure of fusion of the müllerian ducts (uterus didelphys and bicornuate uterus), and failure of the sagittal septum to reabsorb (Fig. 16-12). The congenital uterine anomalies that are most commonly associated with infertility and pregnancy loss include the septate and unicornuate uterus.

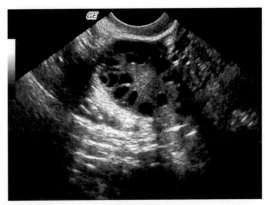

Fig. 16-10 Endovaginal ultrasound of polycystic ovary showing "string of pearls."

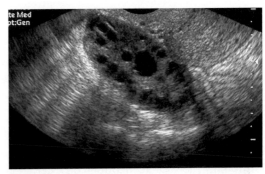

Fig. 16-11 Ovary with increased echogenicity containing multiple, tiny follicles.

Sonographic identification and differentiation of uterine anomalies can be difficult as imaging the uterus in the coronal plane will best show the uterine cavity and the shape of the fundus. Careful transducer angulation may attain this view, but when available, three-dimensional ultrasound can be used to acquire this plane. Identification of the endometrium is also easier when patients undergo imaging in the secretory phase of the menstrual cycle when the endometrium is thick and echogenic.

A close association also exists in the development of the uterus with the excretory system. When a uterine anomaly is identified, the kidneys should also be evaluated for the presence of congenital anomalies, such as a unilateral renal agenesis or **ectopia**.

Uterus Didelphys

Uterus didelphys is a rare, complete duplication of the uterus, cervix, and vagina that results from the complete failure of the müllerian ducts to fuse together.[3,8] Both uteri may be similar in size, or one may be smaller in size. The vaginal duplication may result in one smaller

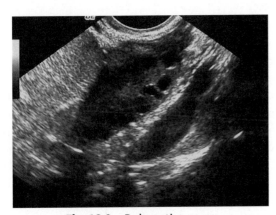

Fig. 16-9 Polycystic ovary.

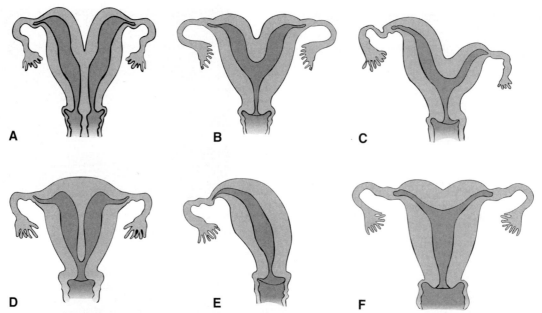

Fig. 16-12 Congenital uterine abnormalities. **A,** Uterus didelphys: double uterus. **B,** Bicornuate uterus. **C,** Bicornuate uterus with rudimentary left horn. **D,** Septate uterus. **E,** Unicornuate uterus. **F,** Arcuate uterus.

vagina (hemivagina) opening within the other vagina, so this anomaly may not be identified on external visual inspection. The condition can be associated with unilateral hematocolpos.[8] The symptoms associated with uterus didelphys when the hemivagina is obstructed include dysmenorrhea beginning shortly after menarche, progressive pelvic pain after menses, and a unilateral pelvic mass.[9]

Sonographic Findings. The appearance with ultrasound is two separate endometrial echo complexes.[2,8] A deep fundal notch is also separated widely with full complement of myometrium (Figs. 16-13 to 16-16).[3,8] Two cervices and vaginas should be visualized. The initial impression of uterus didelphys may suggest a normal uterus with an adjacent pelvic mass, especially if the uteri are asymmetric. This appearance is related to an obstructed hemivagina causing **hematocolpos** or **hematometracolpos.**

Bicornuate Uterus

Bicornuate uterus is a duplication of the uterus entering one cervix or two cervices, with only one vagina. This results from partial fusion of the müllerian ducts during embryologic development. Bicornis bicollis describes the duplication of the cervix and uterus, and bicornis unicollis describes the duplication of the uterus without duplication of the cervix. The cervix fuses normally, and the fundus fails to fuse.[8] Fertility problems can occur

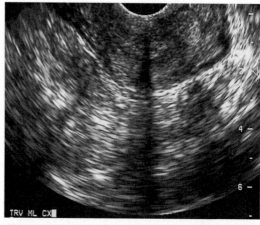

Fig. 16-13 Transverse image of cervix with two cervices.

when one of the horns does not communicate and is rudimentary.[2]

Sonographic Findings. Sonographic examination of the bicornuate uterus will show a deep fundal notch. The endometrial echoes appear as two different complexes widely separated.[2,3,8] This gives the same appearance as uterus didelphys in the fundal region (Figs. 16-17 to 16-21). Differentiation of bicornuate uterus and uterus didelphys can be made with the identification of duplication of the vaginal canal, which will be evident in uterus didelphys.

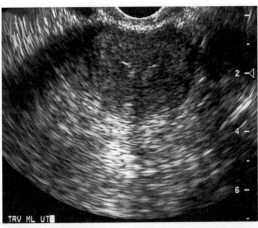

Fig. 16-14 Transverse image of lower uterine segment with uterus didelphys.

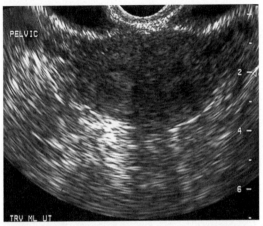

Fig. 16-15 Transverse image at level of uterine corpus that shows uterus didelphys.

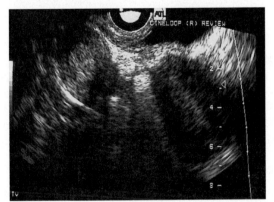

Fig. 16-16 Two fundal horns shown in uterus didelphys.

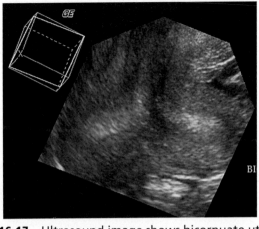

Fig. 16-17 Ultrasound image shows bicornuate uterus with three dimensions. (Courtesy GE Medical Systems.)

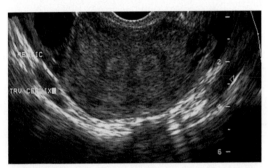

Fig. 16-18 Transverse image of cervical region in patient with bicornis bicollis.

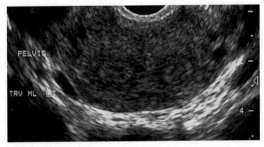

Fig. 16-19 Transverse image of bicornuate uterus at level of uterine corpus.

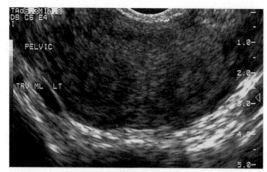

Fig. 16-20 Endovaginal ultrasound shows bicornuate uterus near fundal region. Note widely separated endometria.

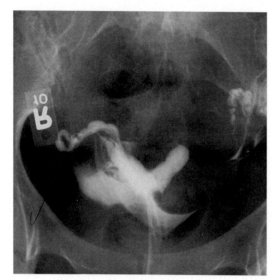

Fig. 16-21 Hysterosalpingogram shows bicornuate uterus.

Septate Uterus

Septate uterus is the most common congenital uterine abnormality.[3] It is the result of a failure in reabsorption of the median septum. Fusion of the müllerian ducts does occur.[2,3,8] This process leaves the uterine cavity completely separated by a thin septum known as uterus septus or a partially reabsorbed septum known as uterus subseptus. The consequence of the anomaly leads to fertility problems; although once the condition is identified, treatment is available. Patients with this defect can have the septum removed via **hysteroscopy.**[2,8] Combination of ultrasound results with a **hysterosalpingography** or magnetic resonance imaging (MRI) to determine whether the abnormality is actually a septate uterus becomes very important.[3,8]

Sonographic Findings. The sonographic appearance of a septate uterus shows a convex, flat, or minimally

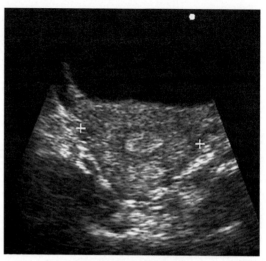

Fig. 16-22 Transverse endovaginal image of lower uterine segment in patient with uterus subseptus.

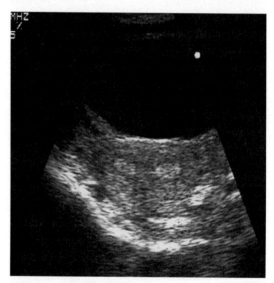

Fig. 16-23 Transverse endovaginal image of fundus in septate uterus shows separation of endometria.

indented fundal contour.[10] Two endometrial echoes appear close together because they are only separated by a thin septum (Figs. 16-22 and 16-23).[8]

Arcuate Uterus

Arcuate uterus is the mildest form of congenital uterine anomalies. It is a minor lack of fusion of the fundal region that results in a slight depression in that area. The endometrium is fairly normal, which is why this anomaly is considered a normal variant.[3,8] Patients with an arcuate uterus have significant second-trimester pregnancy loss and a higher rate of preterm labor when compared with patients with a normal uterus.[11]

Sonographic Findings.   Arcuate uterus is difficult to diagnose with ultrasound. The uterus appears normal with a subtle fundal indentation, and the uterine cavity is slightly concave (Fig. 16-24).

Table 16-1 is a summary of the sonographic findings of uterine anomalies.

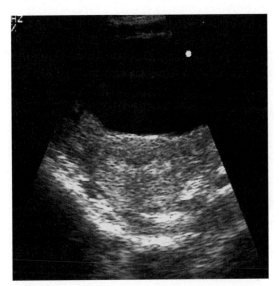

Fig. 16-24   Ultrasound imaging of arcuate uterus with slight indentation of endometrium.

SUMMARY

Pelvic ultrasound combined with accurate patient history and physical examination plays a vital role in diagnosis of possible causes of infertility and other symptoms. Three-dimensional ultrasound may improve the accuracy of diagnosis of the causes of infertility, especially in regards to congenital uterine anomalies, by allowing easier access to the coronal plane of the uterus for better visualization of the contour of the fundal region. When abnormalities are confirmed, surgical and medical treatment options may be available to increase the chances for successful pregnancy.

CLINICAL SCENARIO—DIAGNOSIS

■ The ultrasound findings are consistent with duplication of the cervix and uterus. Additional conversation with the patient reveals that she had a hemivagina that would be consistent with uterus didelphys. A gestational sac is revealed in the right horn without evidence of a live embryo or yolk sac, consistent with her last menstrual period, which was 9 weeks prior. Quantitative pregnancy tests confirm a failed pregnancy.

Table 16-1	*Congenital Uterine Anomalies*	
Uterine Anomalies	**Development**	**Sonographic Findings**
Uterine didelphys	Complete failure of müllerian ducts to fuse	Two separate endometrial echoes, two cervices and vaginas
Bicornuate uterus	Müllerian ducts only partially fused	Two separate endometrial echoes, one or two cervices and one vagina
Septate uterus	Müllerian ducts fuse with failure of reabsorption of median septum	Two close endometrial echoes
Arcuate uterus	Only minor lack of fusion of uterus in fundal region	One normal endometrial echo with slight fundal indentation

CASE STUDIES FOR DISCUSSION

1. A 32-year-old woman from the emergency department is seen for a pelvic ultrasound. Her condition is G4P0040. Three of her pregnancies ended in elective abortions, and the last was a spontaneous abortion. She has pelvic pain isolated to her right lower quadrant. The ultrasound reveals a right ovary containing a mass. The mass has septations with a fluid-debris level (Fig. 16-25). What would be the most likely diagnosis?

2. A 28-year-old woman is seen for pelvic ultrasound. She has had five previous spontaneous abortions and states that she has been trying to start a family for 2 years. The patient is also scheduled for a hysterosalpingogram for evaluation of her uterus. The ultrasound reveals a slight fundal notch in the uterus. The endometrium appears to be duplicated. What diagnosis would be most likely?

3. A 25-year-old woman with a history of **oligomenorrhea,** pelvic pain, and weight gain is seen in the ultrasound department for a pelvic ultrasound. She has never been pregnant but reports that she has been trying to become pregnant for the past year. A pelvic ultrasound reveals a normal uterus and endometrium. The ovaries appear to be slightly enlarged with multiple small follicles (Fig. 16-26). What is most likely diagnosis?

4. A 33-year-old woman with a history of a positive pregnancy test, spotting, and passing blood clots for 1 day arrives from the emergency department for a pelvic ultrasound. She reports a miscarriage 2 years prior. The ultrasound reveals she has a deep fundal notch and a single cervix. Two endometria are identified, with a gestational sac in the right horn (Figs. 16-27 and 16-28). Which uterine anomaly is most likely?

5. A 21-year-old woman is seen for a pelvic ultrasound. She has a history of extreme pain with menstruation. She has had a failed pregnancy but has been unable to conceive again. The ultrasound reveals a normal uterus with a small amount fluid in the cul-de-sac. Her ovaries are shown in Figs. 16-29 and 16-30. What is the most likely diagnosis?

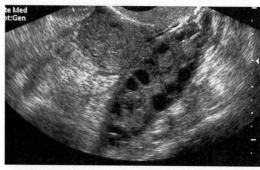

Fig. 16-26 Left ovary contains tiny, multiple follicles that were also shown on right ovary.

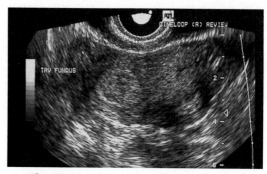

Fig. 16-27 Region of uterine corpus.

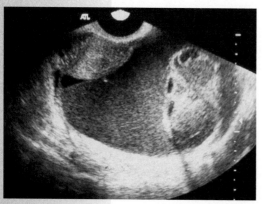

Fig. 16-25 Right ovary contains septations and fluid debris level.

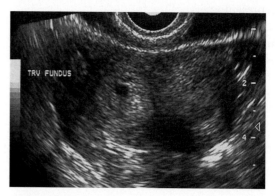

Fig. 16-28 Gestational sac is identified in right uterine horn.

CASE STUDIES FOR DISCUSSION—cont'd

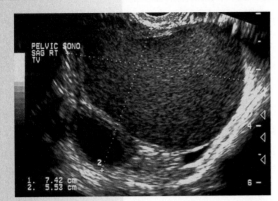

Fig. 16-29 Right ovary shows septations with debris.

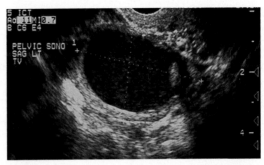

Fig. 16-30 Left ovary with thick walls, septations, and debris.

STUDY QUESTIONS

1. A 32-year-old woman with a history of pelvic pain and amenorrhea is seen. Laboratory values reveal she has an elevated testosterone level. Ultrasound reveals multiple small follicles bilaterally. Which of the following is most likely?
   a. normal ovaries
   b. bilateral ovarian cysts
   c. polycystic ovarian disease
   d. ovarian torsion
   e. endometrioma

2. A 26-year-old woman is seen for an ultrasound. She has been trying to get pregnant for 3 years and has pain and menorrhagia. The pelvic ultrasound reveals a mass in the left lower quadrant. The mass appears to have thick walls, internal echoes, and through transmission. This would most likely represent which of the following?
   a. dermoid
   b. hemorrhagic cyst
   c. polycystic ovarian disease
   d. endometrioma
   e. ovarian torsion

3. A 21-year-old woman is seen for a pelvic ultrasound. The ultrasound reveals a uterus with a deep fundal notch and two separate endometrial echoes. One cervix is noted. What is the most likely abnormality?
   a. uterus didelphys
   b. bicornuate uterus
   c. arcuate uterus
   d. septate uterus
   e. normal uterus

4. A 32-year-old woman with infertility is seen for a pelvic ultrasound. The ultrasound reveals a uterus containing two closely spaced endometrial echoes. The fundus appears flat and smooth. Which of the following is most likely?
   a. arcuate uterus
   b. septate uterus
   c. normal uterus
   d. uterus didelphys
   e. bicornuate uterus

5. A 34-year-old woman is seen for a pelvic ultrasound after a computed tomographic scan shows a large left adnexal mass. She has no symptoms. The ultrasound reveals a 6-cm left adnexal mass. The mass is well defined and contains a fluid-debris level. What is the most likely diagnosis?
   a. ovarian cyst
   b. chocolate cyst
   c. polycystic ovarian disease
   d. ovarian torsion
   e. hydrosalpinx

6. A 14-year-old girl is seen for a pelvic ultrasound. She has had significant pelvic pain associated with her menses. On physical examination, her physician palpated a pelvic mass in the right lower quadrant. The ultrasound reveals a normal uterus with a large pelvic mass in the right lower quadrant, which on

further investigation shows findings consistent with hematometracolpos. What diagnosis is most likely?

a. arcuate uterus
b. septate uterus
c. uterus didelphys
d. endometriosis
e. hydrosalpinx

7. An 18-year-old woman is seen for pelvic ultrasound with a history of intermittent pelvic pain. She reports that she is sexually active but has never been pregnant. The pelvic ultrasound reveals a normal uterus with a slight indentation in the fundus and concave endometrium. What is the best diagnosis?

a. septate uterus
b. arcuate uterus
c. uterus didelphys
d. bicornuate uterus
e. normal uterus

8. A 20-year-old woman has had recurrent pain in the left lower quadrant for the past 4 months corresponding with her menstrual cycles. Her physician palpates a mass in the left lower quadrant and orders a pelvic ultrasound. Ultrasound examination reveals a mass, measuring 6 × 4 cm, adjacent to the iliac artery and vein. It appears to be a well-defined and hypoechoic mass with through transmission. What diagnosis is most likely?

a. hemorrhagic cyst
b. abdominal abscess
c. endometrioma
d. polycystic ovarian disease
e. dermoid

9. A 33-year-old woman arrives for an ultrasound of her pelvis. She reports a history of recurrent first trimester losses. She also has occasional pelvic pain. The ultrasound reveals a slightly indented and convex uterine fundus with two endometrial echoes. What is the best diagnosis?

a. uterus didelphys
b. septate uterus
c. bicornuate uterus
d. arcuate uterus
e. normal uterus

10. A 22-year-old woman with a history of infertility for 1 year is seen for a pelvic ultrasound. Laboratory studies reveal an increase in LH and LH-to-FSH ratio. She is otherwise asymptomatic. Sonographic evaluation of the pelvis reveals a normal uterus. The ovaries are slightly enlarged and increased in echogenicity with multiple follicles present at the periphery. What is the best diagnosis?

a. endometriosis
b. ovarian cysts
c. hemorrhagic ovarian cysts
d. ovarian torsion
e. polycystic ovarian disease

REFERENCES

1. Garcia-Velasco JA, Alvarez M, Palumbo A et al: Rupture of an ovarian endometrioma during the first trimester of pregnancy, *Eur J Obstet Gynecol Reprod Biol* 76:41-43, 1998.
2. Hagen-Ansert SL: *Textbook of diagnostic ultrasonography*, vol 2, ed 5, St Louis, 2001, Mosby.
3. Rumack CM, Wilson SR, Charboneau JW: *Diagnostic ultrasound*, vol 1, ed 2, St Louis, 1998, Mosby.
4. Muzii L, Marana R, Caruana P et al: Postoperative administration of monophasic combined oral contraceptives after laparoscopic treatment of ovarian endometriomas: a prospective, randomized trial, *Am J Obstet Gynecol* 183:588-592, 2000.
5. Mittal S, Kumar S, Kumar A et al: Ultrasound guided aspiration of endometrioma: a new therapeutic modality to improve reproductive outcome, *Int J Gynecol Obstet* 65:17-23, 1999.
6. Milad MP, Cohen L: Preoperative ultrasound assessment of adnexal masses in premenopausal women, *Int J Gynecol Obstet* 66:137-141, 1999.
7. Hunter MH, Sterrett JJ: Polycystic ovary syndrome: it's not just infertility, *Am Fam Physician* 62:1079-1090, 2000.
8. Callen PW: *Ultrasonography in obstetrics and gynecology*, ed 3, Philadelphia, 1994, WB Saunders.
9. Pieroni C, Rosenfeld DL, Mokrzycki ML: Uterus didelphys with obstructed hemivagina and ipsilateral renal agenesis, *J Reprod Med* 46: 133-136, 2001.
10. Homer HA, Li TC, Cooke ID: The septate uterus: a review of management and reproductive outcome, *Fertil Steril* 73:1-14, 2000.
11. Woelfer B, Salim R, Banerjee S et al: Reproductive outcomes in women with congenital uterine anomalies detected by three-dimensional ultrasound screening, *Obstet Gynecol* 98:1099-1103, 2001.

BIBLIOGRAPHY

Berman MC, Craig M, Kawamura DM: *Diagnostic medical sonography: a guide to clinical practice*, ed 2, Philadelphia, 1997, JB Lippincott.
Thomas CL: *Taber's cyclopedic medical dictionary*, ed 18, Philadelphia, 1997, FA Davis.

17 Ovarian Mass

KATHI KEATON BOROK

CLINICAL SCENARIO

■ A 51-year-old woman is seen in the ultrasound department for a pelvic and abdominal ultrasound evaluation. The patient has noticed increasing abdominal girth and has a sensation of pelvic heaviness and a loss of appetite. Laboratory tests ordered by her physician report abnormal liver function tests and elevation of both serum amylase and calcium-125 (CA-125) values.

A transabdominal and transvaginal pelvic ultrasound reveals a multilocular cystic mass in the right ovary that measures 15 cm in its largest dimension. The borders of the cyst are thick and irregular. The mass contains multiple septations and papillary projections, and calcifications are present within some loculations (Fig. 17-1). The abdominal ultrasound reveals multiple hyperechoic masses in the liver (Fig. 17-2). What are the possible diagnoses for these findings?

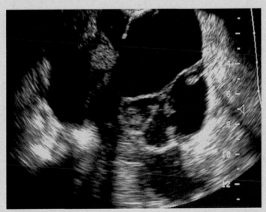

Fig. 17-1 Multiseptated ovarian mass containing papillary projections. Note presence of small calcifications in some septations.

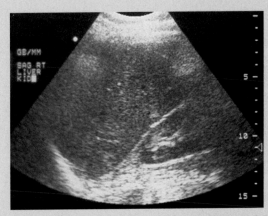

Fig. 17-2 Abdominal sonogram identifies multiple hyperechoic masses in liver.

OBJECTIVES

■ Describe normal ovarian anatomy and function.
■ List patient risk factors for development of ovarian masses.
■ Describe the sonographic features of benign ovarian masses.
■ Discuss the sonographic features of malignant ovarian masses.
■ Identify factors useful in differentiation of ovarian masses.

GLOSSARY OF TERMS ■■■■■■■■■

Amylase: a class of enzymes that catalyze the conversion of starch to sugar

Angiogenesis: the formation of blood vessels

Ascites: an accumulation of fluid in the peritoneal cavity

Avascular: absence or poverty of blood vessels

Broad ligament of the uterus: folds of the peritoneum attached to the uterus and consisting of two layers of peritoneum, between which lie pelvic blood vessels and remnants of the wolffian ducts

Ciliated cells: epithelial cells that possess threadlike projections from their free surfaces

Cortex: the outer layer of an organ

Crenulated: with scalloped projections

Cystadenocarcinoma: a predominantly cystic malignant tumor that arises from the epithelium of a glandular organ

Cystadenoma: a predominantly cystic benign tumor composed of epithelial cells

Ectoderm: the outer layer of cells in a developing embryo; produces structures that include skin and teeth

Encapsulated: enclosed in a sheath

Endoderm: the innermost layer of cells in a developing embryo; produces, among other structures, epithelium of the digestive tract, bladder, vagina, and urethra

Endometrial hyperplasia: an abnormal proliferation of cells of the uterine lining

Epithelium: the layer of cells that form mucous and serous membranes and the surface of the skin

Estrogen: a female sex hormone produced by the ovary

Gastrin: a hormone secreted by the stomach and duodenum

Germ cell: ovum or sperm cell

Graafian follicle: a mature ovum-containing follicle

Granulosa: a layer of cells in the outer wall of a graafian follicle

Haploid: with half the normal number of chromosomes found in normal body cells; germ cells are normally haploid

Hirsutism: hairiness

Hypogastric: relating to the lower middle of the abdomen

Involute: to diminish in size

Ipsilateral: on the same side

Karyotype: chromosomes of a single cell photographed through a microscope

Leiomyoma, or fibroid: a benign fibrous tumor of the uterus

Loculation: division into small spaces or cavities

Luteinization: development of a corpus luteum within a ruptured graafian follicle

Medulla: the central portion of an organ

Meigs' syndrome: ascites and pleural effusion associated with a benign ovarian tumor

Mesoderm: a primary embryologic germ layer that lies between the endoderm and ectoderm; connective tissue arises from the mesoderm

Mesothelial cells: cells of the epithelium of serous membranes

Metrorrhagia: spotting between periods

"Moth-eaten" cyst formation: the sonographic appearance of a Krukenberg's tumor in which a solid mass appears to be permeated with holes, or cystic areas

Mucin: a glycoprotein produced by mucous membranes

Neoplasm: an abnormal new tissue formation

Nodule: a small group of cells

Oocyte: the developing female germ cell

Parenchyma: the essential functional part of an organ

Pedunculated: possessing or supported by a stalk

Progesterone: a hormone produced by the corpus luteum and the placenta; facilitates implantation of a fertilized ovum

Pseudomyxoma peritoneum: a type of tumor that develops in the peritoneum as a result of cells escaped from an ovarian cystadenoma; mucuslike ascites fills the peritoneal cavity in response to tumor papillary adhesions to abdominal wall and intestine

Sebum: a semifluid fatty secretion of the sebaceous glands

Septations: dividing structures

Serous: watery

Signet-ring cell: a cell type typically contained in a mucus-secreting adenocarcinoma

Teratoma: a tumor consisting of one or more of the three primary embryonic germ layers

Theca: a sheath of membrane forming the outer wall of a structure, such as a graafian follicle

Wolffian: embryonic structures that develop into parts of the male genitourinary system

Zollinger-Ellison syndrome: a condition caused by tumors that secrete excess amounts of gastrin; the stomach reacts by secreting excess digestive fluids, and peptic ulcers result

According to statistics from the American Cancer Society, ovarian cancer killed approximately 13,900 women in the United States in 2001. Ovarian masses are usually asymptomatic, so more than 70% of patients with ovarian malignant disease are seen with advanced disease.[1] Although the 5-year survival rate for patients with stage I lesions is 90%, stage IV tumors carry a dismal survival rate of about 5%.[1] Early detection is critical to patient survival.

Pelvic ultrasound plays an important role in the timely detection and evaluation of ovarian masses, many of which are found incidentally during ultrasound for unrelated conditions. Several patient indicators may prompt a pelvic ultrasound, including pain, a palpable mass, gastrointestinal discomfort, or menstrual disturbances. Other indications may include a family history of cancer or patient obesity that limits a physical examination. Family history of ovarian or breast cancer presents the greatest risk factor for ovarian cancer.

A careful ultrasound evaluation of the pelvis provides valuable information regarding the presence and location of a mass, its size, its consistency, and associated findings, such as **ascites.** Doppler ultrasound is still being evaluated as a diagnostic tool, but it can sometimes help to characterize a mass. Generally accepted among investigators is that a low-resistance flow pattern suggests neovascularity like that found in a malignant mass (Fig. 17-3). Flow resistance may be evaluated with the resistive index, which is defined as the systolic peak velocity minus the diastolic peak velocity divided by the systolic peak velocity. The pulsatility index is another useful flow index and is defined as the systolic peak velocity minus the diastolic peak velocity divided by the mean velocity.

Although the diagnosis of a pelvic mass can only be made with certainty by a pathologist, sonographic information—combined with patient history, a physical examination, and laboratory findings—is extremely valuable to a physician during consideration of treatment options. In this chapter, many ovarian masses will be examined, including benign and malignant masses. Not included in this group, however, are **theca** lutein masses, which are discussed in Chapter 21. Polycystic ovary disease is evaluated in Chapter 16.

NORMAL OVARIAN ANATOMY

Ovaries are almond-shaped structures composed of cortical and medullary tissue and covered by **epithelium.** The **cortex** is the site of follicular development, and the **medulla** is the vascular core of the ovary. The ovaries develop **oocytes** and produce **estrogen** and **progesterone.** In postmenopausal women, the ovaries cease to function, at which time they atrophy. Although their positions may vary, the ovaries typically reside in the adnexa anterior to the internal iliac vessels and medial to the external iliac vessels. Ovarian size varies with the phase of a woman's menstrual cycle and with her age. In premenopausal women, ovaries typically measure 1 to 2 cm in length, 3 cm in width, and 2 cm in anteroposterior diameter; in postmenopausal women, they generally measure about 1 cm smaller in all dimensions.[2]

Normal Sonographic Appearance

The ovaries are fairly homogeneous in texture, with an echogenicity similar to that of the uterus (Fig. 17-4). Anechoic follicles may be seen in the ovarian periphery, and the vascular medulla may appear somewhat echogenic compared with the cortex. The ovaries may sometimes be found by scanning along the iliac vessels.

OVARIAN CYSTS
Follicular Cysts

Follicular cysts are among the most common cause of ovarian enlargement in young women. They occur when a dominant, or graafian, follicle fails to either ovulate or regress. The walls of follicular cysts are smooth and thin, with an inner lining of **granulosa** cells and an outer layer of theca interna cells. The cysts contain **serous** fluid, sometimes accompanied by clotted blood. Follicular

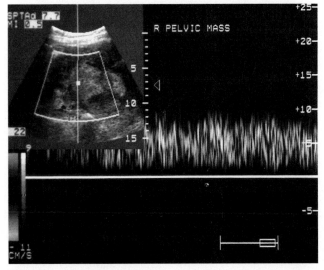

Fig. 17-3 Doppler evaluation of Krukenberg's tumor reveals low-resistance flow pattern characteristic of malignant masses.

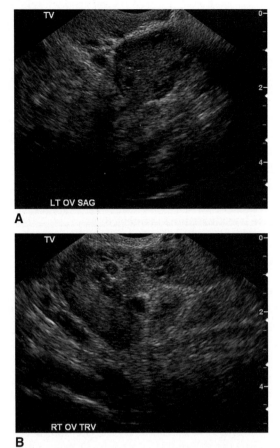

Fig. 17-4 Longitudinal **(A)** and transverse **(B)** images of normal left ovary containing several small follicles. (Courtesy Lori Davis and Natalie Cauffman, Florida Hospital Deland.)

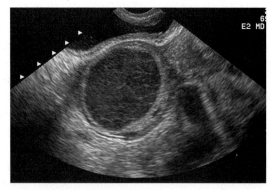

Fig. 17-5 Hemorrhagic follicular cyst. (Courtesy GE Medical Systems.)

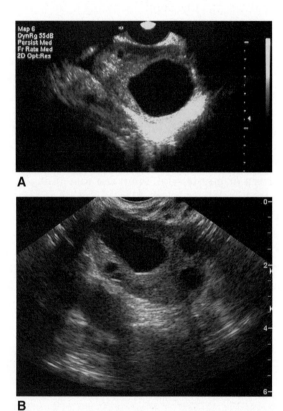

Fig. 17-6 **A,** Enhanced acoustic transmission shown through cyst. **B,** Ovary containing follicular cyst and several small follicles. (**B** Courtesy Lori Davis and Natalie Cauffman, Florida Hospital Deland.)

cysts typically range in size from 3.0 to 8.0 cm^2 but may attain diameters as large as 20.0 cm.[3] They are usually asymptomatic but may produce dull adnexal pressure and pain; precipitation of ovarian torsion causes severe pain. In response to estrogen production by a follicular cyst, menstrual abnormalities may occur. In most cases, these cysts eventually rupture or are resorbed. For a persistent or enlarged cyst, aspiration or surgical removal may be considered.

Sonographic Findings. Follicular cysts most commonly appear as anechoic, thin-walled unilocular structures, but they sometimes contain diffuse, low-level echoes that reflect bleeding into the capsule (Fig. 17-5). Enhanced acoustic transmission through these masses indicates their cystic nature (Fig. 17-6, *A* and *B*). With acute hemorrhage, follicular cysts may become echogenic, raising suspicion of **neoplasm.** Color Doppler sonography may be helpful in distinguishing clot formation in a functional cyst from solid material in a neoplasm.

In contrast to the vascular tissue of a neoplasm, clotted blood in a hemorrhagic cyst is **avascular.** A follow-up sonogram will confirm resolution of a follicular cyst.

Corpus Luteum Cyst

A corpus luteum cyst forms from a ruptured **graafian follicle.** After ovulation, the follicle collapses and many capillaries from the theca interna grow between the granulosa cells, investing them with a rich blood supply

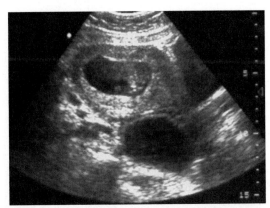

Fig. 17-7 Corpus luteum cyst identified during early pregnancy.

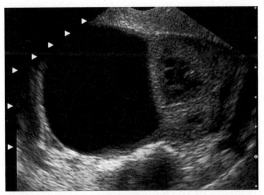

Fig. 17-8 Anechoic corpus luteum shows enhanced through transmission. (Courtesy GE Medical Systems.)

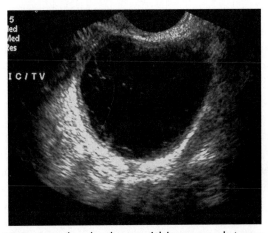

Fig. 17-9 Low-level echoes within corpus luteum cyst suggest hemorrhage. Note enhanced acoustic transmission posterior to cystic structure.

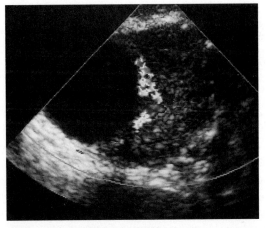

Fig. 17-10 Color Doppler demonstrates vascularity at the rim of this corpus luteum cyst.

to nourish their growth and **luteinization.** Vascular invasion into the newly forming corpus luteum often results in hemorrhage into the cavity of the cyst. A corpus luteum enlarges to 1 cm or more[4] and can be identified transvaginally in most menstruating women during the 14-day luteal cycle that follows ovulation.

The cyst functions to produce progesterone, necessary for maintenance of the endometrial lining in preparation for pregnancy. If pregnancy occurs, the corpus luteum persists and continues to produce hormones to nurture the pregnancy until the placenta is well developed. Once the placenta assumes the task of progesterone production, the corpus luteum begins to **involute.** It usually cannot be identified sonographically after week 16 of pregnancy.[1]

If pregnancy does not occur, the corpus luteum typically regresses and disappears by the beginning of the next cycle. Persistence of the cyst may delay menstruation or cause abnormal bleeding from continued progesterone production.

Sonographic Findings. The sonographic presentation of a corpus luteum cyst is variable. The most common appearance is that of a round hypoechoic or anechoic structure, with enhanced through transmission (Figs. 17-7 and 17-8). Although walls may be thin, they are often thick, hyperechoic, and **crenulated.** Internal echoes may be present because of hemorrhage, or the cyst may have a predominantly solid appearance (Fig. 17-9). Color Doppler sonography is useful for identification of the rich, vascular rim around a corpus luteum cyst (Fig. 17-10; see Color Plate 9), particularly when the cyst is isoechoic to the ovary and difficult to identify with grayscale imaging. Flow around the circumference of a corpus luteum is typically intense and of low resistance, reflecting the prolific **angiogenesis** necessary for development of the corpus luteum.

The variable appearance of a corpus luteum may make sonographic differentiation of a true ovarian abnormality difficult. The patient's history, including age, menstrual timing, and pregnancy status, provides important diagnostic information.

Parovarian Cyst

Parovarian cysts comprise about 10% of adnexal masses.[2] They occur at all ages but are most often found in menstruating women, especially women in their 20s and 30s.[5] Parovarian cysts arise from the tissues of the **broad ligament of the uterus** and are lined with a flat epithelium. They are most often mesothelial and originate from **wolffian** structures. Patients with parovarian cysts are usually asymptomatic but may have pelvic or lower abdominal pain in the presence of a large cyst or in the infrequent instance of cyst rupture or torsion. These cysts are rarely malignant. Because of the low potential for morbidity and mortality, a sonographic diagnosis of parovarian cyst may allow the physician to defer surgery for small asymptomatic masses.

Sonographic Findings. Most parovarian cysts are predominantly cystic, with thin smooth walls and enhanced through transmission. When hemorrhage has occurred, internal echoes may be present. Parovarian cysts vary in size and can become quite large. Distinguishing these cysts sonographically from the simple functional variety is often difficult. Diagnosis depends on identification of the **ipsilateral** ovary near, but separate from, the cyst (Fig. 17-11). Application of gentle hand or transducer pressure may help separate the cystic structure from the ovary. Infrequently, a parovarian cyst may contain a **cystadenoma,** with one or more solid **nodules,** thickened or irregular walls, and occasional **septations.**

CYSTIC/COMPLEX NEOPLASMS

Endometrioma

An endometrioma represents the localized form of endometriosis, a common condition in women, especially during the reproductive years. The etiology of the disorder is unclear, but it is thought to relate to migration of endometrial tissue from the uterus or to primary ectopic development of endometrial tissue outside the uterus.

An endometrioma is a collection of blood lined by endometrium. The walls are usually thick and fibrotic, often adherent to adjacent structures. Endometriomas are frequently multiple. Although usually asymptomatic, these cysts may rupture or undergo torsion. Either event causes pain and may precipitate emergency surgery.

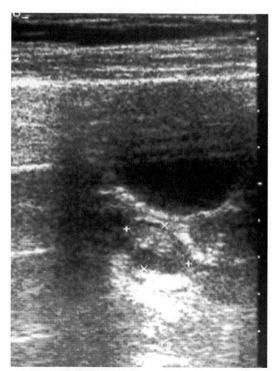

Fig. 17-11 Ipsilateral ovary is clearly shown to be near but separate from parovarian cyst.

Sonographic Findings. Endometriomas are generally well-defined unilocular or multilocular cysts, sometimes showing hyperechoic foci in the cyst walls (Fig. 17-12). Although their echogenicity can range from anechoic to solid, 95% are seen as cysts containing diffuse, low-level echoes (Fig. 17-13).[6] The similarity of the sonographic appearances of endometriomas, hemorrhagic cysts, and abscesses may present a diagnostic challenge, requiring consideration of additional clinical or sonographic factors (Fig. 17-14). Hemorrhagic cysts often produce acute pain, in contrast to endometriomas, which are usually either asymptomatic or produce less intense, more chronic discomfort. In addition, follow-up sonograms show resolution of hemorrhagic cysts, whereas endometriomas tend to persist. Acute illness supports the diagnosis of abscess. Color Doppler sonography may be useful to differentiate an endometrioma from a neoplastic lesion. In contrast to a neoplasm, an endometrioma typically does not have internal vascularity.

Benign Cystic Teratoma

Benign cystic **teratomas** are the most common ovarian neoplasm,[7] constituting 20% of all ovarian tumors[8] and about 95% of **germ cell** tumors.[9] They occur most frequently during the reproductive years.[10] Teratomas are rare before puberty, but they comprise 50% of adolescent adnexal masses.[11] Cystic teratomas, or dermoids, result from an abnormal germ cell. These germ cells, or ova,

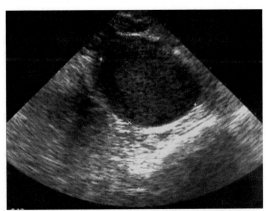

Fig. 17-12 Note presence of calcifications in walls of endometrioma.

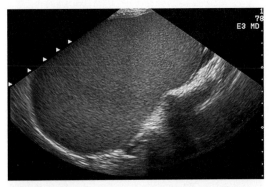

Fig. 17-13 Endometrioma containing diffuse low-level echoes. (Courtesy GE Medical Systems.)

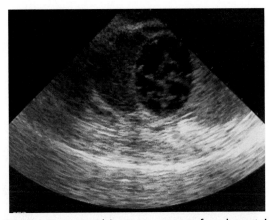

Fig. 17-14 Sonographic appearance of endometrioma sometimes resembles that of hemorrhagic cyst. Follow-up sonograms may be necessary for diagnosis.

usually have a **karyotype** of 23,X, half the normal complement of chromosomes in a body cell. In contrast, most of the germ cells found in a teratoma have a 46,XX karyotype. This finding suggests that teratomas may be caused by failure of a **haploid** ovum to divide appropriately during meiosis. The egg cell duplicates its

chromosomes in preparation for division into two new germ cells but then fails to divide. The resulting cell therefore has twice as many chromosomes as is appropriate and may develop as a dermoidal mass. A familial tendency to produce dermoids has been reported.[10]

Cystic teratomas are unilateral in 80% to 90% of patients[10]; infrequently, multiple cysts may occur within a single ovary. These tumors tend to grow slowly during a woman's reproductive years. At diagnosis, cystic teratomas are relatively small compared with other neoplastic lesions, although they can grow to a diameter of 15 cm. These cysts may be **pedunculated.** Cystic teratomas are usually composed of three germ cell layers: **ectoderm, mesoderm,** and **endoderm,** with ectoderm predominating. Contained within the cyst is pure **sebum,** with varying amounts of fat and one or more dermoid plugs, which may contain hair, teeth, and bone fragments.

Cystic teratomas are commonly asymptomatic, although pain may result in the event of torsion or rupture. Larger lesions may produce an abdominal mass or swelling. Malignant transformation occurs in 1% to 3% of cases.[9,10,12,13] Cystic teratomas are often surgically removed, but because of their typically slow growth rate, patient fertility concerns may be considered. Whenever possible, lesions are excised without removal of the involved ovary; in fact, surgery can sometimes be delayed until patients have completed their families.

Sonographic Findings. Benign cystic teratomas characteristically show an anechoic cystic component and a shadowing density that corresponds to a dermoid plug (Fig. 17-15). Strong acoustic attenuation occurs in the presence of bone, teeth, and hair in the plug, sometimes producing the "tip-of-the-iceberg" sign (Fig. 17-16). This intensely echogenic focus is the cystic teratoma's most defining feature. Other distinctive sonographic features include a fat-fluid level and hyperechoic lines and dots generated by hair (Fig. 17-17, *A* and *B*).

Benign cystic teratomas have variable appearances that may mimic hemorrhagic cysts, endometriomas, primary ovarian neoplasms, and metastatic tumors. Teratomas, however, often have two or more features characteristic of dermoids, and sonographically similar lesions usually have no more than one (Figs. 17-18 and 17-19).

Color Doppler sonography may be helpful in differentiation of benign and malignant cystic teratomas. Blood flow in benign cystic teratomas is typically found only in the periphery because the cyst contains mostly avascular fat and hair. Conversely, malignant teratomas show intratumoral blood flow significantly more frequently than benign teratomas, with the exception of struma ovarii, a rare and typically benign form of cystic teratoma that contains highly vascular thyroid tissue.

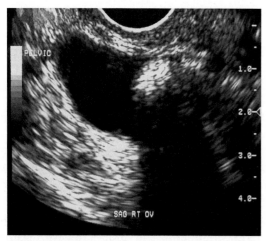

Fig. 17-15 Dermoid plug produces shadowing echo density within cystic structure.

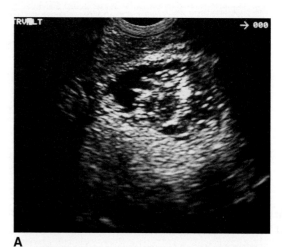

A

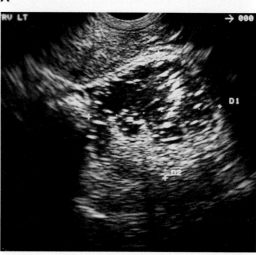

B

Fig. 17-17 **A** and **B,** Hair within mass may present as echogenic lines and dots, and fat-fluid level may be appreciated.

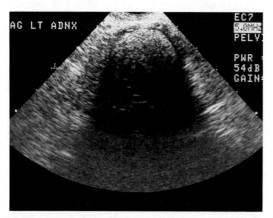

Fig. 17-16 Strongly attenuating tissues in dermoid plug reduce or eliminate sonographic representation of structure distal to its surface, producing characteristic "tip-of-iceberg" sign.

Serous Cystadenoma/Cystadenocarcinoma

Serous lesions comprise 30% of all ovarian neoplasms.[3] Arising from the epithelium, these tumors are lined with **mesothelial, ciliated,** and secretory **cells.** They are bilateral in 12% to 50% of patients[14] and have a tendency to recur. Most serous ovarian lesions are benign serous cystadenomas, which occur with greatest frequency in women between the ages of 30 and 40 years.[14] These lesions are usually filled with serous fluid and are smooth surfaced and movable. Serous cystadenocarcinomas reach peak incidence among women in their 60s and represent the most common ovarian malignant disease. They usually contain bloody fluid and, because of surface papillary projections, may adhere to adjacent organs. Serous **cystadenocarcinomas** are highly malignant, with strong potential for metastases. Treatment for

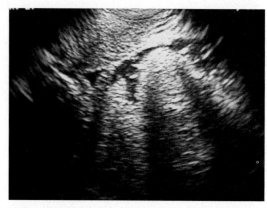

Fig. 17-18 Mostly solid-appearing mass shows two features characteristic of dermoid: *1,* apparent dermoid plug; and *2,* echogenic lines and dots consistent with finding of hair in mass.

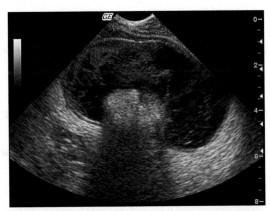

Fig. 17-19 Low-level echoes represent hemorrhage into dermoid. Note presence of dermoid plug and echogenic lines and dots. (Courtesy GE Medical Systems.)

these lesions, therefore, usually includes radical surgery followed by radiotherapy.[15]

Patients with serous ovarian tumors are often asymptomatic but may have **hypogastric** pain, increasing abdominal girth, or a sensation of pelvic heaviness. Pain may accompany abdominal enlargement, particularly in the presence of malignant disease. Patients with serous cystadenocarcinomas may have elevated serum and urine **amylase** values[14]; serum CA-125 levels are elevated in 80% of women with serous ovarian malignant diseases.[4]

Sonographic Findings. Serous cystadenomas typically present sonographically as unilocular anechoic masses. These masses are usually thin walled, containing thin septations and occasional papillary projections into the cyst cavity (Fig. 17-20, *A* and *B*; see Color Plate 10). Benign and semimalignant serous cystadenomas tend to grow slowly but can attain diameters of up to 20 cm,[2] in which case they may fill the pelvis and be mistaken for ascites. Serous cystadenocarcinomas may also become quite large. On sonographic investigation, these tumors typically demonstrate multiple **loculations** and thick septations (Figs. 17-21 and 17-22). Echogenic foci, representing calcifications, are sometimes observed (Fig. 17-23, *A* and *B*). Cyst borders often appear thick and irregular, with internal papillary projections (Fig. 17-24).

Mucinous Cystadenoma/Cystadenocarcinoma

Mucinous tumors are less common than serous tumors, comprising about 20% of ovarian neoplasms.[1] Seventy-five percent to 80% are benign cystadenomas, and 5% to 10% are malignant cystadenocarcinomas.[2] Within

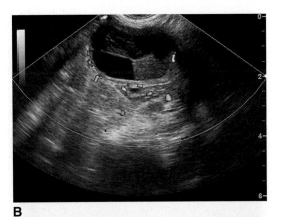

B

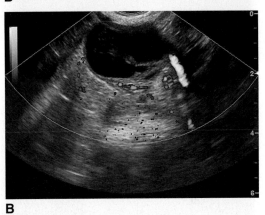

B

Fig. 17-20 **A** and **B,** Serous ovarian tumor containing thin septations and papillary projections. (Courtesy Lori Davis and Natalie Cauffman, Florida Hospital Deland.)

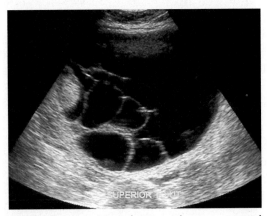

Fig. 17-21 Serous cystadenocarcinoma containing multiple thick loculations and papillary projection. (Courtesy Lori Davis and Natalie Cauffman, Florida Hospital Deland.)

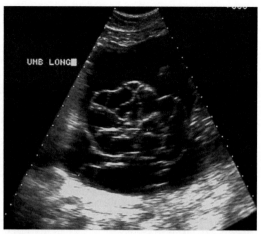

Fig. 17-22 Multiple septations in large malignant serous mass.

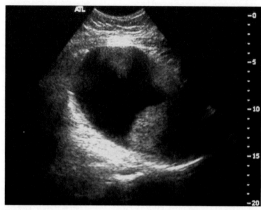

Fig. 17-24 Papillary serous carcinoma. Large solid projection into cystic mass.

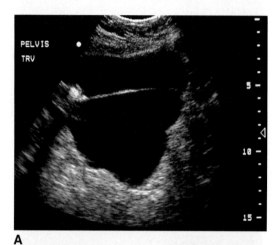

A

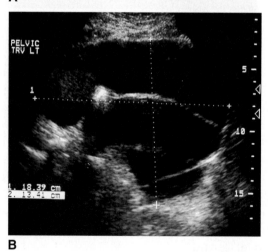

B

Fig. 17-23 **A** and **B,** Large serous cystadenocarcinoma. Note echogenic calcification in septation.

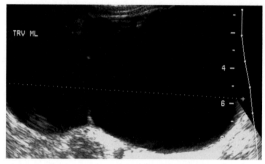

Fig. 17-25 Large mucinous tumor filling pelvic cavity.

the continuum from benign to malignant, about 14% of mucinous ovarian tumors are of borderline malignancy.[2] The benign form occurs most often among women in their 20s to 40s. Malignant mucinous tumors are more common in a slightly older age group, usually occurring during the 30s to the 60s. Borderline tumors reach peak prevalence in women in their 30s.

Mucinous tumors of the ovary are epithelial lesions that contain thick mucinous material within multiple loculations. Mucinous tumors may become extremely large; they are, in fact, among the largest of human tumors (Fig. 17-25). Patients are usually asymptomatic until tumor size becomes sufficient to produce symptoms, at which time they often have abdominal mass or enlargement or edema of the legs from compression of the inferior vena cava. Because of their size, these tumors are prone to undergo torsion and rupture is possible, particularly in the case of malignant tumors. If rupture occurs, mucinous material may spill and accumulate in the abdomen, causing **pseudo-myxoma peritoneum.** Mucinous tumors may produce

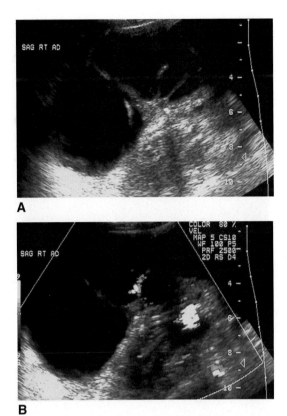

A

B

Fig. 17-26 A, Mucinous cystadenoma containing several thick septations. **B,** Note color flow Doppler demonstration of flow in septation.

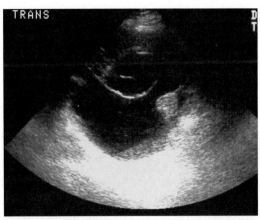

Fig. 17-27 Gravity-dependent low-level echoes identified in borderline malignant mucinous tumor.

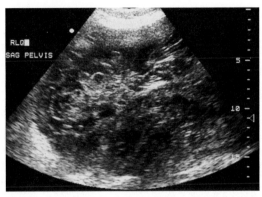

Fig. 17-28 Irregular walls and multiple irregular septations shown in mucinous cystadenocarcinoma.

estrogen or androgens, and those circulating hormones may produce symptoms of **endometrial hyperplasia** or **hirsutism. Gastrin** secretion by functional mucinous tumors may result in **Zollinger-Ellison syndrome,** accompanied by its characteristic symptoms of diarrhea and gastric or duodenal ulcers. Mucinous ovarian tumors are treated with surgery, sometimes combined with radiation therapy or chemotherapy. Patient survival from mucinous cystadenocarcinomas depends largely on stage of disease at detection.

Sonographic Findings. A mucinous ovarian mass presents sonographically as a multiloculated cystic mass with a diameter of up to 15 to 30 cm.[1] Cyst walls and septations are thick, and thick mucoid contents may produce gravity-dependent low-level echoes (Figs. 17-26, A and B, and 17-27). Differing echogenicity may be appreciated in the various compartments. Ninety-five percent of benign mucinous tumors are unilateral.[7] Malignant mucinous cystadenocarcinomas, on the other hand, are more often bilateral and have thicker, more irregular walls and septations (Fig. 17-28). Papillary projections are less frequently observed within mucinous tumors than within serous tumors.

Endometrioid

Endometrioids are epithelial ovarian tumors that occur most frequently among women in their 40s and 50s and are often associated with endometrial adenocarcinoma. About 80% of endometrioids are malignant. Malignant endometrioids comprise 20% to 25% of all ovarian malignant tumors[2] and rank as the second most common epithelial malignant disease. Endometriosis has been linked to several epithelial tumors, including endometrioid. In fact, some studies report endometrioid cancer originating directly from endometriotic tissue in up to 24% of cases.[2] Endometrioids typically measure from 12 to 20 cm and contain blood-stained fluid.[2] Although most are malignant, endometrioids bear a better prognosis than either serous or mucinous cystadenocarcinomas, probably because of diagnosis at an earlier stage.

Sonographic Findings. Endometrioids usually present sonographically as cystic masses that contain

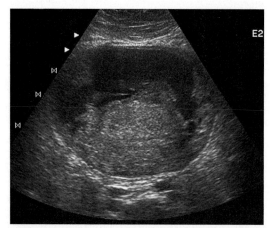

Fig. 17-29 Malignant ovarian tumor containing large papillary projection. (Courtesy GE Medical Systems.)

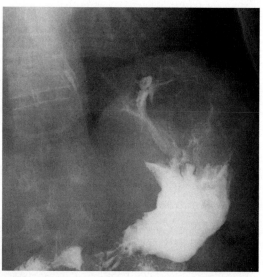

Fig. 17-30 Primary malignant gastric lesion was discovered radiographically after diagnosis of Krukenberg's tumor.

papillary projections (Fig. 17-29). Occasionally, these lesions appear as predominantly solid with areas of hemorrhage or necrosis. Twenty-five percent to 30% of endometrioids are bilateral.[3]

Krukenberg's Tumor

Ovaries are a common site of metastases from a variety of neoplasms, especially those of the breast and of the gastrointestinal tract. Metastatic ovarian tumors typically arise during the reproductive years and comprise 5% to 10% of ovarian neoplasms.[16] Krukenberg's tumors are ovarian metastatic adenocarcinomas that contain **mucin**-secreting **signet-ring cells.** These lesions are produced by primary neoplasms of the gastrointestinal tract, most commonly gastric carcinoma (Fig. 17-30). A Krukenberg's tumor is often discovered before the primary lesion. In addition to surgical removal of the Krukenberg's tumor, the primary malignant disease must be sought and managed.

Krukenberg's tumors are **encapsulated** tumors. They may be cystic, mixed, or solid. Cystic Krukenberg's tumors tend to be the largest and may present as lower abdominal masses. Cystic spaces are filled with serous or mucinous fluid. A correlation appears to exist between the size of a Krukenberg's tumor and its texture. Krukenberg's tumors are typically solid when small, becoming increasingly cystic as size increases, suggesting that these are initially solid tumors that undergo progressive necrosis and hemorrhage as they grow.[17]

Sonographic Findings. Krukenberg's tumors may be solid masses that diffusely infiltrate and increase the bulk of the ovarian **parenchyma,** so the possibility of metastatic lesions should be explored when the ovaries are enlarged, particularly when they are asymmetrically

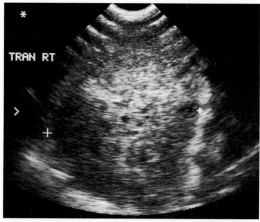

Fig. 17-31 Right ovary diffusely enlarged from infiltration of Krukenberg's tumor. Note less homogeneous echo texture than typical of normal ovarian tissue.

enlarged (Fig. 17-31). Ascites is often an associated finding. Because of the range of tissue complexity of these masses as they develop, Krukenberg's tumors have variable echogenicity and may exhibit a characteristic **"moth-eaten" cyst formation**[17] that correlates with a solid mass infiltrated with cystic areas representing necrosis and hemorrhage (Figs. 17-32 and 17-33, *A* and *B*). This pattern contrasts with primary ovarian lesions, in which usually predominantly cystic lesions contain solid components. Tumor encapsulation provides clear tumor margins. Sonographically distinguishing metastatic Krukenberg's tumors from primary ovarian lesions is sometimes difficult, particularly later in the

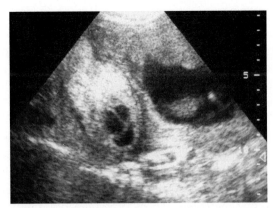

Fig. 17-32 Krukenberg's tumor displaying characteristic "moth-eaten" cyst formation.

course of metastatic disease when Krukenberg's tumors may be more cystic. Factors supporting the diagnosis of Krukenberg's tumor include bilaterality, few adhesions, clear margins, and absence of papillae or irregular septae. Interrogation of these tumors with color Doppler sonography reveals prominent low-resistance flow, characteristic of neoplastic lesions, in the solid portions of these masses (Fig. 17-34).

SOLID NEOPLASMS

Brenner Tumor

Brenner tumors, also known as *transitional cell tumors,* are uncommon solid ovarian masses that represent about 2% of all ovarian neoplasms.[18] These lesions usually occur among women in their 30s to their 70s, with 50 years as the mean age of incidence. Arising from ovarian surface epithelium, these dense fibrous tumors are usually smaller than 2 cm in diameter and rarely exceed 10 cm.[2] Six percent to 7% are bilateral.[2] Brenner tumors are occasionally associated with an ipsilateral neoplasm or cyst, most commonly a mucinous cystadenoma or a cystic teratoma.

Brenner tumors are typically asymptomatic and are discovered as incidental findings. Some of these lesions are functional, however, producing estrogen that may cause endometrial hyperplasia. Patients with these functional Brenner tumors often have resulting **metrorrhagia.** Brenner tumors may also be associated with **Meigs' syndrome.** Although most of these tumors are benign, in rare cases, a Brenner tumor may be malignant.

Sonographic Findings. Most Brenner tumors are unilateral and small, typically measuring less than 1 to 2 cm in diameter.[2] Although these masses are solid, they

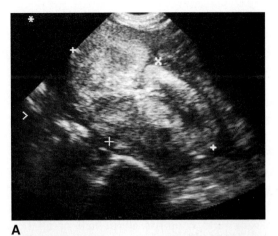

A

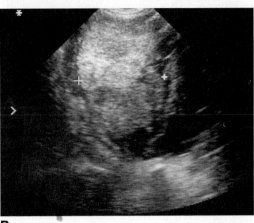

B

Fig. 17-33 **A** and **B,** Krukenberg's tumors often present with variable echo texture.

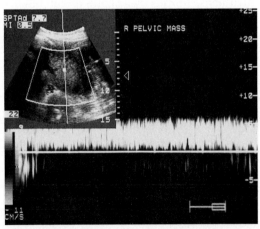

Fig. 17-34 Color Doppler sonography reveals low-resistance flow in Krukenberg's tumor.

may be hypoechoic with no posterior acoustic enhancement (Fig. 17-35). Multiple calcifications may be present. Cystic areas are uncommon but may occur as the result of a coexistent cystadenoma. Brenner tumors may be difficult to differentiate sonographically from other solid pelvic masses, including ovarian fibromas and thecomas and uterine **leiomyomas.**

Fibroma

Fibromas derive from germ cells in the stroma of the ovary and are characterized by abnormalities of chromosome 12.[19] They represent about 4% of all ovarian neoplasms[3] and comprise about half of all sex-cord stromal tumors.[2] These tumors occur at all ages but are most common among menopausal and postmenopausal women. Fibromas consist entirely of mature fibroblastic collagen-producing cells. They vary greatly in size, ranging from microscopic to melon sized.[3,13]

Although small ovarian fibromas are often asymptomatic, larger ones may produce pressure and pain. Large fibromas may be pedunculated and prone to torsion. Tumors that exceed 5 cm in diameter are frequently accompanied by ascites, and about 1% are associated with Meigs' syndrome.[2] Fibromas are always benign, but treatment generally includes removal of the tumor along with the affected ovary.

Sonographic Findings. Fibromas have sonographic findings similar to those of Brenner tumors and pedunculated uterine fibroids. They are typically hypoechoic with marked posterior acoustic attenuation from their dense fibrous tissue component, but areas of cystic degeneration may alter the typical sonographic appearance.[2] Most fibromas are unilateral.[1]

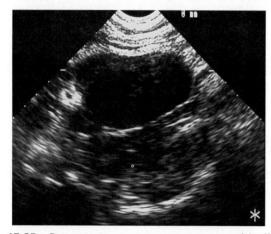

Fig. 17-35 Brenner tumor presents sonographically as hypoechoic mass; its solid nature is suggested sonographically by absence of posterior acoustic enhancement.

Thecoma

Thecomas are members of the family of sex-cord stromal lesions and, like fibromas, are characterized by aberrations in chromosome 12. Thecomas contain a variable combination of thecal and fibroblastic cells; it is the compositional balance of those cell types that distinguishes several members of a group of solid ovarian tumors. When thecal cells predominate, a lesion is classified as a thecoma; more plentiful fibrous tissue results in a classification of fibroma or thecofibroma. Thecomas occur most often in postmenopausal women and represent about 1% of ovarian neoplasms. Most measure about 5 to 10 cm in diameter.[2] Symptoms, when present, usually relate to tumoral estrogen production. These tumors are rarely malignant.

Sonographic Findings. The sonographic profile of thecomas is similar to that of fibromas. Thecomas are almost always unilateral (Fig. 17-36).

Sertoli-Leydig Cell Tumor

Sertoli-Leydig cell tumors (SLCTs) are rare, representing less than 0.5% of all ovarian tumors. More than 90% occur in menstruating women, most commonly in women in their 20s and 30s.[20] SLCTs are sex-cord stromal ovarian lesions derived of testicular cell types. Like other sex-cord tumors, these tumors contain cells with identifiable chromosomal abnormalities. SLCTs often produce testosterone, which results in virilization in about one third of patients.[2] Symptoms of virilization may include loss of secondary sex characteristics, acne, male-pattern balding, deepening of the voice, and clitoral enlargement. Patients may have menstrual disorders or mass-related symptoms, including abdominal swelling and pain. SLCTs occasionally produce estrogen. Laboratory findings may include abnormal quantities of circulating hormones, particularly testosterone. About 10% to 20% of SLCTs are malignant.[3] Prognosis and

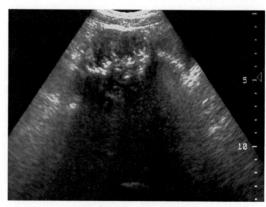

Fig. 17-36 Thecoma.

treatment depend on tumor stage and differentiation. Treatment usually includes removal of the tumor and the affected ovary and tube. For treatment of advanced disease, more aggressive surgery, and sometimes chemotherapy, may be undertaken. Prognosis is generally good.

Sonographic Findings. The diameters of SLCTs typically measure between 5 and 15 cm.[2] Smaller tumors usually appear solid, with an echo texture similar to that of fibroids, and larger tumors are often multiloculated with cystic components. Tumor size generally corresponds to likelihood of malignancy; that is, larger tumors are more commonly malignant.

Table 17-1 is a summary of the pathology and sonographic findings of ovarian masses.

Table 17-1	*Ovarian Lesions*		
Pathology	**Sonographic Appearance**	**Benign Versus Malignant**	**Occurrence**
Follicular cyst	Thin-walled, cystic; up to 20-cm diameter; diffuse low-level internal echoes; echogenic in presence of acute hemorrhage	Benign	Common during reproductive years
Corpus luteum cyst	Hypoechoic or anechoic; enhanced through transmission; up to 5-cm diameter; during pregnancy, thick, hyperechoic, crenulated walls, internal echoes, solid when collapsed	Benign	Identified in most women during luteal phase
Paraovarian cyst	Thin-walled, cystic; variable size; separate from ipsilateral ovary; internal echoes; internal cystadenoma	Rarely malignant	10% of all adnexal masses
Endometrioma	Well-defined unilocular or multilocular; diffuse, low-level internal echoes; up to 15- to 20-cm diameter; often bilateral; hyperechoic foci in walls; anechoic; solid	Benign	Most common in patients with history of infertility
Benign cystic teratoma	Anechoic cystic component; dermoid plug; "tip-of-iceberg" sign; fat/fluid level; hyperechoic lines and dots	1% to 3% undergo malignant transformation	Most common ovarian neoplasm; more frequent during reproductive years
Serous cystadenoma	Anechoic, unilocular; up to 20-cm diameter; thin walls and internal septations; usually unilateral; papillary projections	Benign, semimalignant	Combined with serous cystadenocarcinoma: 30% of ovarian neoplasms; most common in 30s to 40s
Serous cystadenocarcinoma	Multilocular; thick, irregular borders; papillary projections from walls of cysts; multiple thick septae; multiple echogenic foci; often bilateral	Highly malignant	More common in 60s

Continued

Table 17-1	*Ovarian Lesions—cont'd*		
Pathology	**Sonographic Appearance**	**Benign Versus Malignant**	**Occurrence**
Mucinous cystadenoma	Cystic, multilocular; thick walls and septations; up to 15- to 30-cm diameter; gravity-dependent echoes; compartments with differing echogenicity; usually unilateral	85% benign	Combined with mucinous cystadenocarcinomas: 20% of ovarian neoplasms; most common in 20s to 40s
Mucinous cystadenocarcinoma	Appearance similar to mucinous cystadenoma but with thicker, more irregular walls and septations; often bilateral; papillary projections	Malignant	Most common in 30s to 60s
Endometrioid	Cystic mass with papillary projections; 1- to 20-cm diameter; most often bilateral; predominantly solid	80% are malignant	20% to 25% of ovarian malignant diseases; common in 50s to 60s
Krukenberg's tumor	Variable echogenicity; asymmetrically enlarged ovary; few adhesions to other organs; "moth-eaten" cyst; ascites	Malignant	5% to 10% of ovarian neoplasms; most common during reproductive years
Brenner tumor	Hypoechoic; no posterior enhancement; <1- to 2-cm diameter; Meigs' syndrome; calcifications; cystic areas	Very rarely malignant	Uncommon; most common in 40s to 80s
Fibroma, thecoma	Hypoechoic; no posterior enhancement; Meigs' syndrome	Benign	<5% of ovarian neoplasms; most common among menopausal, post-menopausal women
Sertoli-Leydig cell tumor	Predominantly solid; 5- to 15-cm diameter; larger tumors may be multiloculated and cystic	10% to 20% malignant	Rare; most common in 20s to 30s

SUMMARY

Sonographic characterization of ovarian masses provides information valuable in differentiation of benign and malignant masses. Although a final diagnosis can only be reached with microscopic tissue examination, sonographic information—combined with a patient's history and clinical presentation—can suggest a diagnosis and assist the clinician with patient management decisions.

CLINICAL SCENARIO—DIAGNOSIS

◼️ The sonographic appearance of the ovarian mass is suggestive of a cystadenoma or cystadenocarcinoma. Although elevated CA-125 values are often inconclusive, the patient's abnormal value, combined with the cystic ovarian mass, raises suspicion of an epithelial malignant disease, such as a serous or mucinous cystadenocarcinoma. Although papillary projections may be seen in either lesion, they are more common in serous tumors and an elevated serum amylase value further supports that diagnosis. The lesions in the liver suggest metastases. The patient underwent a total abdominal hysterectomy with bilateral salpingoooophorectomy, after which the diagnosis of a serous cystadenocarcinoma was confirmed pathologically. The patient is undergoing radiation therapy and chemotherapy.

CASE STUDIES FOR DISCUSSION

1. A 25-year-old patient is seen for a pelvic ultrasound for left adnexal pain of 2 months. Sonographic examination of the left adnexa reveals a predominantly cystic mass that measures 2 cm in its largest dimension. The walls of the mass are thin and smooth. The mass appears to be pedunculated from the left ovary, but gentle pressure with a transvaginal transducer shows that the mass is actually separate from the ovary. A small multilocular cystic structure is observed within the larger cyst (Fig. 17-37). What is the most likely diagnosis?

2. An apparently healthy 32-year-old patient is seen for a pelvic ultrasound before oral contraceptives are begun. Sonography reveals the presence of two complex masses associated with the left ovary and another arising from the right. The largest of the masses measures 5.4 cm. All of the masses are predominantly cystic but contain multiple low-level echoes (Fig. 17-38). On color Doppler sonog-

raphy, absence of internal vascularity is shown. What is the most likely diagnosis?

3. A 28-year-old patient is referred for a pelvic ultrasound to evaluate a palpable abdominal mass. In addition to feeling pressure from the mass, the patient has diarrhea and hypogastric pain. Sonographic evaluation reveals a 20-cm multilocular cystic mass arising from the right ovary. The mass has thick walls and contains septations and gravity-dependent low-level echoes. Several papillary projections are also noted (Fig. 17-39). What do these findings most likely represent?

4. A 50-year-old patient with metrorrhagia is referred for a pelvic ultrasound. Sonographic evaluation reveals a thick endometrial lining and a 2-cm hypoechoic mass in the left ovary. Acoustic attenuation is observed posterior to the mass. In addition, a significant amount of ascites is present in the pelvis. What are some possible diagnoses?

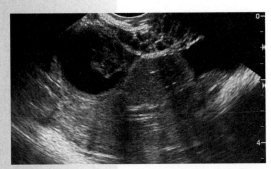

Fig. 17-37 Cystic structure containing small multilocular cystic structure. (Courtesy Lori Davis and Natalie Cauffman, Florida Hospital Deland.)

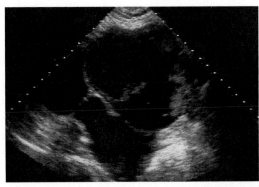

Fig. 17-39 Multiseptated mass containing papillary projections.

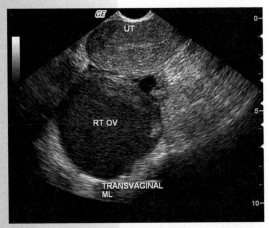

Fig. 17-38 Ovarian mass containing multiple low-level echoes. (Courtesy Lori Davis and Natalie Cauffman, Florida Hospital Deland.)

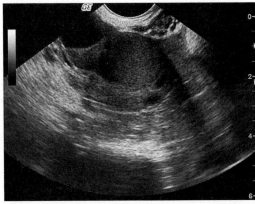

Fig. 17-40 Primarily solid mass arising from left ovary. (Courtesy Lori Davis and Natalie Cauffman, Florida Hospital Deland.)

CASE STUDIES FOR DISCUSSION—cont'd

5. A 26-year-old patient with acute left adnexal pain is referred for a pelvic ultrasound. Her last menstrual period occurred 18 days before her visit. The sonographic evaluation reveals a round, mostly echogenic 2-cm mass arising from the right ovary (Fig. 17-40). Color Doppler sonography shows no flow in the solid portions of the mass. What is the most likely nature of the mass?

STUDY QUESTIONS

1. A patient is seen for an obstetric ultrasound to evaluate the size and dates of her pregnancy. Sonographic parameters determine the gestational age to be 9 weeks, 1 day. Evaluation of the ovaries reveals a round hypoechoic mass in the left ovary. With color Doppler sonography, the sonographer shows a ring of intense low-resistance flow around the circumference of the cyst. The appearance of this mass most suggests which of the following?
   a. endometrioma
   b. corpus luteum cyst
   c. follicular cyst
   d. paraovarian cyst

2. A 46-year-old patient is seen with a 3-month history of midcycle spotting. Transvaginal ultrasound reveals a 2-cm hypoechoic left ovarian mass that attenuates the sound beam. Multiple calcifications are identified within the tumor. This mass most likely represents which of the following?
   a. Brenner tumor
   b. Krukenberg's tumor
   c. endometrioid
   d. benign cystic teratoma

3. A 25-year-old patient is referred for a pelvic ultrasound to locate a "lost" intrauterine contraceptive device (IUD). The IUD is identified appropriately positioned in the uterine cavity. Evaluation of the ovaries results in an incidental finding of a complex right ovarian mass. The mass contains a strongly attenuating echodensity and a cystic component in which echogenic lines and dots are observed. What is the most likely diagnosis of this mass?
   a. Sertoli-Leydig cell tumor
   b. endometrioma
   c. paraovarian cyst
   d. benign cystic teratoma

4. A 34-year-old patient is referred for a pelvic ultrasound because physical examination revealed palpably large ovaries. With ultrasound, the left ovary measures 4.2 cm in length, 5.3 cm in width, and 5.0 cm in anteroposterior diameter. The right ovary measures 5.1 × 6.2 × 4.3 cm. A moderate amount of ascites is identified. These findings most likely point to which of the following?
   a. Brenner tumor
   b. fibroma
   c. Krukenberg's tumor
   d. thecoma

5. A 19-year-old patient is seen for a pelvic sonogram for recent onset of the symptoms of virilization. Her voice has deepened, and she is losing the hair around her temples. Laboratory studies reveal elevated serum testosterone levels. Sonographic evaluation reveals a 6-cm multiloculated mass arising from the left ovary. These findings most suggest which of the following?
   a. Krukenberg's tumor
   b. Sertoli-Leydig cell tumor
   c. serous cystadenoma
   d. mucinous cystadenoma

6. A 47-year-old woman is seen for a follow-up sonographic evaluation of endometriosis. A pelvic ultrasound reveals bilateral predominantly cystic masses, each containing papillary projections. Which of the following is the most likely diagnosis?
   a. serous cystadenoma
   b. mucinous cystadenoma
   c. Krukenberg's tumor
   d. endometrioid

7. A 26-year-old woman with left adnexal pain is seen for a pelvic ultrasound. The ultrasound reveals a round, thin-walled sonolucent structure in the left ovary. Acoustic enhancement is noted posterior to the mass, which measures 2.1 cm in its largest dimension. This most likely represents which of the following?
   a. follicular cyst
   b. corpus luteum cyst

c. paraovarian cyst

d. endometrioma

8. A 52-year-old woman with pelvic pain is referred for a pelvic ultrasound, which reveals a 6-cm right ovarian mass. The mass is hypoechoic and produces marked posterior acoustic shadowing. A small amount of ascites is present. These findings are most suggestive of which of the following?

a. fibroma

b. benign cystic teratoma

c. endometrioid

d. Sertoli-Leydig cell tumor

9. A 33-year-old patient is seen for a pelvic ultrasound. The patient has increasing abdominal girth, despite diet and exercise. Sonographic evaluation reveals what appears to be a large amount of ascites filling the pelvis. On careful evaluation, however, thin septations are discovered throughout the fluid mass and several papillary projections are observed as well. What is the most likely diagnosis?

a. serous cystadenoma

b. mucinous cystadenocarcinoma

c. Brenner tumor associated with Meigs' syndrome

d. paraovarian cyst

10. A 30-year-old patient is referred for a pelvic ultrasound because of a family history of breast cancer. Sonographic evaluation reveals bilateral ovarian masses and ascites. The lesions are predominantly solid with scattered cystic spaces. No papillary projections are observed. Color Doppler sonography reveals low-resistance flow in the solid parts of the masses. What is the most likely diagnosis?

a. endometrioid

b. endometrioma

c. Brenner tumor

d. Krukenberg's tumor

REFERENCES

1. Hagen-Ansert SL: *Textbook of diagnostic ultrasonography*, vol 1, ed 5, St Louis, 2001, Mosby.

2. Callen PW: *Ultrasonography in Obstetrics and Gynecology*, ed 4, Philadelphia, 2000, WB Saunders.

3. Rumack CM, Wilson SR, Charboneau JW: *Diagnostic ultrasound*, vol 1, ed 2, St Louis, 1998, Mosby.

4. Durfee SM, Frates MC: Sonographic spectrum of the corpus luteum in early pregnancy: gray-scale, color, and pulsed Doppler appearance, *J Clin Ultrasound* 27:55-59, 1999.

5. Barloon TJ, Brown BP, Abu-Yousef MM et al: Paraovarian and paratubal cysts: preoperative diagnosis using transabdominal and transvaginal sonography, *J Clin Ultrasound* 24:117-121, 1996.

6. Patel MD, Feldstein VA, Chen D et al: Endometriomas: diagnostic performance of US, *Radiology* 210:739-734, 1999.

7. Patel MD, Feldstein VA, Lipson SD et al: Cystic teratomas of the ovary: diagnostic value of sonography, *AJR Am J Roentgenol* 171:1061-1065, 1998.

8. Lee DK, Kim SH, Cho JY et al: Ovarian teratomas appearing as solid masses on ultrasonography, *J Ultrasound Med* 18:141-145, 1999.

9. Johnson SC, Jordan GL: Sonographic diagnosis of multiple unilateral ovarian teratomas, *J Ultrasound Med* 20:279-281, 2001.

10. Serafini G, Quadri PG, Gandolfo NG et al: Sonographic features of incidentally detected small, nonpalpable ovarian dermoids, *J Clin Ultrasound* 27:369-373, 1999.

11. Teng N, Roberts JA: Adnexal tumors, *eMedicine Journal* 2, 2001, www.emedicine.com/MED/topic2830.htm.

12. Emoto M, Obama H, Horiuchi S et al: Transvaginal color Doppler ultrasonic characterization of benign and malignant ovarian cystic teratomas and comparison with serum squamous cell carcinoma antigen, *Cancer* 88:2298-2304, 2000.

13. Zalel Y, Seidman D, Oren M et al: Sonographic and clinical characteristics of struma ovarii, *J Ultrasound Med* 19:856-860, 2000.

14. Brophy CM, Morris J, Sussman J et al: "Pseudoascites" secondary to an amylase-producing serous ovarian cystadenoma, *J Clin Gastroenterol* 11:703-706, 1989.

15. Tarlowska L, Sikorowa L, Piatkowski Z: Ovarian serous cystadenoma, *Pol Med J* 11:368-379, 1972.

16. Choi BI, Choo IW, Han MC et al: Sonographic appearance of Krukenberg tumor from gastric carcinoma, *Gastrointest Radiol* 13:15-18, 1988.

17. Shimizu H, Yamasaki M, Ohama K et al: Characteristic ultrasonographic appearance of the Krukenberg tumor, *J Clin Ultrasound* 18:698-703, 1990.

18. Ohara N, Teramoto K: Magnetic resonance imaging of a benign Brenner tumor with an ipsilateral simple cyst, *Arch Gynecol Obstet* 265:96-99, 2001.

19. Liang SB, Sonobe H, Taguchi T et al: Trisomy 12 in ovarian tumors of thecoma-fibroma group: a fluorescence in situ hybridization analysis using paraffin sections, *Yuji Pathol Int* 51:37-42, 2001.

20. Lantzsch T, Stoerer S, Lawrenz K et al: Sertoli-Leydig cell tumor, *Arch Gynecol Obstet* 264:206-208, 2001.

BIBLIOGRAPHY

Venes D, Thomas CL: *Taber's cyclopedic medical dictionary*, ed 19, Philadelphia, 2001, Davis.

Berube MS, Neely DJ, DeVinne PB: *The American heritage dictionary*, ed 2, Boston, 1985, Houghton Mifflin.

III OBSTETRICS

18 | Uncertain Last Menstrual Period

JILL HERZOG

CLINICAL SCENARIO

■ A 22-year-old woman is seen by her obstetrician for prenatal care after a positive home pregnancy test. The patient gives the first day of her last menstrual period as 6 weeks and 5 days earlier and has no history of contraception use in the previous 4 months. During a digital pelvic examination, the obstetrician suspects that the uterus is larger than the estimated age of only 6 weeks and 5 days.

Further clinical history reveals that the last menstrual period was of a lighter flow volume than usual for this patient. The patient is sent to the ultrasound department 4 days later for estimation of gestational age. The ultrasound findings suggest a live embryo with a CRL estimating a gestational age of 10 weeks and 2 days. What is the best estimate of gestational age for this pregnancy?

OBJECTIVES

■ Describe the purpose of biometric measurements during the first trimester of pregnancy for estimation of gestational age.

■ Demonstrate appropriate techniques used for accurate first-trimester biometric measurements.

■ Describe the purpose of biometric measurements during the second and third trimesters of pregnancy for estimation of gestational age.

■ Demonstrate appropriate techniques used for accurate second- and third-trimester biometric measurements.

■ Describe additional measurements that may be performed throughout pregnancy for confirmation of gestational age.

■ Describe additional measurements that may be performed for diagnostic purposes during specific gestational age ranges.

■ Identify the technical limitations of delayed biometric imaging in cases of uncertain last menstrual period.

GLOSSARY OF TERMS

Amniocentesis: the procedure of aspiration of amniotic fluid sample with insertion of a needle through the maternal abdomen into the amniotic sac; the sample may be used to evaluate genetic composition, fetal maturity, or metabolic assays

Amnion: thin, smooth innermost membrane of pregnancy enclosing the fetus and the amniotic cavity

Aneuploidy: an abnormal number of chromosomes

Beta hCG: maternal serum test for detection of human chorionic gonadotropin for the diagnosis of pregnancy

Biometry: application of statistics to biologic science, as in assessment of fetal size on basis of statistics

Cesarean section: method of fetal delivery with surgical incision of the uterus

Chorion: the outermost membrane of pregnancy enclosing the amniotic and chorionic cavities; composed of trophoblasts

Chorionic villus sampling: the procedure of aspiration of a sample of chorionic villi found at the area of implantation and the early placenta

Decidua: the endometrial lining during pregnancy

Decidua capsularis: the portion of the decidua that encloses the chorionic cavity

Decidua parietalis: the portion of the remaining decidua other than at the implantation site

Distal femoral epiphysis: the small ossification center of the femur nearest the knee

Ectopic pregnancy: any pregnancy that occurs outside the uterine cavity

Endovaginal imaging: sonographic imaging performed with the introduction of a transducer into the vaginal canal

Gestational age: the age of the pregnancy, most often referred to as the length of time since the first day of the last menstrual period

Hypertelorism: increased distance between the medial borders of the orbital rims

Hypotelorism: decreased distance between the medial borders of the orbital rims

Obstetrician: a physician who treats women during pregnancy and delivery

Oligohydramnios: a markedly decreased amount of amniotic fluid surrounding the fetus

Ossification: the formation of bone substance

Pathology: a condition produced by disease

Pregnancy induction: the process of causing labor and delivery of fetuses with the use of medication

Sonologist: a professional educated to perform ultrasound examinations and interpret the findings

---

For more than three decades, ultrasonography has engraved a mark in the estimation of gestational age. Diagnostic ultrasound plays a role in the management of the pregnant patient whose history leaves the clinician with the task of estimating a due date on the basis of an uncertain last menstrual period (LMP). Advances in equipment and techniques have made sonographic determination of the gestational age possible even earlier in the pregnancy than previously. The acceptance of **endovaginal imaging** in the first trimester has been one of the biggest advances. The gestational sac diameter may be measured before the embryo is seen, but the first-trimester crown-rump length (CRL) is considered the most accurate predictor for gestational age. Early second-trimester **biometry** can also be of predictive value when obtained and interpreted accurately. The patient who does not seek prenatal care until the late third trimester creates the most difficult clinical scenario. This increased difficulty is the result of biologic variations in fetal size later in

the pregnancy that decrease the accuracy of biometry performed for the first time at this advanced gestational age. At any stage in the pregnancy, precise technique must be used to accurately estimate gestational age with sonographic measurements.

FIRST-TRIMESTER BIOMETRY

Before the advent of pregnancy testing and ultrasonography, the LMP was the most identifiable reference point for the beginning of the pregnancy.[1] With advances in prenatal testing, pregnancy is now known to have a duration of approximately 280 days from the first day of the LMP, also referred to as 9 calendar or 10 lunar months. This is also known as *Nägele's rule.*[1-3] The knowledge of an accurate gestational age is needed to manage the pregnancy optimally and reduce the risks of preterm and postterm deliveries[3] and to coordinate elective procedures, such as biochemical screening evaluation, **chorionic villus sampling** (CVS), amniocentesis, and delivery method, such as a repeat **cesarean section** or **pregnancy induction**.[2,4-7] Because many women who potentially become pregnant in any given month may have variable cycle lengths, bleeding in early pregnancy, or inaccurate accounts of menstrual dates, estimation of a due date can be a clinical challenge. Patients who seek prenatal care during the first or second trimester of pregnancy without a strong knowledge of LMP or normal cycle lengths may undergo an ultrasound examination to estimate gestational age with biometric measurements of the structures of pregnancy or the fetus. Among the measurements that may be obtained during the first trimester for dating purposes, with ultrasound techniques, are the gestational sac diameter and the CRL.[1-4,8,9] First-trimester measurements are considered to be reliable indicators because pathologic states and fetal abnormalities have the least impact on fetal size during this time[2] and biologic variation is at a minimum during the first few weeks of pregnancy (Box 18-1).[4]

Gestational Sac

The appearance of an anechoic fluid collection, surrounded by an echogenic ring in the fundal region of the endometrial cavity, is the first sonographic evidence of an intrauterine pregnancy (Fig. 18-1).[2,4,8,10] This echogenic ring is a vital structure of a normal pregnancy because it represents the **chorion** and **decidua capsularis**.[4] Absence of the echogenic ring should prompt suspicion of a pseudogestational sac associated with **ectopic pregnancy** and may warrant clinical correlation with **beta-hCG** levels.[4] As the pregnancy progresses and displacement of the endometrial echo occurs, a second outer echogenic ring may be seen that represents the remainder of the endometrial lining, known as the **decidua parietalis**.[1,4] The appearance of

these two echogenic rings has become known as the double decidual sac sign and may be seen between week 4 and week 6 from the LMP.[1,4,8] The space between the two decidual rings is the unoccupied endometrial cavity that will become obliterated as the pregnancy progresses.

With two scan planes, a measurement made in each of the three dimensions of the gestational sac can be used to calculate a mean sac diameter (MSD). These sac measurements should be made at the interface between the echogenic border and the fluid (see Fig. 18-1).[2,4,10] The introduction of endovaginal ultrasound techniques has allowed the visualization of this normal progression of early pregnancy.[10] With high-frequency endovaginal technique, a pregnancy dating only 4 weeks and 1 or 2 days from the LMP may be visualized as a 2- to 3-mm fluid collection within the uterus (see Fig. 18-1).[4] The MSD should correlate closely with suspected **gestational age**, and any significant variance or suspicion of pregnancy loss should be closely correlated with beta-hCG levels. The MSD is not a true fetal parameter, but its correlation to the estimated gestational age and

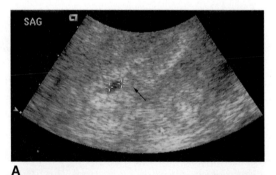

A

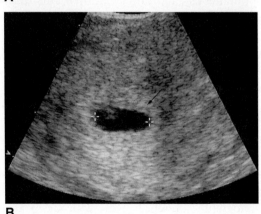

B

Fig. 18-1 A, Tiny 3.8-mm anechoic fluid collection is seen in uterine cavity. **B,** A 1.15-cm gestational sac is seen within uterine cavity. Both sacs are surrounded by echogenic decidua *(arrows)*. Correct caliper placement is shown at fluid interface with echogenic border.

BOX 18-1

First-Trimester Biometry

GESTATIONAL SAC
Mean sac diameter

CROWN-RUMP DIAMETER
Additional Measurements
Yolk sac (2 to 6 mm)
Nuchal translucency (≤3 mm between 10 and
   14 weeks)

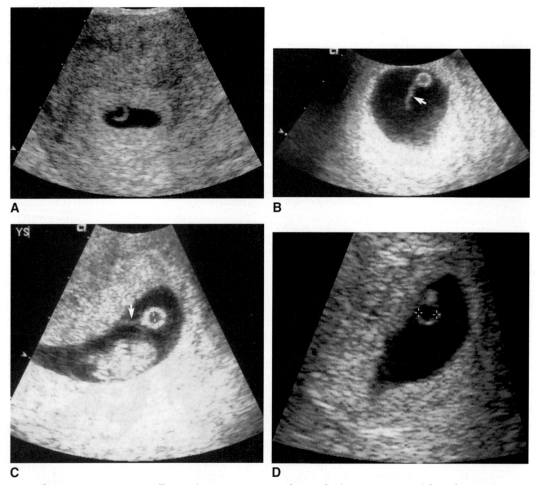

Fig. 18-2 **A** to **D,** Yolk sac is seen as round anechoic structure with echogenic border within gestational sac. **B** and **C,** Vitelline duct may be shown as echogenic line *(arrow)* connecting yolk sac to embryo. **D,** Correct caliper placement is shown for measurement of yolk sac.

growth rate may prove to be valuable in the prediction of spontaneous abortion.[1] Normal first-trimester gestational sac growth rate should be approximately 1 mm per day.[1] During this time of rapid embryologic change, a repeat examination may be performed within a few days to show the progression of the pregnancy and confirm it as normal or abnormal.

Yolk Sac

The sonographically visualized yolk sac is more accurately called the *secondary yolk sac.*[1] Most sonographers and **sonologists** loosely use the term yolk sac in discussion of this second structure of pregnancy to be visualized. The sonographic presence of the yolk sac in an early gestational sac may be considered a predictor of a normally progressing pregnancy even without visualization of the embryo.[4] With endovaginal technique, a gestational sac measuring 8 mm or more should show a yolk sac to be indicative of a normal early pregnancy.[2,4,9]

The secondary yolk sac appears as a round anechoic structure with an echogenic rim (Fig. 18-2).[4] This yolk sac supplies nutrition for the developing embryo through the vitelline duct (see Fig 18-2).[4] The size of the yolk sac is most often measured to be 2 to 6 mm throughout the first trimester, and an abnormally small or large measurement may be indicative of pending loss or fetal abnormality. The yolk sac diameter should be measured with placement of calipers along the inner borders of the echogenic ring (see Fig. 18-2). The yolk sac is also often used to assist in locating the tiny embryo. After the yolk sac is located, close evaluation of adjacent structures will often identify the embryonic disk recognized with the flicker of cardiac activity.

Crown-Rump Length

Once the gestational sac has formed and contains a yolk sac, the next structure of pregnancy visualized with ultrasound is the embryo. The embryonic period is con-

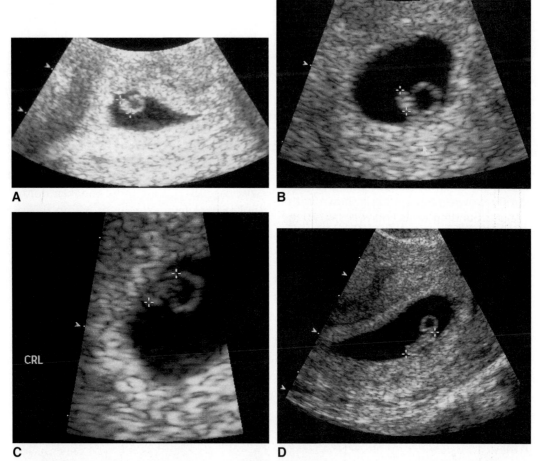

Fig. 18-3 **A** to **D,** Tiny embryo of early pregnancy is visualized adjacent to yolk sac. It has disklike appearance and becomes more evident as pregnancy progresses. Various sizes of embryos are represented as visualized between weeks 5 and 7 from last menstrual period (LMP). **D,** More easily recognized embryo as separate structure near week 7 LMP. Embryo should be measured in its longest axis, excluding yolk sac, as shown with caliper placement in images.

sidered to be week 6 through week 12 of the pregnancy.[4] In the earliest stage of the embryonic period, the yolk sac may be used as a landmark for locating the tiny embryo (Fig. 18-3) and possible cardiac activity. Initially the embryo is found adjacent to the yolk sac and appears on the ultrasound image as a flat, disklike structure (see Fig. 18-3). Faint flickering of this structure, which represents early cardiac activity, may be seen on two-dimensional ultrasound as early as 5.5 weeks (Fig. 18-4). The normal embryonic heart rate (EHR) range is 120 to 180 beats per minute (bpm).[1] If the EHR is 100 bpm or less, it should be compared with the maternal heart rate to ensure that maternal uterine vessels are not being sampled and represented as embryonic cardiac activity.

The embryo should be visualized in a gestational sac that measures 25 mm.[1,4] Evaluation of the embryo must

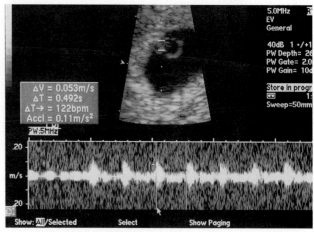

Fig. 18-4 Early embryo shows flicker of cardiac activity and should be measured at rate between 120 and 180 beats per minute.

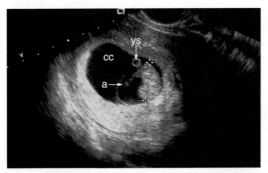

Fig. 18-5 Embryo begins to show C shape by approximately 8 weeks last menstrual period. Caliper placement for accurate crown-rump length is shown with thin amnion *(a)* surrounding fetus and yolk sac *(ys)* in chorionic cavity *(cc)*.

include multiple scan planes to obtain the longest axis for accurate gestational dating. A measurement of the longest axis, excluding the yolk sac, will provide accurate information for estimation of gestational age (Fig. 18-5; see also Fig. 18-3). This measurement may be difficult because of the small size of the embryo early in the pregnancy. By approximately 8 weeks from the LMP, the embryo begins to take on a C-shaped appearance (see Fig. 18-5). An accurate CRL may be found with placement of the calipers at the top of the fetal head (crown) to the bottom of the torso (rump; Fig. 18-6; see also Fig. 18-3). Care must be taken not to include the yolk sac or fetal extremities within this measurement. Any inclusion of these two structures undermines the accuracy of gestational age.

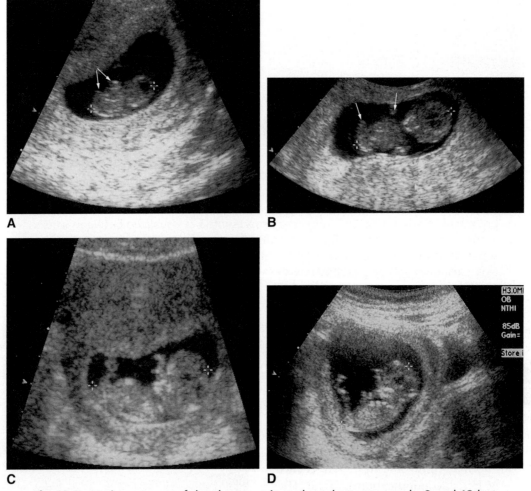

Fig. 18-6 Various stages of development in embryo between weeks 8 and 12 last menstrual period. **A,** Faint demonstration of early limb buds *(arrows)* at 8 weeks 1 day. **B,** Limb buds *(arrows)* are more evident as embryo nears 10 weeks gestational age. Care should be taken not to include extremities in crown-rump length (CRL) measurement. **C** and **D,** Between weeks 11 and 12, embryo begins to take on more humanlike shape as it nears end of first trimester. CRL measurement is shown at all of these ages.

Nuchal Translucency

The final measurement that may be performed during an ultrasound examination in the first trimester is in fact not a measurement for gestational age estimation but rather a secondary measurement and early screening tool for possible fetal aneuploidy. The soft tissues found at the back of the fetal neck in the first trimester have been termed the nuchal translucency.[4,8,11] The thickness of this space has been the source of numerous studies in the past decade. A thickened nuchal translucency has been identified as associated with fetal aneuploidy, most specifically trisomy 21, also known as *Down syndrome*.[4,11] Before the nuchal translucency measurement is used, gestational age must be assessed with the CRL.

Techniques for measurement of the nuchal translucency have been scrutinized and require accuracy and precision both in the caliper placement and in the time of imaging in the pregnancy. The appropriate technique for measurement of the nuchal translucency is placement of the calipers at the fetal skin and the posterior aspect of the nuchal membrane (Fig. 18-7).[4] This technique must be performed with precision because spaces of this small size can be misinterpreted as ab-

normal with even the slightest variation. The **amnion** is often found along the posterior edge of the fetus. With the fetus in the supine position, the amniotic cavity behind the fetus may be confused for the nuchal translucency and measured as abnormally thickened.[4] Sonographer experience in this technique and knowledge of these normal structures are important to prevent inaccurate measurements that may create false-positive results.

Studies performed to determine the validity of the thickened nuchal translucency and a cutoff value for this thickening have generated a narrow window of time for evaluation of the nuchal translucency to be a predictor for fetal chromosomal abnormality. The nuchal translucency is considered to be thickened if measured 3 mm or more between weeks 10 and 14 of the pregnancy.[4] The sonographer should perform the nuchal translucency measurement as part of the first-trimester examination only if the gestational age is within this range. Reporting of the nuchal translucency should not be considered if the CRL suggests gestational age outside of this range.

An additional limitation in the validity of the nuchal translucency is the potentially normal resolution of the thickening, recognized even in cases of fetal **aneuploidy**.[4] This means that resolution of an abnormal measurement earlier in the pregnancy does not rule out an abnormality. Close clinical correlation and patient counseling should be performed in cases of an abnormally thickened nuchal translucency.

SECOND- AND THIRD-TRIMESTER BIOMETRY

After the first 12 weeks of pregnancy, the pregnancy enters the second of three trimesters. The early portion of the second trimester can still yield accurate gestational age with multiple biometric measurements.[4,7] Performance of one long axis measurement of the fetus is no longer acceptable or possible in this trimester, and multiple anatomic structures must be evaluated and measured.

Estimation of gestational age with these measurements is still accurate with the appropriate technique. Through approximately 20 weeks, the primary biometric parameters of biparietal diameter (BPD), head circumference (HC), abdominal circumference (AC), and femur length (FL) have minimal biologic variation unless a pathologic condition is present.[2,4] With identification of sonographic landmarks of fetal anatomy, these measurements may be obtained with

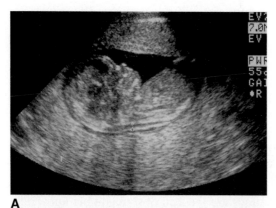

A

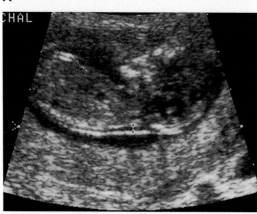

B

Fig. 18-7   A and **B,** Caliper placement for nuchal translucency in first trimester is shown.

BOX 18-2

Second- and Third-Trimester Biometry

PRIMARY PARAMETERS

Biparietal diameter
Head circumference
Abdominal circumference
Femur length

SECONDARY PARAMETERS

Occipitofrontal diameter
Transcerebellar diameter (1 mm per week between
   weeks 15 and 25)
Binocular distance

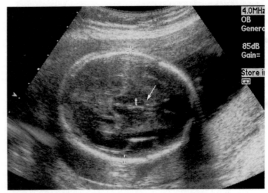

Fig. 18-8 Location for biparietal diameter is shown with visualization of thalamus *(t)* and cavum septum pellucidum *(arrow)*. Caliper placement is shown from outer edge to inner edge of cranium perpendicular to cerebral falx.

consistency and accuracy. In the case of suspected pathology, biometric measurements should be interpreted with only the unaffected anatomy and may be supplemented with the secondary biometric parameters. After mid term, or 20 weeks from the LMP, the fetus enters the growth stage of pregnancy and, considering that all newborns are not the same size, the estimation of gestational age is more challenging. Measurements performed in the late second and third trimesters are more accurate for estimation of gestational size rather than age.[4,8] For this reason, gestational age is more easily determined with fetal biometry in the first half of pregnancy. Any measurement performed to assess gestational age or size should be performed in the same technique used to derive the chart used for this assessment (Box 18-2).[4,8]

Primary Biometric Parameters

Biparietal Diameter. As the patient enters the second trimester of pregnancy, the fetal cranium and intracranial structures become more evident and permit sonographic measurements to be performed with a high level of accuracy. The BPD is considered to be one of the best predictors for gestational age, second only to the CRL performed in the first trimester.[1,2,4,8,9] The BPD is a biometric measurement performed in the transaxial view of the fetal head just above the level of the ears. For this measurement to provide valuable information, it must be performed with an image of the fetal head at a plane that allows visualization of certain intracranial sonographic landmarks.

Once the location of the fetal head is determined, the sonographer should position the transducer scan plane to view the intracranial structures transversely from the lateral aspect of the fetal head. The BPD measurement should be performed perpendicular to the interhemispheric fissure, also known as the *cerebral falx*. The diamond-shaped, hypoechoic thalamus should be seen near the center of the cranium, with the cavum septum pellucidum visualized anteriorly. The cavum septum pellucidum appears as an anechoic to hypoechoic structure anterior to the thalmus identified with the visualized three echogenic lines. The BPD should be calculated at the widest point of the fetal head at this level. Calipers should be placed on the outer edge of the near field cranium and the inner edge of the far field cranium (Fig. 18-8).[1,2,4,8,9,10,12]

The BPD can be an excellent predictor for gestational age, especially in the early second trimester,[3] but it is not without limitations for accuracy. Among these limitations are the lack of sonographer knowledge and precision, fetal head molding, and biologic variation in the third trimester.[2,4,7] The sonographer must be prepared to accurately perform the technique of BPD measurement to obtain the gestational age. Caliper placement should correspond to the technique used for derivation of the chart used to estimate the gestational age.[4] The outer to inner measurement, described previously, is the most common technique used, but it must be performed correctly to be valuable. Fetal head shape may influence the accuracy of the BPD.[1,8] This occurs more commonly in cases of **oligohydramnios** or other sources of fetal crowding. In any circumstance, fetal head shape should be evaluated when the BPD is in an unexpected range. An abnormally widened BPD may be a result of a rounded fetal head, also known as

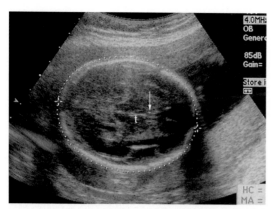

Fig. 18-9 Ellipse measurement of head circumference (HC) around fetal cranium contributes information in estimation of gestational age. HC should be measured at same level as biparietal diameter, with visualization of thalamus *(t)* and cavum septum pellucidum *(arrow)*.

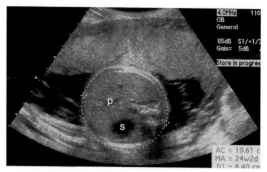

Fig. 18-10 Abdominal circumference is shown with ellipse at level of fetal stomach *(s)* and portal sinus *(p)*.

brachycephaly.[7] An abnormally shortened BPD may be a result of a flattened fetal head, also known as dolichocephaly.[7] With any fetal head shape, the third trimester creates more biologic variation in fetal head size than any other time in the pregnancy. This variation prevents accurate estimation of gestational age during this late stage of the pregnancy.

Head Circumference. The HC equips the interpreting physician with an additional cranial measurement for gestational age assessment. The HC may be calculated with the BPD and the occipitofrontal diameter (OFD). With advances in technology and ultrasound equipment, the HC is now most often performed within the machine with an ellipse measurement. This measurement should be performed at the same transverse image of the fetal head as the BPD. The ellipse tracing should be placed along the outer border of the fetal cranium and should not include the fetal scalp (Fig. 18-9).[4] HC can be of increased value in cases of abnormal fetal head shape because it is least influenced by shape.[1,2]

Abdominal Circumference. Gestational age may also be determined with measurement of the AC of the fetus. This biometric measurement is used in estimation of gestational age but is better used for estimation of fetal size or weight.[1] The AC should be obtained with the true transverse plane of the fetal abdomen at the level of the umbilical vein junction with the left portal vein.[1,2,8] This image should show the fetal stomach along with a hockey-stick–shaped appearance of the portal sinus anteriorly in the fetal abdomen (Fig. 18-10). The accuracy of the angle through the fetal abdomen may be confirmed with the appearance of the three **ossification** centers of the fetal spine seen in a true transverse axis.

The fetal kidneys should not be seen along this level of the transverse fetal abdomen, and inclusion of the kidneys will undermine the accuracy of the measurement for estimation of gestational age.

Once the correct landmarks are visualized and an image is acquired, the AC may be obtained with the ellipse tracing around the edge of the skin surface on the fetal abdomen. (see Fig. 18-10). If the ellipse measurement is not available on the equipment, abdomen diameters may be obtained perpendicular to one another in the anteroposterior (AP) and transverse dimensions of the fetal abdomen. Calculation of the AC may be performed with these two diameters.

The AC measurement also has limitations for assessment of gestational age. Fetal crowding can alter fetal abdomen shape and thus its size. The same conditions that may cause fetal head molding, such as oligohydramnios and advanced gestational age, may influence fetal abdomen circumference. Sonographer recognition of these conditions may prevent false interpretation of gestational age. The fetal abdomen also has a rather large variation during the third trimester because of biologic influences. Fetal AC is influenced more by fetal size than fetal age, especially in the third trimester.[1] Gestational age assessment should not rely heavily on the AC, particularly in the third trimester.

Femur Length. The fetal FL is second to the BPD in accuracy for prediction of gestational age in the second trimester.[2,8] The FL has little biologic variation in the second trimester and is least affected by surrounding structures.[8] For the FL, the sonographer should follow the transverse plane of the fetal torso from the level of the AC to the pelvic region. With scanning inferiorly to the iliac wings, the fetal lower extremities can be visualized. The long axis of the femur should be relatively easy to locate because of its limited range of motion. Once the femur is identified, a pivoting motion or rotation of the transducer should allow demon-

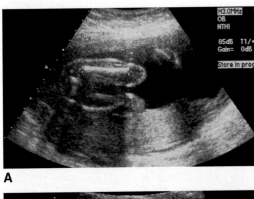

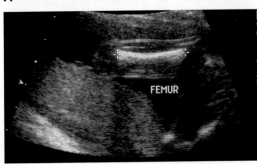

Fig. 18-11 **A** and **B,** Diaphysis of femur is visualized perpendicular to beam, and caliper placement is shown.

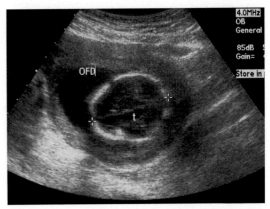

Fig. 18-12 Occipitofrontal diameter may also be measured at level of thalamus *(t)* along interhemispheric fissure or demonstrated with calipers.

stration of its longest axis. The femur closest to the transducer should be used in estimation of gestational age and imaged perpendicular to the beam's axis. Complete fetal anatomic surveys should include visualization of both femurs for the presence of ossification and gross symmetry.

The FL should be measured in the long axis to include only the diaphysis, or shaft, of the femur (Figs. 18-11).[1,2,8] The cartilaginous portion of the femoral head should not be included in the measurement, and the **distal femoral epiphysis,** seen after approximately 32 weeks,[4,7] should not be included. If gestational age is completely unknown, visualization of the distal femoral epiphyses has been used to estimate an age of 32 weeks or more LMP.[4] Accurate performance of the FL can be a valuable predictor of gestational age until the late third trimester. Limitations to this assessment exist, such as biologic influences that may become more evident near term or in cases of suspected skeletal dysplasia. Care should be taken to recognize these limitations to prevent inaccurate assessment of gestational age.

Secondary Biometric Parameters

Occipitofrontal Diameter. The occipitofrontal diameter (OFD) is a secondary biometric measurement that may be used along with the BPD to determine the fetal head shape and size. The OFD is performed at the same transverse image as the BPD, with calipers placed directly on the fetal cranium measuring along the interhemispheric fissure (Fig. 18-12).[1] A comparison of the BPD and OFD measurements will generate the cephalic index with the following formula:

$$CI = \frac{BPD}{OFD} \times 100^1$$

A cephalic index of 76 to 84 is considered to be within the normal range, indicating normal fetal head shape.[1] A cephalic index of more than 84 indicates a brachycephalic shape, and a cephalic index of less than 76 indicates a dolichocephalic shape.

Transcerebellar Diameter. Contents of the posterior fossa in the fetal head should be evaluated for evidence of **pathology,** and the cerebellum may often be used as a secondary biometric measurement to assess gestational age. The cerebellum can be visualized with angling the transducer inferiorly in the posterior skull from the plane of the BPD. This angulation allows visualization of the cerebellum, cerebral peduncles, and the thalamus from posterior to anterior in the fetal cranium. The cerebellum can be identified as two hypoechoic circular structures with echogenic borders, also known as the cerebellar hemispheres, on both sides of the midline. The hemispheres are adjacent to a brightly echogenic wedge between them. This echogenic wedge represents the vermis.

The transcerebellar diameter (TCD) may be measured with placement of the calipers on the most lateral borders of the cerebellar hemispheres (Fig. 18-13).[2] This measurement in millimeters is considered to correlate directly with gestational age between weeks 15 and 25.[1,7,8] The TCD is not considered to be the most accurate of cranial measurements, but in cases of fetal head molding, it may assist in calculation of gestational age.[9,10]

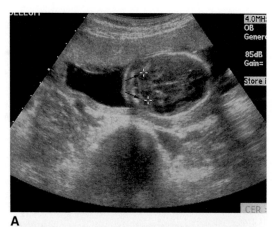

A

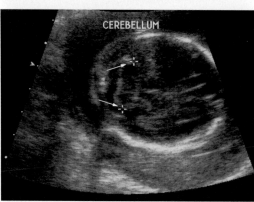

B

Fig. 18-13 **A** and **B**, Visualization of circular cerebellar hemispheres *(arrows)* and echogenic vermis between them shows cerebellum. Calipers show transcerebellar diameter.

Correlation with the TCD and gestational age can also assist in the diagnosis of cerebellar hypoplasia.

Binocular Distance. At any time during a pregnancy, the fetal head may found in an extremely low position within the maternal pelvis. This position may make an accurate BPD technically impossible, even after patient manipulation. If the BPD is unobtainable, the binocular distance may be performed as a secondary parameter in calculation of gestational age.[2,8] Although this is not the method of choice for dating the pregnancy, a measurement from the lateral borders of the fetal orbits in the transverse plane may provide an acceptable substitute. The measurement across the distance of both orbital rims is called the binocular distance. Calipers should be placed at the most lateral border of the orbits (Fig. 18-14). Additional measurements may be performed between each orbital rim and between the medial borders of the orbits. The comparison of these measurements with the binocular distance may assist in diagnosis of facial abnormalities, such as **hypotelorism** and **hypertelorism**.[2]

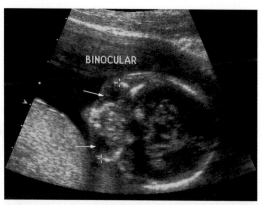

Fig. 18-14 Technically limited intracranial examinations may require use of binocular distance to estimate gestational age. Calipers should be placed on lateral rims of orbits *(arrows)* for accurate measurement.

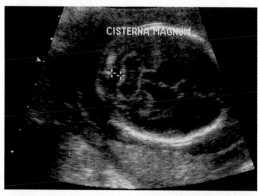

Fig. 18-15 Cisterna magna is identified as anechoic space between posterior skull and cerebellum. Calipers should be placed at midline for accurate anteroposterior measurement.

Miscellaneous Fetal Measurements of the Second and Third Trimesters

Cisterna Magna. The cisterna magna is found in the posterior fossa immediately posterior to the cerebellum. It appears on sonographic images as an anechoic space between the cerebellum and the posterior cranium (Fig. 18-15). The AP thickness of the cisterna magna is not considered to correlate with gestational age, but if abnormal in size, it is found to be an early indication of fetal pathologic conditions. The cisterna magna should measure 1 cm or less in its AP dimension.[1,2] An abnormally thickened cisterna magna has been identified and associated with fetal abnormalities such as ventriculomegaly, cerebellar hypoplasia, and Dandy-Walker malformation. Absence or obliteration of the cisterna magna is a finding associated with fetal spinal dysraphism.[1,4,9]

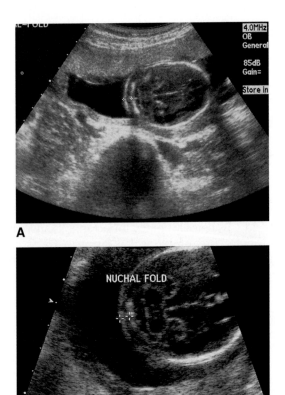

Fig. 18-16 **A** and **B,** Nuchal fold thickness measurement is shown at cerebellar view of posterior fossa and is performed from outer edge of cranium to outer edge of skin surface.

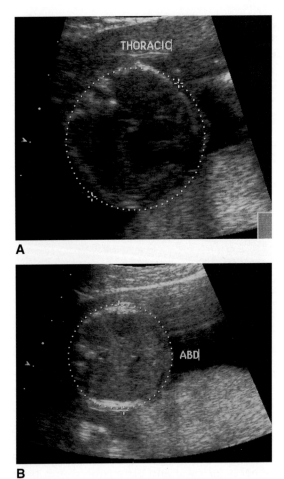

Fig. 18-17 **A,** Thoracic circumference is measured and compared with, **B,** abdominal circumference (AC). Thoracic/AC ratio for this fetus is 0.96 and considered within normal limits to rule out sonographic evidence of fetal pulmonary hypoplasia.

Nuchal Fold. The nuchal fold measurement is the second-trimester counterpart to the nuchal translucency in the first trimester. The nuchal fold is the skin at the posterior edge of the fetal cranium. A measurement of this skin thickness may be taken at the same image plane as the TCD. Calipers must be placed at the midline along the outer edge of the cranium and the outer edge of the fetal skin surface (Fig. 18-16).[4,8,9] Studies have indicated that a nuchal fold thickness of 5 to 6 mm or more between weeks 15 and 19 is associated with trisomy 21, or Down syndrome.[4] For the nuchal fold thickness to be used as a marker for Down syndrome, care must be taken by the sonographer to be certain that fetal head flexion or extension does not influence the measurement. The interpretation of this measurement should be used only in the early second trimester.[4]

Thoracic Circumference. The circumference of the fetal thorax is not used in the assessment of gestational age. The normal fetus has a thoracic circumference slightly smaller in size than the abdomen circumference. The comparison of these two circumferences may provide valuable information regarding possible pathology, especially skeletal dysplasias. An abnormally small thoracic to AC ratio ($<0.94 \pm 0.05$)[2] may assist the clinician in diagnosis of the possibility of pulmonary hypoplasia. The thoracic circumference should be performed in the transverse plane of the fetal chest at the level of the four-chamber fetal heart (Fig. 18-17). At this same image, the heart circumference may be compared with the thoracic circumference. The normal heart circumference is approximately one third of the thoracic circumference.[2] Clinicians place a higher value on chest measurements for diagnosis of potentially lethal fetal abnormalities rather than for gestational dating purposes.

Long Bones. In addition to the femur, all other long bones of the extremities may be measured to assist in management of the pregnancy. These measurements may include the humerus, radius, ulna, tibia, or fibula.

Charts for each bone measurement have been derived. Gestational age determination itself does not rely on the measurement of these other bones, but identification of pathologic conditions may be possible with comparison of all of these measurements.[8] Visualization of these bones to complete a survey of fetal anatomy may provide a challenge to the sonographer. The complexity of this challenge is increased if measurements are needed. Sonographer knowledge of the anatomy is important. In the lower extremities, the smaller fibula is found along the lateral aspect of the lower leg. In the upper extremities, the smaller radius is found along the lateral edge of the forearm and closest to the thumb side of the wrist. This knowledge is necessary to compare measurements with the appropriate chart for accurate diagnosis. A good technique must be used to identify the bones, given the wide range of motion associated with them. Box 18-3 has a review of miscellaneous measurements.

SUMMARY

Accurate sonographic measurements are essential to the clinician in management of pregnancies with a certain or uncertain LMP. Diagnostic ultrasound can be of significant value for assessment of gestational age because of the variability of the female reproductive cycle length. Sonographers must have a thorough knowledge of fetal anatomy and expertise in fetal ultrasonography to provide accurate biometric measurements.[6] Although limitations exist in the prediction of gestational age because of biologic variations or the presence of pathologic conditions, an accurate estimation can be made with strong certainty during the first half of the pregnancy with ultrasonography. Most manufacturers of diagnostic ultrasound equipment have incorporated computerized calculation packages that report a composite gestational age with the primary biometric parameters. Sonographers and sonologists should recognize the importance of evaluation of each biometric parameter individually for avoidance of misinterpretation of gestational age with asymmetric growth. The use of secondary biometric parameters and additional anatomic measurements may assist in determination of a more accurate estimation of gestational age.

The accurate interpretation of the sonographic findings can be of significant value to the clinician in management of a pregnancy with an uncertain LMP. Subsequent ultrasound examinations during the pregnancy may be performed to assess and chart fetal growth. The accuracy of fetal biometry is at its highest level earlier in the pregnancy, and the gestational age for all subsequent examinations performed in the pregnancy should be based on the earliest examination results.

CLINICAL SCENARIO—DIAGNOSIS

■ With consideration that the patient did indicate the reported LMP was lighter in flow than usual, the gestational age should be based on the ultrasound findings. With a closer look at the discrepancy in the estimation based on LMP and the ultrasound estimation for gestational age, a precise 21-day difference was found. This lighter than usual LMP quite possibly was in fact some bleeding associated with implantation. This bleeding is sometimes believed to be the LMP by the patient, although it may not be of the same intensity or duration as her normal menstrual period. In this case, gestational age was considered to be 10 weeks and 2 days, as reported with the ultrasound, and a due date was calculated from this estimation. A follow-up ultrasound was performed at 17 weeks and confirmed the estimated due date and normal fetal growth and anatomy.

CASE STUDIES FOR DISCUSSION ▬▬▬

1. A patient is seen in the ultrasound department for an initial obstetric sonogram for gestational dating without any history of prenatal care. The clinician has estimated that the patient is approximately 30 weeks pregnant based on the clinical examination and the questionable LMP history. The sonographer performs the routine biometric measurements for dating a pregnancy (BPD, HC, AC, FL) and reveals the isolated finding of moderate ventriculomegaly. The calculated gestational age based on all measurements corresponds to 32 weeks 3 days. On closer evaluation of the measurements, the BPD and HC have a 3-week discrepancy from the AC and FL. What additional imaging may be performed to more accurately assess fetal size and estimate gestational age?

2. A patient is referred for an ultrasound for evidence of suspected premature rupture of membranes (PROM) at a gestational age of 23 weeks 4 days. The patient had a prior ultrasound at 10 weeks 3 days. The current examination confirms the diagnosis of PROM with severe oligohydramnios and estimates a gestational age of 21 weeks and 1 day with routine biometric measurements including BPD, HC, AC, and FL. The cephalic index is abnormally low at 70. What other cranial measurements may be performed to assess fetal head size and estimate gestational age more accurately?

3. A patient had a first-trimester ultrasound examination that confirmed a suspected gestational age of 8 weeks and 3 days. Exactly 25 weeks later, the patient returns for an additional examination for a clinical symptom of decreased fetal movement. The second examination shows a gestational age of 29 weeks and 6 days. How should the gestational age be estimated for this pregnancy and its management?

4. A patient is seen in the ultrasound department for a first-trimester examination because of light vaginal spotting. The patient reports an LMP 5 weeks 6 days prior. The ultrasound examination reveals a smooth-walled gestational sac fundally in the uterine cavity measuring 6.5 mm without evidence of a yolk sac or embryo. What is the most likely cause for the sonographic appearance of this gestational sac?

5. A patient is seen during the second trimester of pregnancy for evaluation of an abnormally high alpha fetoprotein (AFP). She gives a strong history of an LMP that would date her pregnancy currently at 17 weeks and 2 days. Routine biometric measurements of the fetus reveal that the estimated gestational age is 21 weeks. Based on all clinical and sonographic findings, what is the estimated gestational age of this pregnancy?

STUDY QUESTIONS

1. The structure of pregnancy that may be used to locate the early embryonic disk is the:
   a. chorionic cavity
   b. amnion
   c. secondary yolk sac
   d. decidua capsularis
   e. chorion

2. The most accurate sonographic measurement for the prediction of gestational age is the:
   a. mean sac diameter
   b. yolk sac diameter
   c. embryonic heart rate
   d. crown-rump length
   e. abdomen circumference

3. In the technically difficult examination, this measurement may be substituted for the unobtainable biparietal diameter in estimation of gestational age:
   a. binocular distance
   b. cistern magna thickness
   c. nuchal fold thickness
   d. nuchal translucency measurement
   e. occipitofrontal diameter

4. The nuchal translucency measurement performed between weeks 10 and 14 should not exceed:
   a. 1 to 2 mm
   b. 3 mm
   c. 4 to 6 mm
   d. 1 to 2 cm
   e. 3 to 4 cm

5. A normal pregnancy has a duration of:
   a. 280 days
   b. 10 calendar months
   c. 9 lunar months
   d. 30 weeks
   e. all of the above

6. This term is used to describe an abnormally flattened fetal head shape:
   a. microcephaly
   b. brachycephaly
   c. dolichocephaly
   d. oligocephaly
   e. cebocephaly

7. The distal femoral epiphyses are normally visualized after what gestational age?
   a. 20 weeks
   b. 28 weeks
   c. 32 weeks
   d. 35 weeks
   e. 40 weeks

8. Which of the following biometric measurements is a better predictor for gestational size rather than gestational age?
   a. biparietal diameter
   b. head circumference
   c. abdominal circumference
   d. femur length
   e. long bone measurements

9. Biometric measurements performed during the third trimester are not as accurate for gestational dating because:
   a. biologic variations in fetal size occur
   b. fetal growth has reached a plateau
   c. fetal long axis can no longer be assessed
   d. sonographic landmarks are no longer visualized
   e. consistent measurement techniques cannot be easily reproduced

10. All of the following are recognized as part of the double decidual sac sign except:
    a. decidua parietalis
    b. amnion
    c. decidua capsularis
    d. chorion
    e. gestational sac

REFERENCES

1. DuBose TJ: *Fetal sonography,* Philadelphia, 1996, WB Saunders.
2. Hagen-Ansert SL: *Textbook of diagnostic ultrasonography,* vol 2, ed 5, St Louis, 2001, Mosby.
3. Taipale P, Hiilesmaa V: Predicting delivery date by ultrasound and last menstrual period in early gestation, *Obstet Gynecol* 97:189-194, 2001.
4. Callen P: *Ultrasonography in obstetrics and gynecology,* ed 4, Philadelphia, 2000, WB Saunders.
5. Roser J: Calculating the EDD, which is more accurate, scan or LMP? *Practising Midwife* 3:28-29, 2000.
6. Lowe SW, Pruitt RH, Smart PT et al: Routine use of ultrasound during pregnancy, *Nurse Pract* 23:60, 63-64, 66, 1998.
7. Sanders RC: *Clinical sonography: a practical guide,* ed 3, Philadelphia, 1998, Lippincott Williams & Wilkins.
8. Berman MC, Cohen HL: *Obstetrics and gynecology,* ed 2, Philadelphia, 1997, Lippincott.
9. Rumack CM, Wilson SR, Charboneau JW: *Diagnostic ultrasound,* vol 2, ed 2, St Louis, 1998, Mosby.
10. Anderhub B: *General sonography: a clinical guide,* St Louis, 1995, Mosby.
11. Lockwood CJ, Bahado-Singh R, D'Alton ME et al: Applying new advances in OB ultrasound, *Contemp OB/GYN* 46:51-52, 55, 59-60, 2001.
12. Curry RA, Tempkin BB: Ultrasonography: an introduction to normal structure and functional anatomy, Philadelphia, 1995, WB Saunders.

BIBLIOGRAPHY

DeLange M: First trimester pregnancy failure: review of sonographic findings and interaction with the patient, *Society of Diagnostic Medical Sonographers, 18th Annual Conference Proceedings,* 2001.

DuBose TJ: Embryonic heart rate and age, *Society of Diagnostic Medical Sonographers, 17th Annual Conference Proceedings,* 2000.

Guariglia L, Rosati P: Transvaginal sonographic detection of embryonic-fetal abnormalities in early pregnancy, *Obstet Gynecol* 96:328-332, 2000.

Pinnette MG: The fetus as a patient, *Society of Diagnostic Medical Sonographers, 17th Annual Conference Proceedings,* 2000.

Thomas CL: *Taber's cyclopedic medical dictionary,* ed 18, Philadelphia, 1997, FA Davis Company.

19

Size Greater than Dates

MICHAEL HARTMAN

CLINICAL SCENARIO

■ A 31-year-old woman is seen in the ultrasound department for a follow-up obstetric sonogram. The patient is of average size and in good health with no history of smoking or alcohol or drug abuse. This is her first pregnancy, and she has had a previous sonographic examination at 12 weeks' gestational age. The current ultrasound measurements and subsequent estimated fetal weight are recorded during this examination. The results are determined to be within normal limits based on the patient's last menstrual period and previous sonogram, which place her at approximately 32 weeks' gestational age. Testing for gestational diabetes at this time falls within the upper limits of normal. The patient goes into labor at the end of her term and has a lengthy and most difficult labor but eventually delivers vaginally an 11-lb, 1-oz baby girl (Fig. 19-1). In addition to the size of the fetus, the placenta was approximately twice the size of normal. What possible explanation could be identified for such an unexpected outcome?

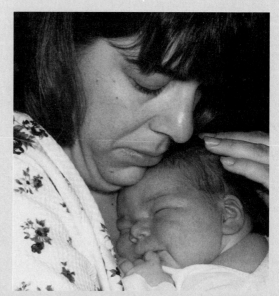

Fig. 19-1 Mother and newborn 3 days after delivery.

OBJECTIVES

■ Define the terms associated with excessive fetal growth.

■ Differentiate between large for gestational age and macrosomia.

■ Identify the common causes of large for gestational age pregnancies.

■ Describe the sonographic appearance of macrosomia.

■ List the risk factors associated with macrosomia.

■ Describe the management of and interventions for suspected macrosomia.

GLOSSARY OF TERMS

Beckwith-Wiedemann syndrome: disorder characterized by macrosomia, omphalocele, and macroglossia associated with normal karyotype

Brachial plexus injury: damage to the nerves that control arm and hand muscles

Cystadenoma: a benign ovarian tumor that often becomes extremely large

Facial palsies: complete or partial loss of voluntary movement of the facial muscles

Gestational diabetes: a temporary type of diabetes that develops in some pregnant women because of an inability to produce enough insulin to keep blood sugar within a safe range

Hydatidiform mole: a benign form of gestational trophoblastic disease involving the conversion of the chorionic villi

Hydrops fetalis: abnormal accumulation of fluid in fetal tissue and organs, leading to anemia and a decreased ability of the blood to carry oxygen

Marshall-Smith syndrome: a disorder characterized by unusually quick physical growth and bone development before birth associated with respiratory difficulties, mental retardation, and certain physical characteristics

Morbidity: a diseased state or frequency of disease

Mortality: a fatal outcome or death rate

Regression models: tables used to determine gestational age and weight on the basis of measurements

Ruvalcaba-Myhre syndrome: a rare inherited disorder characterized by excessive growth before and after birth, an abnormally large and narrow head, and benign subcutaneous growths (hamartomas)

Shoulder dystocia: condition in which the fetal shoulders become impacted behind the symphysis pubis

Sotos' syndrome: also known as *cerebral gigantism*. A syndrome that is characterized by an enlarged head circumference accompanied by increased birth weight; mental retardation may also be present

Trophoblastic disease: tumors that arise from an abnormal proliferation of the chorionic villi

Weaver syndrome: a disorder of large birth size, accelerated growth and skeletal maturation, associated with limb, craniofacial, neurologic, and other abnormalities

Obstetric ultrasound examinations are frequently requested because the patient's size is greater than the size expected for gestational age (size greater than dates). This is based on the patient's last menstrual period (LMP) and the physical examination that may include a fundal height measurement. The fundal height measurement is performed with external palpation of the uterus and measurement of the distance from the symphysis pubis to the uterine fundus. The fundal height roughly correlates in centimeters with the gestational age in weeks. This measurement is not highly accurate and may not always be a reflection of excessive fetal growth and can also be affected by multiple factors, including the technique of the clinician, maternal weight, fetal position, an increase in amniotic fluid, and the size of the placenta. In addition, size greater than dates may be suspected when the patient has had a significant weight gain. The uterus may also present large for dates when leiomyomas are present or when ovarian masses mimic an enlarged uterus or hamper the ability to accurately measure the uterus. This chapter explores the possible results and outcomes when a patient is seen for an obstetric sonogram for size greater than dates.

EXCESSIVE FETAL GROWTH

Excessive fetal growth is typically divided into two categories with fetal weight in the determination. *Large for gestational age* (LGA) is a term suggested when the estimated fetal weight is greater than the 90th percentile for gestational age.[1] In contrast, the subsequent chapter discusses the term small for gestational age (SGA), which is suggested when the estimated fetal weight is less than the 10th percentile for gestational age.[2] Macrosomia is determined when the estimated fetal weight is greater than or equal to 4500 g.[2] Appropriate fetal growth is clinically significant and a direct indicator of fetal well being. Identification of fetuses that are not growing appropriately is important because as fetal growth discrepancy becomes greater, whether from macrosomia or growth restriction, the risk of perinatal **morbidity** and **mortality** is significantly elevated.

Estimation of Fetal Weight

The estimation of fetal weight is simply that—an estimation. A multitude of variables contributes to fetal weight discrepancies. The very nature of the process for determination of fetal weight involves much variability in that sonographic measurements of the fetal head, abdomen, and femur bones, regardless of the degree of care and accuracy by the sonographer, are assigned a weight approximation on the basis of previous research data. Even the best sonographic determination of fetal weight has been estimated to be as much as 10% discrepant of the actual weight.[3] This potential discrepancy percentage will not appreciably affect a fetus of average size with regard to the determination of fetal weight. However, in cases of LGA, it can result in a significant discrepancy of several hundred grams.[3] One study showed that for a confidence level of 90% that a newborn would actually weigh more than 4000 g, one must estimate the sonographic fetal weight at 4750 g.[4]

The most reliable formula used to determine the estimated fetal weight incorporates all fetal parameters, such as biparietal diameter, head circumference, abdominal circumference (AC), and femur length.[5] It should be understood by all concerned that the accuracy of this determination is not without limitation and ranges of discrepancy.[3] Patients and their families need to be properly educated with regard to the degree of accuracy in the estimation of fetal weight with sonographic examination.

Calculation Software. Most current ultrasound equipment provides the sonographer with the ability to record a multitude of obstetric measurements and perform calculations during the examination. Because of the variety of **regression models** available, it is important to know which is being used to obtain consistency within the laboratory.[2] With regard to diversity, it is also important to understand the obstetric population with which one is working and to make appropriate adjustments to the regression models when necessary.[2]

Pregnancy Dating. Critical information used in the proper dating of a pregnancy includes an accurate LMP date and the performance of an early baseline sonogram for later comparison. However, in about 20% to 40% of all pregnancies, the correct menstrual age is uncertain because of unknown or unclear LMP dates.[6] Accurate assessment of the fundal height of the uterus during physical examination in cases of maternal obesity may also be extremely difficult. In addition, pregnancy dating and the determination of estimated fetal weight involve the following basic assumptions:

Menstrual cycles last 28 days
Women ovulate 14 days into their menstrual cycles
Fertilization occurs within 24 hours of ovulation
Implantation occurs within 2 days of fertilization
Pregnancies last 280 days (menstrual dating)
Babies weigh 7.5 lbs at delivery
Fetal growth is constant

These assumptions are simply averages calculated over time and across multiple populations. Just one of these assumptions may significantly impact the calculation of pregnancy dating. Taken together, a much wider potential range of error exists. For these reasons, an early baseline sonographic examination is a most reliable indicator of fetal age that may be referenced throughout the duration of the pregnancy.

Macrosomia

The term *macrosomia* is defined simply as an abnormally large size of the body. In this case, the term refers to the entire fetus, neonate, or newborn as body size infers the inclusion of the whole being. Fetal macrosomia complicates more than 10% of all pregnancies in the United States.[7] With respect to delivery, any fetus that is too large for the maternal pelvis through which it must pass is macrosomic.[8] The most straightforward approach to the sonographic determination of macrosomia is to use the estimated fetal weight.[1]

Risk Factors. The major risk factor for macrosomia is **gestational diabetes,** which accounts for up to 40% of all cases.[2] Among diabetic mothers, the prevalence rate of macrosomia is 25% to 42% versus 8% to 10% among nondiabetic mothers.[9] Despite the higher frequency in diabetic mothers, nondiabetic mothers account for up to 60% of macrosomic cases due to their majority versus the smaller diabetic mother population.[10] Macrosomia is associated with enlargement of the placenta (Fig. 19-2; see Color Plate 11).[11] A placental thickness obtained at a right angle to its long axis measuring greater than 3 cm before 20 weeks gestation or greater than 5 cm before 40 weeks is considered abnormal.[12]

Time of delivery is an important factor to consider. One study showed an increased incidence of macrosomia from 1.7% at 36 weeks' gestation to 21% at 42 weeks' gestation.[13] Chronic and progressing macrosomia is in direct proportion to an elevated risk of associated conditions, and women who have previously delivered a macrosomic infant are at an increased risk in future pregnancies.[2] Primary perinatal complications include **shoulder dystocia,** soft tissue trauma, humeral and clavicular fractures, **brachial plexus injury** and **facial**

palsies, meconium aspiration, prolonged labor, and asphyxial injuries.[1] Shoulder dystocia (Fig. 19-3) occurs when the arm of the fetus prevents or complicates delivery and may result in serious traumatic injury. Because many of these injuries are unpredictable events, available evidence suggests that planned interventions on the basis of estimates of fetal weight may not significantly reduce the incidence of shoulder dystocia and the adverse outcomes attributable to fetal macrosomia.[14] However, because evidence strongly suggests an increased risk of prenatal complication for pregnancies in excess of 4500 g, the option for cesarean delivery should be considered with fetal macrosomia in diabetic patients with small pelvic structures and in any pregnancy where macrosomia is a concern.

The sonographic fetal AC measurement has been determined to be helpful in identification of potential macrosomic infants. One study reports a less than 1% incidence rate of infant birth weights greater than 4500 g with AC measured less than 35 cm. The incidence rate significantly increased to 37% in cases where the AC was greater or equal to 38 cm.[15] Macrosomic infants of diabetic mothers usually have organomegaly, especially a disproportional enlargement of the heart, liver, adrenals, and adipose tissue.[16]

Hydrops fetalis is also associated with macrosomia and may present sonographically with one or more of the following[1]: increased placental thickness, increased thickness of scalp or body wall greater than 5 mm (Figs. 19-4 and 19-5), hepatosplenomegaly, pleural and pericardial effusions, ascites, and structural fetal anomalies.

Prenatally diagnosed syndromes associated with macrosomia include **Beckwith-Wiedemann, Marshall-Smith, Ruvalcaba-Myhre, Sotos',** and **Weaver syndromes.**[3] Other risk factors for macrosomia include prolonged gestation and maternal obesity.[2] Pregnancies that extend beyond the normal term length tend to eventually fall under the macrosomic category simply because of continued growth before delivery.

INCREASED FUNDAL HEIGHT

Other factors contribute to a patient with size greater than dates. Multiple gestation (Fig. 19-6) may present with an increased fundal height on clinical examination, and the cause for the increased size is easily clarified

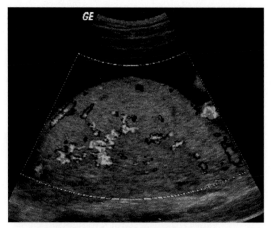

Fig. 19-2 Enlarged placenta.

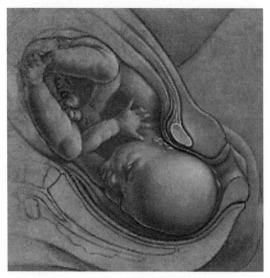

Fig. 19-3 Fetal position leads to potential shoulder dystocia at delivery.

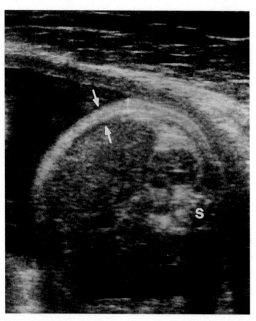

Fig. 19-4 Increased subcutaneous fat (*arrows*) of body wall thickness. *S,* Spine.

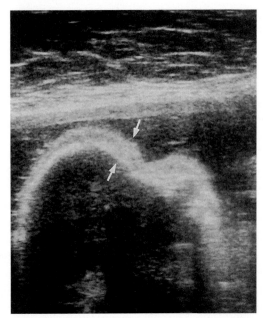

Fig. 19-5 Increased subcutaneous fat (*arrows*) on scalp.

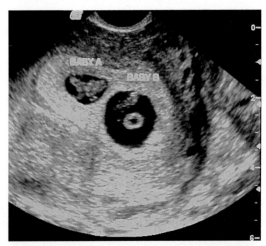

Fig. 19-6 Increased uterine size was noted clinically in 7-week, 1-day twin gestation.

with sonographic examination. Complications of multiple gestations may contribute significantly to a discrepancy. Conjoined twins (Fig. 19-7, *A* and *B*) are a potentially lethal complication that may be identified when a sonographic evaluation is performed because of an increased fundal height. Twin-to-twin transfusion syndrome is a serious condition in monozygotic twins where fetal size discrepancy is shown. Because of arteriovenous shunting of blood within a shared placenta, the recipient twin sonographically displays an increase (while the donor twin shows a decrease) in size and amniotic fluid.

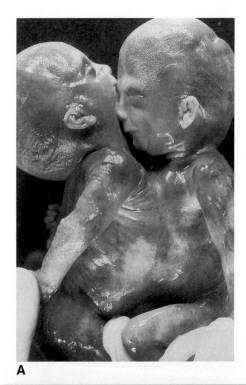

A

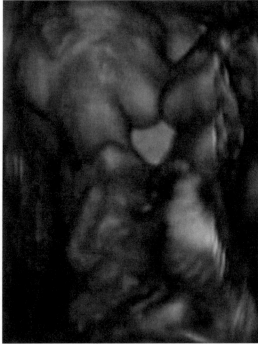

B

Fig. 19-7 **A,** Thoracoomphalopagus conjoined twins, gross specimen. **B,** Thoracoomphalopagus conjoined twins, three-dimensional ultrasound images.

Another complication of pregnancy that may present with a size-date discrepancy is gestational **trophoblastic disease,** also known as *molar pregnancy.* Patients also frequently have hyperemesis. The most common form, the benign **hydatidiform mole** (Fig. 19-8), appears sonographically as an inhomogeneous or complex mass within the uterus without the presence of a fetus. Gestational trophoblastic disease is discussed in detail in Chapter 21.

Polyhydramnios may contribute to an increased fundal height with singleton pregnancies as well. Frequently, a subjective assessment will raise suspicion of polyhydramnios when noting that the fetus looks like a "small fish in a big fishbowl." Two methods used to quantify the amount of amniotic fluid have been defined and are useful for the less experienced sonographer and for following patients over time. The single-pocket assessment can be performed with identification of the largest vertical pocket of amniotic fluid and measurement of the anterioposterior depth. Polyhydramnios would be indicated when the pocket exceeds 8 cm (Fig. 19-9), and oligohydramnios would be indicated when the pocket is less than 2 cm.[5] The

amniotic fluid index (AFI) may also be used to assess amniotic fluid. The method involves dividing the maternal uterus into four quadrants and adding the anterior to posterior measurements of the amniotic fluid in each of the quadrants. The total is normally equal to 13 cm, plus or minus 5 cm.[17] Increasing AFI correlates linearly with increasing birth weight. One study reports more than double the risk of a macrosomic infant birth with an AFI greater than 15 and a risk of more than six times with an AFI greater than 18.[18] Although several studies have been conducted in recent years to identify a more accurate assessment of the upper and lower limits of normal amniotic fluid levels to define clinically significant polyhydramnios, less than exact correlations have been the result. It continues to be a nonspecific finding but one that warrants further investigation as more than 100 fetal anomalies are associated with this condition, including diabetes (Fig. 19-10).[3]

Genetic constitution, such as familial physical traits like parental stature, need to be considered in cases of suggested macrosomia.[8] Larger parents are more likely to produce larger than average-sized babies, whereas smaller parents tend to have a propensity toward smaller than average-sized babies.

In addition, a history of size greater than dates may not actually relate to the pregnancy. Leiomyomas (fibroids) are benign uterine tumors that can be significant in size, contributing to an increased fundal height (Fig. 19-11). They can also increase in size during pregnancy. Leiomyomas (see Chapter 13) typically appear as well-defined masses of variable echogenicity within the myometrium. Sonographic evaluation of a patient with an increased fundal height may also reveal ovarian enlargement, which may be from an ovarian

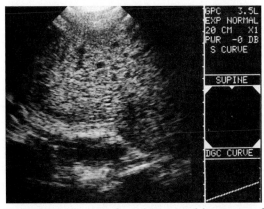

Fig. 19-8 Patient seen for ultrasound because of size greater than dates. Sonogram reveals molar pregnancy.

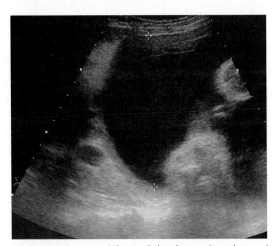

Fig. 19-9 Patient with polyhydramnios has single pocket measurement of more than 10 cm.

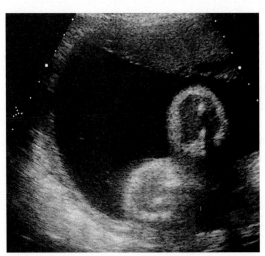

Fig. 19-10 Polyhydramnios noted in patient was result of diabetes.

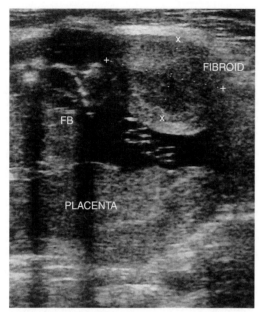

Fig. 19-11 Fibroid identified in image was contributing factor in patient having increased fundal height.

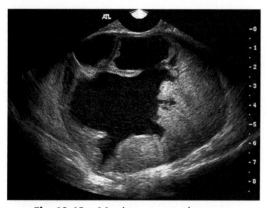

Fig. 19-12 Mucinous cystadenoma.

cyst or neoplasm (see Chapter 17) such as a benign cystic teratoma or **cystadenoma**. The sonographic appearance of a cyst should be anechoic and thin-walled and exhibit enhancement. Teratomas and cystadenomas (Fig. 19-12) often have a complex appearance, although a teratoma often has a characteristic shadowing from the presence of calcifications.

SUMMARY

Determination of the cause (Table 19-1) for size greater than dates can be evaluated with diagnostic medical sonography. However, this imaging method continues to have limitations based on the myriad of variables

relative to the complexity of pregnancy and fetal development. Although sonographic estimations of fetal weight have shown poor accuracy in the prediction of macrosomia,[19,20] use of a combination of specific maternal and fetal characteristics has shown the ability to more accurately estimate birth weight. Some of the significant predictors of term birth weight are gestational age, parity, fetal gender, maternal height, maternal weight, and third-trimester maternal weight gain rate.[21] In addition, three-dimensional ultrasound and magnetic resonance imaging are expected to generate estimates of fetal weight that are more accurate than those for two-dimensional ultrasound or clinical estimates.[22] Ultrasound continues to be used in the determination of fetal weight and can also be useful in evaluation of the anatomic structures of the fetus and mother to identify other possible causes for a size greater than dates presentation.

Table 19-1	Causes for Size Greater than Dates
Diagnosis	**Sonographic Findings**
LGA	Fetal weight >90th percentile
Macrosomia	Fetal weight 4500 g
Hydrops fetalis	Fluid in two body cavities (ascites, pericardial effusion, pleural effusion) or skin edema plus fluid in one body cavity; also associated placentomegaly, hepatosplenomegaly, structural anomalies
Multiple gestation	More than one fetus, one or more placentas
Molar pregnancy	Heterogeneous mass within uterine cavity, no fetus; associated with large, bilateral, multilocular ovarian cysts
Polyhydramnios	Single pocket, >8 cm; AFI, >18 cm
Leiomyomas	Well-defined lesions of variable echogenicity

AFI, Amniotic fluid index; *LGA*, large for gestational age.

CLINICAL SCENARIO—DIAGNOSIS

◼ Sonographic examinations with normal results were performed at 12 and 32 weeks' gestation. Although the patient underwent evaluation for glucose levels during these examinations, she was not monitored for gestational diabetes throughout the final 2 months of pregnancy. Labor was difficult and lengthy because of the large size of the baby. The newborn was evaluated and found to have a significantly enlarged liver and spleen, tissue swelling, jaundice, and a mild heart murmur. No indication of fetal tissue swelling or organomegaly was seen during the second ultrasound examination most likely because these conditions had not manifested to a noticeable degree. These findings, along with the massive size of the placenta at delivery, lead to a diagnosis of macrosomia resulting from gestational diabetes. The associated conditions completely resolved during the first few weeks of the newborn's life (Fig 19-13).

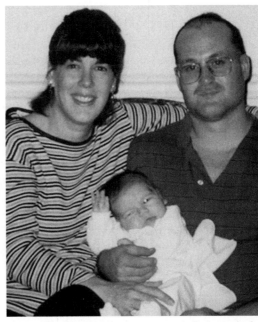

Fig. 19-13 Mother (with gestational diabetes), father, and newborn (with macrosomia) 1 month after delivery.

CASE STUDIES FOR DISCUSSION

1. A patient is seen for an ultrasound examination at 33 weeks, 2 days' gestational age, with second-trimester ultrasound, with a fundal height measurement of 40 weeks' gestation. Sonographic examination reveals a single fetus measuring 34 weeks' gestational age. Scalp edema, increased subcutaneous fat, ascites (Fig. 19-14, *A* and *B*), and pleural effusions are noted. An enlarged placenta measuring 5.3 cm and a diaphragmatic hernia are also identified. What is the most likely diagnosis?

2. A 41-year-old woman is seen for an obstetric ultrasound for increased fundal height at 28 weeks' gestation with first trimester ultrasound. Sonographic examination reveals an omphalocele (Fig. 19-15) and macroglossia. The estimated fetal weight is difficult to ascertain because of the distortion of the abdomen, although the measurements do reveal that the fetus is LGA. Chromosomal analysis excludes the possibility of aneuploidy, and maternal levels of glucose are tested excluding gestational

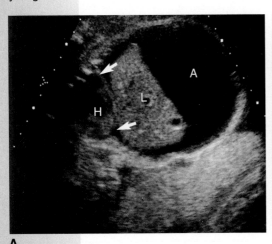

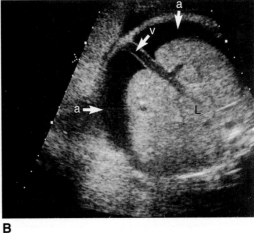

A **B**

Fig. 19-14 **A,** Sagittal abdomen. *A,* Ascites; *H,* heart; *L,* liver. **B,** Transverse abdomen. *a,* Ascites; *v,* ductus venosus.

CASE STUDIES FOR DISCUSSION—cont'd

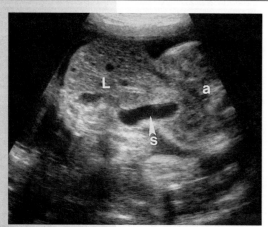

Fig. 19-15 Omphalocele. *a,* Abdomen; *S,* stomach; *L,* liver.

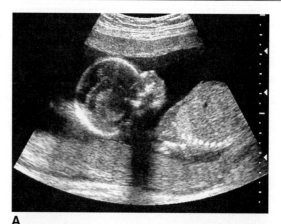

A

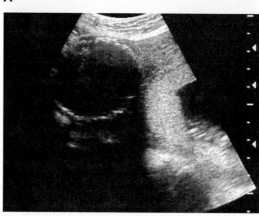

B

Fig. 19-16 A, Sagittal view of uterus shows single fetus measuring 16 weeks, 1 day gestational age. **B,** Well-defined, calcified lesion is noted at uterine fundus.

diabetes. What is the most likely cause of the increased fundal height?

3. A patient is seen for ultrasound at 16 weeks' gestation with LMP. The patient explains that her physician thought her uterus was consistent with a 22-week gestation and thought he might be palpating the fetal head at the top of the uterus. Sonographic evaluation of the pregnancy shows a single fetus in the breech position (Fig. 19-16, *A*) measuring 16 weeks, 1 day. A calcified lesion (Fig. 19-16, *B*) at the fundal region of the uterus is also identified and appears to be contiguous with the myometrium. What is the most likely cause of the size-date discrepancy?

4. A patient is seen for obstetric ultrasound at 15 weeks, 2 days with LMP and 21 weeks with fundal height measurement. The ultrasound reveals the finding in Fig. 19-17. What is the most likely cause of the size-date discrepancy?

5. A 25-year-old woman is seen for an obstetric ultrasound at 24 weeks' gestation with LMP for increased fundal height.

The ultrasound reveals the finding in Fig. 19-18 in addition to absence of the fetal calvarium and brain. What is the cause of the size-date discrepancy?

CASE STUDIES FOR DISCUSSION—cont'd

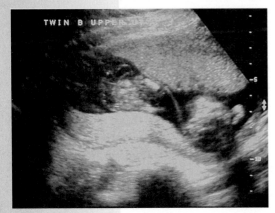

Fig. 19-17 Transverse view of pregnancy consistent with 15-week, 2-day gestation.

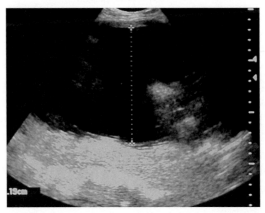

Fig. 19-18 An 11.2-cm, single pocket measurement of amniotic fluid is identified in 24-week gestation.

STUDY QUESTIONS

1. A 24-year-old woman with a history of reduced fetal movement is seen for an obstetric sonogram. There is no indication of bleeding, pain, or other complications. Based on a previous, unremarkable sonogram in the first trimester, the pregnancy should currently measure 37 weeks' gestation. The patient is 5 feet, 11 inches in height, and the father is 6 feet, 7 inches in height. The average age by ultrasound is 40 weeks' gestational age. The remainder of the examination is unremarkable. What is the most likely diagnosis?
   a. abnormally increased growth
   b. hydrops fetalis
   c. normal growth from tall parents
   d. high suspicion for anomaly

2. A 29-year-old woman is seen for an obstetric sonogram for an increased fundal height at 27 weeks' gestation with last menstrual period. The ultrasound examination reveals two fetuses sharing a single placenta. Baby A measures 28 weeks and shows mild polyhydramnios. Baby B measures 25 weeks and shows moderate oligohydramnios. What is the most likely diagnosis?
   a. normal twin pregnancy
   b. Marshall-Smith syndrome
   c. trophoblastic disease
   d. twin-to-twin transfusion syndrome

3. A patient is seen for obstetric ultrasound at 24 weeks' gestation with last menstrual period and a reported fundal height measurement of 28 weeks. The ultrasound reveals a single fetus measuring 24 weeks, 1 day. The remainder of the examination is unremarkable. What is the most likely cause of the size-date discrepancy?
   a. low accuracy of fundal height measurement
   b. incorrect fetal ultrasound measurements
   c. polyhydramnios
   d. an undiagnosed anomaly

4. A 21-year-old woman is seen in the ultrasound department for an obstetric examination with an indication of large for gestational age at 28 weeks by first-trimester ultrasound. The ultrasound shows a fetus measuring 28 weeks. The amniotic fluid index is 25 cm. What is the most likely diagnosis?
   a. oligohydramnios
   b. polyhydramnios
   c. macrosomia
   d. hydrops fetalis

5. A 24-year-old woman is seen for an obstetric sonogram with a history of irregular periods. Based on the date of her last menstrual period, the pregnancy should measure 14 weeks. The sonogram shows a single fetus at 18 weeks' gestational age with no

other remarkable findings. What is the most likely diagnosis?

a. inaccurate last menstrual period date
b. macrosomia
c. gestational diabetes
d. hydatidiform mole

6. A 29-year-old woman is seen for an obstetric ultrasound at 35 weeks' gestation. She has a history of gestational diabetes in two prior pregnancies. Sonograms at 11 weeks and 23 weeks have confirmed gestational age and have been otherwise unremarkable. The current examination reveals an average age with ultrasound of 38 weeks, 4 days. The placenta appears generous in size, measuring 6.2 cm. What is the most likely diagnosis?

a. inaccurate last menstrual period date
b. hydrops
c. microsomia
d. poor nutrition
e. macrosomia

7. A 27-year-old woman is seen for an obstetric ultrasound for increased fundal height at 32 weeks' gestation. She has had a previous, unremarkable sonogram at 10 weeks' gestation. The current examination reveals a gestational age measurement of 34 weeks. Enlargement of the liver, spleen, and placenta is identified in addition to ascites and bilateral pleural effusions. What is the most likely diagnosis?

a. Beckwith-Wiedemann syndrome
b. Ruvalcaba-Myhre syndrome
c. hydrops fetalis
d. Weaver syndrome

8. A 31-year-old woman is seen for an obstetric sonogram with a history of a prolonged gestation. There is no indication of complications. Based on a previous, unremarkable first-trimester sonogram, the pregnancy should measure 43 weeks at this examination, which is confirmed. The remainder of the examination is unremarkable. What is the most likely diagnosis?

a. abnormal growth
b. hydrops fetalis
c. large for gestational growth
d. normal growth for length of pregnancy
e. gestational diabetes

9. An 18-year-old woman is seen by her family practitioner with a history of a positive home pregnancy

test and an unknown last menstrual period date. The physician measures a fundal height of 25 cm. This would correlate with a gestational age of:

a. 20 weeks
b. 22 weeks
c. 25 weeks
d. 28 weeks
e. 30 weeks

10. A 22-year-old woman is seen for an obstetric ultrasound at 16 weeks' gestation (with last menstrual period) for increased uterine size and absent heart tones. The sonogram shows a large heterogeneous mass within the uterus. No identifiable fetus or amniotic fluid can be detected. What is the most likely diagnosis?

a. fetal demise
b. hydatidiform mole
c. hydropic placenta
d. Ruvalcaba-Myhre syndrome

REFERENCES

1. Callen PW: *Ultrasonography in obstetrics and gynecology,* Philadelphia, 2000, WB Saunders.
2. Sauerbrei EE, Nguyen KT, Nolan RL: *A practical guide to ultrasound in obstetrics and gynecology,* Philadelphia, 1998, Lippincott-Raven.
3. McGahan JP, Goldberg BB: *Diagnostic ultrasound: a logical approach,* Philadelphia, 1998, Lippincott-Raven.
4. Watson WJ, Seed JW: Sonographic diagnosis of macrosomia. In Divon MY, editor: *Abnormal fetal growth,* New York, 1991, Elsevier.
5. Hagen-Ansert SL: *Textbook of diagnostic ultrasonography,* St Louis, 2001, Mosby.
6. Bowie JD, Andreotti RF: Estimating gestational age in utero, *Radiol Clin North Am* 20:325, 1980.
7. Zamorski MA, Biggs WS: Management of suspected fetal macrosomia, *Am Fam Physician* 63:302-306, 2001.
8. Deter RL, Hadlock FP: Use of ultrasound in the detection of macrosomia: a review, *J Clin Ultrasound* 13:519, 1985.
9. Mintz MC, Landon MB: Sonographic diagnosis of fetal growth disorders, *Clin Obstet Gynecol* 31:44, 1988.
10. Manning FA: General principles and applications of ultrasonography. In *Maternal-fetal medicine,* ed 4, Philadelphia, 1999, WB Saunders.
11. Elchalal U, Ezra Y, Levi Y et al: Sonographically thick placenta: a marker for increased perinatal risk: a prospective cross-sectional study, *Placenta* 21:268-272, 2000.
12. Dudley NJ, Fagan DG, Lamb MP: Short communication: ultrasonographic placental grade and thickness: associations with early delivery and low birthweight, *Br J Radiol* 66:175-177, 1993.

13. Boyd ME, Usher RH, Mclean FH: Fetal macrosomia: prediction, risks, proposed management, *Obstet Gynecol* 61:715, 1983.

14. Sacks DA, Chen W: Estimating fetal weight in the management of macrosomia, *Obstet Gynecol Surv* 55:229-239, 2000.

15. Gilby JR, Williams MC, Spellacy WN: Fetal abdominal circumference measurements of 35 and 38 cm as predictors of macrosomia: a risk factor for shoulder dystocia, *J Reprod Med* 45:936-938, 2000.

16. Morris FH: Infants of diabetic mothers: fetal and neonatal pathophysiology, *Perspect Pediatr Pathophysiol* 8:223, 1984.

17. Phelan JP, Smith CV, Broussard P et al: Amniotic fluid volume assessment with the four quadrant technique at 36-42 weeks gestation, *J Reprod Med* 32:540, 1987.

18. Myles TD, Nguyen TM: Relationship between normal amniotic fluid index and birth weight in term patients presenting for labor, *J Reprod Med* 46:685-690, 2001.

19. Combs CA, Rosenn B, Miodovnik M et al: Sonographic EFW and macrosomia: is there an optimum formula to predict diabetic fetal macrosomia? *J Matern Fetal Med* 9:55-61, 2000.

20. Landon MB: Prenatal diagnosis of macrosomia in pregnancy complicated by diabetes mellitus, *J Matern Fetal Med* 9:52-54, 2000.

21. Nahum GG, Stanislaw H, Huffaker BJ: Accurate prediction of term birth weight from prospectively measurable maternal characteristics, *J Reprod Med* 44:705-712, 1999.

22. O'Reilly-Green C, Divon M: Sonographic and clinical methods in the diagnosis of macrosomia, *Clin Obstet Gynecol* 43:309-320, 2000.

BIBLIOGRAPHY

Dirckx JH: *Stedman's concise medical dictionary for the health professions*, ed 4, Philadelphia, 2001, Williams and Wilkins.

20

Size Less than Dates

FRANKLYN C. CHRISTENSEN and CHARLOTTE HENNINGSEN

CLINICAL SCENARIO

■ A 39-year-old woman, G1 P0, is seen at the high-risk obstetric clinic for an ultrasound evaluation of the fetus. She is a professional in a high-stress career who works 70 to 80 hours a week. On her last prenatal visit, the uterine fundal height measured 30 cm and lagged behind the gestational age of 33 weeks, 4 days. She had a prior ultrasound at 16 weeks that confirmed the gestational age was consistent with her last menstrual period. The prior ultrasound also failed to reveal any obvious fetal congenital anomalies, and a genetic amniocentesis showed normal fetal chromosomes. Her medical history is significant for type I diabetes mellitus since the age of 12 years, and her condition is well controlled

with an insulin pump. During her pregnancy, blood pressures have been normal and she has always had a trace of proteinuria.

The current ultrasound examination reveals a single viable fetus in the vertex presentation. Fetal biometry shows an average ultrasound age of 31 weeks, 5 days, and the amniotic fluid index is 6.7 cm. The estimated fetal weight is at the 8th percentile for gestational age. The placenta is posterior-fundal and unremarkable. Her blood pressure is 149/100 mm Hg, and her urine dipstick test reveals significant protein. She also has a severe headache. What are the possible explanations for these findings?

OBJECTIVES

■ Describe the clinical scenarios for an explanation of a finding of size less than dates.

■ Describe the sonographic appearance and technique for a diagnosis of oligohydramnios.

■ Describe the sonographic appearance of the more common renal diseases associated with size less than dates.

■ Describe clinical conditions, the basic physiology, and sonographic findings to understand and make a diagnosis of intrauterine growth restriction.

■ Describe the role of ultrasound in the diagnosis of premature rupture of membrane.

GLOSSARY OF TERMS ▬

Beat-to-beat variability: the normal variation of the fetal heart rate seen from the autonomic nervous system control of the fetal heart

Chorioamnionitis: infection that involves the chorion, amnion, and amniotic fluid

Chronic hypertension: in pregnancy, represents persistent elevated blood pressures identified before pregnancy or before 20 weeks' gestation

Cyanotic heart disease: any heart abnormality or disease that results in cyanosis

Cytomegalovirus: a group of herpes viruses that infects humans and other animals causing development of characteristic inclusions in the cytoplasm or nucleus; may cause flulike symptoms; congenital infection may cause malformation, fetal growth deficiencies, and death

Diabetes mellitus type 1: a medical disease marked by the immune destruction of pancreatic cells that produce insulin, resulting in a decrease or lack of secretion of insulin by the pancreas

Karyotype: the chromosome characteristics of an individual cell or of a cell line presented as a systematized array of chromosomes from a photomicrograph of a single cell nucleus arranged in pairs in descending order of size

Nonsteroidal antiinflammatory drugs: drugs used for pain, such as ibuprofen and indomethacin

Preeclampsia: development of hypertension with proteinuria or edema or both as the result of pregnancy or the influence of a recent pregnancy; usually occurs after 20 weeks' gestation

Premature rupture of membranes: rupture of the amniotic membranes before the onset of labor

Prune-belly syndrome: a condition associated with bladder outlet obstruction consisting of laxity of the abdominal wall, cryptorchidism, and a urethral obstruction, such as posterior urethral valves

Pyelectasis: dilation of the renal pelvis

Sickle cell anemia: a decrease of oxygen material, such as hemoglobin, from an autosomal dominant disease characterized by crescent-shaped or sickle-shaped erythrocytes and accelerated breaking of erythrocytes

Systemic lupus erythematosus: a connective tissue autoimmune disorder characterized by skin lesions and disseminated vital organ involvement with antinuclear antibodies present

---

Measurement of the uterine fundal height during every prenatal visit after 20 weeks' gestation is an integral part of obstetric care. It is a simple, safe, inexpensive, and reasonably accurate method to screen for fetal growth and amniotic fluid volume abnormalities. Longitudinal studies have shown that symphysis to fundus measurements correctly identify only 40% of small for gestational age (SGA) fetuses.[1] Therefore, standard of care is to order or perform an obstetric ultrasound when the uterine fundal height is in discordance with the estimated gestational age.

When evaluating a pregnant woman considered to have size less than dates, a medical history, vital signs, social and family history, and recent symptomatology are warranted. Some patients may have decreased fetal movement that would suggest the finding of oligohydramnios. Others may be found to have recently elevated blood pressure or a history of vascular disease, such as pregestational **diabetes mellitus** or **systemic lupus erythematosus** (SLE). Family history may reveal prior cases of neonates with renal abnormalities or a tendency for small babies. Evaluation of social habits, such as work, nutrition, and the use of alcohol or recreational drugs, can be extremely useful. In general, a carefully performed obstetric ultrasound together with pertinent clinical data will yield an accurate diagnosis.

OLIGOHYDRAMNIOS

Oligohydramnios is a decrease in the volume of amniotic fluid, and its diagnosis is most frequently made with ultrasound. Amniotic fluid volume results from a balance between what enters and exits from the amniotic cavity. From 20 weeks' gestation to term, most of the amniotic fluid is a result of fetal urination and respiratory secretions. The incidence of oligohydramnios varies according to the criteria used for diagnosis. When a maximal vertical pocket (MVP) of less than 2 cm is used, the incidence rate is 3%[2]; but when an amniotic fluid index (AFI) of less than 5 cm is used, the incidence rate of oligohydramnios is 8%.[3] No consensus exists in the literature as to which sonographic method for amniotic fluid volume measurement is best.

Oligohydramnios can be a result of decreased fetal urinary production or excretion or can result from amniotic fluid loss (Fig. 20-1) from **premature rupture**

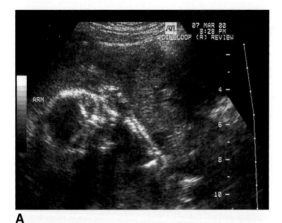

A

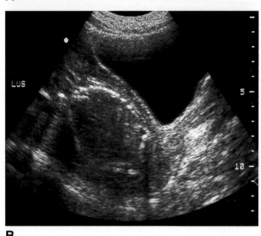

B

Fig. 20-1 Severe oligohydramnios is noted in fetus at 20 weeks, 3 days' gestational age. Note lack of fluid around, **A**, fetal head and, **B**, abdomen. Fetus is in breech position. Single pocket of amniotic fluid measuring 0.9 cm is identified. Patient had reported abdominal pain and leaking fluid.

of membranes (PROM). Ruptured membranes may be suggested with the finding of decreased amniotic fluid on ultrasound and a fetus that is of an appropriate size without structural anomalies. Fetal anomalies, medication or drug use by the mother (**nonsteroidal anti-inflammatory drugs** [NSAIDs], angiotensin-converting enzyme [ACE] inhibitors, cocaine), maternal medical disease, placental insufficiency, and chromosome alterations can all explain a finding of oligohydramnios.

Sonographic Findings

Most clinicians use some form of objective measurement to estimate the amniotic fluid volume. The MVP involves a survey of the entire amniotic cavity and measurement of the deepest pocket of amniotic fluid, free of umbilical cord or fetal parts. The criteria for

definition of oligohydramnios vary, but a deepest pocket of less than 2 cm is most widely accepted.[2]

The AFI is calculated with adding the deepest pocket of fluid measured from each of the four quadrants of the uterus. Measurement of pockets of fluid devoid of umbilical cord or fetal parts is preferable. The AFI must be measured with the patient supine, orienting the transducer in the maternal sagittal plane, measuring the sonographic planes perpendicular to the floor, and using the umbilicus and linea nigra as landmarks to divide the uterus into four quadrants.[3]

Whenever the diagnosis of oligohydramnios is made, a targeted ultrasound examination of the fetus should follow. Malformation or features of urinary obstruction are searched for, such as an empty bladder that does not fill after 1 hour of observation. Absence of the kidneys (renal agenesis) or multicystic kidneys is often found. Urinary outlet obstruction with a distended fetal bladder may also be identified, suggesting the presence of posterior urethral valves (PUVs).

FETAL RENAL ANOMALIES
Renal Agenesis

Renal agenesis is the congenital absence of one or both kidneys from the complete lack of formation. The incidence rate of renal agenesis is one in 3000 births and one in 240 stillbirths.[4,5] It is 2.5 times more common in males than in females. Bilateral absence of the kidneys is more common in twins than in singletons. An increased incidence is not seen with advanced maternal age or maternal medical disease.

Renal agenesis is a developmental anomaly that occurs at 4 to 6 weeks of embryonic life.[6] Three main embryologic events are necessary for normal formation of the kidneys.[7] Failure of one of the steps in renal formation, the development of the metanephros, results in complete absence of the kidney. Because of the absence of fetal urination, women with a fetus with bilateral renal agenesis will have oligohydramnios, clinically identified as size less than dates. In unilateral renal agenesis, one of the kidneys does not develop and the contralateral fetal kidney undergoes compensatory hypertrophy. This hypertrophy occurs prenatally.[8] Because renal function exists in the presence of unilateral renal agenesis, the amniotic fluid volume is usually within normal limits.

Sonographic Findings. The sonographic criteria for the diagnosis of bilateral renal agenesis (Fig. 20-2, *A*) are (1) presence of severe oligohydramnios or anhydramnios after 14 to 16 weeks' gestation and (2) failure

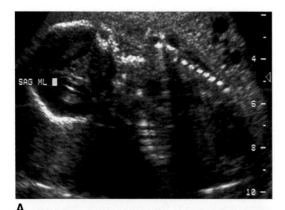

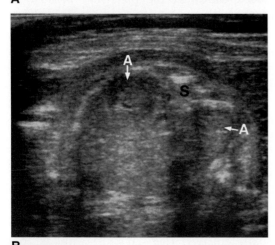

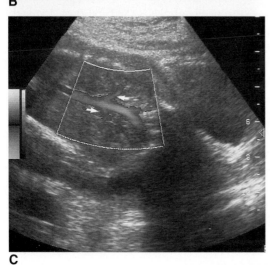

Fig. 20-2 **A,** Renal agenesis was confirmed in fetus in breech position with severe oligohydramnios. Neither bladder nor renal arteries were identified. **B,** Renal agenesis in 29-week fetus shows enlarged adrenal glands *(A)* occupying renal spaces. Oligohydramnios and absent bladder confirmed diagnosis. **C,** Normal renal arteries. Power Doppler maps out renal arteries bilaterally in growth-restricted fetus with oligohydramnios, confirming presence of kidneys that are poorly visualized.

to visualize the fetal kidneys and the urinary bladder.[9] After 26 to 28 weeks' gestation, preterm PROM or placental dysfunction may be the cause for the low or absent amniotic fluid volume. The accuracy of ultrasound for the antenatal diagnosis of renal agenesis in the second and third trimesters has been documented.[10]

First-trimester diagnosis of renal agenesis is rare because at that point in gestation, amniotic fluid volume is often not reduced. The fetal kidneys may be visualized from 10 weeks' gestation with a transvaginal ultrasound examination. In contrast to the fetal adrenals, that are relatively hypoechogenic, the fetal kidneys appear as bilateral echogenic masses with a similar density to that of the fetal lungs. The fetal adrenal glands have served as a source of false-negative diagnoses in cases of renal agenesis (Fig. 20-2, *B*). They may appear enlarged and be confused for fetal kidneys. However, adrenal hypertrophy has been found not to occur, and the false-negative diagnosis of renal agenesis is related to a change in the normal adrenal shape and not to any enlargement of the fetal adrenal gland.[9]

Difficulty may arise in identification of the fetal kidneys in the presence of oligohydramnios. Color or power Doppler imaging is recommended as an adjunct in the diagnosis of bilateral renal agenesis. Color Doppler will identify the renal arteries (Fig. 20-2, *C*; see Color Plate 12) in most cases,[11] and renal agenesis is strongly suspected when the renal arteries are not identified with this technique.

Autosomal Recessive Polycystic Kidney Disease

Large bright or hyperechogenic kidneys are sometimes seen when a routine ultrasound examination is performed or when a woman is referred later in gestation for some other indication, such as size less than dates. The finding of enlarged hyperechogenic kidneys should stimulate detailed examination of the fetus. Obstructive uropathy must be considered when the bladder is enlarged, with or without ureteral dilation. When associated with other abnormalities, syndromes or chromosomal alterations should be considered and karyotyping should be offered.

If the fetus appears to have isolated hyperechogenic kidneys with a normal **karyotype,** then the diagnosis lies between renal dysplasia, autosomal recessive polycystic kidney disease (ARPKD), autosomal dominant polycystic kidney disease (ADPKD), nephrocalcinosis, or rarely, a variant of normal (renal cystic diseases are also discussed in Chapters 7 and 9). A detailed family history, together with ultrasound evaluation of the

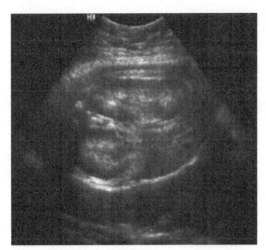

Fig. 20-3 Enlarged echogenic kidneys are noted bilaterally. Note absence of amniotic fluid also identified in association with autosomal recessive polycystic kidney disease.

parents' kidneys, is helpful in diagnosis because both ARPKD and ADPKD can present with oligohydramnios.

ARPKD occurs in approximately one in 40,000 births.[12] This type of polycystic kidney disease is characterized by bilateral enlargement of the kidneys with numerous microscopic corticomedullary cysts. Liver changes including bile duct proliferation with portal fibrosis are also invariably present, although they may not be evident on fetal ultrasound.[13] The locus of the gene for ARPKD has been defined on the short arm of chromosome 6, and prenatal diagnosis is reliable in nearly 80% of cases when certain criteria are met.[14] Genetic material/DNA saved from the first fetus affected with ARPKD is invaluable to facilitate early prenatal diagnosis in subsequent pregnancies.

Sonographic Findings. Typical in utero presentation of ARPKD is the finding of enlarged hyperechogenic kidneys with loss of corticomedullary differentiation (Fig. 20-3). This is presumably the result of numerous small cysts that are undetectable with ultrasound and the oligohydramnios often associated to the renal dysfunction. Increased echogenicity has been identified as early as 12 to 16 weeks' gestation. However, an accurate diagnosis of ARPKD may be difficult early in pregnancy because the size of the fetal kidneys may still be normal. Evidence of renal enlargement and marked echogenicity is usually present by 24 weeks' gestation, although occasionally the diagnosis cannot be made until the third trimester or after birth.[15] Marked oligohydramnios is a common finding, and its presence is associated with an extremely high perinatal mortality rate because of associated pulmonary hypoplasia.

Multicystic Dysplastic Kidneys

Dysplastic kidneys can be of any size, ranging from normal-size or small kidneys (with or without cysts) to massive kidneys distended with multiple large cysts up to 9 cm in diameter. The latter are commonly termed *multicystic dysplastic kidneys* (MCDKs). The incidence rate of unilateral dysplasia is one in 3000 to 5000 births. It occurs with less frequency in the bilateral form, with an incidence of one in 10,000.[16] Prenatal diagnosis of unilateral dysplastic kidneys is variable; however, bilateral MCDKs are more likely to be diagnosed earlier in the pregnancy because of the associated finding of oligohydramnios.

A strong association exists between MCDK and obstruction: MCDKs are usually attached to atretic ureters. A detailed examination of the fetus should be performed to identify contralateral renal anomalies (Fig. 20-4, *A*) or associated extrarenal anomalies, including heart, spine, extremities, face, and umbilical cord. Extrarenal anomalies are identified in 35% of cases and are more prevalent with bilateral MCDK.[17]

Sonographic Findings. The classic presentation of MCDK is a multiloculated abdominal mass consisting of multiple thin-walled cysts that do not appear to connect. The cysts are distributed randomly, the kidney is usually enlarged (Fig. 20-4, *B*) with an irregular outline, and no renal pelvis can be shown. Parenchymal tissue between the cysts is usually hyperechogenic.

In the unilateral form, oligohydramnios is not common, but in the bilateral form, a decreased or absent amount of amniotic fluid volume is likely and the bladder will not be visualized. Bilateral severe MCDKs may be difficult to distinguish from renal agenesis because it is not uncommon for MCDKs to decrease in size as pregnancy progresses. Evaluation of other anatomic structures may be limited as the result of severe oligohydramnios. Color Doppler can be useful in determination of the diagnosis of MCDK because the renal artery is always small or absent and the Doppler waveform, when identified, is markedly abnormal.

Hydronephrosis

Hydronephrosis is a dilation of the renal collecting system. It may be accompanied by dilation of the ureters with or without dilation of the bladder dependent on the level of obstruction. The severity of hydronephrosis can be defined as mild, moderate, or severe. Mild hydronephrosis is described as dilation of the renal pelvis, moderate hydronephrosis is described as dilation of the renal pelvis and calyces, and severe hydro-nephrosis is described as gross dilation of the collecting

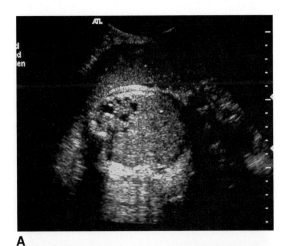

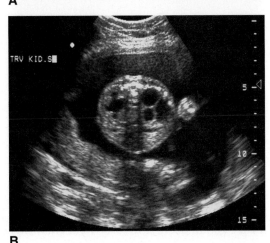

Fig. 20-4 A, Unilateral cystic dysplasia was noted in association with contralateral renal agenesis. Note absence of amniotic fluid surrounding fetus. **B,** Unilateral multicystic dysplastic kidney is identified in fetus with contralateral ureteropelvic junction obstruction. Normal amount of amniotic fluid is seen.

system with a decrease in the renal parenchyma. It should also be noted that mild **pyelectasis** has been associated with Down syndrome.[18] Oligohydramnios may accompany hydronephrosis when the obstruction is severe, bilateral, or associated with a serious contralateral anomaly. The most common congenital obstructive genitourinary anomalies include ureteropelvic junction (UPJ) obstruction, ureterovesical junction (UVJ) obstruction, and PUVs. The purpose of the sonographic examination encompasses the identification of the renal obstructive disorder and the level of obstruction because this effects the treatment options and the prognosis for the fetus.

Ureteropelvic Junction Obstruction. Ureteropelvic junction obstruction is the most common cause of congenital hydronephrosis. This may occur from an arrest or hypoplasia of the development of the junction of the renal pelvis and the proximal ureter. UPJ obstructions are bilateral in 30% of cases but when unilateral may be accompanied by a contralateral anomaly, including MCDK, renal agenesis, or duplication. Extrarenal anomalies have also been associated with UPJ obstruction, including cardiovascular and central nervous system anomalies.[18]

Sonographic findings. UPJ obstruction can be diagnosed when the renal pelvis is dilated (Fig. 20-4, *B*). There is absence of ureteral dilation, and the bladder appears normal. With an isolated UPJ obstruction, the amniotic fluid should also be within normal limits.

Ureterovesical Junction Obstruction. Ureterovesical junction obstruction describes an obstruction at the junction of the distal ureter and bladder and is usually accompanied by duplication of the ureters. The ureter inserting into the upper pole is typically obstructed because that ureter inserts into an ectopic ureterocele in the bladder, resulting in a dilated upper pole of the kidney contiguous with a dilated ureter.

Sonographic findings. The diagnosis of a UVJ obstruction can be made when hydronephrosis is identified with accompanying hydroureter (Fig. 20-5, *A*). The identification of the dilated ureter helps to make the differentiation between a UPJ (in which the ureter is not distended) and UVJ obstruction. The bladder should appear normal in size, and the ectopic ureterocele (Fig 20-5, *B*) may be identified, although in utero identification of the ureterocele may be difficult because of its small size.

Posterior Urethral Valves. Posterior urethral valves are the most common of bladder outlet obstructions resulting from the development of abnormal valves in the posterior urethra. It is accompanied by bilateral hydronephrosis and hydroureters. It is seen most commonly in males and may also be accompanied by **prune-belly syndrome.** When identified early in pregnancy, patients may be offered prenatal vesicoamniotic shunting to decompress the bladder and kidneys and provide a pathway for fluid from the fetus into the amniotic cavity, which may also aid in fetal lung development and reduce fetal growth restriction anomalies.

Sonographic findings. The ultrasonographic appearance of PUV may vary. The fetal bladder may be grossly dilated, and the dilated proximal urethra may also be identified showing a "keyhole" appearance (Fig. 20-6). A distended bladder may be noted, with significant bladder wall thickening, or spontaneous bladder decompression can occur with accompanying

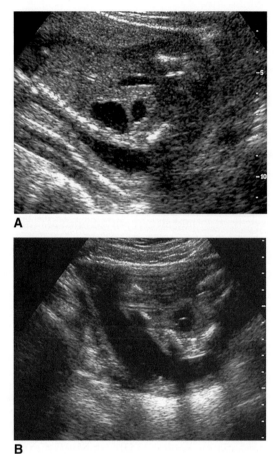

Fig. 20-5 **A,** Dilated right renal pelvis is identified in addition to dilated ureter, confirming diagnosis of ureterovesical junction obstruction. **B,** Ectopic ureterocele was also noted in fetal bladder.

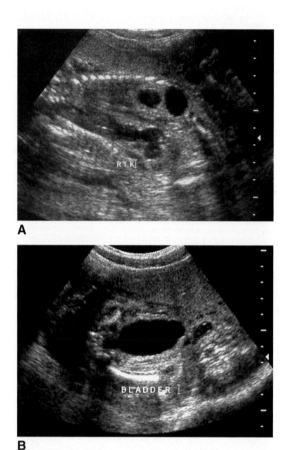

Fig. 20-6 **A,** Bilateral severe hydronephrosis is identified in male fetus with posterior urethral valves. **B,** Keyhole bladder appearance can be seen. Note lack of amniotic fluid surrounding fetus.

urinary ascites. Bilateral hydronephrosis and hydroureters also are identified in the fetus, and severe oligohydramnios may also be seen depending on the gestational age. In cases in which PUV is suspected, the gender should also be documented because PUV is typically identified in males.

INTRAUTERINE GROWTH RESTRICTION

Intrauterine growth restriction (IUGR) is generally defined as a birth weight or fetal weight less than the 10th percentile at any given gestational age. However, constitutional factors such as the gender of the infant, race of the mother, parity, body-mass index, and environmental factors can all affect the distribution of normal birth weight in any population. These factors must be considered when evaluating fetal growth for a mother referred for size less than dates. In general, standards for fetal growth have been incorporated with

ultrasound computer software and different programs exist that can be applied to a variety of geographic locations.

The term *intrauterine growth restriction* is erroneously used on occasion as a substitute for the original term *small for gestational age*. SGA describes a population of fetuses with a weight below the 10th percentile without reference to the cause. Fetal growth restriction describes a subset of these SGA fetuses with weight below the 10th percentile as a result of a pathologic process from a variety of maternal, fetal, or placental disorders. The use of the term *intrauterine growth retardation* is no longer recommended because it implies a component of mental retardation.

IUGR has traditionally been subdivided into two growth restriction patterns: symmetric and asymmetric. In the symmetric form, both the fetal head and the abdomen are proportionately decreased. In the asymmetric form, a greater decrease in abdominal size is seen. Approximately 20% to 30% of all IUGR cases are symmetric, with the remaining 70% to 80% IUGR cases asymmetric. It is now recognized that the timing of the pathologic insult is of more importance than the actual nature of the underlying pathologic process. For example, hypertensive complications of pregnancy resulting in placental insufficiency occurring late in the second trimester could result in asymmetric IUGR. However, hypertensive complications affecting placental function early in the pregnancy will result in symmetric IUGR.

The causes for IUGR are many and have been divided in three categories according to fetal, placental, and maternal factors.[19] The most common fetal factors associated with IUGR include chromosomal alterations, fetal infections (i.e., toxoplasmosis, cytomegalovirus), multiple pregnancies, and fetal malformations. Placental factors may include tumors and placental or umbilical cord accidents or abnormalities.

Maternal Diseases Associated with Intrauterine Growth Restriction

Although many maternal factors may contribute to a growth-restricted fetus, not all of them involve maternal medical disease. Factors such as race and height/weight and nutritional factors, such as low prepregnancy weight and poor weight gain, may negatively affect fetal growth. A poor obstetric history, including previous stillbirth, preterm birth, or IUGR, has been associated with an elevated risk for a growth-restricted infant with the next pregnancy. Environmental factors such as cigarette smoking, substance abuse, intake of certain medications, and high altitude may also negatively affect the rate of fetal growth.

In general, maternal diseases that compromise oxygen availability or cause endothelial vascular damage are associated with fetal growth restriction. Hypoxic conditions, such as **sickle cell anemia,** severe lung disease, and **cyanotic heart disease,** are associated with IUGR.[20] Women with renal failure or after renal transplantation can have a severely growth restricted fetus. Chronic vascular diseases such as insulin-dependent diabetes mellitus and **chronic hypertension** have long been known to cause fetal growth disorders. **Preeclampsia** itself, or superimposed on chronic vascular conditions, may cause fetal growth failure, especially when the onset is before 37 weeks' gestation.[21] The finding of IUGR in the context of preeclampsia makes that condition severe and is considered an indication for delivery. Other conditions that are commonly seen in association with IUGR include collagen vascular disorders such as

SLE and the presence of antiphospholipid antibodies (antiphospolipid antibody syndrome).

Sonographic Findings. Ultrasonography is the method of choice for diagnosis and evaluation of fetuses with possible IUGR. The finding of a significant discrepancy in some or all of the fetal biometric parameters when these are compared with measurements expected based on gestational age is consistent with the diagnosis of fetal growth restriction. Biometric parameters commonly measured include the biparietal diameter (BPD), head circumference (HC), abdominal circumference (AC), and femur length (FL). A variety of formulas are then used to calculate an estimated fetal weight. Sonographic prediction of fetal weight is not completely accurate, which is why the evaluation and management of fetuses suspected to have IUGR is based on serial ultrasound examinations.

Symmetric IUGR is characterized by measurements of the fetal head, abdomen, and femur that are all below the expected values for a given gestational age. In asymmetric fetal growth restriction, the AC is smaller than expected, but fetal head and femur measurements are appropriate for gestational age. However, the ultrasound differentiation of these two patterns of IUGR does not provide an etiology. Although historically symmetric IUGR has been associated with intrinsic insults such as chromosomal alterations or fetal infections and asymmetric IUGR has been associated with extrinsic insults such as placental insufficiency, the onset of the fetal insult is more important than the insult itself. An extrinsic insult that occurs early in gestation may cause symmetric IUGR. Mixed patterns of fetal growth restriction are also possible, limiting even further the clinical utility of separating IUGR into two distinct patterns.

When the diagnosis of IUGR is made, a careful anatomic survey of the fetus should be performed. Oligohydramnios is a common component of IUGR when placental function is insufficient. Normal or increased amniotic fluid volume in the context of IUGR should prompt the search for fetal congenital anomalies and should give suspicion of the presence of a chromosomal alteration. Pulsed Doppler assessment of umbilical artery blood flow may reveal abnormalities in true cases of IUGR. An increase in the ratio of systolic to diastolic flow in the umbilical artery (S:D ratio) is indicative of rising placental resistance. Diastolic flow may eventually disappear (Fig. 20-7) or may even reverse in direction toward the fetus. These findings may be ominous when considering continued in utero fetal well-being.[22]

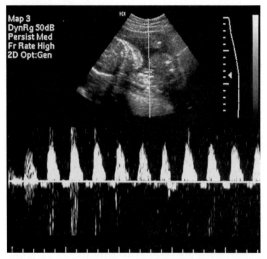

Fig. 20-7 Flow reversal is noted in Doppler of umbilical cord. Fetus was severely growth restricted and in apparent distress, resulting in early delivery.

PREMATURE RUPTURE OF MEMBRANES

Premature rupture of membranes is rupture of amniotic membranes before the onset of labor. When this happens before 37 weeks, it is called *preterm PROM.* PROM occurs in approximately 10% of all pregnancies at term and between 0.7% to 2.0% of pregnancies before 37 weeks' gestation.[23] Most women with PROM at term go into spontaneous labor within the first 24 hours. However, when preterm PROM occurs, the latency period (time from rupture of membranes to labor) may be long. The likelihood of pulmonary hypoplasia is dependent both on the gestational age at which rupture occurs and on the amount of residual amniotic fluid volume and duration of oligohydramnios. Patients with preterm PROM have a higher risk of **chorioamnionitis** and of a cesarean delivery.

Sonographic Findings

Ultrasound findings in PROM are the same as those described in the oligohydramnios section of this chapter (see Fig. 20-1). Even when there appears to be convincing evidence of PROM, the fetal urinary bladder should be imaged and documented to exclude renal agenesis as the primary cause.

SUMMARY

Evaluation of pregnant women referred for size less than dates can sometimes become a challenge for the sonographer and physician. Measurement of the amniotic fluid volume, careful examination of the fetus for congenital anomalies associated with oligohydramnios such as fetal kidney disorders (ARPKD, MCDK, PUV), and a detailed history and physical examination will many times reveal the diagnosis (Table 20-1). Fetal growth restriction is better evaluated with serial ultrasound examinations measuring fetal biometric parameters and comparing them with the expected measurements for a given gestational age. When the estimated fetal weight is found to be less than the 10th percentile, IUGR is diagnosed. In conjunction with clinical data such as severe hypertension, diabetes with vascular disease, or the presence of preeclampsia, an ultrasound examination may provide the necessary tools to decide on expectant management of the pregnancy or to proceed with delivery of the fetus.

CLINICAL SCENARIO—DIAGNOSIS

■ This 39-year-old patient has a long history of type I diabetes mellitus. Her age could be a factor in that she is at an increased risk of having a child with a chromosomal abnormality that could be associated with fetal growth restriction. However, that was ruled out by the genetic amniocentesis. No congenital anomalies in the fetus are suspected because a fetal anatomic survey was performed at 16 weeks of gestation. She is a busy professional and may not be ingesting enough water for adequate hydration. This could explain the low amniotic fluid volume of 6.7 cm. However, the most important factors in this patient are her elevated blood pressure, headache, and worsening proteinuria. These findings are consistent with the diagnosis of preeclampsia. The IUGR suggests that the preeclampsia is severe, and delivery of the fetus is indicated.

Table 20-1	*Causes for Size Less than Dates*
Diagnosis	**Sonographic Findings**
Oligohydramnios	MVP, <2 cm; AFI, <5 cm
Renal agenesis	Absence of kidneys and bladder; severe oligohydramnios; absence of renal arteries shown with Doppler
ARPKD	Large echogenic kidneys bilaterally; absence of bladder; severe oligohydramnios
MCDK	Multiple large cysts that do not connect; usually unilateral with normal fluid; when bilateral, associated with severe oligohydramnios and absence of bladder
Hydronephrosis	Dilatation of renal collecting system
UPJ obstruction	Dilatation of renal collecting system without dilatation of ureter; amniotic fluid is usually normal
UVJ obstruction	Dilatation of renal collecting system and ureter; may identify ectopic ureterocele; amniotic fluid is usually normal
PUV	Grossly distended bladder; bilateral hydronephrosis and hydroureter; severe oligohydramnios; male gender
IUGR	Fetal weight, <10th percentile
PROM	Oligohydramnios

AFI, Amniotic fluid index; *ARPKD,* autosomal recessive polycystic kidney disease; *IUGR,* intrauterine growth restriction; *MCDK,* multicystic dysplastic kidney; *MVP,* maximal vertical pocket; *PROM,* premature rupture of membranes; *PUV,* posterior ureteral valves; *UPJ,* ureteropelvic junction; *UVJ,* ureterovesical junction.

CASE STUDIES FOR DISCUSSION

1. A 21-year-old woman at 27 weeks' gestation is seen for an ultrasound after hospitalization for leaking fluid vaginally. The fetus is in the vertex presentation, and biometric parameters are consistent with her menstrual dates. The AFI is 3.2 cm, and the fetal anatomy is suboptimally visualized (Fig. 20-8, *A* and *B*). The fetal bladder is identified, and power Doppler shows renal arteries (Fig. 20-8, *C*). What is the most likely diagnosis?

2. A 28-year-old woman is referred for an ultrasound evaluation at approximately 27 weeks' gestation with fundal height measurement. She reports that she has had no prenatal care for this pregnancy. The ultrasound shows a single fetus measuring 30 weeks, 5 days' gestational age. No amniotic fluid is identified (Fig. 20-9, *A*), and the patient denies leaking fluid. Power Doppler is used (Fig. 20-9, *B*). What is the most likely diagnosis?

3. A 25-year-old woman is seen for a follow-up obstetric ultrasound at 29 weeks' gestation to rule out placenta previa. A first trimester ultrasound at 7 weeks, for a history of spotting, confirmed the gestational age. The ultrasound reveals a unilateral fetal abdominal mass consisting of multiple thin-walled cysts that do not appear to connect (Fig. 20-10). The AFI is 12.2 cm. The placenta is fundal in location without evidence of previa. The remainder of the examination is unremarkable. What are the most likely diagnosis and prognosis?

4. A 37-year-old woman, G1 P0, is seen at 29 weeks, 5 days with first-trimester ultrasound at a fetal diagnostic center for decreased fundal height. The patient also reveals that she has been previously diagnosed with fibroids. The ultrasound examination reveals multiple large fibroids (Fig. 20-11, *A* and *B*). Fetal biometry reveals an ultrasound age consistent with 23 weeks, 4 days, and there is also a decreased amount of amniotic fluid. Doppler of the umbilical cord reveals the finding in Fig. 20-11, *C*. The fetal anatomy is suboptimally visualized because of the oligohydramnios, but no gross abnormalities are identified. What is the most likely diagnosis?

5. A 24-year-old woman is seen at a maternal fetal center at 17 weeks' gestation for an abnormal ultrasound in the

obstetrician's office. The ultrasound reveals an extremely distended bladder (Fig. 20-12, *A*). The renal pelvices are also noted to be dilated bilaterally, and the remainder of the examination is within normal limits. The gender is male (Fig. 20-12, *B*). What are the most likely diagnosis and outcome for this fetus?

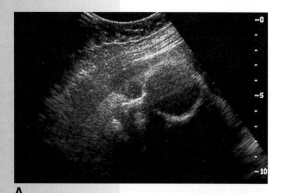

A

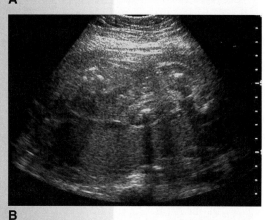

B

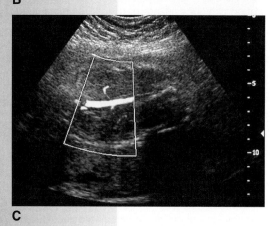

C

Fig. 20-8 **A,** Fetal head is visualized in vertex position. **B,** No amniotic fluid is identified around head or abdomen. **C,** Power Doppler of aorta and renal arteries is noted.

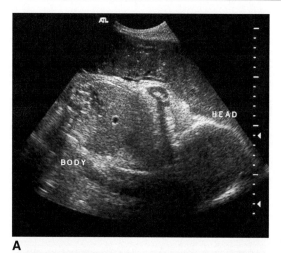

A

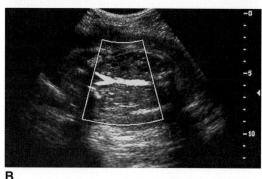

B

Fig. 20-9 **A,** Single fetus is noted in vertex position. No evidence of amniotic fluid is seen. **B,** Power Doppler of aorta and bifurcation is identified.

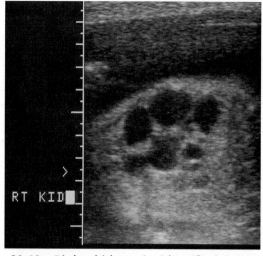

Fig. 20-10 Right kidney is identified in image. Normal amniotic fluid is seen.

CASE STUDIES FOR DISCUSSION—cont'd

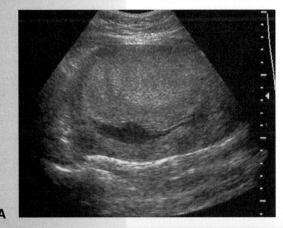

A

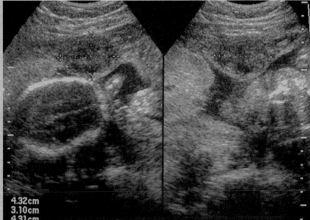

B

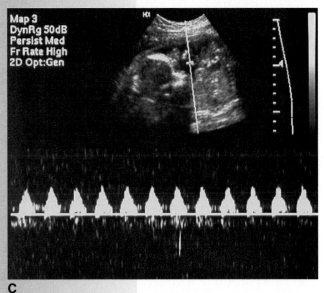

C

Fig. 20-11 A, Image of placenta shows large retroplacental fibroid. **B,** Decrease in amniotic fluid is also identified in longitudinal and transverse image of another fibroid. **C,** Doppler analysis shows lack of diastolic flow.

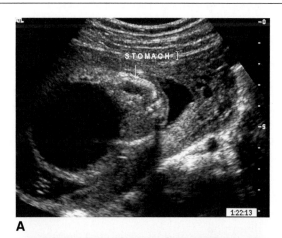

A

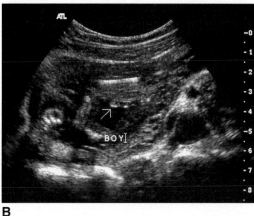

B

Fig. 20-12 A, Huge cystic mass is noted in fetal abdomen. **B,** Gender is male.

STUDY QUESTIONS

1. A 41-year-old woman is seen for size less than dates. She is at 31 weeks gestation confirmed with a 9-week early ultrasound. The fetus appears structurally normal, and the estimated fetal weight is at the ninth percentile for gestational age. The amniotic fluid index (AFI) is 6.1 cm. She had a history of a coldlike virus during pregnancy, and laboratory tests confirm a positive test for toxoplasmosis. She declines genetic amniocentesis. Three weeks later she is delivered for an AFI of 4.3 cm. This is consistent with which one of the following?
   a. intrauterine growth restriction
   b. intrauterine growth restriction with oligohydramnios
   c. oligohydramnios
   d. a severe renal anomaly
   e. small for gestational age

2. A 30-year-old woman is evaluated because of size less than dates and decreased fetal movement. She is at 26 weeks' gestation. Ultrasound reveals oligohydramnios and bright, large uniformly echogenic kidneys. These findings represent which one of the following?
   a. autosomal dominant polycystic kidney disease
   b. autosomal recessive polycystic kidney disease
   c. multicystic dysplastic kidneys
   d. fetal renal hyperplasia
   e. bilateral renal tumors

3. A routine ultrasound examination is performed in a pregnant woman at 21 weeks' gestation. Ultrasound reveals a multiloculated left abdominal mass that contains multiple thin-walled cysts. The amniotic fluid volume appears normal. Fetal growth is appropriate for gestational age, and no other anomalies are identified. What is the diagnosis?
   a. Meckel-Gruber syndrome
   b. autosomal dominant polycystic kidney disease
   c. unilateral autosomal recessive polycystic kidney disease
   d. unilateral multicystic dysplastic kidney
   e. severe hydronephrosis

4. An obstetric ultrasound is performed on a 37-year-old woman referred for size less than dates. She is currently at 34 weeks' gestation. She reports normal fetal activity. She has trace protein in the urine, and her blood pressure is elevated at 150/102 mm Hg.

She has no apparent edema. A review of her medical record shows her blood pressure has been elevated since her first prenatal visit at 10 weeks. The ultrasound shows a fetus with intrauterine growth restriction and oligohydramnios. What is the diagnosis?
   a. mild preeclampsia
   b. severe preeclampsia
   c. systemic lupus erythematosus
   d. chronic hypertension
   e. diabetes mellitus

5. A 34-year-old woman states that 4 weeks ago she had a flulike illness. The ultrasound examination shows mild dilation of the lateral ventricles in the fetal brain and intracerebral calcifications. According to her last menstrual period, she is at 22 weeks' gestation. The fetal biometry shows the following: BPD: 19 weeks, 4 days; HC: 19 weeks, 6 days; AC: 19 weeks, 2 days; and FL: 20 weeks, 0 days. An amniocentesis is performed. Fetal karyotype is normal and the presence of cytomegalovirus (CMV) in the amniotic fluid is confirmed. Which of the following terms best represents the above findings:
   a. microcephaly
   b. ventriculomegaly-CMV syndrome
   c. symmetric intrauterine growth restriction
   d. asymmetric intrauterine growth restriction
   e. intrauterine growth restriction

6. A 22-year-old woman with type I diabetes known to have diabetic nephropathy and retinopathy receives a follow-up ultrasound examination at 32 weeks' gestation for evaluation of fetal growth. The amniotic fluid index is within normal limits. The fetal biometry is as follows: BPD: 31 weeks, 4 days; HC: 32 weeks, 0 days; AC: 27 weeks, 5 days; and FL: 31 weeks, 2 days. Which of the following terms best describes the previously mentioned findings?
   a. asymmetric intrauterine growth restriction
   b. symmetric intrauterine growth restriction
   c. fetal growth retardation
   d. fetal nephropathy syndrome
   e. diabetic growth restriction syndrome

7. An ultrasound examination is performed on an 18-year-old woman. She is at 20 weeks' gestation and has been referred for size less than dates and an elevated maternal serum alpha fetoprotein. The

detailed ultrasound reveals oligohydramnios and large kidneys containing multiple large cysts. The most likely diagnosis is?

a. autosomal dominant polycystic kidney disease
b. autosomal recessive polycystic kidney disease
c. multicystic dysplastic kidneys
d. nephrocalcinosis
e. renal dysplasia

8. A young woman is seen in the labor and delivery unit with a severe headache. Her blood pressure is taken at 196/115 mm Hg, and she has significant proteinuria and edema. She is diagnosed with severe preeclampsia. She is at 35 weeks' gestation, and the fetal heart rate tracing shows decreased beat-to-beat variability. An ultrasound examination shows oligohydramnios with an amniotic fluid index of 2.2 cm. The placenta is grade 3. The average ultrasound age is 34 weeks, 3 days. Which of the following best explains the nonreassuring fetal heart rate tracing and the oligohydramnios?

a. fetal chromosomal abnormality
b. cord accident
c. placental insufficiency
d. hypertension
e. fetal congenital anomaly

9. A 26-year-old woman is seen for ultrasound at 25 weeks, 2 days' gestational age for decreased fundal height. The amniotic fluid index measures 12.9 cm, and fetal biometry is consistent with the gestational age earlier confirmed with 6-week ultrasound examination. Survey of the fetal anatomy reveals a dilated renal pelvis and ureter on the left kidney. The right kidney is within normal limits, and the bladder is unremarkable. Which of the following is the most correct diagnosis?

a. hydronephrosis
b. ureteropelvic obstruction
c. ureterovesical junction obstruction
d. posterior ureteral valves
e. urethral atresia

10. A patient is seen for ultrasound at 32 weeks' gestation without prior prenatal care. The fetal biometry confirms a single fetus measuring an average age of 31 weeks, 2 days. Fetal anatomic survey reveals right kidney with moderate dilation of the renal pelvis and calyces. The bladder and contralateral kidney appears within normal limits, and the remainder of the examination is unremarkable. The amniotic

fluid index is 15.1 cm. What is the most likely diagnosis?

a. hydronephrosis
b. multicystic dysplastic kidneys
c. posterior ureteral valves
d. ureteropelvic obstruction
e. ureterovesical junction obstruction

REFERENCES

1. Walraven GE, Mkanje RJ, van Roosmalen J et al: Single pre-delivery symphysis-fundal height measurement as a predictor of birthweight and multiple pregnancy, *Br J Obstet Gynaecol* 102:525-529, 1995.
2. Chamberlain PF, Manning FA, Morrison I et al: Ultrasound evaluation of amniotic fluid. I. The relationship of marginal and decreased amniotic fluid volumes to perinatal outcome, *Am J Obstet Gynecol* 150:245-249, 1984.
3. Phelan JP, Ahn MO, Smith CV et al: Amniotic fluid index measurements during pregnancy, *J Reprod Med* 32:601-604, 1987.
4. Cardwell MS: Bilateral renal agenesis: clinical implications, *South Med J* 81:327-328, 1988.
5. Whitehouse W, Mountrose U: Renal agenesis in non-twin siblings, *Am J Obstet Gynecol* 116:880-882, 1973.
6. Kaffe S, Godmilow L, Walker BA et al: Prenatal diagnosis of bilateral renal agenesis, *Obstet Gynecol* 49:478-480, 1977.
7. Wax JR, Prabhakar G, Giraldez RA et al: Unilateral renal hypoplasia and contralateral renal agenesis: a new association with 45,x/46, xy mosaicism, *Am J Perinatol* 11:184-186, 1994.
8. Hartshorne N, Shepard T, Barr M: Compensatory renal growth in human fetuses with unilateral renal agenesis, *Teratology* 44:7-10, 1991.
9. Droste S, Fitzimmons J, Pascoe-Mason J et al: Size of the fetal adrenal in bilateral renal agenesis, *Obstet Gynecol* 76:206-209, 1990.
10. Romero R, Cullen M, Grannum P et al: Antenatal diagnosis of renal agenesis with ultrasound, *Am J Obstet Gynecol* 151:38-43, 1985.
11. Sepulveda W, Corral E, Sanchez J et al: Sirenomelia sequence versus renal agenesis: prenatal differentiation with power Doppler ultrasound, *Ultrasound Obstet Gynecol* 11:445-449, 1998.
12. Zerres K, Mucher G, Becker J et al: Prenatal diagnosis of autosomal recessive polycystic kidney disease (ARPKD): molecular genetics, clinical experience, and fetal morphology, *Am J Med Genet* 76:137-144, 1998.
13. Jung J, Benz-Bohm G, Kugel H et al: MR cholangiography in children with autosomal recessive polycystic kidney disease, *Pediatr Radiol* 29:463-466, 1999.

14. Gagnadoux MF, Attie T, Amiel J et al: Prenatal diagnosis of autosomal recessive polycystic kidney disease, *Arch Pediatr* 9:942-947, 2000.

15. Wisser J, Hebisch G, Froster U et al: Prenatal diagnosis of autosomal recessive polycystic kidney disease (ARPKD) during the early second trimester, *Prenat Diagn* 15:868-871, 1995.

16. Wool AS, Winyard PJ: Advances in the cell biology and genetics of human kidney malformations, *J Am Soc Nephrol* 9:1114-1125, 1995.

17. Lazebnick N, Bellinger MF, Ferguson TE et al: Insights into the pathogenesis and natural history of fetuses with multicystic dysplastic kidney disease, *Prenat Diagn* 19:418-423, 1999.

18. Angtuaco TL, Collins B, Quirk JG: The fetal genitourinary tract, *Semin Roentgenol* XXXIV:13-28, 1999.

19. Lin CC, Santolaya-Forgas J: Current concepts of fetal growth restriction. Part I: causes, classification and pathophysiology, *Obstet Gynecol* 92:1044-1055, 1998.

20. Patton DE, Lee W, Cotton DB et al: Cyanotic maternal heart disease in pregnancy, *Obstet Gynecol Surv* 45:594-600, 1990.

21. Xiong X, Mayes D, Demiaczuk N et al: Impact of pregnancy-induced hypertension on fetal growth, *Am J Obstet Gynecol* 180:207-213, 1999.

22. Reed KL, Anderson CF, Shenker L: Changes in intracardiac Doppler blood flow velocities in fetuses with absent umbilical artery diastolic flow, *Am J Obstet Gynecol* 157:774-779, 1987.

23. King JC, Mitzner W, Butterfield AB et al: Effect of induced oligohydramnios on fetal lung development, *Am J Obstet Gynecol* 154:823-830, 1986.

Bleeding with Pregnancy

CHARLOTTE HENNINGSEN and LENNARD D. GREENBAUM

CLINICAL SCENARIO

◼ A 21-year-old woman is seen in the emergency department at 14 weeks' gestation with vaginal bleeding. An obstetric ultrasound is ordered to rule out miscarriage (Fig. 21-1). What is the most likely diagnosis?

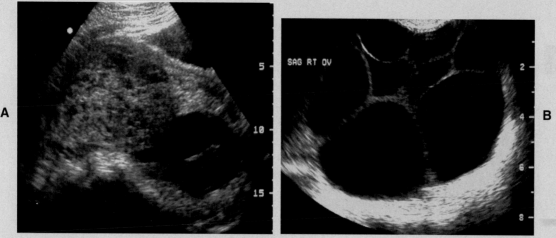

Fig. 21-1   A, Mass with multiple cystic spaces is seen within uterus. B, Ovaries are enlarged and multilocated as shown in right ovary.

OBJECTIVES

◼ List the various causes of bleeding with pregnancy.

◼ Differentiate the most common causes of bleeding in the first trimester of pregnancy from the most common causes of bleeding in the second and third trimesters of pregnancy.

◼ Explain the beta human chorionic gonadotropin levels that are used in diagnosis of ectopic pregnancy, gestational trophoblastic disease, and pregnancy failure.

◼ List the causes of bleeding in the second and third trimesters of pregnancy and differentiate the sonographic findings.

◼ Identify Doppler findings identified with a variety of the causes of bleeding with pregnancy.

◼ Describe the patient symptoms and sonographic findings associated with retained products of conception.

GLOSSARY OF TERMS ■■■■■

Anembryonic pregnancy, or blighted ovum:
  occurs when a gestational sac is devoid of an embryo
Aneuploid: abnormal chromosome pattern
Dyspnea: difficulty in breathing
Exsanguination: bleeding to death
Heterotopic pregnancy: the presence of two or more
  implantation sites that occur simultaneously, with
  one intrauterine and one extrauterine pregnancy

Idiopathic: of unknown cause
Karyotype: chromosomal make-up of an individual
Micrognathia: small chin
Multiparous: defines a woman who has given birth
  more than once
Syndactyly: fusion of the extremities or digits
Trophoblast: tissue that arises from the blastocyst
  that contributes to the development of the placenta

Sonography is a diagnostic tool frequently used in the evaluation of bleeding in pregnant patients. In the first trimester, the viability of the pregnancy is a primary concern; however, patient symptoms and laboratory tests may also lead to a search for an ectopic pregnancy or gestational trophoblastic disease. In the second and third trimesters of pregnancy, the most common causes of bleeding include placenta previa and abruptio placenta, although other conditions, including placenta accreta, may be seen with similar symptoms. Furthermore, ultrasound examination may be used in the investigation of abnormal bleeding after delivery. A thorough search with ultrasound and knowledge of the sonographic findings specific to these various conditions can lead to the correct diagnosis and appropriate treatment.

FIRST-TRIMESTER BLEEDING
Subchorionic Hemorrhage

Subchorionic hemorrhages are low-pressure hemorrhages that occur most commonly in the first trimester of pregnancy. They often result from the implantation of the fertilized ovum into the uterus. These areas of hemorrhage are seen between the uterine wall and the membranes and are not associated with the placenta, which distinguishes subchorionic hemorrhage from abruptio placenta. Patients may have spotting or bleeding with or without uterine contractions. Subchorionic hemorrhage may spontaneously regress or may lead to spontaneous abortion (SAB); the larger hematomas are more likely to result in the loss of the pregnancy.[1]

Sonographic Findings. Sonographic examination of a subchorionic hemorrhage reveals blood, which may initially be echogenic and progressively become anechoic (Fig. 21-2), located adjacent to the gestational sac and at the margin of the placenta. The lack of vas-

cularity identified with color Doppler can help differentiate hematoma from a neoplasm.[2] When the hemorrhage is anechoic, it may resemble a second gestational sac.

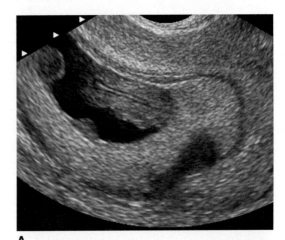

A

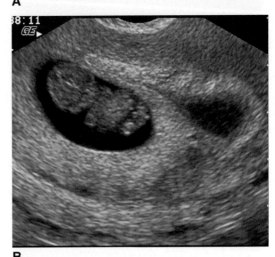

B

Fig. 21-2 Subchorionic hemorrhages are shown in, **A,** 8-week gestation and, **B,** 10-week gestation. (**A** and **B** Courtesy GE Medical Systems.)

Abortion

Threatened abortion (TAB) is characterized by bleeding and cramping in the first trimester and is seen in one third of pregnancies.[3] TAB may lead to a missed abortion (MAB), in which embryonic death occurs without expulsion of the products of conception, or SAB, in which expulsion of the products of conception occurs. Approximately 15% of pregnancies end in a SAB.[4] Pregnancy loss is often **idiopathic** but may occur in **aneuploid** fetuses or as the result of maternal endocrine or vascular disorders, anatomic factors, or immunologic disease.[5]

Correlation between the serum beta human chorionic gonadotropin (beta-hCG) and the findings in the uterus can be used to confirm whether or not the sonographic milestones of a first-trimester pregnancy are met. The gestational sac may be identified as early as 4.5 weeks by last menstrual period (LMP) and should grow about 1 mm per day.[6] With endovaginal technique, the yolk sac should be visualized by the time the mean sac diameter reaches 8 mm and the embryo should be visualized when the mean sac diameter is greater than 16 mm (Fig. 21-3).[7] The embryo with cardiac activity is noted by 6.5 weeks. The normal heart rate in the first trimester is 90 to 170 beats per minute (bpm).[8] Embryonic bradycardia is associated with a poor prognosis. The embryo also grows at a rate of 1 mm per day. Failure to meet any of the milestones mentioned carries a poor prognosis for the pregnancy.[6]

Sonographic Findings. A primary role of sonography in the evaluation of pregnancy in the first trimester is confirmation of viability. If the crown-rump length measures greater than 5 mm and cardiac activity is not seen, the diagnosis of embryonic death can be made with confidence.[6] Failure to meet other first-trimester sonographic milestones should be noted. A subchorionic hemorrhage may also lead to pregnancy loss. Ultrasound may be used to follow bleeding with pregnancy to monitor viability, to confirm fetal death, and to determine when dilation and curettage (D&C) is necessary.

Ectopic Pregnancy

Ectopic pregnancy is defined as a pregnancy located outside of the normal location and is a leading cause of maternal death in the first trimester.[9,10] A history of ectopic pregnancy also affects the future fertility of a patient and increases the risk of a repeat ectopic pregnancy. In addition to a history of ectopic pregnancy, risk factors include a history of pelvic inflammatory disease (PID), tubal surgery, maternal congenital anomalies, defective zygote, fertility treatments, and intrauterine device (IUD) usage. The increased usage of assisted reproductive technology (ART) has not only increased the incidence rates of ectopic pregnancies and multiple gestations but has also increased the incidence rate of heterotopic pregnancies.

The most common location of an ectopic pregnancy is in the fallopian tube, with a reported incidence rate of approximately 95% of ectopic pregnancies.[8] Ectopic pregnancies have also been identified in the cervix, ovary (Fig. 21-4, *A*), uterine cornu, broad ligament, and abdomen. Interstitial or cornual pregnancy (Fig. 21-4, *B*), also rare, occurs in 1.1% to 6.3% of ectopic pregnancies.[11] This type of ectopic pregnancy is located in the interstitial portion of the fallopian tube, which is located in the wall of the uterine cornu, and may result in massive hemorrhage, with rupture leading to serious

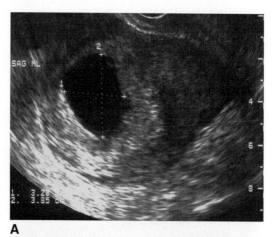

A

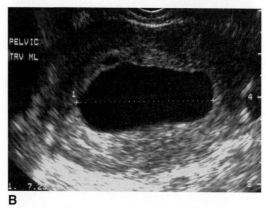

B

Fig. 21-3 Endovaginal images of, **A,** longitudinal and, **B,** transverse uterus show large empty gestational sac. This 32-year-old pregnant woman was seen with bleeding in first trimester. Findings were consistent with anembryonic pregnancy.

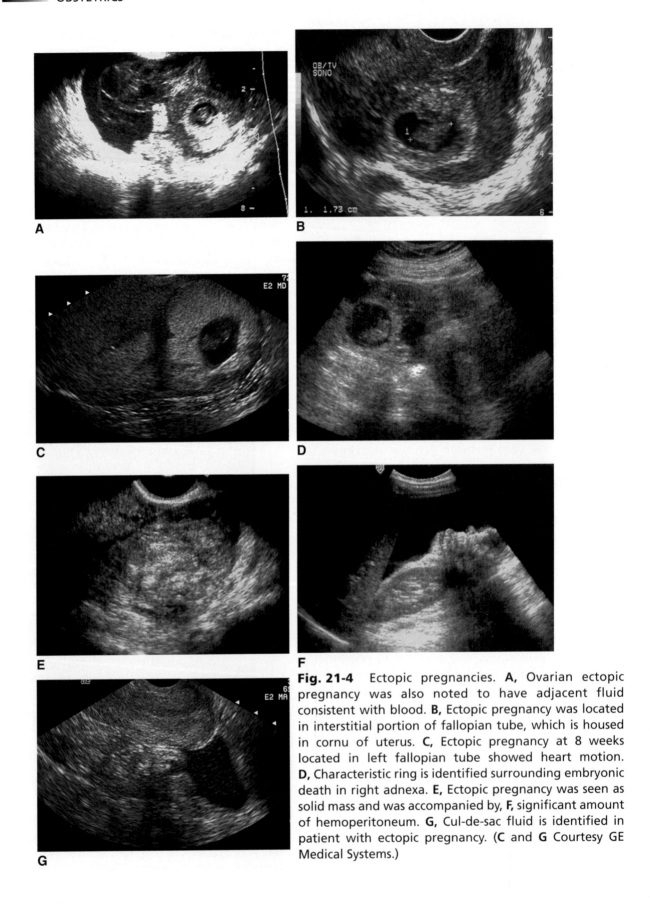

Fig. 21-4 Ectopic pregnancies. **A,** Ovarian ectopic pregnancy was also noted to have adjacent fluid consistent with blood. **B,** Ectopic pregnancy was located in interstitial portion of fallopian tube, which is housed in cornu of uterus. **C,** Ectopic pregnancy at 8 weeks located in left fallopian tube showed heart motion. **D,** Characteristic ring is identified surrounding embryonic death in right adnexa. **E,** Ectopic pregnancy was seen as solid mass and was accompanied by, **F,** significant amount of hemoperitoneum. **G,** Cul-de-sac fluid is identified in patient with ectopic pregnancy. (**C** and **G** Courtesy GE Medical Systems.)

complications, possible hysterectomy, and even death.[12] Cervical pregnancies are rare and account for 1:1000 to 1:18,000 pregnancies but can lead to massive hemorrhage that may necessitate hysterectomy to stop the bleeding.[13,14] Cervical pregnancy may have an ultrasound appearance that is similar to a SAB because a gestational sac is identified within the cervix. Ovarian pregnancies are also rare, occur in less than 3% of ectopic pregnancies, and may be indistinguishable from other ovarian pathologies.[8] Abdominal pregnancies account for approximately 1% of ectopic pregnancies and usually occur in the pelvis, although implantations have also been reported in the upper abdomen, including in the liver.[15]

The clinical symptoms of ectopic pregnancy include bleeding, pain, and a palpable adnexal mass. These symptoms are nonspecific and may even be seen in patients who are not pregnant. In addition, fewer than 50% of patients with an ectopic pregnancy have this clinical triad.[10] Women with an ectopic pregnancy may also be asymptomatic or have symptoms more suggestive of a TAB. The ultrasound findings paired with quantitative beta-hCG levels assist clinicians in confirmation of an intrauterine pregnancy (IUP) or assessment of the risk of an ectopic pregnancy. A gestational sac should be identified in the uterus if the beta-hCG level is 1000 to 2000 mIU/ml (international reference preparation).[7] The absence of an IUP in the presence of these beta-hCG levels suggests an increased risk of ectopic pregnancy. With normal pregnancy, the beta-hCG levels should double every 2 days until they plateau. However, in the presence of an ectopic pregnancy, the levels rise more slowly, although a nonviable pregnancy could also be seen with this finding.

Sonographic Findings. The most specific ultrasound finding diagnostic of ectopic pregnancy is that of an extrauterine gestational sac that contains a living embryo (Fig. 21-4, C). Likewise, ectopic pregnancy is generally excluded in the presence of a living IUP, although **heterotopic pregnancy** should be considered in patients who undergo ART. In the absence of an extrauterine embryo, other positive sonographic findings in combination or isolation may suggest ectopic pregnancy.

The uterus may be consistent with a normal nongravid uterus or may have a decidual reaction or pseudogestational sac. A pseudogestational sac does not show the low-resistant, peritrophoblastic flow with Doppler that accompanies a normal IUP. A pseudogestational sac also lacks the "double-sac sign" that represents the chorionic villi and endometrial cavity seen with early IUPs.[10]

The adnexa should also be carefully evaluated for signs of ectopic pregnancy. A live extrauterine pregnancy is infrequently identified, but an extrauterine gestational sac has been identified in greater than 71% of ectopic pregnancies.[8] An echogenic adnexal ring (Fig. 21-4, D) may be seen with or without the presence of a yolk sac. A peritrophoblastic flow pattern may aid in distinguishing the adnexal ring from an ovarian cyst. However, a corpus luteum may also show a similar flow pattern. A hematosalpinx may also be identified if the fallopian tube is distended with blood. An ectopic may also be seen as a complex mass (Fig. 21-4, E and F).

A thorough investigation may reveal an empty uterus and normal-appearing adnexa. Identification of cul-de-sac fluid (Fig. 21-4, G) is suggestive of ectopic pregnancy, whether in the presence or absence of other positive sonographic findings. Hemoperitoneum may appear anechoic, complex, or echogenic. When ultrasound does not show an IUP or a finding suggestive of ectopic pregnancy, clinical correlation determines when surgical, medical, or expectant management is appropriate.

Gestational Trophoblastic Disease

Gestational trophoblastic disease describes a spectrum of diseases of the **trophoblast** that can be benign, malignant, or malignant/metastatic and includes the complete hydatidiform mole, hydatidiform mole with coexistent fetus, partial mole, invasive mole, and choriocarcinoma. Risk factors include maternal age and a previous history of a molar pregnancy.

Molar Pregnancy. The complete hydatidiform mole is of paternal origin and devoid of maternal chromosomes, which results in a 46,XX **karyotype** without fetal development. The incidence rate of complete molar pregnancy in the United States is 1:2000.[16] Most partial moles are characterized by triploidy with a 69,XXX or 69,XXY karyotype of which 23 chromosomes are of the maternal contribution and 46 chromosomes are of the paternal contribution. A partial mole may be accompanied by a fetus or fetal tissue. Partial moles with a complete fetus occurs in 0.005% to 0.01% of pregnancies.[16] The complete hydatidiform mole may also coexist with a normal fetus as the result of a twin gestation, although the prevalence rate of this rare event is 1:22,000 to 1:100,000.[16]

Clinical findings associated with molar pregnancy most commonly include vaginal bleeding, which may prompt evaluation of the beta-hCG that is markedly elevated (>100,000 IU/ml[9]) in the presence of molar pregnancy. Maternal serum alpha fetoprotein (AFP) levels will be markedly low in pregnancies complicated by complete hydatidiform mole.[17] In addition to abnormal laboratory findings, the patient may have symptoms of hyperemesis, preeclampsia, thyrotoxicosis, or respiratory distress.[17] Clinical examination may reveal a uterus that is greater in size than the expected gestational age and bilateral ovarian enlargement consistent with theca lutein cysts.[18,19]

Molar pregnancies are usually treated with evacuation of the mole followed by serial beta-hCG level tests to ensure that levels fall to normal, which should occur within 10 to 12 weeks. Increasing beta-hCG levels may indicate molar invasion.

Sonographic findings. The complete hydatidiform mole appears as an echogenic mass within the uterus that contains multiple cystic areas (representing the hydropic chorionic villi) and that has been described as having a snowstorm appearance (Fig. 21-5, *A*). In addition, no fetus or fetal parts are identified. Early first-trimester findings may be nonspecific, simulating a MAB or **anembryonic pregnancy,** or may appear as an echogenic mass within the uterus.[8]

A partial mole has an identifiable placenta, although placental enlargement with cystic spaces that represent the hydropic villi is demonstrated. A fetus or fetal tissue will be identified (Fig. 21-5, *B*), but many instances of partial mole will spontaneously abort within the first trimester. When a fetus is present, a careful search for structural defects should be performed because triploid fetuses are usually present. Fetal defects associated with triploidy included intrauterine growth restriction (IUGR), heart defects, **micrognathia,** hand abnormalities such as **syndactyly,** and ventriculomegaly.

A complete hydatidiform mole with a coexistent fetus (Fig. 21-5, *C*) is seen as a normal fetus and placenta with a concurrent molar pregnancy.[20,21] Differentiation of this versus a molar pregnancy is important because of the varying malignant potentials between these two entities. Although a complete mole with coexistent fetus has the same malignant potential as does a solitary hydatidiform mole, a partial mole does not have malignant potential.

In addition to the findings within the uterus, hyperstimulation of the ovaries may occur as a result of the greatly increased beta-hCG levels. Bilateral theca lutein cysts have been documented in up to 50% of molar pregnancies. These enlarged ovaries may rupture or torque, causing severe pain. The sonographic description of theca lutein cysts includes enlarged ovaries that contain multiple large cysts, giving them a "soap-bubble" appearance.[19]

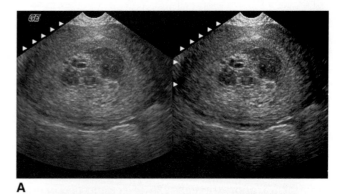

A

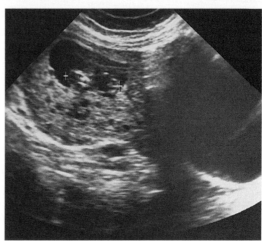

B

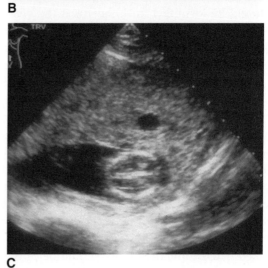

C

Fig. 21-5 **A,** Complete hydatidiform mole is identified in image. **B,** Suprapubic scan shows gravid uterus. There is a small, dead, growth-retarded fetus of approximately 12-week size. The placental tissue is large and has multiple vesicular spaces consistent with hydropic villi. There is no normal placenta. **C,** Molar pregnancy with rare coexistent fetus. (**A** Courtesy GE Medical Systems.) Hagen-Ansert S: Textbook of diagnostic ultrasound, ed 5, St Louis, 2001, Mosby.

Invasive Hydatidiform Mole. Invasive mole, also known as *chorioadenoma destruens*, occurs when the hydropic villi of a partial or complete mole invade the uterine myometrium and even penetrate through the uterine wall. Considered an invasive form of gestational trophoblastic disease, invasive mole may occur during the development of a molar pregnancy or may develop after the evacuation of a mole. Clinical symptoms typically become apparent after the evacuation of a molar pregnancy, when the patient is seen with heavy bleeding. Sonography may be used to assist in the diagnosis of this extension of molar pregnancy and may be used to follow the response to treatment.[19]

Sonographic findings. Sonographic evaluation of the uterus reveals areas of increased echogenicity within the uterus. These focal areas may also appear heterogeneous and contain cystic areas.

Choriocarcinoma. Choriocarcinoma is a malignant tumor that arises from the trophoblastic epithelium. Considered a malignant metastatic form of gestational trophoblastic disease, choriocarcinoma most commonly metastasizes to the lung, liver, and brain.[19] Choriocarcinoma may develop after a molar pregnancy but also may occur after a normal pregnancy, SAB, or ectopic pregnancy and may be seen weeks, months, or several years after a pregnancy. The benign hydatidiform mole and mole with coexistent fetus are considered to have a malignant potential, whereas the partial mole does not have a malignant potential. Clinical symptoms most commonly include vaginal bleeding, but patients may also have **dyspnea**, abdominal pain, and neurologic symptoms.

Sonographic findings. Sonographic evaluation of these neoplasms often reveals a complex mass because of hemorrhage and necrosis. Metastatic lesions may also be identified, and computed tomography (CT) or magnetic resonance imaging (MRI) may be used in evaluation of the extent of the metastatic disease.[19]

SECOND-TRIMESTER BLEEDING
Placenta Previa

Placenta previa is defined as a placenta that is near or covering the internal cervical os. Placenta previa has been reported in one of 200 pregnancies and may lead to serious hemorrhage, increasing maternal morbidity and fetal mortality.[8] Identification of placenta previa is important in prediction of the mode of delivery so that a cesarean section (C-section) can be scheduled to avoid emergency surgery. Placenta previa has been classified

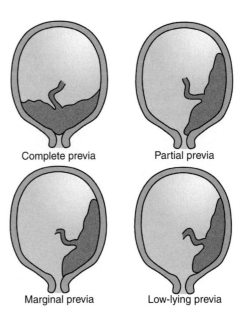

Complete previa   Partial previa

Marginal previa   Low-lying previa

Fig. 21-6 Types of placenta previa.

into varying degrees (Fig. 21-6) to include low-lying placenta, partial previa, and complete previa. A low-lying placenta is within 2 cm of the os, a partial previa partially covers the os, and a complete previa extends completely across the internal cervical os. Sonography is used in the identification of the location of the placenta and in following patients to monitor for placental "migration."

The low-lying placenta and partial previa may migrate and alleviate the need for C-section. This process, which has been defined as trophotropism, describes the atrophy of the placenta in the region of the lower uterine segment with differential growth of other regions of the placenta toward more vascular-rich sites.[22] Research has suggested that a placenta previa that is likely to need C-section is one that overlaps the internal cervical os by 20 mm in the third trimester.[22]

Patients who are at increased risk for placenta previa include those with advanced maternal age, **multiparous** women, and those with a prior history of C-section. The most common symptom of placenta previa is painless bleeding in the third trimester, but patients may be asymptomatic.

Sonographic Findings. The following three defined methods exist for imaging of the lower uterine segment for identification of the location of the placenta in relationship to the internal os: transabdominal imaging (Fig. 21-7), translabial imaging, and endovaginal imaging. Endovaginal imaging is considered the gold standard for diagnosis of placenta previa.[23] With transabdominal imaging, false-positive results may occur from an over-

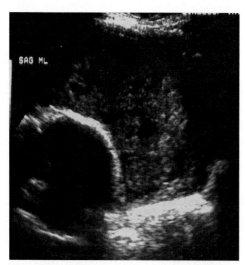

Fig. 21-7 Placenta is identified as presenting part in lower uterine segment of uterus. Patient had history of prior cesarean section and was also at risk for placenta accreta, which was confirmed at time of delivery.

distended bladder, myometrial contractions, and shadowing of the cervix from the fetal head or other overlying fetal parts.[24]

Vasa Previa

Vasa previa describes vessels of fetal origin that completely or partially cover the internal cervical os. Vasa previa occurs in 1:1200 to 1:5000 pregnancies and can lead to fetal **exsanguination** from compression or tearing of the vessels during labor.[25] The most common presentation of vasa previa is dark vaginal bleeding with rupture of the membranes. Associated fetal heart deceleration or demise may also be noted.

Vasa previa may arise from velamentous cord insertion or marginal cord insertion or from the connecting vessels of an accessory or bilobed placenta. Vasa previa has also been seen with increased frequency in association with multiple gestations and low-lying placentas. Prenatal diagnosis can improve fetal and maternal outcome with closer attention to preterm labor, limiting of maternal activity, and planned elective C-section.[25,26]

Sonographic Findings. An obstetric ultrasound should include visualization of the umbilical cord insertion into the placenta. Endovaginal ultrasound should be used in patients with risk factors for vasa previa, including patients in whom the placental cord insertion is not identified because of the limitations of transabdominal imaging that may be associated with maternal size or position of the maternal bladder. Color Doppler or power Doppler (Fig. 21-8; see Color Plate

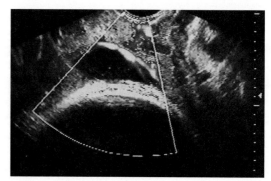

Fig. 21-8 Vessels are clearly shown covering internal os and are enhanced with power Doppler imaging.

13) will usually be needed for confirmation of the diagnosis.

Abruptio Placenta

Abruption of the placenta is defined as a placenta that prematurely separates, which can lead to preterm delivery, IUGR, and fetal death. Abruptio placenta affects less than 1% of pregnancies and is suspected when a patient has bleeding, significant abdominal pain, and uterine contractions.[27] Patients may have such classic and severe symptoms that emergency delivery is necessary and diagnostic imaging is not used.[28]

Placental abruptions may be classified as marginal or retroplacental. Retroplacental abruptions are considered high-pressure bleeds and are associated with maternal hypertension, vascular disease, and cocaine abuse.[29] Conversely, marginal abruptions (Fig. 21-9, *A*) are considered low-pressure bleeds that have mild symptoms or that may be clinically silent.

Sonographic Findings. The sonographic findings suggestive of abruptio placenta include the visualization of hemorrhage in the retroplacental region (Fig. 21-9, *B*). However, blood may drain through the cervix rather than collecting beneath the placenta, precluding sonographic diagnosis.[27]

Placenta Accreta

Placenta accreta refers to an abnormal placental attachment to the uterus as the result of an abnormal or absent deciduas basalis. The three classifications used include *placenta accreta*, which refers to the attachment of the chorionic villi to the myometrium; *placenta increta*, which occurs when the villi invade the myometrium; and *placenta percreta*, which refers to invasion through the myometrium into or through the uterine serosa.[30] *Placenta accreta*, the generic terminology used to describe pathologic adherence of the placenta, occurs in up to 1:2500 deliveries.[31] Risk factors include prior C-section,

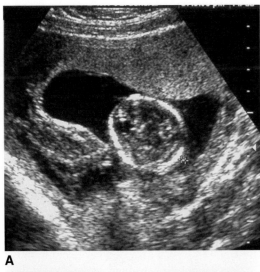

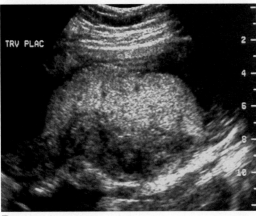

Fig. 21-9 **A,** Patient with marginal abruption was seen with bleeding. She was placed on bedrest, and hemorrhage resolved. Remainder of pregnancy was uneventful. **B,** Abruptio placenta occurred in 30-year-old woman who was seen at emergency department with abdominal pain, bleeding, and unknown last menstrual period. Fetal heart motion was identified, although fetal movement was absent. Fetal death was confirmed next day.

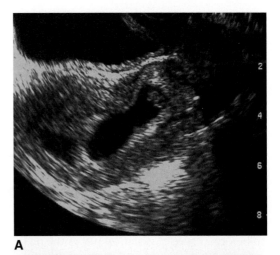

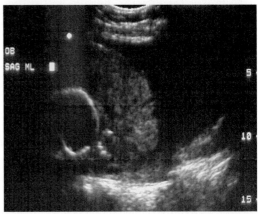

Fig. 21-10 This 34-year-old patient had history of two prior cesarean sections and was seen with bleeding in first trimester. Ultrasound **(A)** shows irregularity in anterior uterine wall with thinning of myometrium in region. In early second trimester, placenta previa was identified **(B)** in addition to multiple venous lakes. Patient had massive blood loss at time of delivery.

placenta previa, multiparity, advanced maternal age, D&C, prior manual removal of the placenta, endometritis, and adenomyosis.[32] A history of C-section plus the identification of placenta previa carries a 25% chance of placenta accreta.[33] Because of the association of placenta previa, patients may have bleeding. Patients with placenta percreta invading the bladder may also have hematuria.

Complications of placenta accreta include significant hemorrhage, which leads to maternal morbidity and mortality. In fact, placenta accreta is a leading predisposing factor of profound obstetric hemorrhage (Fig. 21-10) that leads to pregnancy-related death.[34] In

addition, hysterectomy may be necessary in cases of severe blood loss as may bladder resection in cases where placenta percreta invades the bladder wall.

Sonographic Findings. Sonographic protocol should include a survey of the retroplacental complex when patients have a history of prior C-section and placenta previa. The hypoechoic retroplacental complex represents the decidua basalis and uterine myometrium and should measure 9.5 mm in thickness.[30] Placenta accreta is suggested with a thinning or loss of the retroplacental complex (see Fig. 21-7). Large venous lakes within the placental substance may also be identified, and a disruption of the linear echogenic interface between the uterine serosa and posterior bladder wall may be shown. Ultrasound may also show the projection of the placenta into or through the bladder wall. Color Doppler or power Doppler may be useful in definition of the hypervascularity of the venous lakes and the border between the placenta and retroplacental complex.

Cervical Incompetence

Cervical incompetence occurs in 0.05% to 2% of deliveries and may lead to recurrent pregnancy loss in the second and third trimesters of pregnancy.[35] Cervical incompetence may be diagnosed when the cervix is dilated in the absence of contractions of the uterus.[36] Studies have shown that a cervical length of less than 25 mm before 27 weeks' gestation places the pregnancy at increased risk for preterm delivery and subsequent neonatal morbidity.[37] Risk factors include a previous preterm delivery and a prior second trimester miscarriage and, to a lesser extent, low maternal age (<20 years), cigarette smoking, vaginal bleeding, and multiple pregnancy terminations.[35] Other risk factors, including diethylstilbestrol exposure, cervical cone biopsy, and prior cervical trauma, have been documented.[36] Sonography can be used in evaluation of the cervix in women at high risk of preterm delivery. The sonographic findings, patient history, and symptoms can then be used in the development of a management plan that may include expectant management, cerclage placement, or bed rest. Intervention with identification of a shortened cervix can improve the perinatal outcome.

Sonographic Findings. Obstetric ultrasound protocol includes imaging of the lower uterine segment of the uterus and documentation of the cervical length (Fig. 21-11). Transabdominal imaging of the cervix may be limited, and endovaginal or translabial imaging should then be used to ensure adequate resolution. Translabial imaging may be used, but because of the increased resolution with endovaginal imaging, it may be reserved for patients with active bleeding or premature rupture of membranes.[38] In addition, ultrasound may be used to follow a patient for evaluation of the success of a cerclage.

Measurements of the cervical length should be from the internal to external cervical os. The mean cervical length with endovaginal imaging is 3.2 cm to 4.8 cm.[7] Cervical incompetence should be considered when the cervix measures less than 3 cm. The application of fundal pressure or scanning with the patient standing may aid in identification of patients who would otherwise go without diagnosis. In addition, imaging of the cervix at the beginning of the ultrasound examination may identify those patients with a cervix that may return

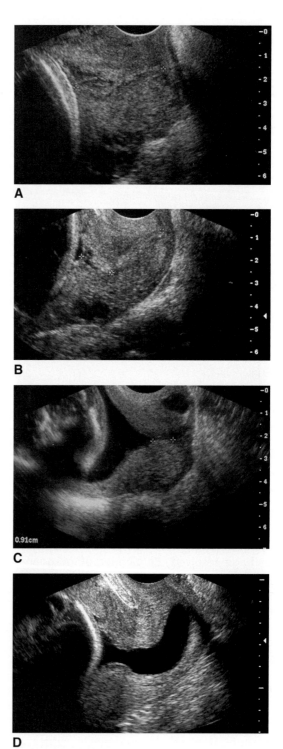

Fig. 21-11 **A,** Example of normal cervix measuring 3.8 cm imaged with endovaginal technique. **B,** Normal cervix was not straight, so two sets of calipers were used to derive correct measurement of 4.4 cm. **C,** Patient was seen with cervical length of 0.91 cm. She underwent cerclage placement and was placed on bedrest. **D,** Patient was seen with open cervix.

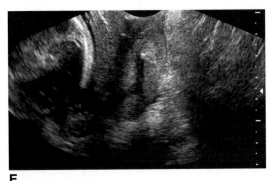

Fig. 21-11, cont'd E, One week later, with cerclage placement and bedrest, closed cervix is identified.

to a normal length during the course of an obstetric ultrasound. Cervical changes may also include identification of beaking or funneling of the cervix.

POSTPARTUM BLEEDING

Retained Products of Conception

Postpartum hemorrhage is the most common complication of the uterus after delivery. Abnormal postpartum bleeding is defined as heavy bleeding after the first 24 hours and may be evaluated sonographically for diagnosis of retained products of conception.[39] In addition, products of conception may be retained after abortion. The patient may undergo conservative treatment, but when conservative treatment fails, D&C or hysteroscopy may be necessary.[40]

Sonographic Findings. An echogenic mass within the endometrial cavity in a postpartum uterus suggests retained products of conception (Fig. 21-12). Post-abortion sonographic findings may also include bony remnants that are highly echogenic and shadow. Importantly, retained placental tissue may have a similar appearance to blood clots (Fig. 21-13), so a positive finding may be relatively insignificant and resolve without further intervention.[40]

SUMMARY

Sonography can be used to aid in the diagnosis of the multiple causes of abnormal bleeding that vary depending on the gestational age. Sonographic findings can assist in the development of a treatment plan that may prevent further complications and decrease maternal morbidity and mortality and when feasible, lower perinatal morbidity and mortality as well.

Table 21-1 is a summary of the pathology for bleeding with pregnancy.

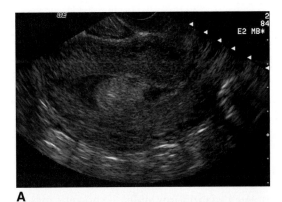

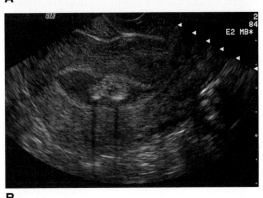

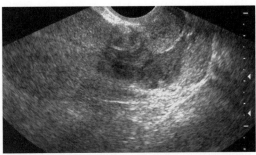

Fig. 21-12 Retained products of conception. **A,** Echogenic mass is identified within endometrium. **B,** Some bony remnants with shadowing are also identified. (**A** and **B** Courtesy GE Medical Systems.)

Fig. 21-13 Patient with persistent bleeding after cesarean section. Large hematoma is identified within uterus and extending into uterine excision site.

CLINICAL SCENARIO—DIAGNOSIS

■ This patient was seen with the typical sonographic appearance of a molar pregnancy with associated theca lutein cysts. Although the quantitative beta-hCG levels were not available at the time of the sonographic evaluation, they were later reported as being excessively elevated, and the mole was evacuated.

Table 21-1	*Causes for Bleeding with Pregnancy*
Diagnosis	**Sonographic Findings**
Subchorionic hemorrhage	Area of variable echogenicity adjacent to gestational sac
Missed abortion	Embryonic death without expulsion of products of conception
Spontaneous abortion	Uterus devoid of products of conception
Ectopic pregnancy	Variable appearance including: absence of normally placed gestational sac, extrauterine live embryo, ring sign, cul-de-sac fluid, uterine decidual reaction, hematosalpinx
Complete hydatidiform mole	Echogenic mass with multiple cystic areas in uterus; theca lutein cysts
Partial mole	Placental enlargement with cystic spaces; fetus or fetal parts
Mole with coexistent fetus	Normal fetus with normal placenta plus large placenta mass with cystic spaces
Placenta previa	Placenta partially or completely covering internal cervical os
Vasa previa	Vessels partially or completely covering internal os
Abruptio placenta	Variable amount of blood at margin of placenta or retroplacental; blood may appear echogenic to anechoic
Placenta accreta	Thinning of retroplacental complex; large venous lakes; disruption of uterine serosa; placental mass extending from uterus into bladder; placental hypervascularity

CASE STUDIES FOR DISCUSSION

1. A 30-year-old woman, G3 P2, is seen with bleeding at 31 weeks' gestation. She also has a history of two prior cesarean sections. Sonographic evaluation shows the finding in Fig. 21-14. What are the important considerations for this patient at the time of delivery?

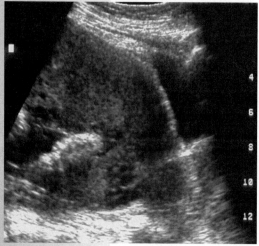

Fig. 21-14 Longitudinal image of lower uterine segment shows placenta on anterior and posterior walls of uterus.

2. A 28-year-old woman is seen with pelvic pain and significant vaginal bleeding after a medical abortion. The ultrasound findings are shown in Fig. 21-15. What is the most likely cause of the bleeding?

3. A 25-year-old woman is seen with positive home pregnancy test results, bleeding, and left lower quadrant pain. Clinical history also reveals multiple episodes of PID in the past. The ultrasound findings are revealed in Fig. 21-16. What is the most likely diagnosis?

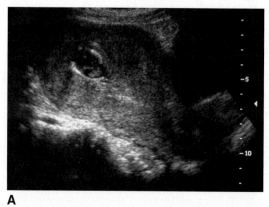

A

Fig. 21-15 A, Transabdominal and,

CASE STUDIES FOR DISCUSSION—cont'd

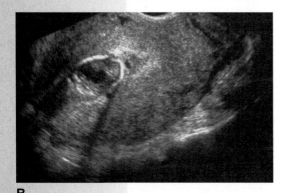

B, endovaginal images of longitudinal uterus shows well-circumscribed structure of mixed echogenicity located within endometrium. Small amount of cul-de-sac fluid is also identified.

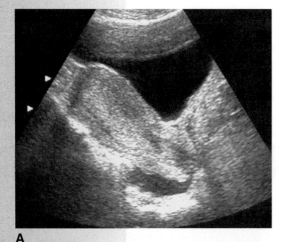

B

Fig. 21-16 **A,** Longitudinal images of uterus reveal echogenic decidual reaction within endometrium and cul-de-sac fluid. **B,** Right and left ovary were identified, and ring sign was also identified in left adnexa.

4. A 40-year-old woman, G10 P4, is seen with bleeding and cramping at 6 weeks' gestation by last menstrual period. The ultrasound reveals a small gestational sac containing a yolk sac consistent with a 5.5-week gestation. Another ultrasound is performed 10 days later for persistent bleeding and cramping. The findings are shown in Fig. 21-17. What is the most likely diagnosis?

5. A 24-year-old woman, G2 P1, is seen at 8 weeks' gestation with bleeding. Obstetric ultrasound is ordered and reveals the findings in Fig. 21-18. The ovaries are identified and are within normal limits. What is the most likely diagnosis?

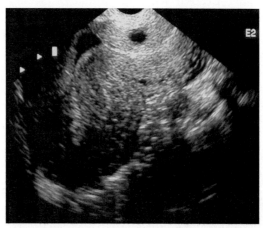

Fig. 21-17 Ultrasound examination reveals uterus without evidence of pregnancy. Small amount of fluid is seen in distal portion of endometrium. Nabothian cyst is incidentally noted in anterior cervix. Adnexae are unremarkable.

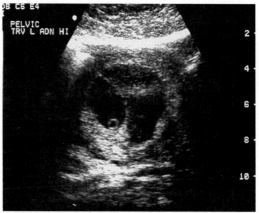

Fig. 21-18 Transverse view of uterus shows gestational sac and yolk sac. Live embryo with heart rate of 162 bpm is noted. Crown-rump length corresponding to 8²/₇ weeks is also identified. Hypoechoic crescent-shaped structure is identified at left lateral margin of gestational sac.

STUDY QUESTIONS

1. A 32-year-old woman is seen for ultrasound with positive pregnancy test results and pelvic pain. She has a history of pelvic inflammatory disease and reveals that she had difficulty becoming pregnant. The ultrasound reveals an empty uterus and a moderate amount of cul-de-sac fluid. This is most suspicious for which of the following?
   a. ectopic pregnancy
   b. missed abortion
   c. molar pregnancy
   d. spontaneous abortion
   e. threatened abortion

2. A 30-year-old pregnant woman is seen at the emergency department at 32 weeks' gestation with knifelike abdominal pain and bleeding. Ultrasound reveals a large hypoechoic collection of fluid in the retroplacental region that appears to be expanding in size during the sonographic examination. This would be consistent with which of the following?
   a. marginal abruption
   b. placenta previa
   c. placental abruption
   d. subchorionic hemorrhage
   e. vasa previa

3. A 25-year-old woman, G2 P1, is seen at the emergency department at 10 weeks' gestation with vaginal bleeding. Laboratory test results reveal a beta-hCG level of 257,000 IU/ml. An ultrasound examination is ordered to confirm which of the following?
   a. abruptio placenta
   b. ectopic pregnancy
   c. molar pregnancy
   d. placenta previa
   e. threatened abortion

4. A patient is seen with heavy bleeding 5 days after an uncomplicated delivery. Ultrasound reveals an enlarged postpartum uterus with an echogenic mass. This suggests which of the following?
   a. partial mole
   b. placenta accreta
   c. placenta percreta
   d. retained products of conception
   e. retroplacental hemorrhage

5. An 18-year-old woman is seen by her gynecologist with a 2-week history of spotting. She reports that she had positive urine pregnancy test results after a missed period 6 weeks ago. Endovaginal ultrasound examination of the uterus reveals an embryo, without a heartbeat, with measurements consistent with a 7-week gestation. This would be consistent with which of the following?
   a. abruption
   b. missed abortion
   c. spontaneous abortion
   d. subchorionic hematoma
   e. threatened abortion

6. A 40-year-old woman is seen by her obstetrician with bleeding and excessive nausea and vomiting. Clinical examination reveals a uterus consistent with a 14-week gestation that is inconsistent with her predicted 10-week gestation with last menstrual period. An ultrasound is performed and reveals a viable fetus with a crown-rump length consistent with a 9.5-week gestation. A normal placenta is identified with an adjacent large echogenic mass that contains small cystic lesions. This would be most suggestive of which of the following?
   a. choriocarcinoma
   b. complete hydatidiform mole
   c. complete mole with coexistent fetus
   d. invasive mole
   e. partial hydatidiform mole

7. A 35-year-old woman, G4 P3, is seen for an obstetric ultrasound with bleeding at 34 weeks' gestation. Endovaginal ultrasound reveals the placenta across the lower uterine segment and extending along the anterior and posterior uterine wall. This would be consistent with which of the following?
   a. complete previa
   b. low-lying placenta
   c. partial previa
   d. placenta accreta
   e. placenta increta

8. A 22-year-old pregnant woman is seen in the ultrasound department with heavy bleeding and cramping. She is 8 weeks pregnant by last menstrual period, which was confirmed with a 6-week ultrasound after an episode of spotting. The ultrasound reveals an empty uterus. This would be most consistent with which of the following?
   a. ectopic pregnancy
   b. missed abortion
   c. molar pregnancy

  d. spontaneous abortion
  e. threatened abortion

9. A 36-year-old woman, G5 P4, is seen for an obstetric ultrasound at 31 weeks' gestation for late prenatal care. Patient history includes two prior cesarean sections and otherwise uneventful pregnancies. The sonographer notes an anterior placenta with partial previa. The sonographer should also look for which of the following abnormal findings?
  a. abruptio placenta
  b. partial mole
  c. placenta accreta
  d. subchorionic hemorrhage
  e. vasa previa

10. A patient is seen with pain and spotting at 7 weeks' gestation. Ultrasound confirms a viable intrauterine pregnancy consistent with the patient's last menstrual period. A mild to moderate amount of cul-de-sac fluid is identified, and an adnexal ring sign is imaged in the left adnexal region. Which of the following diagnoses most accurately describes the sonographic finding described?
  a. cornual ectopic
  b. heterotopic gestation
  c. mole with coexistent fetus
  d. spontaneous abortion
  e. tubal pregnancy

REFERENCES

1. Seki H, Kuromaki K, Takeda S et al: Persistent subchorionic hematoma with clinical symptoms until delivery, *Int J Gynecol Obstet* 63:123-128, 1998.
2. Sepulveda W, Aviles G, Carstens E et al: Prenatal diagnosis of solid placental masses: the value of color flow imaging, *Ultrasound Obstet Gynecol* 16:554-558, 2000.
3. Sieroszewski P, Suzin J, Bernaschek G et al: Evaluation of first trimester pregnancy in cases of threatened abortion by means of Doppler sonography, *Ultraschall Med* 22:208-212, 2001.
4. Brigham SA, Conlon C, Farquharson RG: A longitudinal study of pregnancy outcome following idiopathic recurrent miscarriage, *Hum Reprod* 14:2868-2871, 1999.
5. Jirous J et al: A correlation of the uterine and ovarian blood flows with parity of nonpregnant women having a history of recurrent spontaneous abortions, *Gynecol Obstet Invest* 52:51-54, 2001.
6. Ball RH: The sonography of pregnancy loss, *Semin Reprod Med* 18:351-355, 2000.
7. Callen PW: *Ultrasonography in obstetrics and gynecology,* ed 4, Philadelphia, 2000, WB Saunders.
8. Hagen-Ansert SL: *Textbook of diagnostic ultrasonography,* ed 5, St Louis, 2001, Mosby.
9. Gracia CR, Barnhart KT: Diagnosing ectopic pregnancy: decision analysis comparing six strategies, *Obstet Gynecol* 97:464-470, 2001.
10. Botash RJ, Spirt BA: Ectopic pregnancy: review and update, *Appl Radiol* January:7-12, 2000.
11. Hafner T, Aslam N, Ross JA et al: The effectiveness of non-surgical management of early interstitial pregnancy: a report of ten cases and review of the literature, *Ultrasound Obstet Gynecol* 13:131-136, 1999.
12. Lawrence A, Jurdovic D: Three-dimensional ultrasound diagnosis of interstitial pregnancy, *Ultrasound Obstet Gynecol* 14:292-293, 1999.
13. Su YN, Shih JC, Chiu WH et al: Cervical pregnancy: assessment with three-dimensional power Doppler imaging and successful management with selective uterine artery embolization, *Ultrasound Obstet Gynecol* 14:284-287, 1999.
14. Pascual MA, Ruiz J, Tresserra F et al: Cervical ectopic twin pregnancy: diagnosis and conservative treatment, *Hum Reprod* 16:584-586, 2001.
15. Delabrousse E, Site O, Le Mouel A et al: Intrahepatic pregnancy: sonography and CT findings, *AJR Am J Roentgenol* 173:1377-1378, 1999.
16. Albers E, Daneshmand S, Hull A: Placental pathology casebook, *J Perinatol* 21:72-75, 2001.
17. Jauniaux E, Bersinger NA, Gulbis B et al: The contribution of maternal serum markers in the early prenatal diagnosis of molar pregnancies, *Hum Reprod* 14:842-846, 1999.
18. Gemer O, Segal S, Kopmar A et al: The current clinical presentation of complete molar pregnancy, *Arch Gynecol Obstet* 264:33-34, 2000.
19. Jauniaux E: Ultrasound diagnosis and follow-up of gestational trophoblastic disease, *Ultrasound Obstet Gynecol* 11:367-377, 1998.
20. Montes-de-Oca-Valero F, Marcara L, Shaker A: Twin pregnancy with a complete hydatidiform mole and co-existing fetus following in-vitro fertilization, *Hum Reprod* 14:2905-2907, 1999.
21. Winter TC, Brock BV, Fligner CL et al: Coexistent surviving neonate twin and complete hydatidiform mole, *AJR Am J Roentgenol* 172:451-453, 1999.
22. Oppenheimer L, Holmes P, Simpson N et al: Diagnosis of low-lying placenta: can migration in the third trimester predict outcome? *Ultrasound Obstet Gynecol* 18:100-102, 2001.
23. Ghourab S: Third-trimester transvaginal ultrasonography in placenta previa: does the shape of the lower placental edge predict clinical outcome? *Ultrasound Obstet Gynecol* 18:103-108, 2001.
24. Rosati P, Guariglia L: Clinical significance of placenta previa detected at early routine transvaginal scan, *J Ultrasound Med* 19:581-585, 2000.

25. Catanzarite V, Maida C, Thomas W et al: Prenatal sonographic diagnosis of vasa previa: ultrasound findings and obstetric outcome in ten cases, *Ultrasound Obstet Gynecol* 18:109-115, 2001.

26. Oyelese Y: Placenta previa and vasa previa: time to leave the Dark Ages, *Ultrasound Obstet Gynecol* 18:96-99, 2001.

27. Glantz C, Purnell L: Clinical utility of sonography in the diagnosis and treatment of placental abruption, *J Ultrasound Med* 21:837-840, 2002.

28. Arabin B, van Eyck J, Laurini RN: Hemodynamic changes with paradoxical blood flow in expectant management of abruptio placentae, *Obstet Gynecol* 91:796-798, 1998.

29. Gerig JL, Luna JA, Parsons L et al: Transient recurrent venous phenomenon: a variant of marginal placental abruption? *J Diagn Med Sonogr* 14:255-262, 1998.

30. Isaacs DL, Rouse GA, DeLange M et al: The sonographic appearance of placenta accreta, *J Diagn Med Sonogr* 14:15-20, 1998.

31. Hull AD, Salerno CC, Saenz CC et al: Three-dimensional ultrasonography and diagnosis of placenta percreta with bladder involvement, *J Ultrasound Med* 18:853-856, 1999.

32. Russ PD, Tomaszewski G, Coffin C: Pelvic varices mimicking placenta percreta at sonography, *J Diagn Med Sonogr* 16:183-188, 2000.

33. Hudon L, Belfort MA, Broome DR: Diagnosis and management of placenta percreta: a review, *Obstet Gynecol Surv* 53:509-517, 1998.

34. Chou MM, Ho ESC, Lee YH: Prenatal diagnosis of placenta previa accreta by transabdominal color Doppler ultrasound, *Ultrasound Obstet Gynecol* 15:28-35, 2000.

35. Macdonald R, Smith P, Vyas S: Cervical incompetence: the use of transvaginal sonography to provide an objective diagnosis, *Ultrasound Obstet Gynecol* 18:211-216, 2001.

36. Wong G, Levine D: Sonographic assessment of the cervix in pregnancy, *Semin Ultrasound CT MR* 19:370-380, 1998.

37. Althuisius SM, Dekker GA, Hummel P et al: Final result of the Cervical Incompetence Prevention Randomized Cerclage Trial (CIPRACT): therapeutic cerclage with bed rest versus bed rest alone, *Am J Obstet Gynecol* 185:1106-1112, 2001.

38. Hertzberg BS, Livingston E, DeLong DM et al: Ultrasonographic evaluation of the cervix, *J Ultrasound Med* 20:1071-1078, 2001.

39. Edwards A, Ellwood DA: Ultrasonographic evaluation of the postpartum uterus, *Ultrasound Obstet Gynecol* 16:640-643, 2000.

40. Wolman I, Gordon D, Yaron Y et al: Transvaginal Sonohysterography for the evaluation and treatment of retained products of conception, *Gynecol Obstet Invest* 50:73-76, 2000.

BIBLIOGRAPHY

Habana A, Dokras A, Giraldo JL et al: Cornual heterotopic pregnancy: contemporary management options, *Am J Obstet Gynecol* 182:1264-1270, 2000.

22

Multifetal Gestation

TAMARA SALSGIVER

CLINICAL SCENARIO

■ A 23-year-old woman is seen for obstetric ultrasound to check the fetal growth in a twin gestation. According to the last normal menstrual period, she is expected to be at 19 weeks' gestational age. The ultrasound confirms twins and documents a monochorionic diamniotic gestation (Fig. 22-1; see Color Plate 14). Both fetuses are male, with twin "A"

measuring 16.7 weeks with a low amniotic fluid volume and twin "B" measuring 19.3 weeks with a normal amniotic fluid volume. The cord Doppler on twin A shows a reversal of diastolic flow with a normal flow direction. No specific fetal anomalies are identified. What is the significance of these findings?

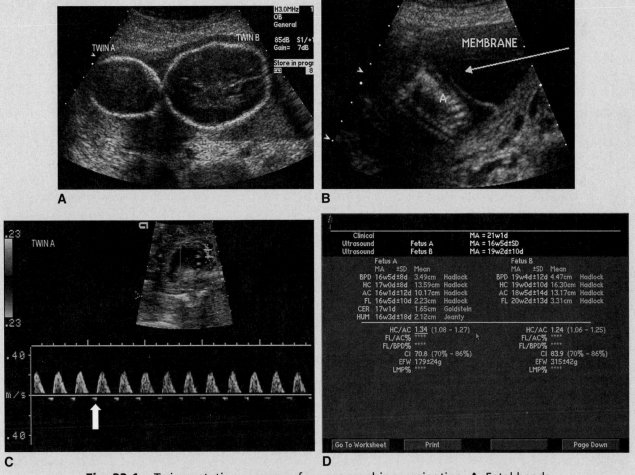

Fig. 22-1 Twin gestation was seen for sonographic examination. **A,** Fetal heads and, **B,** separating membrane are identified. **C,** Umbilical Doppler of twin A. **D,** Fetal biometry for twins A and B.

OBJECTIVES ■

■ Discuss the role of ultrasound in evaluation of a multifetal gestation.

■ Discuss the embryology and incidence of multifetal gestations.

■ Describe the sonographic criteria used in evaluation of the zygosity, chorionicity, and amnionicity in a multifetal gestation.

■ Describe the sonographic approach used in the assessment of gestational age, fetal growth, amniotic fluid, and anatomy in a multifetal gestation.

■ Describe the sonographic findings associated with the more common complications that affect multifetal gestations, including hydramnios, premature labor, intrauterine growth restriction, vanishing twin phenomenon, fetus papyraceus, conjoined twinning, twin-twin transfusion syndrome, and twin reversed arterial perfusion sequence.

GLOSSARY OF TERMS ■

Acardia: a rare congenital anomaly in which the heart is absent; condition is sometimes seen in a conjoined twin whose survival depends on the circulatory system of its twin

Alpha fetoprotein: a glycoprotein synthesized by the embryonic liver that is measured in the mother's blood to screen for neural tube defects or chromosomal abnormalities

Anastomosis: a connection between two vessels

Amnion: a membrane, continuous with and covering the fetal side of the placenta, that forms the outer surface of the umbilical cord

Amnionicity: refers to the number of amniotic membranes

Beta human chorionic gonadotropin: a laboratory test used for quantification of the amount of circulating human chorionic gonadotropin, which is the "pregnancy hormone" secreted by the placental trophoblastic cells that keeps the corpus luteum producing progesterone once conception occurs

Chorion: the outermost extraembryonic membrane composed of trophoblast lined with mesoderm; it gives rise to the placenta and persists until birth as the outer of the two layers of membrane surrounding the amniotic fluid and the fetus

Chorionicity: refers to the number of chorionic membranes, which relates to the number of placentas that will develop

Cleavage: a series of repeated mitotic cell divisions that occurs in an ovum immediately after fertilization

Diamniotic: a twin pregnancy with two separate amniotic membranes (sacs)

Dichorionic: a twin pregnancy with two separate chorionic membranes (placentas)

Discordant growth: refers to twins with a marked difference in size (>20% difference in weight) at birth; condition is usually caused by an overperfusion of one twin and an underperfusion of the other twin and usually affects monochorionic twins

Fetal hydrops: refers to fluid accumulation in serous cavities or edema of soft tissue in the fetus

Gestational age: the age of a fetus, usually expressed in weeks, dating from the first day of the mother's last normal menstrual period; conceptual age plus 2 weeks

High-order multiple pregnancy: pregnancy with three or more fetuses

Hydramnios, or polyhydramnios: an abnormal condition of pregnancy characterized by an excess of amniotic fluid

Hyperemesis gravidarum: an abnormal condition of pregnancy characterized by protracted vomiting, weight loss, and fluid and electrolyte imbalance

Intrauterine growth restriction: an abnormal process in which the development and maturation of the fetus are impeded or delayed more than two deviations below the mean for gestational age, gender, and ethnicity

In vitro fertilization: a method of fertilization of human ova outside the body with collection of the mature ova and placement in a dish with a sample of spermatozoa; after an incubation period of 48 to 72 hours, the fertilized ova are injected into the uterus through the cervix

Monoamniotic: a twin pregnancy with sharing of one amniotic membrane (sac)

Monochorionic: a twin pregnancy with sharing of one chorionic membrane (placenta)

GLOSSARY OF TERMS—cont'd ▰▰▰

Monozygotic: pertaining to or derived from one zygote

Multifetal: more than one fetus

Oligohydramnios: an abnormally small amount or absence of amniotic fluid

Ovulation induction: the process of stimulation of the development of follicles on the ovary

Placental abruption: a separation of the placenta in a pregnancy of 20 weeks or more or during labor before delivery of the fetus

Placental insufficiency: a decreased function of the placenta sufficient to compromise fetal nutrition and oxygen

Placenta previa: a condition of pregnancy in which the placenta is implanted abnormally in the uterus so that it impinges on or covers the internal os of the uterine cervix

Placentation: refers to the formation of the placenta

Preeclampsia: an abnormal condition of pregnancy characterized by the onset of acute hypertension after 24 weeks' gestation; the classic triad of preeclampsia is hypertension, proteinuria, and edema

Stuck twin: a diamniotic pregnancy in which one fetus remains pressed against the uterine wall in a severely oligohydramniotic sac while the other twin is in a severely hydramniotic sac

Triple screen: a laboratory test that measures not only alpha fetoprotein but also human chorionic gonadotropin and estriol; this test is more accurate than testing of alpha fetoprotein alone and screens for additional genetic problems

Twin embolization: a situation in which fetal death of a twin in the second or third trimester results in the fetus passing a clot through the placental circulation to the other twin

Yolk sac: a structure that develops in the inner cell mass of the embryo and expands into a vesicle with a thick part that grows into the cavity of the chorion; after it supplies the nourishment of the embryo, the yolk sac usually disappears during the seventh week after conception

Zygote: a combined cell produced by the union of a spermatozoa and an oocyte at the completion of fertilization until the first cleavage

Zygosity: refers to the number of oocytes released from an ovary and fertilized by spermatozoa

---

The incidence rate of twin and high-order multiple gestations has increased fivefold over the past 20 years.[1] In the past 5 years alone, twin births in the United States occurred at a rate of approximately one in 34 pregnancies, and triplet rates approximated only one in 602.[1] The rates of quadruplet and quintuplet births were lower, with rates of 1 in 8021 and 1 in 52,712 pregnancies, respectively.[1] This increase is thought to be the result of the widespread use of assisted reproductive technology (e.g., **ovulation induction, in vitro fertilization**) and an aging maternal population.[1] Identification of **multifetal** pregnancies is important because of the significantly increased risk for both mother and fetus. Early identification of these pregnancies allows careful screening for complications. Of greatest risk are high-order multiple pregnancies and gestations in which the fetuses share a single placenta.

Before the use of ultrasound in evaluation of obstetric patients, as many as 60% of twins went undiagnosed prenatally.[2] **Placentation** had to be determined postpartum, which meant fetuses at greatest risk for complications could not receive effective management. The use of ultrasound for imaging revolutionized the care of patients with multifetal pregnancies. With sonography, demonstration of the form of twinning that has occurred, assessment of fetal growth and well-being, and screening for common complications are now possible during and throughout the pregnancy. Patient evaluation for a multifetal gestation should be initiated whenever a history of ovulation induction exists, a patient measures large for **gestational age,** two separate heart beats are heard, or laboratory screening tests, such as **beta human chorionic gonadotropin** (beta-hCG), maternal serum **alpha fetoprotein, triple screen,** are abnormally elevated.[2]

As standard imaging protocols for multifetal gestations in the first, second, and third trimesters are discussed, it should be kept in mind that the major causes of adverse outcome are prematurity and **intrauterine growth restriction** (IUGR).[3] **Placental insufficiency** leading to IUGR or **discordant growth** is an especially high risk in monochorionic pregnancies.

IMAGING PROTOCOL

With evaluation of a multifetal pregnancy, establishment of the type of twinning that has occurred is important. This evaluation is best accomplished by counting the number of fetuses, placentas, and amniotic sacs. Determination of fetal gender is also important because twins of opposite gender are unquestionably dizygotic and are, therefore, at a lower risk. Twins of the same gender are of indeterminate **zygosity**. In this case, establishment of **chorionicity** and **amnionicity** is important. Amnionicity and chorionicity are best determined by counting the number of fetal poles, chorionic sacs, and amniotic membranes, which is easiest to accomplish in the first trimester when the number of **yolk sacs** can be evaluated and the **amnion** can clearly be differentiated from the **chorion**. A note of caution: the presence of a multifetal pregnancy should only be determined after 6 weeks' gestational age because a high risk of undercounting gestational numbers exists before this age.[4]

In the first trimester, counting should begin with the number of gestational sacs. When scanning through the rectus abdominis muscles, one should watch for a refraction artifact. This artifact may cause a single gestational sac to appear sonographically as twin gestational sacs; twin gestational sacs should always be confirmed with scanning in two planes. Once a fetal pole can be identified (~6 to 7 weeks' gestational age), the number of fetal poles along with the presence or absence of cardiac activity should be documented. Each fetal pole should be labeled as fetus A, fetus B, fetus C, etc., with the fetus closest to the cervix labeled as A, the second closest as B, then C, etc. Documentation of the number of yolk sacs identified is also important because this may indicate the number of amnions that are present before the amniotic membrane can be seen clearly.[5] Once the amniotic membrane can be seen sonographically (~7 to 8 weeks' gestational age),[5] the number of amnions identified should be documented. The early amniotic membrane is best visualized surrounding the dorsal aspect of the fetus.

A **dichorionic, diamniotic** gestation exists when two separate gestational sacs are identified.[3] Sonographic determination of whether the twins are dizygotic or monozygotic is not possible unless opposite fetal genders can be confirmed later in the pregnancy, which would differentiate this as a dizygotic twinning.

A **monozygotic** pregnancy that is monochorionic and diamniotic exists if only one gestational sac with two yolk sacs and two fetal poles is identified.[5]

A monozygotic pregnancy that is most likely **monochorionic** and **monoamniotic** exists when only one gestational sac with one yolk sac and two fetal poles is identified.[5]

A second- or third-trimester pregnancy is much more difficult to evaluate than a first-trimester pregnancy because the fetuses have grown significantly and determination of which extremities belong to which fetus can be difficult. In the second and third trimester, the number of fetuses should be determined by counting the number of fetal heads. Complete scanning through the uterus in two planes is important so the number of fetuses is not undercounted. With evaluation of fetal dates and anatomy, it is important to begin at the fetal head and follow the fetal trunk to the extremities. This minimizes the confusion of fetal measurements. Determination of chorionicity and amnionicity after the first trimester is also considerably more difficult because the gestational sacs have grown closer together, making it difficult to distinguish whether there is a single chorionic sac or two separate sacs. At this point, chorionicity and amnionicity must be determined by checking the fetal gender, counting the number of placental sites, and evaluating the interfetal membrane.[3,5]

Evaluation of Fetal Gender

If two fetuses of opposite gender (i.e., one male and one female fetus) are identified, they are unquestionably dizygotic twins and the gestation is dichorionic and diamniotic.

If two fetuses of the same gender (i.e., two female fetuses or two male fetuses) are identified, they are of indeterminate zygosity. They may be either dizygotic or monozygotic twins, and therefore, chorionicity and amnionicity cannot be concluded from this information alone. The amnionicity and chorionicity must be carefully evaluated with a look at the placental sites and the interfetal membrane.

Evaluation of Placental Sites

A dichorionic, diamniotic gestation exists if two separate placentas can clearly be identified.

With identification of only one placenta, the placenta should be scanned through carefully because two placentas in close proximity may fuse, sonographically appearing as one. For better evaluation of the placenta, the fetal umbilical cords should be followed to where they insert into the placenta. Once the two cord insertion sites can be seen in the same plane, one should look for the presence of an interfetal membrane. If no membrane exists between the cord insertion sites (Fig. 22-2, *A*), the twins are most likely monozygotic

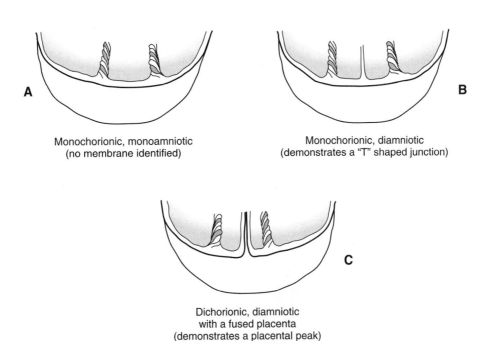

Fig. 22-2 **A,** No membrane is identified between two umbilical cord insertion sites, which represents monochorionic, monoamniotic placentation. **B,** Intertwin membrane is followed to its junction with placenta. When junction appears flat or T shaped, a true monochorionic placentation that is diamniotic is indicated. **C,** Thick, four-layer membrane is followed to its junction with placenta where triangular extension of placental tissue is noted. This represents twin peak sign, which indicates dichorionic placentation in which placentas have fused together.[3,5]

and the gestation is monochorionic and monoamniotic. If an interfetal membrane can be found, one should look at the point where the membrane meets the placenta. If the placental tissue extends a short distance along the membrane forming a triangular peak (Fig. 22-2, *B*), the gestation is most likely dichorionic and diamniotic.[3,5] If the point where the membrane meets the placenta is flat, with more of a T-shaped appearance (Fig. 22-2, *C*), a true monochorionic gestation that is diamniotic would be indicated.[5]

Evaluation of the Interfetal Membrane

If only one placenta is seen and a membrane separating the two fetuses cannot be identified, most likely a **monozygotic** pregnancy that is monochorionic and monoamniotic exists.

If the interfetal membrane is greater than 2 mm in thickness or four distinct layers (amnion-chorion-chorion-amnion) can be differentiated within the membrane, the gestation is most likely dichorionic and diamniotic.[5] The chorionicity should be confirmed with evaluation of the placenta/membrane junction.

If the interfetal membrane is less than 1 mm in thickness and only two layers (chorion-amnion) can be identified, the pregnancy is most likely monozygotic

and monochorionic and diamniotic.[5] The chorionicity should be confirmed with evaluation of the placenta/membrane junction.

It is important to note that high-order multiple gestations occur as combinations of monozygotic and dizygotic twinning. For example, a patient undergoing in vitro fertilization may have two embryos placed in the uterine cavity; both may implant and one may split, resulting in triplets that are trichorionic (three placentas) or dichorionic, with two fetuses sharing one placenta and one fetus with its own placenta. From this example, it is evident that many combinations can occur. In the face of a high-order multifetal gestation, each gestational sac should be evaluated individually. Once again, the number of gestational sacs, the number of fetal poles, the presence or absence of cardiac activity, and the number of amniotic membranes identified should be documented.

EMBRYOLOGY OF TWINNING

The zygosity, chorionicity, and amnionicity can better be understood with a look at the embryology of twinning (Fig. 22-3). Twins arise from one of two scenarios: either two ova are released by the mother in

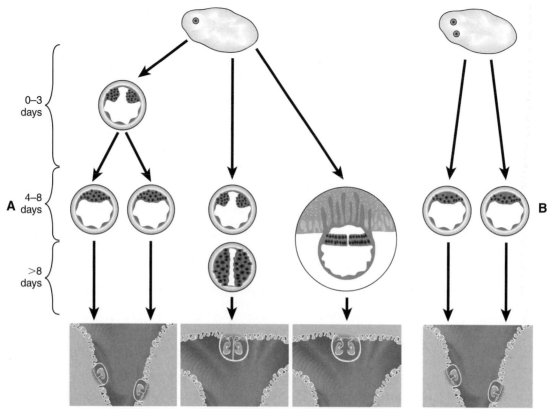

Fig. 22-3 Embryology of twinning. **A,** Monozygotic twinning: single ovum is fertilized and divides, forming two separate embryos. Division occurring before day 4 results in dichorionic, diamniotic gestation.[2,5] Division occurring between days 4 and 8 results in monochorionic, diamniotic gestation. Division occurring after day 8 results in monochorionic, monoamniotic gestation. **B,** Dizygotic twinning: two separate ova are released in same cycle and fertilized, resulting in dichorionic, diamniotic gestation.

the same menstrual cycle and fertilized by separate spermatozoa or one ovum is released and fertilized by a single spermatozoa, subsequently splitting to form two separate embryos (Table 22-1).

Dizygotic, or fraternal, twins are siblings who were conceived at the same time. They are completely individual and have separate placentas and separate amniotic sacs. They are, therefore, always dichorionic and diamniotic. Dizygotic twins can be of the same gender or have opposite genders. Approximately 70% of twins are dizygotic,[3] and only half of these have opposite genders.[3,5] In a case in which the twins are of the same gender, gender alone does not aid in the differentiation of dizygotic and monozygotic twins.

Monozygotic, or identical, twins result from the fertilization of a single ovum. Only 30% of twins are monozygotic.[3] They are genetically identical and are, therefore, always the same gender. Their chorionicity and amnionicity are determined by the time at which

cleavage occurs. As a general rule, once tissue has differentiated, it is no longer capable of division.[2,5] The chorion normally differentiates at 4 days after conception, and the amnion differentiates around day 8.[2,5] If cleavage occurs before day 4, the pregnancy is dichorionic and diamniotic.[2,5] If cleavage occurs between days 4 and 8, the pregnancy is monochorionic and diamniotic. Cleavage after day 8 results in a pregnancy that is monochorionic and monoamniotic.[2,5] Very rarely, cleavage may occur as late as 13 days after conception, resulting in an incomplete separation of the twins. These twins, known as *conjoined twins,* are physically fused and often share internal organs.[2,5] Most monozygotic twins are monochorionic and diamniotic.[3] Twins that share a placenta are not only at risk for preterm birth, IUGR, and fetal anomalies but are also subject to complications that are unique to monochorionic twins. These complications center on the fact that the placenta may have a vascular **anastomosis** between the circulations of the

Table 22-1	*Embryology of Twinning*		
Twinning	**Chorionicity**	**Etiology**	**Sonographic Findings**
Monozygotic	Dichorionic, diamniotic	Single conception dividing 0 to 3 days after conception	Two completely separate gestational sacs identified in first trimester; two separate placentas identified in second or third trimester with membrane identified between fetuses. In condition in which placentas have fused, identification of twin peak sign can identify dichorionic placentation.
	Monochorionic, diamniotic	Single conception dividing 4 to 8 days after conception	One gestational sac identified in first trimester with two distinct yolk sacs and membrane identified between embryos; single placenta identified in second or third trimester with membrane identified between fetuses.
	Monochorionic, monoamniotic	Single conception dividing >8 days after conception	One gestational sac identified in first trimester with single yolk sac and no membrane identified between embryos; single placenta identified in second or third trimester with no membrane identified between fetuses or umbilical cord insertions into placenta.
Dizygotic	Dichorionic, diamniotic	Two separate oocytes fertilized by two separate spermatozoa	Two completely separate gestational sacs identified in first trimester; two separate placentas identified in second or third trimester with membrane identified between fetuses. In condition in which placentas have fused, identification of twin peak sign can identify dichorionic placentation. Opposite fetal genders (one male, one female) can confirm dizygotic twins.

two fetuses. The anastomosis may be artery-to-artery, artery-to-vein, or vein-to-vein.[3,5] Monochorionic twins with vascular anastomosis may have twin-twin transfusion syndrome, twin reversed arterial perfusion (TRAP) sequence, or **twin embolization** develop. An additional complication, cord entanglement, may occur with monochorionic/monoamniotic twins.[2,3,5]

COMPLICATIONS
Hydramnios and Oligohydramnios

The term *hydramnios* is used to describe an excessive accumulation of amniotic fluid, and the term *oligohydramnios* is used to describe a decreased amount of amniotic fluid. Any disturbance in the normal amount of amniotic fluid warrants a careful search for fetal abnormalities. The assessment of amniotic fluid is more challenging in multifetal gestations than in singleton

pregnancies. In a diamniotic pregnancy, a subjective evaluation of amniotic fluid (Fig. 22-4) should be made. (Do both amniotic sacs appear to be of equal size with an adequate amount of amniotic fluid?)

A quantitative assessment of amniotic fluid volume in a diamniotic gestation can be difficult and may be evaluated with measurement of the single largest vertical pocket within each gestational sac or with a traditional four-quadrant amniotic fluid index (AFI).[5] The AFI in a diamniotic gestation can be accomplished with dividing each sac (rather than the uterus) into four quadrants and measuring the quadrants within the sac in the same manner that the uterine quadrants would be measured in a singleton gestation. In a diamniotic pregnancy in which the larger twin is in a sac with excessive amniotic fluid and the smaller twin is in a sac with a low amount of amniotic fluid, the smaller fetus may appear to be "stuck" to the uterine wall and is

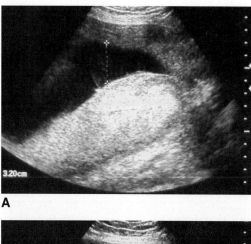

A

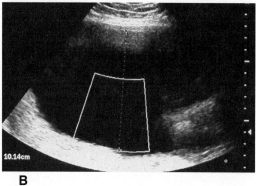

B

Fig. 22-4 Amniotic fluid levels in sacs of diamniotic pregnancy vary greatly from, **A,** one sac (single pocket of 3.2 cm) to, **B,** other (single pocket of 10.1 cm).

known as a *stuck twin*. This may be a case of twin-twin transfusion syndrome.[3,5]

Premature Labor

Prematurity and low birth weight are major contributing factors to the increased morbidity and mortality found in multifetal gestations.[5] The average length of pregnancy for a singleton gestation is 39 weeks, but twin, triplet, and quadruplet gestations normally average 35, 33, and 29 weeks, respectively.[5] Premature labor in multifetal gestations is thought to occur because of an increased uterine volume. Twin pregnancies are five times more likely than singleton pregnancies to be complicated by premature labor, and the risk for triplet gestations is 10 times higher.[5] The role of sonography in these patients is evaluation of the cervical length for thinning. As in a singleton pregnancy, a cervical length of less than 2.5 cm or a "funneling" at the internal cervical os would be considered significant.[5]

Intrauterine Growth Restriction

The birth weight of twins statistically averages 10% less than the birth weight of singletons of comparable gestational age. Because 25% to 30% of twins are considered

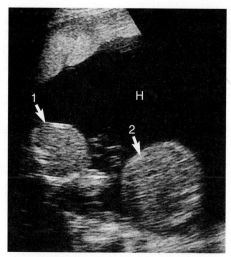

Fig. 22-5 Discordant growth is shown in comparison of abdominal sizes of twins.

to have growth restriction, evaluation of fetal measurements and growth for any discordance is important.[5] With universally accepted fetal biometric measurements (biparietal diameter [BPD], head circumference [HC], abdominal circumference [AC], and femur length [FL]), the estimated fetal weight for each twin should be calculated and compared with norms for the gestational age. A fetal weight below the 10th percentile is suggestive of IUGR, especially in the setting of oligohydramnios.[2,5] Of concern would be any noticeable discordance in estimated fetal weight between the twins. The growth of twins is considered discordant (Fig. 22-5) if the difference in their birth weights is greater than 20% of the larger twin's weight.[2,5] Other factors that have been reported as predictive of discordance include a difference in BPD of 6 mm, a difference in AC of 20 mm, and a difference in FL of 5 mm.[2] If the growth of the twins is not as expected, the cause of the growth disturbance should be investigated.

ABNORMAL TWINNING
Vanishing Twin

Multifetal pregnancies are at an increased risk for spontaneous loss of one or more embryos, especially in the first trimester. With the increased resolution available with transvaginal ultrasound, multifetal pregnancies can be confirmed as early as 6 weeks' gestational age. Statistically, however, only 30% to 60% of the early twin pregnancies detected sonographically result in the birth of twins.[3,5] In approximately 20% of twin gestations diagnosed in the first trimester, one twin dies, leaving behind an empty sac. This twin and its gestational sac

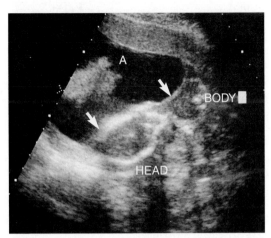

Fig. 22-6 Death of twin *(arrows)* resulted in it being flattened against uterine wall like paper doll.

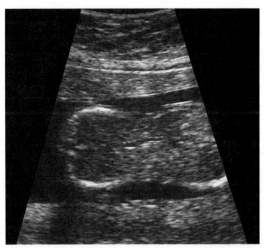

Fig. 22-7 Image shows conjoining of omphalopagus twins.

may be completely reabsorbed, disappearing altogether. This is known as a *vanishing twin*.[3] When the death of a twin occurs later, the fetus may not completely reabsorb but persists as fetus papyraceus.

Fetus Papyraceus

Fetal papyraceus may be defined as a twin fetus that has died in utero, early in development, and has been pressed flat against the uterine wall (Fig. 22-6) by the living fetus. In this case, co-twin demise in a diamniotic pregnancy results in reabsorption of the amniotic fluid around the dead twin. The dead twin appears as an amorphous structure along the wall of the uterus. Little or no amniotic fluid is seen in the sac surrounding this fetus. Provided the twins are dichorionic, the surviving twin can continue to grow unaffected. If, however, co-twin death occurs in a monochorionic pregnancy, death of the co-twin may result in embolization of thrombus across the placental vascular anastomosis to the surviving twin. This may result in renal, hepatic, and cerebral damage in the surviving twin.[5,6] The surviving twin should be checked for signs of twin embolization syndrome. Twin embolization syndrome in the surviving twin may manifest as ventriculomegaly, porencephalic cysts, diffuse cerebral atrophy, microcephaly, hepatic and splenic infarcts, gut atresias, renal cortical necrosis, pulmonary infarcts, facial anomalies, and terminal limb defects.[5,6]

Conjoined Twins

Conjoined twins are monozygotic twins that are physically united at birth. This is a rare anomaly that occurs in only one of 50,000 to 100,000 births.[5] Conjoined twins result from a late and incomplete division of the embryonic disk.[2,5] Most cases of conjoined twins have symmetry of the joined regions and are classified by the part at which they are joined. For example, twins who are joined at the head are termed *craniopagus* ("cranio" pertaining to the head, and "pagus" meaning joined or fused). *Thoracopagus* twins are joined at the thorax, and *omphalopagus* twins (Fig. 22-7) are joined at the anterior mid trunk. Conjoined twins should be suspected when monoamniotic twins do not move away from each other and can be confirmed when fusion of the fetal parts is identified. Evaluation with color-flow Doppler may be helpful. With assessment of a set of conjoined twins, evaluation of the degree of organ sharing and screening for additional malformations are important.

Twin-Twin Transfusion Syndrome

Twin-twin transfusion syndrome is caused by a shunting of blood from one twin to the other. This occurs in approximately 5% to 30% of monochorionic twins and results from an arteriovenous communication in the shared placenta.[3] The "donor" twin pumps blood from its arterial system into the venous system of the "recipient" twin. The donor twin receives less blood and is usually growth restricted, hypovolemic, and anemic. The recipient twin, on the other hand, receives too much blood and, although it may be normal in size, is often macrosomic and hypervolemic. The extra work placed on the recipient twin's heart by all of the extra blood flow can result in **fetal hydrops** or heart failure.[2] Monochorionic twins should be evaluated with serial examinations for growth because placental insufficiency and twin-twin transfusion syndrome are often not apparent until later in the gestation.[5]

Sonographic findings suggestive of twin-twin transfusion syndrome would include the identification of a true monochorionic pregnancy and a marked discrepancy in fetal size (>20% of the larger twin's weight), with the smaller twin in a sac with oligohydramnios and the larger twin in a sac with hydramnios (see Figs. 22-4 and 22-5).[6] Often the amniotic fluid surrounding the smaller twin is so low that the twin appears to be stuck to the uterine wall. Turning the mother on her side to see whether the stuck twin will drop away from the uterine wall may assist in making the diagnosis. The identification of a fold in the amniotic membrane may also be helpful in differentiation of a discrepancy in amniotic fluid volume between the two gestational sacs.

Twin Reversed Arterial Perfusion Sequence

Twin reversed arterial perfusion (TRAP) sequence is a rare condition that complicates approximately 1% of monochorionic pregnancies. The exact pathogenesis is unknown, but the condition is thought to occur because of paired artery-to-artery and vein-to-vein anastomosis within the shared placenta.[3,6] This altered placental circulation leads to reversed blood flow in the umbilical artery, allowing venous blood to be pumped from a healthy twin to another twin who is usually malformed. The malformed twin receives unoxygenated blood directly from the healthy twin rather than oxygenated blood from the placenta. This retrograde perfusion interferes with the normal cardiac development of the malformed twin. The malformed twin is known as an *acardiac parabiotic twin* or an **acardiac** *twin* because the upper half of the body is usually poorly developed. Often, the head, cervical spine, heart, and upper limbs are absent or severely malformed. Gross skin thickening (Fig. 22-8) of the upper trunk and neck areas with possible cystic hygroma may be seen.[5,6] The unoxygenated blood flowing to the malformed twin is retrograde flow coming through the umbilical arteries to the internal iliac arteries, thus supplying a limited amount of oxygen and nutrients to the torso and lower extremities of the fetus. This limited blood supply allows development of only the lower half of the body. Clubbing of the feet or absent toes is common.[5,6] TRAP sequence should be suspected with a twin in which the lower extremities and torso can be seen (and often are moving) but the entire fetus cannot be "laid out," sonographically speaking. Doppler identification of reversed flow in the umbilical arteries and vein of the acardiac twin will confirm the diagnosis.[5] A single umbilical artery is seen in 50% of patients affected by the TRAP sequence.[5]

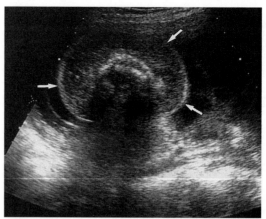

Fig. 22-8 Acardiac twin showed severe skin thickening and was grossly malformed.

MATERNAL COMPLICATIONS

Multifetal gestations carry an increased risk for the mother as well as the fetuses. Maternal complications associated with a multifetal gestation include **hyperemesis gravidarum** (excessive nausea and vomiting leading to dehydration), **preeclampsia** (pregnancy-induced hypertension with swelling), premature labor, placental abnormalities such as **placenta previa** and **placental abruption,** gestational diabetes, and maternal anemia.[1,2,7] In addition, cesarean delivery is often necessary. In patients with maternal complications, ultrasound is useful in establishing gestational age, following fetal growth, and documenting placental location.

SUMMARY

Multifetal gestations are occurring with increasing frequency. Because of the higher risk associated with multifetal gestations and the unique complications that affect these pregnancies, proficiency with the unique approach to sonographic evaluation is important. Zygosity, chorionicity, and amnionicity are most accurately determined in the first trimester. Following these pregnancies sonographically throughout the second and third trimester, however, is important because complications such as IUGR, preterm birth, and fetal anomalies occur at an increased rate in multifetal gestations. Careful screening also allows the identification of complications specific to monozygotic twins, such as twin-twin transfusion syndrome, twin embolization, conjoined twinning, TRAP sequence, and cord entanglement (Table 22-2).

Table 22-2	*Abnormal Twinning*	
Abnormality	**Etiology**	**Sonographic Findings**
Vanishing twin	Early embryonic death of one twin	Early multifetal gestation confirmed sonographically with disappearance of one twin.
Fetus papyraceus	Fetal death of one twin in diamniotic gestation with reabsorption of amniotic fluid around dead twin	Multifetal gestation in which one fetal pole appears as amorphous structure along wall of uterus. Little or no amniotic fluid is seen in sac surrounding fetus. Surviving fetus is usually unaffected.
Conjoined twins	Monozygotic twins that are physically united at birth; usually results from late and incomplete cleavage	Monochorionic, monoamniotic gestation in which twins do not move away from each other and fusion of fetal parts can be identified. Degree of organ sharing should be assessed along with continued screening for additional fetal malformations.
Twin-twin transfusion syndrome	Monochorionic gestation in which there is arteriovenous communication in shared placenta, resulting in shunting of blood from donor twin to recipient twin	Monochorionic gestation with marked discrepancy in fetal size (>20% of larger twin's estimated fetal weight). Smaller twin shows oligohydramnios, and larger twin shows hydramnios.
Twin reversed arterial perfusion sequence	Monochorionic gestation in which there is paired artery-to-artery and vein-to-vein anastomosis; altered placental circulation leads to reversal of blood flow in umbilical artery with development of malformed recipient twin	Monochorionic gestation in which one twin is acardiac with poorly developed upper body. Head, cervical spine, heart, and upper limbs may be absent or severely deformed. Lower half of body may show activity. Clubbing of feet is common. Can be confirmed by documenting reversed flow in umbilical vessels of acardiac twin.

CLINICAL SCENARIO—DIAGNOSIS

■ In this particular case, as discussed at the beginning of this chapter, it is apparent that the twins' growth is discordant. An obvious discrepancy exists in fetal size. The estimated fetal weight of twin A is well below the tenth percentile for the gestational age. This, along with the low amniotic fluid volume and reversal of diastolic flow in the cord Doppler, is suspicious for growth restriction in twin A. Compared with the estimated fetal weights of the twins, discordance is estimated at 43%. In a monochorionic pregnancy, discordance in fetal growth with the smaller twin in an oligohydramniotic sac raises the consideration of twin-twin transfusion syndrome versus IUGR of the smaller twin.

One week after the initial scan on this patient, an amniocentesis was performed to remove fluid from twin B's amniotic sac as an initial treatment of twin-twin transfusion syndrome and oligohydramnios of twin A. A specimen of fluid from twin A's sac was also obtained for karyotyping. The karyotype was normal (46,XY). The patient was referred to an out-of-state facility for laser photocoagulation of the communicating vessels; however, no communicating vessels were found. Three weeks later, twin A had no amniotic fluid and had died in utero. The twins were delivered at 26 weeks' gestational age. Twin B died 1 week later. Twin-twin transfusion syndrome was suspected.

CASE STUDIES FOR DISCUSSION

1. A 21-year-old woman is seen for a screening obstetric ultrasound. A previous ultrasound at 8 weeks documented a dichorionic, diamniotic gestation. The patient is now at 25 weeks' gestational age with her LMP. The ultrasound confirms a dichorionic gestation (Fig. 22-9; see Color Plate 15). Twin A is a female fetus measuring 25.1 weeks with a normal cord Doppler. Twin B is a male fetus measuring 20.8 weeks with an absence of diastolic flow on the cord Doppler. No specific fetal anomalies are identified; however, the amniotic fluid around twin B appears low. What is the significance of these findings?

2. A 35-year-old woman is seen for a first-trimester obstetric ultrasound (Fig. 22-10) with measurement large for dates. With the LMP, she is at approximately 8.5 weeks' gestational age. Two fetal poles with good cardiac activity are identified in a single chorionic sac. Two separate yolk sacs are identified, and two amnions can be seen. What is the significance of these findings?

3. A 28-year-old woman is seen for a first-trimester obstetric ultrasound with a history of cramping and vaginal bleeding. With the LMP, she is at approximately 6.5 weeks' gestational age. Two fetal poles (Fig. 22-11) with good cardiac activity are identified in a single chorionic sac. A single yolk sac is identified; however, it is too early to see the amnion. No evidence is found of subchorionic hemorrhage. What is the significance of these findings?

4. A 24-year-old woman is seen for a second-trimester obstetric ultrasound with a markedly elevated alpha fetoprotein. The ultrasound documents a twin gestation that is monochorionic and monoamniotic. Twin A is a normal, viable fetus (Fig. 22-12, *A*) measuring 24.2 weeks. Cardiac activity is normal at 168 bpm. The umbilical cord

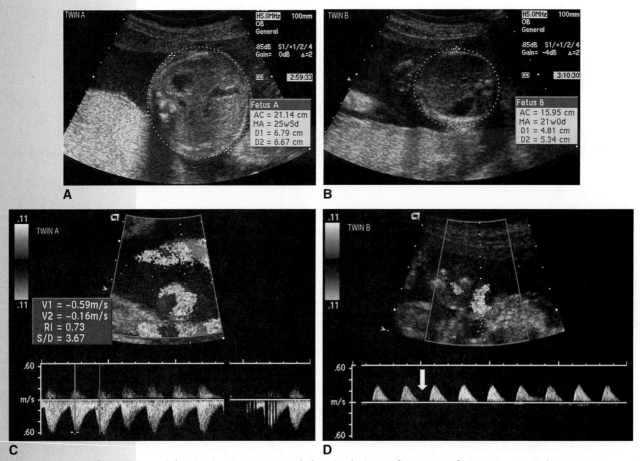

Fig. 22-9 Dichorionic pregnancy. Abdominal circumferences of, **A,** twin A and, **B,** twin B are identified, and umbilical Dopplers of, **C,** twin A and, **D,** twin B are documented.

in twin A appears to be enlarged. Twin B (Fig. 22-12, *B* and *C*) is seen with no head, heart, or upper torso. Twin B does, however, have a lower pelvis and both femurs. Active movement of fetus B is noted throughout the examination. Twin B's umbilical cord insertion site appears small but does have color flow within it. What is the most likely diagnosis?

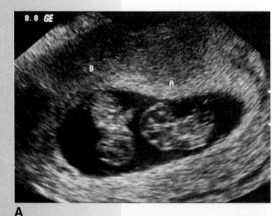

A

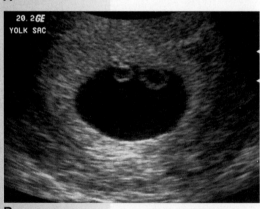

B

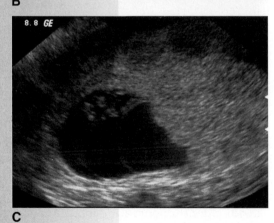

C

Fig. 22-10 **A,** Twin gestation in first trimester is identified. **B,** Two yolk sacs and, **C,** amnions are shown.

5. A 23-year-old woman is seen for a second-trimester obstetric ultrasound. A monochorionic, diamniotic twin gestation was documented on a first-trimester ultrasound examination at 8 weeks. The patient is now approximately 18 weeks with LMP. A monochorionic, diamniotic twin gestation (Fig. 22-13) is confirmed with fetal biometric measurements consistent with 18 weeks' gestational age. Twin B appears normal, with no fetal anomalies identified. Twin A, however, has enlarged ventricles, measuring 1.2 cm. There is a suspected posterior fossa cyst. The spine appears normal. What is the most likely diagnosis?

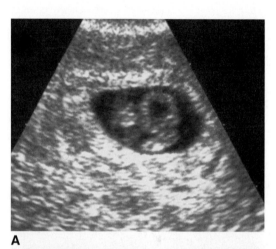

A

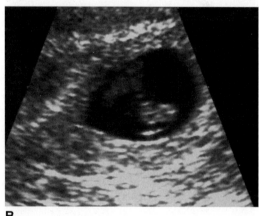

B

Fig. 22-11   Early twin gestation is identified with, **A** and **B,** two embryos and, **A,** one yolk sac.

CASE STUDIES FOR DISCUSSION—cont'd

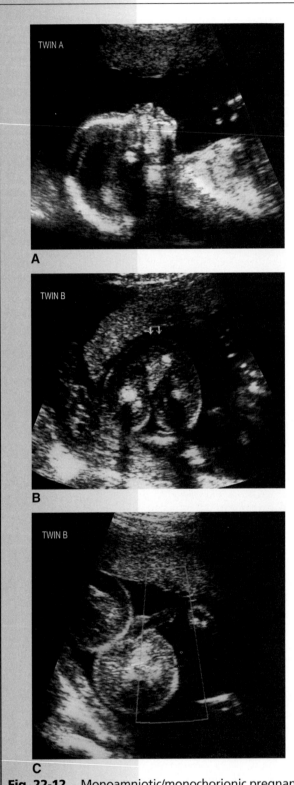

Fig. 22-12 Monoamniotic/monochorionic pregnancy is identified. **A,** Twin A appears structurally normal. **B** and **C,** Twin B is grossly malformed.

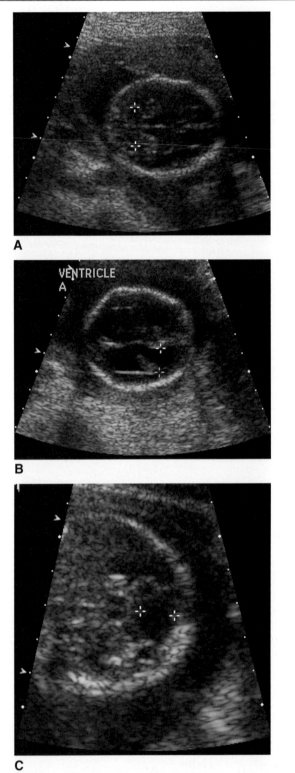

Fig. 22-13 Monchorionic/diamniotic pregnancy is imaged at 18 weeks' gestation. **A,** Posterior fossa of twin B is documented. **B,** Enlarged ventricles are identified in twin A. **C,** Posterior fossa is documented.

CASE STUDIES FOR DISCUSSION—cont'd

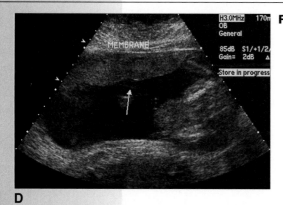

Fig. 22-13, cont'd   **D,** Thin membrane separates twins.

STUDY QUESTIONS

1. Which of the following pregnancies presents the greatest risk of fetal morbidity and mortality?
   a. dizygotic, dichorionic, diamniotic
   b. monozygotic, dichorionic, diamniotic
   c. monozygotic, monochorionic, diamniotic
   d. monozygotic, monochorionic, monoamniotic
   e. all present with an equal risk

2. Monozygotic twins result from the fertilization of two separate oocytes.
   a. true
   b. false

3. Which of the following would most likely result when cleavage occurs later than 13 days after conception?
   a. triplets
   b. quadruplets
   c. conjoined twins
   d. diamniotic twins
   e. dichorionic twins

4. When a single placenta is visualized, which of the following may help distinguish between a dichorionic pregnancy and a true monochorionic pregnancy?
   a. fetal gender
   b. identification of a chorionic peak
   c. thickness of the intertwin membrane
   d. number of layers forming the intertwin membrane
   e. all of the above

5. A 1-week difference in gestational age between fetuses of a multifetal gestation is suggestive of discordant growth.
   a. true
   b. false

6. An acardiac twin can be confirmed with sonographically determining the direction of the blood flow in the umbilical artery.
   a. true
   b. false

7. Which of the following is specifically associated with a monozygotic pregnancy?
   a. conjoined twinning
   b. acardiac parabiotic twinning
   c. twin embolization syndrome
   d. twin-twin transfusion sequence
   e. all of the above

8. Evaluations of fetal growth and amniotic fluid are the most effective means of screening for intrauterine growth restriction.
   a. true
   b. false

9. Which of the following twinning types would be indicated in a dichorionic, diamniotic pregnancy in which the fetal gender is the same?
   a. dizygotic
   b. monozygotic
   c. indeterminate

10. Chorionicity can usually be determined as early as 6 weeks' gestational age.
    a. true
    b. false

REFERENCES

1. Martin JA, Hamilton BE, Ventura SJ et al: Births: final data for 2000. *National vital statistics report*, vol 50, no 5, Hyattsville, Maryland, National Center for Health Statistics, 2002.
2. Hagen-Ansert SL: *Textbook of diagnostic ultrasonography*, vol 2, ed 5, St Louis, 2001, Mosby.
3. Rumack CM, Wilson SR, Charboneau JW: *Diagnostic ultrasound*, vol 2, ed 2, St Louis, 1998, Mosby.
4. Doubilet PM, Benson CB: Appearing twin: undercounting of multiple gestations on early first trimester sonograms, *J Ultrasound Med* 17:199, 1998.
5. Callen PW: *Ultrasonography in obstetrics and gynecology*, ed 4, Philadelphia, 2000, WB Saunders.
6. Sanders RC: *Structural fetal abnormalities: the total picture*, Philadelphia, 1996, Mosby.
7. Deutchman M: *Obstetric ultrasound principles and techniques on CD-ROM*, Nashville, 2001, Healthstream.

BIBLIOGRAPHY

Anderhub B: *General sonography: a clinical guide*, St Louis, 1995, Mosby.

McGahan JP, Goldberg BB: *Diagnostic ultrasound: a logical approach on CD-ROM*, Philadelphia, 1997, Lippincott Williams & Wilkins.

Nyberg DA, Mahony BS, Pretorius DH: *Diagnostic ultrasound of fetal anomalies: text and atlas*, Chicago, 1990, Yearbook Medical Publishers, Inc.

23 Elevated Alpha Fetoprotein

ARMANDO FUENTES and CHRISTOPHER MICHAEL RICKETTS

CLINICAL SCENARIO

■ A 26-year-old woman is seen for an ultrasound at 19 weeks' gestation with no significant medical history. The pregnancy has been uncomplicated until now. She had a routine maternal serum alpha fetoprotein test at 18 weeks' gestation, which was reported as 3.8 multiples of the median. An earlier sonogram during the pregnancy confirmed the dating. The information was given to her the previous day at her physician's office, and fetal heart tones were auscultated.

Sonographic evaluation reveals an appropriately grown infant. The transverse cranial image appears to have scalloping of the frontal bones (Fig. 23-1, *A*) within the parietal bones, giving the appearance of a lemon. The lateral ventricles measure 13 mm. A transverse view of the lumbosacral region reveals the lateral processes of the spine that appear to form a V shape (Fig. 23-1, *B*) for approximately four vertebral bodies. What is the most likely diagnosis?

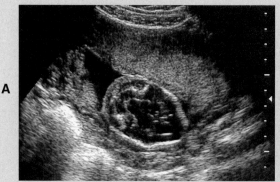
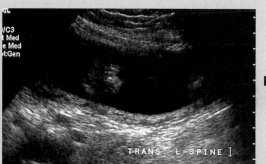

Fig. 23-1 **A,** Fetal head shows lemon shape. **B,** Transverse spine shows V shape.

OBJECTIVES

■ Describe the clinical use of serum alpha fetoprotein as a screen for various fetal anomalies.

■ Describe the appropriate diagnostic approach to a patient with an elevated alpha fetoprotein value.

■ Identify potential pregnancy complications in the setting of an unexplained elevated alpha fetoprotein value.

■ Identify the sonographic appearance of neural tube disorders commonly associated with an elevated alpha fetoprotein value.

■ Identify fetal abdominal wall anomalies associated with elevated alpha fetoprotein values.

■ Describe the sonographic appearance of abdominal wall defects commonly associated with an elevated alpha fetoprotein value.

■ Differentiate sonographic features of limb-body wall complex and amniotic band syndrome.

GLOSSARY OF TERMS

Arnold-Chiari malformation: constellation of cranial findings associated with spina bifida aperta, with scalloping of the frontal bones, banana-shaped cerebellum, and ventriculomegaly

Dysraphism: describes the presence of spine separation, also known as *spina bifida*

Meckel-Gruber syndrome: autosomal recessive disorder involving polycystic kidneys, encephalocele, polydactyly, and cardiac defects

Meconium: initial material passed from the fetal bowels that consists of amniotic fluid debris and cells sloughed from the lining of the gastrointestinal tract during the intrauterine period

Mid gut: refers to the primordium of the small intestine, appendix, ascending colon, and most of the duodenum and transverse colon

Multiples of the median, or multiples of the mean: a statistical measure used for reporting maternal serum alpha fetoprotein results; a composite measure of an individual's laboratory results compared with matched norms

Neural tube: refers to the spinal cord and intracranial contents (brainstem, cerebellum, and cerebrum)

Pentalogy of Cantrell: omphalocele, defective sternum, ventral diaphragmatic defect, anterior pericardial deficiency, and intrinsic cardiac disease

Placental abruption: premature separation of the placenta from the uterus, interrupting the blood supply to and thus endangering the fetus

Preeclampsia: abnormal maternal blood pressure elevation during the last half of pregnancy, accompanied by proteinuria (protein in the urine) and edema

Tetralogy of Fallot: congenital heart defect consisting of ventricular septal defect, pulmonic stenosis, overriding aorta, and right ventricular hypertrophy

Wharton's jelly: gelatinous matrix surrounding the umbilical vessels as they course between the placenta and fetus

Maternal serum alpha fetoprotein (MSAFP) testing has been used since the 1970s for identification of pregnancies at risk for fetal **neural tube** defects (NTDs).[1,2] The use of this noninvasive method of identification of pregnancies at risk has been expanded to include chromosomal abnormalities, anterior abdominal wall defects, and various other fetal anatomic conditions. Whereas obstetric management in the recent past would recommend amniocentesis for further evaluation of the abnormally elevated MSAFP, current sonographic technology provides informative and reliable diagnostic information. This chapter focuses on various etiologies responsible for an elevated MSAFP and their associated sonographic findings.

Alpha fetoprotein (AFP) is a protein synthesized in the yolk sac and later in the fetal liver.[3] The functional role of this protein in fetal development is uncertain. AFP levels reach a peak concentration in fetal serum at the end of the first trimester, and AFP is filtered by the fetal kidney and appears in amniotic fluid.[4] It is also detected in the fetal spine, gastrointestinal tract, liver, and kidneys. The appearance of AFP in the maternal circulation is mainly a result of diffusion across the placenta and the amnion. Any anomalous communi-

cation between the fetal stores of AFP (e.g., spine, gastrointestinal tract, or skin disruption) and the amniotic fluid would result in an abnormally elevated MSAFP value.[5] The optimal period for assessment of MSAFP is between the fifteenth and eighteenth week of gestation. MSAFP elevations occur commonly in the setting of fetal demise, multiple gestations, and a pregnancy misdated at an earlier gestational age. When these situations do not explain the abnormal AFP value seen, then a search for anatomic abnormalities is warranted.

Abnormalities in MSAFP levels are compared with matched norms and reported in terms of **multiples of the median** (MoM). Data from various studies indicate that major fetal anomalies are present in 30% to 58% of patients with MSAFP levels of 5.0 MoM or greater.[6,7] When a cutoff of 2.5 MoM is used, MSAFP screening detects approximately 88% of anencephalic fetuses and 79% of babies with open spina bifida. When no explanation can be determined for an elevated AFP value, despite sonographic and perhaps chromosomal investigation, 20% to 38% of pregnancies have adverse outcomes. These include low birth weight, prematurity, intrauterine growth restriction, **preeclampsia,** and **placental abruption.**[8]

NEURAL TUBE DEFECTS

Neural tube defects (NTDs) are thought to occur as a result of abnormal embryologic cell migration and failure of fusion of the neural tube between 20 to 24 days of conception. Defects in the neural tube primarily include anencephaly, spina bifida, and encephalocele.[9] During development, the neural groove forms in the primitive neural plate; lateral neural folds surround these structures. The folds fuse in the midline over the neural groove to form the neural tube. Rostral neuropore closure typically antedates posterior closure, with the normal process completed before 24 days after conception. Anencephaly occurs as a result of failed closure of one of the anterior neuropores. Likewise, failure of the posterior neuropores to close results in spina bifida, which may be open (meninges exposed) or closed (overlying skin intact).[10] Encephalocele is an intermediate lesion wherein the skull is incompletely formed with varying amounts of brain tissue extruding into the defect.[11] Because up to 20% of spina bifida lesions are closed, not all NTDs will be detected on MSAFP screening. Elevations in AFP occur because of communications between the nervous system and amniotic fluid.[12] The most severe elevations are seen in the setting of anencephaly and severe open spinal defects where large areas of neural tissue are exposed.[13]

A large geographic and ethnic variance in NTD incidence is seen, with the highest incidence in the British Isles (4.5/1000) and very low incidence among people of Japanese and African ancestry (0.6/1000 and 0.2/1000, respectively).[14] In addition, females tend to have higher neural defects (anencephaly and upper spine), whereas males tend to have lower spinal defects.[15] The incidence rate in the United States is 1/1000 to 2/1000.[15]

Considerable evidence implicates abnormal homocysteine metabolism in the development of NTDs. The presence of NTDs has been associated in the conversion of homocysteine to methionine as folate deficiency and the mutation 677T in the N(5),N(10)-methylenetetrahydrofolate reductase gene (MTHFR).[16,17] Supplementation with folic acid during the periconceptional phase and early pregnancy decreases the incidence of NTDs by 71%.[18]

Anencephaly

Anencephaly is a common NTD that occurs in up to 1.2 per 1000 births in the United States and in 3.5 per 1000 births in the United Kingdom.[19] It comprises almost half of open NTDs.[20] Pathologically, anencephaly is characterized by necrotic remnants of partially devel-

oped cerebrum that subsequently degenerated, which are covered by a vascular membrane known as the *cerebrovasculosa.*[14] Because there is complete communication with the amniotic milieu, AFP levels are extremely elevated (>5.0 MoM).[6,7]

Sonographic Findings. Sonographic diagnosis is not technically difficult, although confirmation may not occur until the second trimester when cranial ossification is complete. In fact, appropriately timed ultrasonography yields nearly a 100% detection rate.

The typical fetus with anencephaly shows absence of the cranial vault. As mentioned previously, the forebrain is degenerated and replaced by an angiomatous mass covered by the vascular cerebrovasculosa (Fig. 23-2, *A*). In addition, because the frontal bone is absent, the orbits protrude outward, giving a "frog's eye" appearance (Fig. 23-2, *B*) of the fetal face. Also, significant widening of the upper cervical spine (**dysraphism**) may be noted. Concomitant anomalies are common and

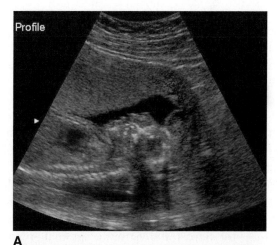

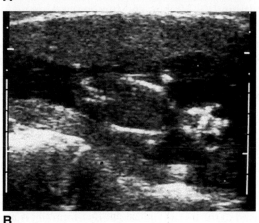

Fig. 23-2   A, Fetal profile with absent calvarium and cerebrovasculosa. **B,** Image of anencephaly shows typical froglike appearance. (**A** Courtesy GE Medical Systems.)

include spina bifida, craniorachischisis, cleft lip/palate, clubfoot, and omphalocele.

Because the swallowing reflex is disrupted from poor neural development, polyhydramnios is seen in 85% of gestations after 25 weeks.[21]

Spina Bifida

Spina bifida is a failure of the fetus's spine to close properly. Literally, *spina bifida* means a "spine, which is cleft or split in two." The two main types of spina bifida are spina bifida aperta and spina bifida occulta.

In spina bifida aperta, a disruption of the skin and subcutaneous tissues is seen over the area of the spine where the incomplete closure occurs. As a result, the meninges protrude out of the vertebral defect and are exposed to the amniotic milieu. With the absence of nervous tissue extruding into the meningeal sac, the lesion is termed a meningocele. Ninety percent of the time, however, nervous tissue is incorporated into the lesion; in this setting, the appropriate term is *meningomyelocele.*[22] When nerve tissue is involved in the defect, varying degrees of neurologic impairment result, ranging from mild anesthesia to complete paralysis. In addition, cranial abnormalities noted may result in an elongated medulla and fourth ventricle, which in conjunction with the cerebellum extend through the foramen magnum into the upper cervical canal, producing hydrocephalus. This constellation of signs is termed the *Arnold-Chiari malformation.* Hydrocephalus will be seen in 70% to 90% of infants with myelomeningocele.[23]

The AFP contained within the spinal cord and blood vessels leaks into the amniotic fluid and subsequently diffuses into the maternal circulation. The most common locations for spina bifida anomalies are the thoracolumbar, lumbar, and lumbosacral areas. Also, a wide variation is seen in the size of the lesions, resulting in higher MSAFP values in large defects.

In the setting of spina bifida occulta, the overlying skin and subcutaneous structures are intact. As a result, diagnosis may be difficult and subtle external clues may be the only indicators of disease. These clues include subcutaneous lipomas, tufts of hair, and pigmented or dimpled skin overlying the lesion. Because the lesion is contained within the overlying skin and subcutaneous tissue, no abnormal leakage of AFP is seen, and as a result, MSAFP is not elevated. Because no nerve tissue is involved in the lesion, neurologic development is normal.

Sonographic Findings. During normal development, the fetal spine may be visualized in the early second trimester. Complete evaluation of the spine involves viewing of spinous structures in the longitudinal and transverse aspects, from the nuchal origin to the distal sacrum. As the spine develops, it forms from three ossification centers, corresponding to the vertebral body and the neural arch on either side. In the transverse cut, the ossification centers assume an O shape because the two posterior elements tilt toward the midline. If the pedicle ossification centers assume a splayed V-, C-, or U-shaped appearance (Fig. 23-3, *A* and *B*) when viewed in the transverse section, the diagnosis of spina bifida should be considered. In contrast to an occulta, however, the overlying skin will be disrupted (Fig. 23-3, *C*), with either a thin-walled cyst (meningocele) or a nerve tissue–containing sac (myelomeningocele) protruding into the surface defect. In addition, abnormal curvature of the spine (kyphosis, lordosis, or scoliosis) may be observed. The top-most level of vertebral misalignment defines the level of the lesion.

Sonographic diagnosis of spina bifida aperta requires a detailed understanding of not only spinal anomalies but also of fetal intracranial anatomy (Fig. 23-3, *D* and *E*). As mentioned previously, the intracranial anomaly known as the Arnold-Chiari malformation often accompanies spina bifida aperta. The Arnold-Chiari malformation is characterized by cerebral ventriculomegaly, decreased intracranial pressure leading to frontal bone collapse (lemon sign), abnormal curvature of the cerebellum as it is impacted into the posterior fossa (banana sign), decreased cerebellar size, failure to visualize the cerebellum, and an obliteration of the cisterna magna.[24] Various authors have documented a 1% prevalence rate of false-positive cranial findings, specifically the lemon sign.[25,26]

Anomalies associated with spinal defects are microcephaly, cephaloceles, cleft lip and palate, hypotelorism, and hypertelorism.[27]

Regarding prognosis with spina bifida, the quoted mortality rate is 25%. Of the survivors, 25% are completely paralyzed, 25% are almost completely paralyzed, 25% need intensive rehabilitation, and 25% have no significant lower limb dysfunction.[24] Neonatal neurologic sequelae depend on the severity and location (Fig. 23-4) of the spina bifida defect. Multiple anomalies, involvement of the thoracic cavity, and craniorachischisis all carry worse prognoses than an isolated lumbosacral defect.

Encephalocele

Encephaloceles, or cephaloceles, as the name implies, are defects in the fetal cranium. The reported incidence rate is one in 5000 to 10,000 births.[14] As with spinal defects, variations of cephaloceles exist. Encephaloceles,

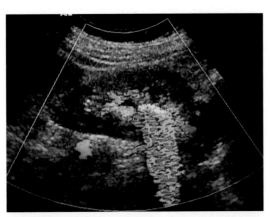

Plate 1 Sagittal image of right kidney with large calculi. Multiple colors are seen posterior to stone. This is called *twinkle sign.*

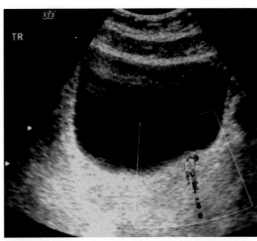

Plate 2 Multiple colors are seen posterior to left ureteral stone. This is called *twinkle sign.*

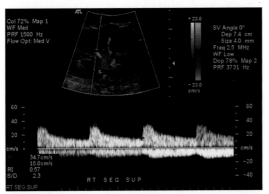

Plate 3 Right kidney segmental artery Doppler. (Courtesy Cindy Rapp, Radiology Imaging Associates, Greenwood Village, Colorado.)

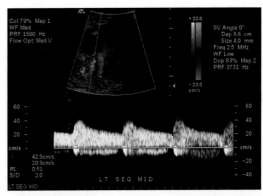

Plate 4 Left kidney segmental artery Doppler. (Courtesy Cindy Rapp, Radiology Imaging Associates, Greenwood Village, Colorado.)

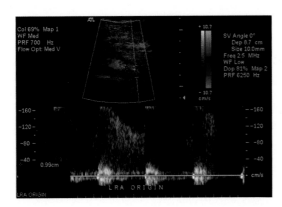

Plate 5 Left main renal artery Doppler evaluation shows high velocities caused by renal artery stenosis. (Courtesy Cindy Rapp, Radiology Imaging Associates, Greenwood Village, Colorado.)

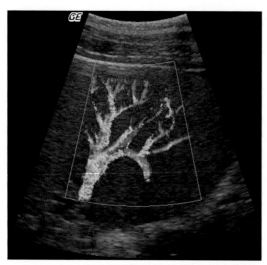

Plate 6 Normal splenic vasculature. (Courtesy GE Medical Systems.)

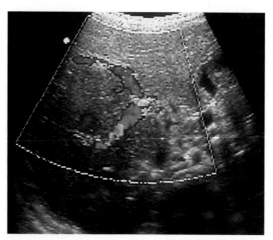

Plate 7 Hepatoblastoma. Surrounding portal veins are displaced around mass.

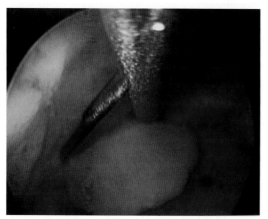

Plate 8 Gynecologist removing endometrial polyp during hysteroscopy.

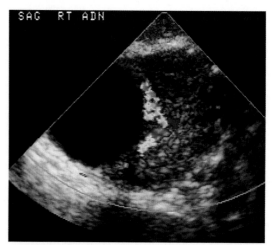

Plate 9 Color Doppler demonstrates vascularity at rim of this corpus luteum cyst.

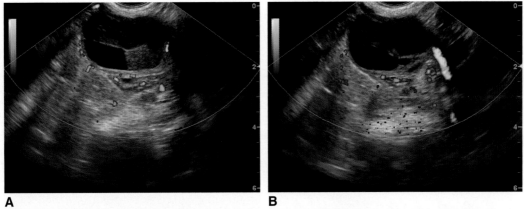

A B

Plate 10 **A** and **B,** Serous ovarian tumor containing thin septations and papillary projections. (Courtesy Lori Davis and Natalie Cauffman, Florida Hospital Deland.)

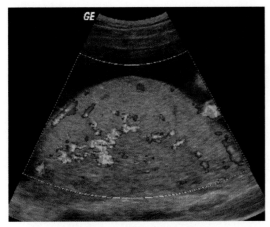

Plate 11 Enlarged placenta.

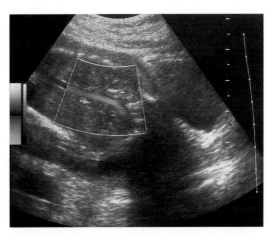

Plate 12 Normal renal arteries. Power Doppler maps out renal arteries bilaterally in growth-restricted fetus with oligohydramnios, confirming presence of kidneys that are poorly visualized.

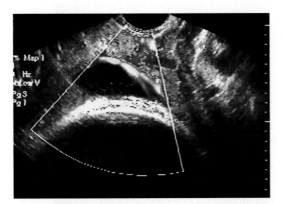

Plate 13 Vessels are clearly shown covering internal os and are enhanced with power Doppler imaging.

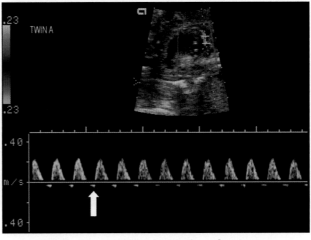

Plate 14 Umbilical Doppler of twin A.

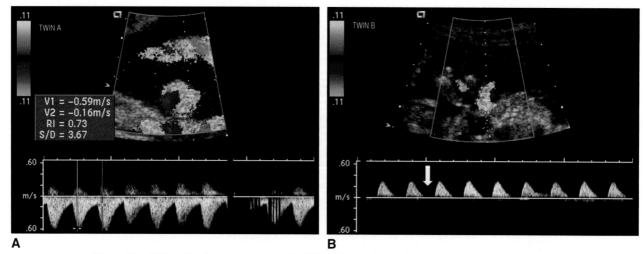

Plate 15 Dichorionic pregnancy. Umbilical Dopplers of, **A,** twin A and, **B,** twin B are documented.

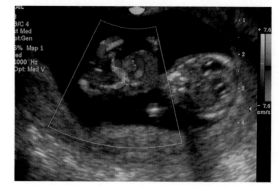

Plate 16 Color Doppler is used to clarify anomaly.

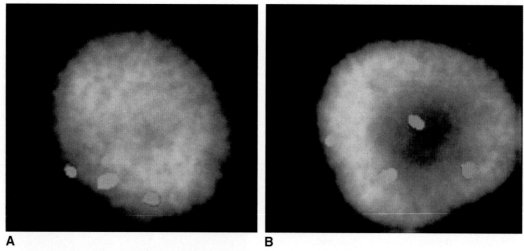

Plate 17 Chromosomal analysis reveals female with trisomy 13. Fluorescence in situ hydridization analysis shows, **A,** two copies of X chromosome coded in green and two copies of chromosome 18 coded in blue. **B,** Two copies of chromosome 21 are coded in red and three copies of chromosome 13 are coded in green.

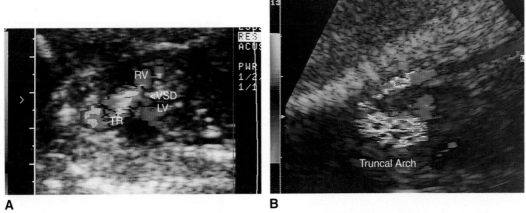

A

B

Plate 18 Color Doppler imaging shows single large vessel arising from both ventricles. Multiple cusps within large vessel may be deformed and dysplastic, resulting in moderate to significant aortic insufficiency. *LV,* Left ventricle; *RV,* right ventricle; *TR,* tricuspid regurgitation; *VSD,* ventricular septal defect.

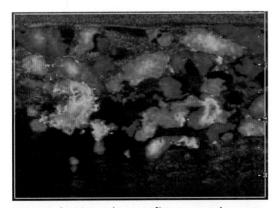

Plate 19 Color Doppler confirms vascular nature of varicoceles. (Courtesy Cindy Rapp, Radiology Imaging Associates, Greenwood Village, Colorado.)

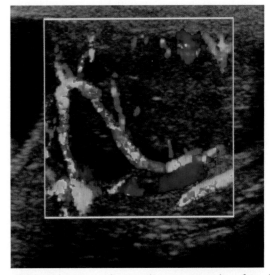

Plate 20 Color Doppler outlines example of embryonal cell carcinoma. (Courtesy Cindy Rapp, Radiology Imaging Associates, Greenwood Village, Colorado.)

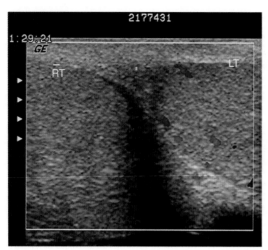

Plate 21 Lack of blood flow is shown in right testis in patient with testicular torsion.

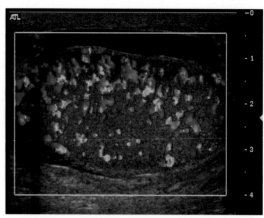

Plate 22 Color Doppler evaluation of left hemiscrotum. (Courtesy Cindy Rapp, Radiology Imaging Associates, Greenwood Village, Colorado.)

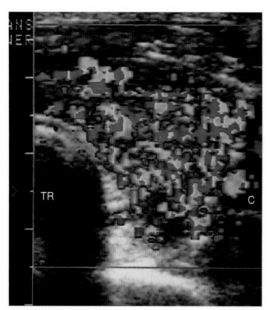

Plate 23 Color Doppler of thyroid inferno seen with Graves' disease.

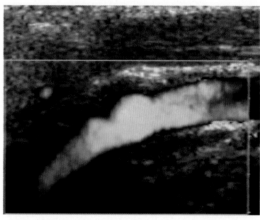

Plate 24 Internal carotid artery from patient with fibromuscular dysplasia. Note peapod appearance of artery. (Courtesy Doug Marcum, Orlando Ultrasound Associates, Inc., Orlando, Florida.)

Plate 25 Color flow is used to show flow in saphenofemoral junction.

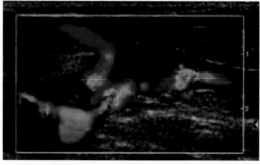

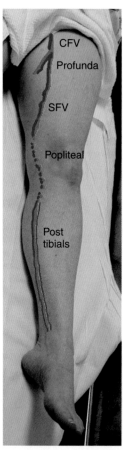
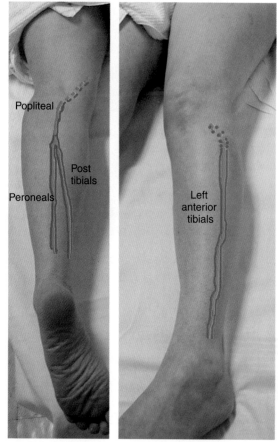

Plate 26 Vascular anatomy identified at anterior and medial aspect of leg.

Plate 27 Vascular anatomy identified at posterior *(left)* and lateral *(right)* aspects of lower leg.

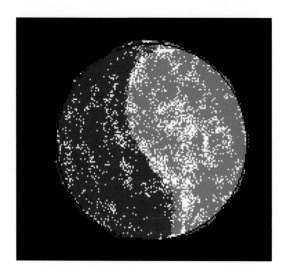

Plate 28 Yin Yang sign shows swirling blood flow pattern.

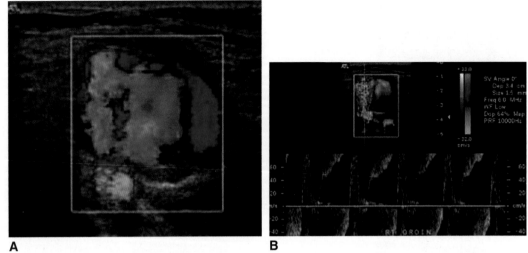

Plate 29 A, Pseudoaneurysm shows Yin Yang sign with color flow Doppler. **B,** Spectral analysis also shows turbulent flow.

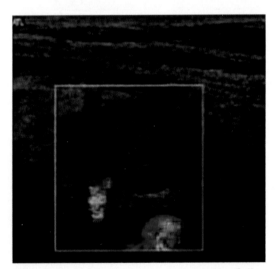

Plate 30 Ultrasound may be used to monitor follow-up.

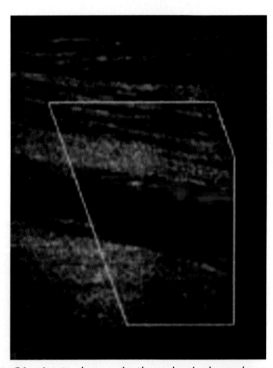

Plate 31 Acute deep vein thrombosis shows homogeneous, low-level echoes.

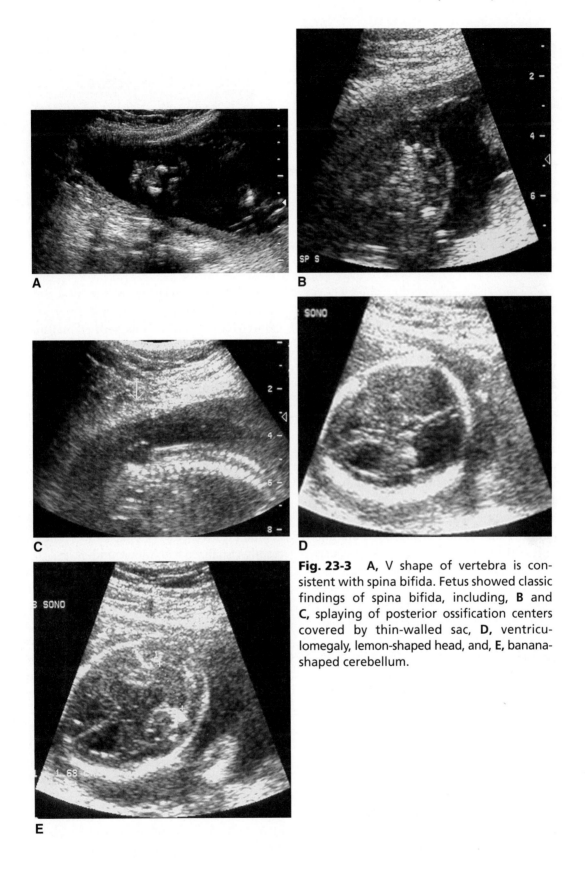

Fig. 23-3 **A,** V shape of vertebra is consistent with spina bifida. Fetus showed classic findings of spina bifida, including, **B** and **C,** splaying of posterior ossification centers covered by thin-walled sac, **D,** ventriculomegaly, lemon-shaped head, and, **E,** banana-shaped cerebellum.

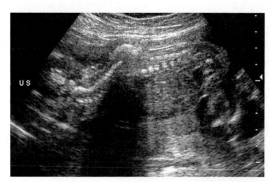

Fig. 23-4 Large spinal defect involved thoracic spine. Outcome for infant was predicted to be extremely poor.

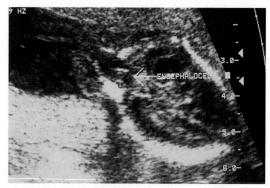

Fig. 23-5 Brain tissue herniating through defect in calvarium is identified in fetus with encephalocele.

also called *meningoencephaloceles,* are defects into which brain tissue herniates, whereas meningoceles are defects through which only meninges herniate. A meningohydroencephalocele describes the situation where brain tissue, meninges, and ventricles protrude through the skull defect.

The most common location for an encephalocele is the midline occipital area, although encephaloceles have been described arising from the parietal, frontal, and nasopharyngeal bones.[28] Encephaloceles are integral to diagnosis of the **Meckel-Gruber syndrome** and are commonly associated with the amniotic band syndrome.

Sonographic Findings. Given the nature of the defect, encephaloceles are seen as an extracranial mass (Fig. 23-5), and depending on the size, location, and presence or absence of brain tissue, encephaloceles may appear cystic or solid. A paracranial cystic structure implies a meningocele, whereas a solid or complex structure implies an encephalocele. When ventricle is implicated into the paracranial defect, a meningohydroencephalocele is present.

Ventriculomegaly is one of the most commonly associated abnormalities. Traction on intracranial contents may be observed, which as a consequence may result in an overall decreased calvarium size (microcephaly).

Documentation of a cranial defect is necessary for accurate diagnosis of a cephalocele. In contrast, a cystic hygroma, usually arising from the fetal neck, may be a difficult distinction if the cranial defect is very small (i.e., a few millimeters).[29] Other distinguishing features of cystic hygromas are internal septations, thick walls, and accompanying soft-tissue edemas.

Long-term sequelae are related to the presence of brain tissue in the defect. The overall mortality rate is 40% (11% for meningoceles and 71% for encephalo-

celes), with a dismal 80% of survivors showing some evidence of neurologic and intellectual impairment.[30] Conversely, 60% of infants with cranial meningoceles have normal intelligence.[31]

ABDOMINAL WALL DEFECTS

Abdominal wall defects are the second most common cause of elevated AFP values. These defects are described as congenital defects that result in protrusion of the stomach or intestines through incomplete closure of the abdominal wall. Complex defects that result in herniation of the heart through the thoracoabdominal wall include **pentalogy of Cantrell,** limb-body wall complex (LBWC), and ectopia cordis.[32] These defects are readily visualized with ultrasound.

Abdominal wall defects are relatively common and occur in approximately one in 2000 live births.[33] The etiology and pathogenesis vary among the different defects. During embryologic development at the 22- to 28-day period, the fetus undergoes intricate invaginations to assume a more human shape. What begins as a cylinder folds in the cranial, rostral, and lateral directions to take a form with discernable cephalad and caudad aspects. When the cranial folding goes awry, complex defects of the thorax and upper abdomen result, known in toto as the pentalogy of Cantrell. Abnormal lateral folding leads to midline omphaloceles, and completely anomalous body folding may result in the rare but devastating body-stalk deformities.[12]

Modern sonographic technology provides valuable tools to help differentiate the various abdominal wall defects. In fact, one recent review indicated a near 100% specificity and sensitivity for ultrasound detection of abdominal wall defects in high-risk populations.[34]

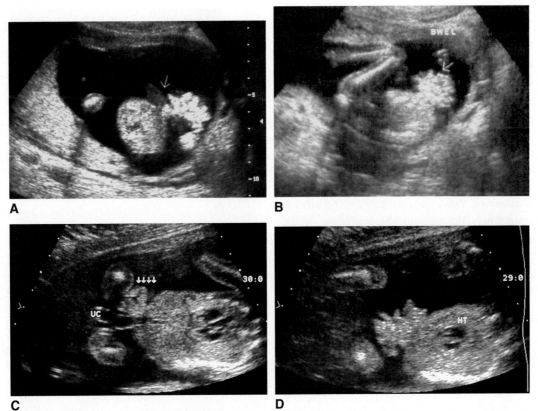

Fig. 23-6   Gastroschisis was identified in fetus at 18.5 weeks' gestation. **A,** Umbilical cord *(arrow)* can be identified adjacent to, **B,** free-floating bowel. Patient was seen with AFP of 7.7 multiples of mean. Sonographic evaluation was performed on patient seen in emergency department with abdominal pain at 20 weeks' gestation. **C** and **D,** Free-floating bowel was noted adjacent to umbilical cord.

Gastroschisis

Gastroschisis is a full-thickness abdominal wall defect that occurs in one of 10,000 live births.[33] The abdominal wall defect usually lies to the right of the umbilicus and is small (2 to 4 cm in size), with small bowel extruding into the amniotic cavity. Because the defect involves all layers of the abdominal wall, an open communication exists between the amniotic milieu and the intraabdominal space, with no protective layer over the herniated bowel. Herniation of liver or stomach through this defect is uncommon. One consequence is greater extrusion of AFP into the amniotic space and therefore into maternal circulation. Indeed, the average MSAFP level with a gastroschisis is 7.0 MoM, as compared with an omphalocele (discussed subsequently) where the average level is 4.1 MoM.[35] Associated anomalies are uncommon with gastroschisis and occur only 7% to 30% of the time.[36,37] Most gastroschisis defects occur spontaneously with no increased incidence of chromosomal abnormalities.[38] In contrast, intrauterine

growth restriction accompanies gastroschisis in up to 77% of cases.[36] Intrauterine fetal death complicates as many as 4.6% of cases.[39]

Various theories exist regarding the cause of gastroschisis. The commonly described vascular obliteration theory states that premature atrophy of the right umbilical vein causes an ischemia-necrosis sequence in the abdominal wall to the right of the umbilical cord. As a result, skin breakdown allows bowel to herniate into the amniotic cavity.[32,38]

Perinatal management of patients with gastroschisis has evolved, with current evidence supporting vaginal delivery as both safe and effective. Indeed, research indicates no survival benefit from de facto cesarean delivery.[40,41]

Sonographic Findings.   The hallmark of gastroschisis is free-floating bowel (Fig. 23-6) originating from the right of the umbilicus. Early in the course of gastroschisis, bowel appears normal with evidence of peristaltic activity. After prolonged exposure to the caustic effects of urine in amniotic fluid, bowel reacts by thickening and developing what is known as a peel. Bowel edema and luminal dilation develop later in the clinical course from mechanical obstruction at the site of the defect. The bowel becomes dilated and thickened. Dilation may also occur from atresia at sites of ischemia, necrosis, and stricture formation. As a result, the bowel wall assumes a more hyperechoic appearance, and peristalsis becomes less noticeable.[34] In some cases, destructive forces on the bowel cause a perforation, with leakage of **meconium** into the amniotic fluid. When this occurs, amniotic fluid appears to have echogenic debris floating freely throughout the amniotic cavity. Bowel perforation in the setting of gastroschisis carries a 50% mortality rate.[32] Although fetal growth may be impaired, difficulty in obtaining accurate abdominal wall circumference may tend to underestimate fetal weight.

Omphalocele

Omphaloceles are defects in the abdomen that result in a herniation of the intraabdominal contents into the umbilical stalk and covering with peritoneum and amnion (Fig. 23-7). During normal development, the **mid gut** herniates into the umbilical stalk, providing room in the abdominal cavity for gut rotation and vascular development. This process normally concludes by week 12 of development, with return of the herniated structures into the abdominal cavity and approximation of the umbilical stalk with overlying skin and subcutaneous tissue. When this process does not occur, the result is an omphalocele.[42] Abnormal embryologic lateral folding mentioned at the beginning of this section is one prevailing theory and more easily explains situations when large defects exist, such as those with liver herniation.[43]

Omphalocele abdominal wall defects occur more frequently than gastroschisis, with an incidence rate of one in 4000 live births.[32] Because omphaloceles involve herniation into the umbilical stalk, abdominal contents are covered by the cord's structures, namely the overlying amnion and gelatinous **Wharton's jelly.** With these protective layers covering the bowel, less AFP extrudes out into the amniotic fluid and the MSAFP is typically lower than that seen with gastroschisis.[37]

Anomalies accompany omphaloceles in 50% to 88% of cases and can involve virtually every organ system.[44] Cardiac defects occur 30 times more frequently in the setting of body fold defects and are reported to accompany omphaloceles 50% of the time.[45] Chromosomal anomalies also frequently accompany omphaloceles. In fact, up to 15% of fetuses with an abdominal folding

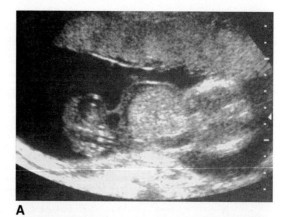

A

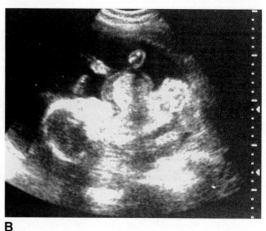

B

Fig. 23-7   **A** and **B,** Transverse and sagittal images of fetus show large omphalocele. Umbilical cord is noted to insert into middle of defect. Patient consented to amniocentesis, which revealed normal karyotype.

defect have a chromosomal anomaly, with 50% with trisomy 18, 39% with trisomy 13, and 12% with trisomy 21.[36,44]

As with gastroschisis, current thought supports vaginal delivery in the absence of massive abdominal herniation. Unfortunately, an isolated omphalocele carries a 10% to 15% mortality rate.[36] Amniotic fluid abnormalities, either polyhydramnios or oligohydramnios, complicate up to one third of omphaloceles and confer a poor outcome.[45] When one or more anomalies accompany an omphalocele, the mortality rate approaches 80%.

Sonographic Findings. The ultrasound diagnosis of omphalocele primarily involves identification of a central abdominal mass enclosed in membrane arising from the mid line. Because the process of normal mid gut herniation may not be completed until gestational week 12, diagnosis before this time may be difficult. Often, the umbilical vessels can be seen inserting into the apex of the sac. In the absence of free-floating bowel,

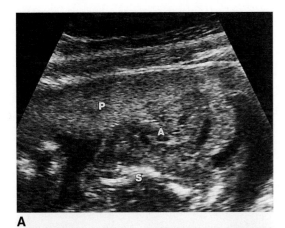

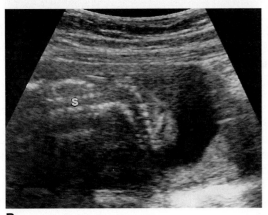

Fig. 23-8 **A,** Abdominal wall defect and, **B,** severe scoliosis are seen in fetus.

presence of a sac covering the abdominal contents may be inferred. Because no contact exists between the bowel and amniotic fluid, bowel wall does not encounter the caustic urine and develop an inflammatory thickened wall. Intraabdominal ascites and ascites in the omphalocele sac may also be seen. Given the strong association with other anomalies, a systematic evaluation of fetal anatomy is necessary.

Limb-Body Wall Complex

Limb-body wall complex is a universally fatal condition that results from abnormal body folding during development at 22 to 28 days' gestation.[46] Primary features are a large anterior abdominal wall defect, short umbilical cord, NTD, facial clefting, and limb defects. MSAFP levels are predictably high given the extent of fetal organ exposure to amniotic fluid. The incidence rate varies from one in 7500 to one in 200,000 but carries no recurrence risk.[47,48]

Sonographic Findings. The appearance (Fig. 23-8) of this major body stalk anomaly characteristically involves extensive thoracic, abdominal, facial, limb, and spine abnormalities. Authors have reported scoliosis in 77% of LBWC cases; these same authors conclude that scoliosis in the setting of any anterior abdominal wall defect should raise one's suspicion for LBWC.[49] Neural tube defects are often extensive and involve the lower spine. In addition, one recent study reported a single umbilical artery in 87.5% of patients with LBWC.[50] The umbilical cord is short or difficult to visualize, and free-floating amniotic bands may be identified. Because LBWC arises from complete failure body folding, other common anomalies include cephaloceles, exencephaly, and diaphragmatic hernias.

AMNIOTIC BAND SYNDROME

Amniotic band syndrome (ABS) is a developmental disorder in which fibrous remnants of amnion constrict the fetus.[51] Bands of varying sizes and shapes affect the fetus in any imaginable configuration and location. Fetal consequences range from simple constriction bands to devastating head clefting. Most commonly, amniotic bands affect limbs and cause amputation, constrictions with edema, and clubfoot, the latter especially in the setting of oligohydramnios.[52] The condition is associated with elevation of AFP in the second trimester. One common theory on the cause of ABS was proposed by Torpin in the 1960s.[53,54] He postulated that the amnion prematurely separates from the chorion. Subsequent to this, amniotic fluid exudes through the more permeable chorion, resulting in oligohydramnios. When the bands of amnion are brought in closer contact with the fetus because of fluid leakage, fetal structures become entangled. Developmental anomalies then arise from the constricting bands through deformation forces.[53,54] ABS occurs from 7.8 in 10,000 to 178 in 10,000, with an equal distribution between males and females.[55] There is no association with chromosomal abnormalities.[56]

Sonographic Findings

Because ABS is a condition in which segments of the amnion directly deform the fetus, sheets or bands of tissue will be evident proceeding from the edge of the amniotic sac to the fetus (Fig. 23-9). This most commonly results in constrictions but may also result in facial clefting, amputations, and clubfoot deformities. The facial clefting can have unusual demarcations involving the orbits and cranium.[57] Evidence of edema around the band increases suspicion for ABS. Confounding structures that may mimic as ABS include uterine synechia and velamentous cord insertion.

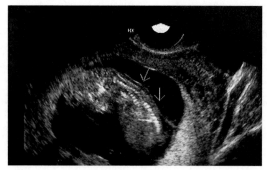

Fig. 23-9 Amniotic band can be identified extending along back of fetus with acrania.

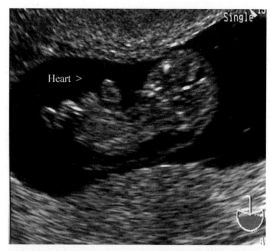

Fig. 23-10 Beating heart was identified extending into amniotic cavity in first-trimester fetus. Indication for ultrasound was recurrent pregnancy losses.

ECTOPIA CORDIS

Ectopia cordis is an abnormality in the cephalic folding sequence during embryologic development. Failure of the fetal chest to form around and enclose the heart results in either part or all of the heart existing outside of the chest cavity. Errors in cephalic folding can also result in other anomalies, such as an epigastric omphalocele, defective sternum, ventral diaphragmatic defects, and anterior pericardial deficiency.[34] This constellation of anomalies is known as the *pentalogy of Cantrell*, with the combination of ectopia cordis and omphalocele as the hallmark.[58] Intrinsic cardiac anomalies also often coexist with the pentalogy of Cantrell.[59] Recent reports indicate an incidence rate of 0.079 per 10,000 or 7.9 per million.[60] Associations with trisomy 13 and 18 and Turner's syndrome have been made.[61] The prognosis is usually fatal.

Sonographic Findings

Ectopia cordis is easily shown with visualization of the fetal heart outside of the chest cavity (Fig. 23-10). A wide spectrum of anomalies exists, from a partial eventration of the heart to complete evisceration of abdominal and thoracic contents. When an omphalocele accompanies ectopia cordis, the abdominal wall defect is usually in the epigastrium.[34] The most common cardiac abnormalities seen are atrial septal defects, ventricular septal defects, and **tetralogy of Fallot.**[60]

SUMMARY

Elevation in the MSAFP can be seen in a variety of fetal anomalies. The presence of AFP in fetal circulation and its subsequent diffusion into the maternal circulation has lent itself as a primary tool for prenatal testing. The presence of any disruption of fetal integrity usually

Table 23-1	*Abnormal Alpha Fetoprotein*	
Elevated		**Decreased**
Wrong dates		Wrong dates
Multiple gestation		Down syndrome
Anencephaly		Trisomy 18
Spina bifida aperta		
Encephalocele		
Gastroschisis		
Omphalocele		
Limb-body wall complex		
Ectopia cordis		
Amniotic band syndrome		
Maternal liver tumors		

results in an elevation of AFP in the mother. Table 23-1 lists anomalies associated with increased and decreased levels of AFP. Defects involving the spine and abdominal wall have been the earliest anomalies involved in major prenatal screening programs. Ultrasonography and AFP measurements are a powerful tool for elucidating various etiologies with determination of the presence or absence of fetal anatomic anomalies. When a fetal abnormality is found, sonographic information is valuable in determination of prognosis and assistance in prenatal management.

CLINICAL SCENARIO—DIAGNOSIS

■ The case describes a lemon-shaped head, along with an elevated MSAFP value. The image of the fetal head in Fig. 23-1, *A*, also shows a banana-shaped cerebellum with obliteration of the cisterna magna. The transverse view of the lumosacral region indicates a widening of the transverse processes of the spine along with a cleft in the skin and soft tissues overlying this area. The most likely diagnosis is an open NTD. The history of an earlier sonogram confirms the gestational age used to calculate the AFP level. Fetal heart tones were auscultated and indicated a live fetus, as elevation of AFP can also be seen in fetal death. The presence of enlarged lateral ventricles also indicates the probability of an Arnold-Chiari malformation.

CASE STUDIES FOR DISCUSSION

1. A 17-year-old woman is seen for an elevated AFP level at 19 weeks' gestation. Ultrasound evaluation reveals a normally growing fetus based on femur length and abdominal circumference. The cranium cannot be visualized. Significant protrusion of the fetal orbits is seen (Fig. 23-11). What is the most likely diagnosis?

2. A 42-year-old woman is seen for ultrasound evaluation to determine gestational age. The patient reports no complications during the pregnancy but does have irregular menstrual periods. Sonographic evaluation reveals the umbilical cord inserting into a protrusion on the anterior abdominal wall, and the vessels can be traced across and then away from the protrusion (Fig. 23-12, *A* and *B;* see Color Plate 16). The contents in the protrusion appear to be homogeneous. Three-dimensional sonography is also used to document the anomaly. What is the diagnosis, and what other anatomic areas are important to visualize?

3. Ultrasound evaluation of a 21-year-old obese woman at 15 weeks' gestation is performed for an elevated AFP value. Ultrasound evaluation is normal. No obvious abnormalities are noted. The gestational age is calculated at 21 weeks' gestation with all parameters. What is the next step in the management?

4. A 33-year-old woman is seen for evaluation of an elevated AFP value at 20 weeks' gestation. A cross section of the cranium indicates a protrusion of inhomogeneous material (Fig. 23-13) at the posterior aspect of the fetal head. What is the most likely diagnosis?

5. A 30-year-old woman is seen for evaluation of an elevated AFP value. The dating is accurate. Sonographic evaluation is performed at 18 weeks' gestation. Images obtained reveal a midline cleft lip, the cardiac structure beating outside of

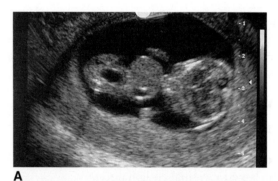

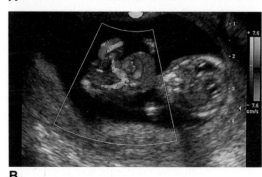

Fig. 23-12   **A,** View of fetus shows defect. **B,** Color Doppler is also used to clarify anomaly.

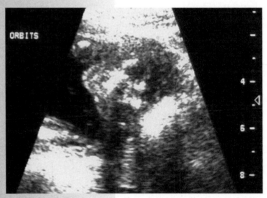

Fig. 23-11   Fetal face is identified. Notice lack of visible calvarium.

CASE STUDIES FOR DISCUSSION—cont'd

the chest cavity, and a large protrusion of the abdominal contents (Fig. 23-14, *A*) into a sac anteriorly. Severe kyphoscoliosis is seen (Fig. 23-14, *B*). What are the most likely diagnosis and prognosis?

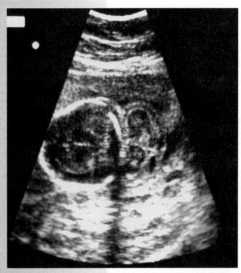

Fig. 23-13 Mass of inhomogeneous material protrudes from posterior aspect of fetal head.

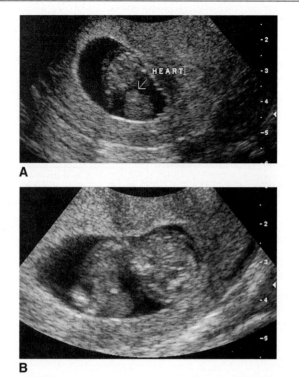

Fig. 23-14 **A,** Heart is identified in anterior abdominal wall defect. **B,** Spine is severely curved.

STUDY QUESTIONS

1. A 27-year-old woman has an alpha fetoprotein value of 4.5 MoM at 19 weeks' gestation. Sonographic evaluation reveals a 24-week viable gestation with normal anatomy. The most likely explanation is:
   a. laboratory error
   b. inaccurate dating
   c. vanishing twin in the first trimester
   d. anterior cranial encephalocele
   e. macrosomia

2. A 20-year-old woman has an ultrasound at another location that revealed the lateral ventricles measuring 15 mm and is referred to a maternal-fetal center. The patient declined alpha fetoprotein testing. Sonographic evaluation may reveal which one of the following findings?
   a. ventricular septal defect
   b. open neural tube defect
   c. atrial septal defect
   d. tetralogy of Fallot
   e. spina bifida occulta

3. A patient is seen for evaluation at 16 weeks' gestation for an alpha fetoprotein (AFP) of 4.0 MoM. Which of the following ultrasound findings would suggest a recalculation of the AFP?
   a. sonographic dating of 26 weeks
   b. sonographic dating of 11 weeks
   c. twin gestation
   d. sonographic dating of 19 weeks
   e. fetal death

4. Sonographic evaluation at 19 weeks' gestation reveals an appropriately growing infant with bilateral clubbed feet. Which of the following conditions may be associated with this finding?
   a. ectopia cordis
   b. tetralogy of Fallot
   c. amniotic band syndrome
   d. gastroschisis
   e. omphalocele

5. A 34-year-old woman is seen for ultrasound for an elevated alpha fetoprotein value at 18 weeks' gestation. The sonographer identifies a large protrusion of abdominal contents contained within a membrane. What is the most likely diagnosis?

a. amniotic band syndrome
b. diaphragmatic hernia
c. gastroschisis
d. omphalocele

6. A 22-year-old woman is seen for an alpha fetoprotein level of 5.0 MoM at 15 weeks' gestation. Ultrasound evaluation reveals only free-floating bowel anterior to the abdomen. The most likely diagnosis is?

a. omphalocele
b. limb-body wall complex
c. gastroschisis
d. anterior encephalocele
e. ectopia cordis

7. Which of the following is not associated with an Arnold-Chiari malformation?

a. ventriculomegaly
b. spina bifida occulta
c. lemon sign
d. encephalocele
e. banana sign

8. Alpha fetoprotein is produced by which organ?

a. brain
b. lung
c. liver
d. heart
e. kidneys

9. A sonographic evaluation at 10 weeks' gestation reveals an anterior abdominal wall defect. The most likely diagnosis at this gestational age is?

a. gastroschisis
b. omphalocele
c. limb-body wall complex
d. amniotic band syndrome
e. none of the above

10. A 27-year-old woman is seen for an elevation of the alpha fetoprotein (AFP) at 3.0 MoM. The ultrasound images reveal an appropriately grown singleton fetus. No abnormalities are noted. The placenta has a subchorionic hypoechoic area. The most likely explanation for the elevated AFP is?

a. spina bifida occulta
b. retroplacental clot

c. inaccurate dating
d. placenta previa
e. clinically insignificant amniotic band syndrome

REFERENCES

1. Ross HL, Elias S: Maternal serum screening for fetal genetic disorders, *Obstet Gynecol Clin North Am* 24:33-47, 1997.
2. Aitken DA, Crossley JA: Neural tube defects/alpha-fetoprotein/Down's syndrome screening, *Curr Opin Obstet Gynecol* 9:113-120, 1997.
3. Gitlin D, Perricelli A, Gitlin GM: Synthesis of feto-protein by liver, yolk sac, and gastrointestinal tract of the human conceptus, *Cancer Res* 32:979-982, 1972.
4. Gitlin D: Normal biology of alpha-fetoprotein, *Ann N Y Acad Sci* 259:7-16, 1975.
5. Glick PL, Pohlson EC, Resta R et al: Maternal serum alpha-fetoprotein is a marker for fetal anomalies in pediatric surgery, *J Pediatr Surg* 23:16-20, 1988.
6. Crandall BF, Robinson L, Grau P: Risks associated with an elevated maternal serum alpha-fetoprotein level, *Am J Obstet Gynecol* 165:581-6, 1991.
7. Larson JM, Pretorius DH, Budorick NE et al: Value of maternal serum alpha-fetoprotein levels of 5.0 MOM or greater and prenatal sonography in predicting fetal outcome, *Radiology* 189:77-81, 1993.
8. Robinson L, Grau P, Crandall BF: Pregnancy outcomes after increasing maternal serum alpha-fetoprotein levels, *Obstet Gynecol* 74:17-20, 1989.
9. Golden JA, Chernoff GF: Intermittent pattern of neural tube closure in two strains of mice, *Teratology* 47:73-80, 1993.
10. Van Allen MI, Kalousek DK, Chernoff GF et al: Evidence for multi-site closure of the neural tube in humans, *Am J Med Genet* 47:723-743, 1993.
11. Moore KL: *The developing human: clinically oriented embryology*, ed 4, Philadelphia, 1988, WB Saunders.
12. Brock DJ, Sutcliffe RG: Alpha-fetoprotein in the antenatal diagnosis of anencephaly and spina bifida, *Lancet* 2:197-199, 1972.
13. Argo K: Prenatal diagnosis of congenital anomalies. In Hagen-Ansert S, editor: *Diagnostic ultrasonography*, vol 2, ed 4, St Louis, 1995, Mosby.
14. Greenberg F, James LM, Oakley GP Jr: Estimates of birth prevalence rates of spina bifida in the United States from computer-generated maps, *Am J Obstet Gynecol* 145:570-573, 1983.
15. Seller MJ: Sex, neural tube defects, and multisite closure of the human neural tube, *Am J Med Genet* 58:332-336, 1995.
16. Christensen B, Arbour L, Tran P et al: Genetic polymorphisms in methylenetetrahydrofolate reductase and methionine synthase, folate levels in red blood cells, and risk of neural tube defects, *Am J Med Genet* 84:151-7, 1999.

17. Botto LD, Yang Q: 5,10-Methylenetetrahydrofolate reductase gene variants and congenital anomalies: a HuGE review, *Am J Epidemiol* 151:862-77, 2000.

18. Czeizel AE, Dudas I: Prevention of the first occurrence of neural-tube defects by periconceptional vitamin supplementation, *N Engl J Med* 327:1832-1835, 1992.

19. Hobbins JC, Grannum PA, Berkowitz RL et al: Ultrasound in the diagnosis of congenital anomalies, *Am J Obstet Gynecol* 134:331-345, 1979.

20. Main DM, Mennuti MT: Neural tube defects: issues in prenatal diagnosis and counselling, *Obstet Gynecol* 67:1-16, 1986.

21. Goldstein RB, Filly RA: Prenatal diagnosis of anencephaly: spectrum of sonographic appearances and distinction from the amniotic band syndrome, *AJR Am J Roentgenol* 151:547-550, 1988.

22. Chervenak FA, Duncan C, Ment LR et al: Perinatal management of meningomyelocele, *Obstet Gynecol* 63:376-380, 1984.

23. Pilu G: Ultrasound evaluation of the fetal neural axis. In Callen PW, editor: *Ultrasonography in obstetrics and gynecology*, ed 4, Philadelphia, 2000, WB Saunders.

24. Campbell J, Gilbert WM, Nicolaides KH et al: Ultrasound screening for spina bifida: cranial and cerebellar signs in a high-risk population, *Obstet Gynecol* 70:247-250, 1987.

25. Van den Hof MC, Nicolaides KH, Campbell J et al: Evaluation of the lemon and banana signs in one hundred thirty fetuses with open spina bifida, *Am J Obstet Gynecol* 162:322-327, 1990.

26. Ball RH, Filly RA, Goldstein RB et al: The lemon sign: not a specific indicator of meningomyelocele, *J Ultrasound Med* 12:131-134, 1993.

27. Jeanty P, Romero R: Is there a neural tube defect? In Jeanty P, Romero R, editors: *Obstetrical ultrasound*, New York, 1984, McGraw-Hill.

28. Chervenak FA, Isaacson G, Mahoney MJ et al: Diagnosis and management of fetal cephalocele, *Obstet Gynecol* 64:86-91, 1984.

29. Nicolini U, Ferrazzi E, Massa E et al: Prenatal diagnosis of cranial masses by ultrasound: report of five cases, *J Clin Ultrasound* 11:170-174, 1983.

30. Nyberg DA, Mahony BS, Pretorious DH: *Diagnostic ultrasound of fetal anomalies: text and atlas*, St Louis, 1990, Mosby.

31. Lorber J: Results of treatment of myelomeningocele. An analysis of 524 unselected cases, with special reference to possible selection for treatment, *Dev Med Child Neurol* 13:279-303, 1971.

32. Lockwood C: Congenital anomalies. In Eden RFB, editor: *Assessment and care of the fetus: physiological, clinical, and medicolegal principles*, vol 1, Norwalk, Conn, 1990, Appleton & Lange.

33. Carpenter MW, Curci MR, Dibbins AW et al: Perinatal management of ventral wall defects, *Obstet Gynecol* 64:646-651, 1984.

34. Lennon CA, Gray DL: Sensitivity and specificity of ultrasound for the detection of neural tube and ventral wall defects in a high-risk population, *Obstet Gynecol* 94:562-566, 1999.

35. Palomaki GE, Hill LE, Knight GJ et al: Second-trimester maternal serum alpha-fetoprotein levels in pregnancies associated with gastroschisis and omphalocele, *Obstet Gynecol* 71:906-909, 1988.

36. deVries PA: The pathogenesis of gastroschisis and omphalocele, *J Pediatr Surg* 15:245-251, 1980.

37. Moore TC: Gastroschisis and omphalocele: clinical differences, *Surgery* 82:561-568, 1977.

38. Torfs CP, Curry CJ: Familial cases of gastroschisis in a population-based registry, *Am J Med Genet* 45:465-467, 1993.

39. Lindham S: Omphalocele and gastroschisis in Sweden 1965-1976, *Acta Paediatr Scand* 70:55-60, 1981.

40. Segel SY, Marder SJ, Parry S et al: Fetal abdominal wall defects and mode of delivery: a systematic review, *Obstet Gynecol* 98:867-873, 2001.

41. Bethel CA, Seashore JH, Touloukian RJ: Cesarean section does not improve outcome in gastroschisis, *J Pediatr Surg* 24:1-4, 1989.

42. Langman J: Caudal part of the foregut. In Langman J, editor: *Medical embryology*, ed 3, Baltimore, 1975, Williams & Wilkins.

43. Seashore JH: Congenital abdominal wall defects, *Clin Perinatol* 5:61-77, 1978.

44. Hughes MD, Nyberg DA, Mack LA et al: Fetal omphalocele: prenatal US detection of concurrent anomalies and other predictors of outcome, *Radiology* 173:371-376, 1989.

45. Greenwood RD, Rosenthal A, Nadas AS: Cardiovascular malformations associated with omphalocele, *J Pediatr* 85:818-821, 1974.

46. Goldstein I, Winn HN, Hobbins JC: Prenatal diagnostic criteria for body stalk anomaly, *Am J Perinatol* 6:84-85, 1989.

47. Van Allen MI, Curry C, Walden CE et al: Limb-body wall complex: II. Limb and spine defects, *Am J Med Genet* 28:549-565, 1987.

48. Potter EL, Craig JM: *Pathology of the fetus and infant*, ed 3, Chicago, 1975, Year Book.

49. Patten RM, Van Allen M, Mack LA et al: Limb-body wall complex: in utero sonographic diagnosis of a complicated fetal malformation, *AJR Am J Roentgenol* 146:1019-1024, 1986.

50. Negishi H, Yaegashi M, Kato EH et al: Prenatal diagnosis of limb-body wall complex, *J Reprod Med* 43:659-664, 1998.

51. Miller ME, Graham JM Jr, Higginbottom MC et al: Compression-related defects from early amnion rupture: evidence for mechanical teratogenesis, *J Pediatr* 98:292-297, 1981.

52. Higginbottom MC, Jones KL, Hall BD et al: The amniotic band disruption complex: timing of amniotic rupture and variable spectra of consequent defects, *J Pediatr* 95:544-549, 1979.

53. Torpin R: Amniochorionic mesoblastic fibrosis strings and amniotic bands, *Am J Obstet Gynecol* 91:65, 1965.

54. Torpin R: *Malformations caused by amnion rupture,* Springfield, Ill, 1968, Charles C Thomas.

55. Buyse ML: *Birth defects encyclopedia.* Cambridge, England, 1990, Blackwell Scientific.

56. Burton DJ, Filly RA: Sonographic diagnosis of the amniotic band syndrome, *AJR Am J Roentgenol* 156:555-558, 1991.

57. Wehbeh H, Fleisher J, Karimi A et al: The relationship between the ultrasonographic diagnosis of innocent amniotic band development and pregnancy outcomes. *Obstet Gynecol* 81:565-568, 1993.

58. Cantrell JR, Haller JA, Ravitch MM: A syndrome of congenital defects involving the abdominal wall, sternum, diaphragm, pericardium, and heart, *Surg Gynecol Obstet* 107:602-614, 1958.

59. Toyama WM: Combined congenital defects of the anterior abdominal wall, sternum, diaphragm, pericardium, and heart: a case report and review of the syndrome, *Pediatrics* 50:778-792, 1972.

60. Khoury MJ, Cordero JF, Rasmussen S: Ectopia cordis, midline defects and chromosome abnormalities: an epidemiologic perspective, *Am J Med Genet* 30:811-817, 1988.

61. Ghidini A, Sirtori M, Romero R et al: Prenatal diagnosis of pentalogy of Cantrell, *J Ultrasound Med* 7:567-572, 1988.

24 Genetic Testing

CHARLOTTE HENNINGSEN and AHMED AL-MALT

CLINICAL SCENARIO

■ A 36-year-old woman, G3 P2002, is seen at 26 weeks' gestation for an obstetric ultrasound for late prenatal care. The ultrasound reveals the findings in Fig. 24-1. The patient is then referred to a maternal-fetal center for counseling and elects to have amniocentesis. What does the amniocentesis reveal?

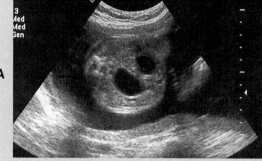
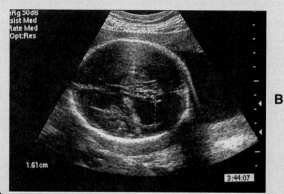
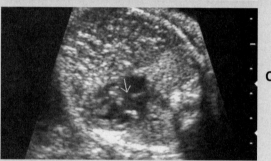

Fig. 24-1 **A,** This 26-week gestation is seen with ultrasound finding of double-bubble sign, which is consistent with duodenal atresia. **B,** Ventriculomegaly is also identified, in addition to, **C,** atrial septal defect.

OBJECTIVES

■ Describe the methods of noninvasive biochemical testing for assessment of risk of aneuploidy.

■ List the methods of invasive testing for chromosomal analysis.

■ Describe the anomalies associated with an increased nuchal translucency.

■ List the soft findings associated with chromosomal anomalies.

■ Describe the sonographic findings suggestive of trisomies 21, 13, and 18 and triploidy and 45,X.

GLOSSARY OF TERMS

Aneuploidy: an abnormal number of chromosomes

Chromosomes: found in the nucleus of a cell; contain DNA and genetic information

Clinodactyly: a finger or toe that is abnormally curved inward or outward

Cyclopia: one orbit or fusion of two orbits

Cystic hygroma: cystic lesions that occur with lymphatic obstruction, usually located at the posteriolateral aspect of the neck

Diaphragmatic hernia: displacement of abdominal contents into the thorax through a defect (usually left-sided) in the diaphragm

Duodenal atresia: abnormal development of the proximal duodenum that leads to an obstruction that presents sonographically as a double-bubble sign

Epicanthal fold: a fold of skin at the inner aspect of the eyelid

Holoprosencephaly: a anomaly characterized by absent or incomplete fusion of the forebrain; the most severe form results in fusion of the cerebrum, thalamus, with absence of the falx and a single ventricle; severe facial anomalies are associated with this abnormality

Hydrops: a condition of fluid overload that is diagnosed when fluid is identified in two body cavities or one body cavity with anasarca (skin edema)

Hypotelorism: closely spaced eyes

Karyotype: the pattern of chromosomes in an individual

Meningomyelocele: an open defect in the bony spine through which meninges and spinal cord protrude

Micrognathia: a small chin

Microphthalmia: small eyes

Mosaicism: the presence of two or more karyotypically distinct cell lines in the same tissue or individual

Oligohydramnios: a decrease in amniotic fluid

Omphalocele: herniation of abdominal contents through a defect at the base of umbilical cord

Polydactyly: extra digits

Polyhydramnios: an excess of amniotic fluid

Pyelectasis, or hydronephrosis: dilation of the renal pelvis

Radial ray defect: characterized by hypoplasia or aplasia of the radius

Syndactyly: fusion of digits

Talipes: clubfoot; an abnormal deviation of the foot relative to the leg

TORCH infections: *t*oxoplasmosis, *o*ther, *r*ubella, *c*ytomegalovirus, *h*erpes simplex; a group of infections that may have adverse affects on the fetus

Translocation: rearrangement of genetic material in which a part of a chromosome may be located on another chromosome

Trophoblast: tissue that develops into the placenta

Multiple well-established prenatal screening tests are used to identify the risks of chromosomal anomalies and a myriad of additional fetal abnormalities. Prenatal diagnosis can be assisted with screening blood tests, sonographic evaluation, and genetic testing. Noninvasive pregnancy screening is designed to identify those pregnancies at increased risk for abnormalities so that a targeted ultrasound and amniocentesis can be offered to those who will most benefit. Screening blood tests include pregnancy-associated plasma protein A (PAPP-A), free beta human chorionic gonadotropin (beta-hCG), hCG, alpha fetoprotein (AFP), unconjugated estriol (E_3), and dimeric inhibin A; and definitive genetic testing may be accomplished through chorionic villus sampling (CVS), amniocentesis, and fetal cord blood sampling. In addition to these biochemical screening tests, ultrasound may also be used to search for anomalies when maternal serum testing reveals an increased risk and to confirm or correct gestational age, as this is the most common cause of abnormal serum screening tests. Other factors that affect screening tests include multiple gestations and fetal viability. When a chromosomal anomaly is suspected or has been confirmed with genetic testing, ultrasound may be used to search for specific abnormalities (Table 24-1), so that the patient may be accurately counseled regarding prognosis, treatment, and pregnancy options.

MATERNAL SERUM SCREENING

First-Trimester Screening

Pregnancy-associated Plasma Protein A. Pregnancy-associated plasma protein A is a first-trimester biochemical screening test that is evaluated

Table 24-1	*Sonographic Findings Associated with Chromosomal Anomalies*
Chromosomal Anomaly	**Sonographic Findings**
Trisomy 21	Increased nuchal thickening, duodenal atresia, heart defects (atrioventricular canal, tetralogy of Fallot, ventricular septal defect, etc.), GI defects (duodenal atresia, esophageal atresia), cystic hygroma, ventriculomegaly, limb anomalies (absent middle phalanx of fifth digit, sandal gap toes, clinodactyly), pyelectasis, echogenic intracardiac focus
Trisomy 18	Clinched hands, choroids plexus cysts, omphalocele, talipes, rocker bottom foot, micrognathia, heart defects, CNS anomalies, absent radius, congenital diaphragmatic hernia, hydrops, IUGR, polyhydramnios, GU anomalies
Trisomy 13	CNS anomalies (holoprosencephaly, Dandy-Walker malformation, meningomyelocele, etc.), omphalocele, facial anomalies, polydactyly, talipes, heart defects, GI anomalies, GU anomalies, cystic hygroma, absent radius, polyhydramnios, IUGR
Turner's syndrome	Cystic hygroma, hydrops, heart defects, renal anomalies, oligohydramnios, female gender
Triploidy	Partial mole, heart defects, GI anomalies, GU anomalies, CNS anomalies, abnormal extremities, facial anomalies, syndactyly of third and fourth digits, IUGR, oligohydramnios

CNS, Central nervous system; *GI,* gastrointestinal; *GU,* genitourinary; *IUGR,* intrauterine growth restriction.

from maternal serum. PAPP-A is produced by the **tro-phoblast** of the placenta and is decreased in pregnancies affected by Down's syndrome and trisomy 18.[1]

Free Beta Human Chorionic Gonadotropin. Free beta-hCG is a glycoprotein hormone derived from the placenta. hCG has alpha and beta subunits, and the beta subunit peaks at 8 to 10 weeks' gestation then falls to a plateau. The free beta-hCG levels in trisomy 21 pregnancies are increased.

Multiple Marker Screening. Multiple marker screening in the first trimester has been used to increase the sensitivity in detection of trisomy 21. The combination of nuchal translucency (NT) measurements, PAPP-A, and free beta-hCG has a reported sensitivity of 89%.[2]

Second-Trimester Screening

Triple Screen. The triple screen is a biochemical test most commonly drawn from maternal serum that evaluates AFP, hCG, and E_3. This second-trimester screening test is used between 15 and 20 weeks' gestation for evaluation of risk for neural tube defects (and other fetal anomalies), as discussed in Chapter 23, and chromosomal anomalies, including Down's syndrome.[3] AFP is a glycoprotein produced in the yolk sac and fetal liver, E_3 is a hormone produced by the fetal liver and the placenta, and hCG is produced in the placenta. These biochemicals are found in amniotic fluid and are circulated into the maternal blood and may be tested in maternal serum or evaluated from amniotic fluid. When hCG is elevated and AFP and E_3 are decreased, an increased risk exists for Down's syndrome (trisomy 21). The triple screen detects approximately 60% of fetuses with Down's syndrome but also has an approximately 5% false-positive rate.[3] When the hCG, AFP, and E_3 are all decreased, the pregnancy is at increased risk for trisomy 18.

Quadruple Screen. The quadruple screen adds dimeric inhibin A (a protein derived from the placenta) to the triple test, increasing the detection rate of Down's syndrome to 76%[4] and improving the false-positive rate.[3] Unlike the serum markers used in the triple test, dimeric inhibin A values are independent of gestational age. Because the quadruple screen does include the hCG, AFP, and E_3, an accurate gestational age is imperative. Ultrasound may be used to define gestational age so that risk factors for trisomy 21 can be recalculated.

GENETIC TESTING

Genetic testing in pregnancy is performed for identification of the absence or presence of a normal **karyotype**. A human karyotype will contain 46 **chromosomes:** 22 pairs of autosomes and a pair of sex chromosomes. The chromosome analysis of a male fetus will reveal 46,XY, and a female fetus will reveal 46,XX. Chromosome analysis may detect additions, deletions, breaks, **translocations,** and mutations in the karyotype.

Genetic abnormalities may be dominant, usually inherited by one parent, and carry a 50% risk of transmission to the fetus. Or they may be recessive, inherited from both parents, and carry a 25% risk of transmission to the fetus. Anomalies may also be X-linked and transmitted by the mother to the male fetus. A mosaic includes genetic defects in a portion of cells with the other portion appearing normal.

Genetic testing in pregnancy is accomplished with CVS, amniocentesis, and cordocentesis. These testing procedures are performed with ultrasound guidance, and sterile technique is observed.

Chorionic Villus Sampling

Chorionic villus sampling is performed between 10 and 12 weeks' gestation and follows a sonographic examination that confirms gestational age and viability. CVS is a technique that extracts the chorionic villi from the trophoblast in the placenta with ultrasound guidance and a transabdominal or transcervical approach. The advantages of CVS when compared with amniocentesis include the access to genetic information earlier in pregnancy and earlier results, which lower the complication rate and psychologic burden when termination is elected.[5]

DNA analysis from CVS can be used to identify genetic defects, although they may be confined to the placenta when **mosaicism** is identified and amniocentesis may be necessary to determine whether the abnormal chromosome pattern is also in the fetus. In addition, CVS does not evaluate AFP, which is in the amniotic fluid, and therefore will not screen for open neural tube defects. Fetal limb-reduction abnormalities have been associated with CVS performed before 10 weeks' gestation.[6] Fetal loss rates are similar to those associated with second trimester amniocentesis.[7]

Amniocentesis

An alternative to CVS is early amniocentesis, which may be performed between 12 and 15 weeks' gestation. Although early amniocentesis alleviates the risk of an additional invasive procedure for placental mosaicism, failed attempts may occur when tenting of the amniotic membranes results from the lack of fusion of the amnion to chorion at this stage in pregnancy. Early amniocentesis does allow for testing of AFP, unlike CVS. The fetal loss rate may vary with the gestational age, although studies have found the loss rate to be increased over that of second-trimester amniocentesis and early

amniocentesis has also been associated with **talipes.**[3,4] Early amniocentesis is performed in a similar manner to second trimester amniocentesis.

Amniocentesis to rule out genetic defects is usually performed between 15 and 18 weeks' gestation, with a fetal loss rate of 0.8% in the United States.[8] The procedure usually includes an ultrasound evaluation to screen for abnormalities, growth, and viability. Amniocentesis is performed transabdominally with ultrasound guidance to extract amniotic fluid from the gestational sac that is transported for analysis. Results of the chromosomal analysis are usually available between 1 and 3 weeks and are considered the gold standard for detection of chromosomal anomalies.[9,10]

Conventional chromosomal analysis requires up to 3 weeks to culture and evaluate the chromosomes from amniotic fluid (Fig. 24-2, *A*), which adds additional stress to patients who are at increased risk for **aneuploidy** based on biochemical tests, maternal serum testing, or advanced maternal age. Fluorescence in situ hybridization (FISH) allows for limited analysis of uncultured amniotic fluid, with results available with 24 hours.[10,11] The FISH assay typically evaluates for numeric anomalies of chromosomes 21, 13, 18, X, and Y by adding a fluorescent match colored with dye to the fetal cells. The number of colored signals (Fig. 24-2, *B* and *C*; see Color Plate 17) represents the number of copies of certain chromosomes. The information obtained is more limited than with a cultured analysis, but the results can be obtained more quickly regarding the most common aneuploidies. A complete cultured analysis should be completed to confirm the findings.

In addition to genetic analysis, second- and third-trimester amniocentesis may also evaluate AFP levels and **TORCH** titers for evidence of fetal infections. Amniocentesis may also be used to reduce fluid levels in patients with severe **polyhydramnios** and may be used in the late third trimester to evaluate lung maturity when early delivery should be considered. Whenever an invasive procedure is performed, $Rh_o(D)$ immune globulin (RhoGam) should be administered to Rh-negative females to prevent sensitization in future pregnancies.

CHROMOSOMAL ANOMALIES
Nuchal Translucency

NT is an elevation of the skin, which contains fluid, at the posterior and lateral region of the neck. When identified, it can be reliably measured from 11 to 14 weeks gestation for evaluation for fetal aneuploidy. It is

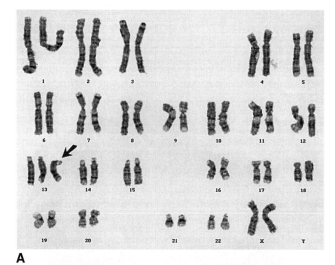

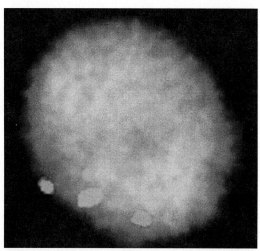

B

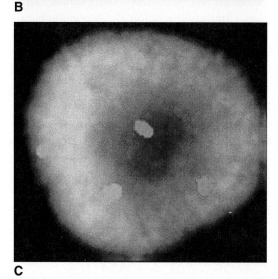

C

Fig. 24-2 **A,** Chromosomal analysis reveals female with trisomy 13. Fluorescence in situ hybridization analysis shows, **B,** two copies of X chromosome coded in green and two copies of chromosome 18 coded in blue. **C,** Two copies of chromosome 21 are coded in red and three copies of chromosome 13 are coded in green.

important to note that normal and abnormal NTs may spontaneously resolve and that resolution does not affect the associated risks for anomalies. An increased NT has been associated with trisomy 21, in addition to other chromosomal anomalies, including trisomy 18, trisomy 13, and 45,X. Increased NT may be isolated or part of "spacesuit" **hydrops,** where the skin line is separated by fluid along the entire body.[11] Spacesuit hydrops suggests an increased risk of aneuploidy in addition to NTs that contain septations or are of increased echogenicity. In the presence of normal chromosomes, NT has been associated with numerous abnormalities, including congenital heart defects, congenital **diaphragmatic hernia,** abdominal wall defects, and neural tube defects; multiple syndromes have also been identified.[12] In the absence of identifiable structural defects, an increased NT has been associated with a poor pregnancy outcome, including spontaneous abortion and fetal death.[13]

Sonographic Findings. An increased NT can be confirmed when the lucency measures 3 mm or more.[7] The technique includes obtaining an image of the fetus in a midsagittal plane (Fig. 24-3) without the presence of flexion or extension of the fetal head.[14] High-resolution equipment with the ability to measure .001-mm structures should be used.[12] The image should be magnified for ease in caliper placement. The measurement should be obtained with measurement of the actual lucency from inside the skin to the back of the neck. The amnion should be identified and excluded from this measurement.

Controversial Findings

A sonographic evaluation of a fetus may identify an anomaly that should precipitate a thorough search for additional anomalies, suggesting that a syndrome or chromosomal anomaly may be the cause. Multiple ultrasound markers for chromosomal anomalies exist

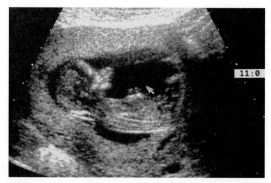

Fig. 24-3 Nuchal translucency measured 2.2 mm and was within normal limits.

that when isolated are often insignificant, including choroid plexus cysts, echogenic intracardiac focus (EIF), renal **pyelectasis,** and echogenic bowel (Table 24-2). When coupled with abnormal maternal serum screening, advanced maternal age (≥35 years old), or additional positive ultrasound findings, an amniocentesis should be offered for chromosomal analysis.

Choroid Plexus Cysts. Choroid plexus cysts have been identified in 0.4% to 3.6% of pregnancies and are usually an insignificant finding that resolves spontaneously.[15] Choroid plexus cysts have been associated with aneuploidy, most specifically trisomy 18. Because choroid plexus cysts (Fig. 24-4) are usually an insignificant finding, targeted ultrasonography for additional anomalies, maternal age, and maternal

Table 24-2	*Soft Markers for Aneuploidy Causes for Size Greater Than Dates*
Sonographic Finding	**Associated Chromosomal Anomaly**
Choroid plexus cysts	Trisomy 18
Echogenic intracardiac focus	Trisomy 21; trisomy 13
Renal pyelectasis	Trisomy 21
Echogenic bowel	Trisomy 21 (may be associated with fetal infections and cystic fibrosis)

serum testing should be considered when deciding whether amniocentesis is warranted.

Echogenic Intracardiac Focus. An EIF is a common finding identified in 5% of fetuses.[16] Although generally considered a normal variant, EIF has also been associated with trisomy 21 and trisomy 13. In most instances, the EIF will be located in the left ventricle (Fig. 24-5), which may be less significant than when identified in the right ventricle or bilaterally.[17] The EIF is identified on the four-chamber view of the heart and should have a similar echogenicity to fetal bone.[18] As with choroid plexus cysts, other factors such as maternal age, maternal serum testing, and presence of other anomalies should be considered when deciding whether amniocentesis is appropriate.

Renal Pyelectasis. Mild renal pyelectasis is another common finding that has questionable significance, although it has been associated with trisomy 21. Mild pyelectasis (Fig. 24-6) is defined as a dilated renal pelvis of 4 mm or more in the anteroposterior (AP) diameter.[8] Furthermore, many cases will resolve by the third trimester. Multiple studies have shown that approximately 25% of fetuses with trisomy 21 will show pyelectasis[16]; however, as an isolated finding, pyelectasis generally does not warrant amniocentesis.

Echogenic Bowel. Echogenic bowel has been identified in 0.2% to 1.4% of fetuses in the second trimester. It may be an isolated finding with no significance but has been associated with aneuploidy (most commonly trisomy 21), cystic fibrosis, and intrauterine infections.[19] In addition, echogenic bowel has also been identified with pregnancies affected by intrauterine growth restriction, placental insufficiency, and perinatal death.[20] Echogenic bowel (Fig. 24-7) can be diagnosed when the echogenicity of bowel is similar to bone. Results of maternal infection titers and cystic fibrosis

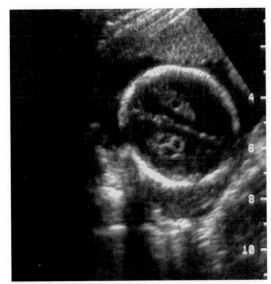

Fig. 24-4 Multiple choroid plexus cysts were identified bilaterally. No other abnormalities were identified.

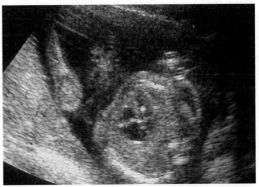

Fig. 24-5 Echogenic intracardiac focus is noted in left ventricle of fetus with abnormal triple screen.

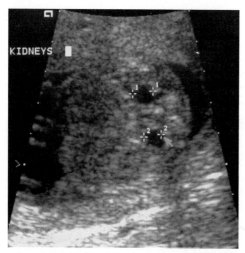

Fig. 24-6 Mild pyelectasis was noted bilaterally in fetus with trisomy 21. Right anteroposterior (AP) diameter of renal pelvis measured 6.7 mm, and left AP diameter measured 5.6 mm. Atrioventricular canal defect was also identified.

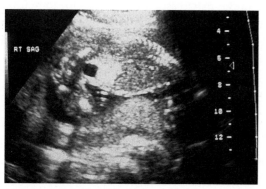

Fig. 24-7 Echogenic bowel may be associated with trisomy 21.

carrier testing should be factored into the decision to offer amniocentesis.

Trisomy 21

Down's syndrome, also known as *trisomy 21*, is most commonly characterized by an extra twenty-first chromosome, although Down's syndrome may also occur with mosaics and translocations. It is the most common chromosomal anomaly, occurring in 1:700 births and resulting in mild to moderate retardation and a variety of other anomalies, including cardiac anomalies that may be life threatening.[21] An increased risk exists in women who are of advanced maternal age, but trisomy 21 may affect fetuses in women of all ages.

Trisomy 21 infants have a characteristic appearance that includes **epicanthal folds,** a round head, flattened nasal bridge, small ears, redundant skin at the back of the neck, and a protruding tongue.[5] Anomalies may be identified in these children, including heart defects, gastrointestinal defects, limb anomalies, **cystic hygroma,** and hydrops.

Sonographic Findings. Sonographic evaluation and diagnosis of Down's syndrome has been challenging because many of the findings are nonspecific and there may also be an absence of any positive findings. Sonographic findings (Fig. 24-8) that have been identified as more significant for trisomy 21 include a thickened nuchal fold (≥6 mm). This measurement should be taken of the skin thickness at the back of the neck at the level of the transcerebellar measurement and is most effective when taken between 15 and 20 weeks' gestation. Other findings include an atrioventricular canal defect, **duodenal atresia** that presents as a double-bubble sign, ventriculomegaly, and hypoplasia or aplasia of the middle phalanx of the fifth digit (Fig. 24-9). Decreased humoral and femoral lengths and a sandal gap appearance of the foot (a gap between the first and second digits) may also be associated with trisomy 21. Small ears, **clinodactyly,** and single umbilical artery may also be identified. A number of soft findings may suggest trisomy 21, including renal pyelectasis, EIF, and echogenic bowel; however, in isolation, these findings are generally insignificant. The sensitivity of ultrasound detection of trisomy 21 is reported between 59.2% and 91.0%.[22] Combination of ultrasound findings with maternal serum screening and maternal age risk factors may improve the detection of trisomy 21.

Trisomy 18

Trisomy 18, also known as *Edwards' syndrome,* is a severe anomaly characterized by an extra chromosome 18 that occurs in 3:10,000 live births. Trisomy 18 is associated with defects that affect multiple organ systems and is seen in increased frequency in women of advanced maternal age. Many trisomy 18 fetuses spontaneously abort, and 90% of infants born live die within the first year. Survivors have profound mental and physical disabilities.[21]

One of the characteristic features of trisomy 18 is a persistently clenched hand (Fig. 24-10), and the second digit may overlap the remaining digits. Patients may have choroid plexus cyst, **omphalocele,** talipes (Fig. 24-11), low-set ears, and **micrognathia.** Other associated anomalies include those of the cardiovascular system, extremities, gastrointestinal system, genitourinary system, and central nervous system.

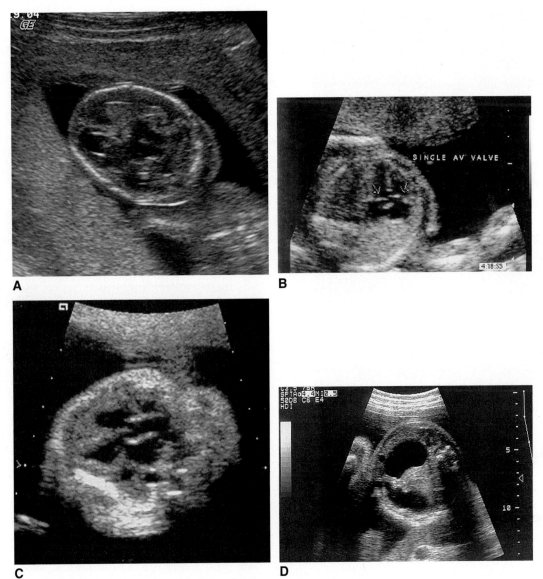

Fig. 24-8 **A,** Thickened nuchal fold is identified in fetus with trisomy 21. Heart defects that may be identified in association with trisomy 21 include, **B,** atrioventricular canal defects and, **C,** tetralogy of Fallot, which is shown in this image documenting characteristic overriding aorta. **D,** Duodenal atresia was identified in patient whose karyotype revealed trisomy 21. (**A** Courtesy GE Medical Systems.)

Sonographic Findings. Sonographic findings (Fig. 24-12) associated with trisomy 18 are evident in 77% to 97% of fetuses.23 Identification of clenched hands with choroids plexus cysts suggests this anomaly. Other findings that may be identified include rocker bottom **feet, omphalocele, congenital heart defects, micrognathia,** a strawberry-shaped head, talipes, **radial ray defects, hydronephrosis,** agenesis of the corpus callosum, and congenital diaphragmatic hernia. Severe intrauterine growth restriction, hydrops, and polyhydramnios may also be identified.

Trisomy 13

Trisomy 13, also known as *Patau's syndrome,* is seen with karyotype revealing an extra chromosome 13 and occurs in 1:5000 births.[21] Women of advanced maternal age are at risk for a pregnancy affected by trisomy 13. This severe chromosomal anomaly is characterized by multiple anomalies that occur across most organ systems, with many spontaneously aborting in utero and most live births resulting in death within the first month. Survivors have severe mental and physical deficits and seizure disorder.

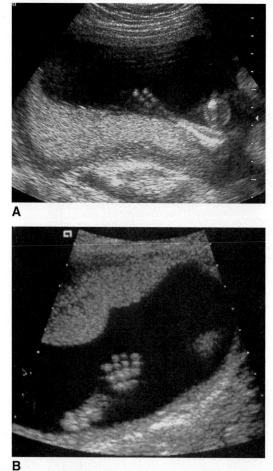

Fig. 24-9 Middle phalanx of fifth digit may be hypoplastic or absent in presence of trisomy 21. **A,** Normal-appearing fifth digit is identified. **B,** Absent middle phalanx noted in fetus with trisomy 21.

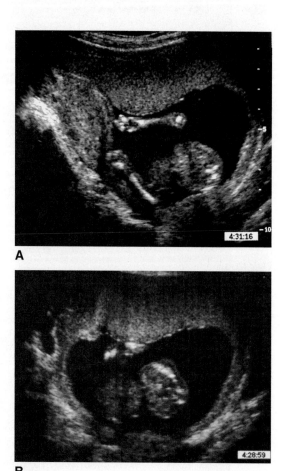

Fig. 24-10 Patient was seen for amniocentesis at 17 weeks' gestation for advanced maternal age. Ultrasound examination revealed, **A,** persistently clinched hands and, **B,** omphalocele. Heart defect was also suspected. Chromosomal analysis revealed trisomy 18.

Characteristic features suggestive of trisomy 13 include **holoprosencephaly** (Fig. 24-13), facial anomalies (Fig. 24-14), **polydactyly,** heart defects, and omphalocele. A variety of anomalies of the central nervous system, gastrointestinal system, cardiovascular system, genitourinary system, and extremities may also occur.

Sonographic Findings. The sonographic identification of trisomy 13 has a sensitivity of 90% to 100%.[21] The sonographic findings of holoprosencephaly and associated facial anomalies (**cyclopia, hypotelorism, microphthalmia,** cleft lip and palate) suggest trisomy 13, although holoprosencephaly may be an isolated anomaly. Other sonographic findings include talipes, polydactyly (Fig. 24-15, *A* and *B*), microcephaly, echogenic kidneys, and agenesis of the corpus callosum.[5] **Meningomyelocele,** renal anomalies, cystic hygroma, omphalocele, EIF (Fig. 24-15, *C* and *D*), and radial ray

defects may also be identified. Mild ventriculomegaly and polyhydramnios may also be found.

Turner's Syndrome

Turner's syndrome is also expressed as 45,X and is characterized by the absence of a sex chromosome. The occurrence rate of Turner's syndrome is 1:5000 to 10,000 births and is not associated with advanced maternal age.[5] Many fetuses spontaneously abort, although infants who are live born usually have normal intelligence.

Fetuses with Turner's syndrome often have large cystic hygromas and associated hydrops. Female infants have a characteristic webbed neck, are short in stature, and are infertile. Congenital heart defects and renal anomalies may also be present.

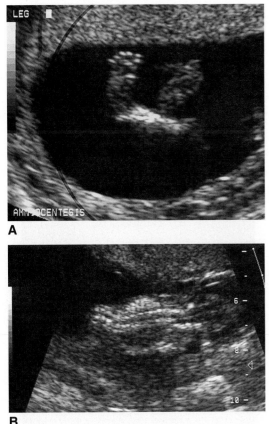

A

B

Fig. 24-11 Patient was seen at maternal-fetal center after abnormal ultrasound in obstetrician's office. At 16 weeks, 1 day gestational age, **A,** talipes and, **B,** abnormal curvature of spine were noted. Additional findings included absent radii with clubbed hands. Two weeks later, patient returned for evaluation of fetal heart, which revealed ventricular septal defect. Patient consented to amniocentesis, which diagnosed trisomy 18.

Sonographic Findings. A cystic hygroma (Fig. 24-16) with hydrops suggests Turner's syndrome. Congenital heart defects, specifically coarctation of the aorta, short femurs, and renal anomalies, may also be identified. **Oligohydramnios** may also be present.[5]

Triploidy

Triploidy is a profoundly severe anomaly characterized by an extra set of chromosomes that is most commonly caused by two sperm fertilizing the ova. Triploid fetuses (Fig. 24-17, *A*) frequently spontaneously abort and are often associated with a partial mole (see Chapter 21).[9]

Multiple anomalies involving the gastrointestinal tract, cardiovascular system, central nervous system, and genitourinary tract may be identified. Facial anomalies and abnormalities of the extremities may also be noted.

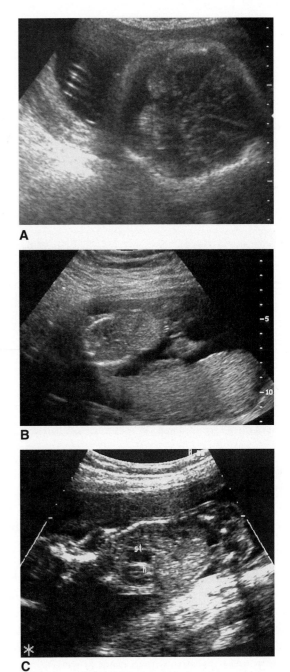

A

B

C

Fig. 24-12 Sonographic findings that may be associated with trisomy 18 include central nervous system anomalies. **A,** Dandy-Walker malformation was identified in fetus of young woman who declined amniocentesis. Diagnosis of trisomy 18 was made at birth. **B,** Omphalocele and, **C,** congenital diaphragmatic hernia may be associated with trisomy 18 and other chromosomal anomalies.

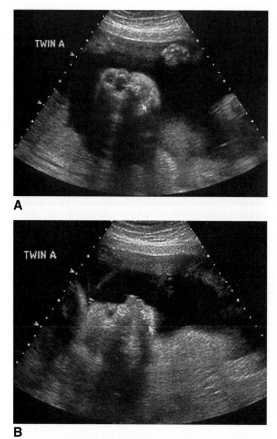

Fig. 24-13 Holoprosencephaly and trisomy 13 were confirmed in fetus with, **A,** cyclopia and, **B,** absent nose.

Sonographic Findings. **Syndactyly** of the third and fourth digits strongly suggests triploidy. In addition, omphalocele (Fig. 24-17, *B*), renal anomalies, meningomyelocele, agenesis of the corpus callosum, holoprosencephaly, and hydrocephalus may be identified. Low-set ears, micrognathia, facial clefts, and talipes may also been seen. Severe intrauterine growth restriction, oligohydramnios, and a large placenta containing multiple cystic spaces may be present as well.[5]

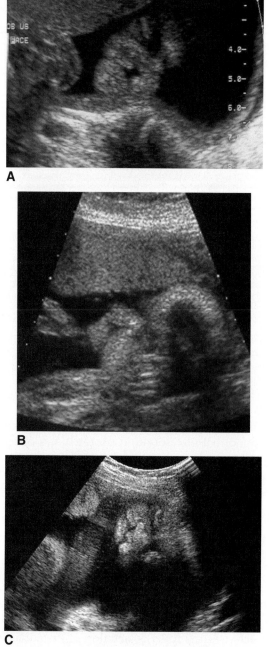

Fig. 24-14 **A** and **B,** Median clefts and, **C,** bilateral clefts may be associated with aneuploidy.

CLINICAL SCENARIO—DIAGNOSIS

■ The amniocentesis revealed trisomy 21, which would be expected in a fetus with the combination of duodenal atresia, ventriculomegaly, and heart defect. The patient returned at 35 weeks with absence of fetal movements. Sonographic examination confirmed fetal death.

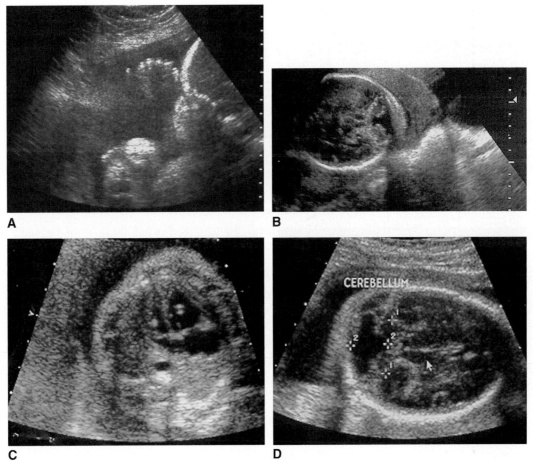

Fig. 24-15 **A,** Polydactyly was noted in fetus that also had, **B,** Dandy-Walker malformation. Chromosomal analysis confirmed trisomy 13. **C,** Bilateral and multiple echogenic foci were identified in fetus in addition to, **D,** Dandy-Walker malformation.

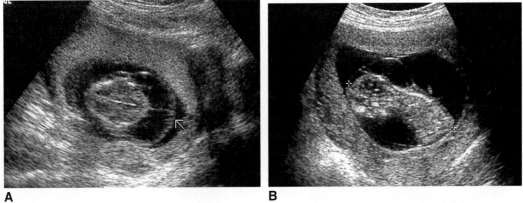

Fig. 24-16 **A,** Cystic hygroma is identified in fetus with Turner's syndrome. **B,** Another fetus with nuchal translucency of 13 mm was diagnosed with Turner's syndrome after amniocentesis.

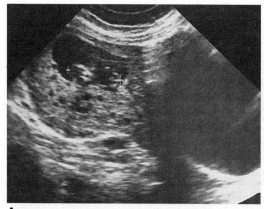

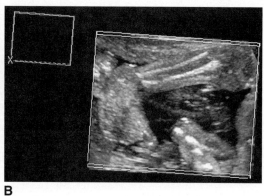

A

B

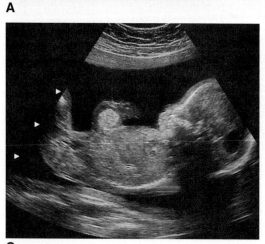

C

Fig. 24-17 **A,** Partial mole may be seen with severely growth-retarded fetus and enlarged placenta containing multiple cystic spaces. Fetal death was confirmed during examination. Other findings that may be associated with triploidy include, **B,** talipes and, **C,** omphalocele. (**B** and **C** Courtesy GE Medical Systems.)

CASE STUDIES FOR DISCUSSION

1. A 30-year-old woman is seen for ultrasound after an abnormal triple test at 17²/₇ weeks' gestation. The ultrasound reveals the finding in Fig. 24-18. What is the primary concern for this pregnancy?

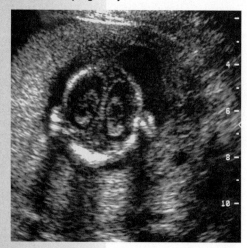

Fig. 24-18 Bilateral choroids plexus cysts are identified.

2. A 24-year-old woman is seen for an obstetric ultrasound for uncertain last menstrual period. The ultrasound reveals the findings in Fig. 24-19. What is the most likely diagnosis?

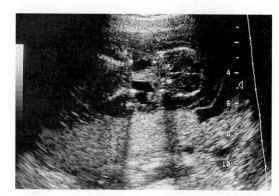

Fig. 24-19 Cystic hygroma is identified at lateral aspects of neck. Diffuse edema is identified around fetal head and extended to fetal body.

CASE STUDIES FOR DISCUSSION—cont'd

3. A 35-year-old woman is seen for ultrasound at 28 weeks' gestation for decreased fundal height. The patient had a first-trimester ultrasound at 7 weeks' gestation for vaginal spotting. The ultrasound reveals an amniotic fluid index of 28.2 cm, an average ultrasound age of 25 weeks and 4 days, and the findings in Fig. 24-20. What is the most likely diagnosis?

4. A 25-year-old woman is referred to a maternal-fetal center for the finding in Fig. 24-21. A targeted ultrasound is performed and confirms the finding, and the rest of the examination is unremarkable. An amniocentesis is performed and reveals which chromosomal anomaly?

5. A 21-year-old woman is seen at 22²/₇ weeks' gestation for size and dates. Identification of multiple fetal anomalies prompted a referral to a maternal-fetal center. During the ultrasound examination, the anomalies in Fig. 24-22 were identified, in addition to a ventricular septal defect; and an amniocentesis was performed. What is the most likely result of the amniocentesis?

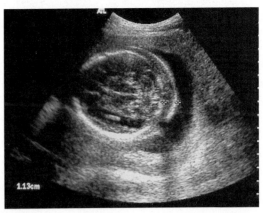

Fig. 24-21   Nuchal thickening is identified in fetus at 19²/₇ weeks' gestation.

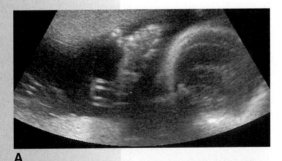

A

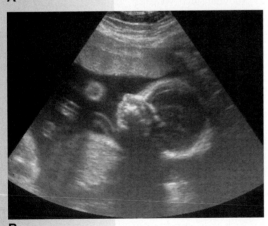

B

Fig. 24-20   Fetus showed, **A,** persistently clinched hand and, **B,** micrognathia.

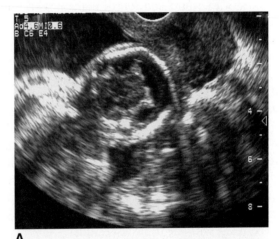

A

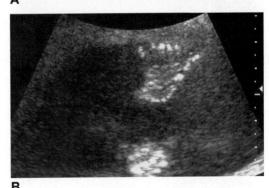

B

Fig. 24-22   **A,** Single ventricle is identified consistent with holoprosencephaly. **B,** Polydactyly and heart defect are also identified in fetus.

STUDY QUESTIONS

1. The quadruple screen includes all of the following biochemical markers except which?
   a. alpha fetoprotein
   b. unconjugated estriol
   c. human chorionic gonadotrophin
   d. inhibin A
   e. pregnancy-associated plasma protein A

2. A 25-year-old woman is seen for an ultrasound at 18 weeks' gestation after abnormal triple screen results. The sonographer identifies a nuchal fold measuring 7 mm. The remainder of the examination is unremarkable. What is the most likely diagnosis?
   a. a normal fetus
   b. trisomy 13
   c. trisomy 18
   d. trisomy 21
   e. triploidy

3. Fusion of the third and fourth digits is associated with which of the following chromosomal anomalies?
   a. triploidy
   b. trisomy 13
   c. trisomy 18
   d. trisomy 21
   e. Turner's syndrome

4. A 32-year-old woman is seen for obstetric ultrasound with abnormal triple test results that revealed a decrease in human chorionic gonadotrophin, unconjugated estriol, and alpha fetoprotein. Which of the following abnormalities will be most useful to correlate with the triple test results?
   a. clinched hands
   b. cystic hygroma
   c. polydactyly
   d. syndactyly
   e. thickened nuchal fold

5. In which of the following invasive procedures is tenting of the membranes most likely to occur?
   a. amniocentesis
   b. chorionic villus sampling
   c. cordocentesis
   d. early amniocentesis
   e. lung maturity testing

6. A 36-year-old woman with a history of vaginal bleeding is seen for an obstetric ultrasound at 12 weeks' gestation. The ultrasound reveals a nuchal translucency measuring 4.8 mm. This suggests which of the following?
   a. aneuploidy
   b. cardiac anomalies
   c. poor pregnancy outcome
   d. trisomy 21
   e. all of the above

7. A 42-year-old woman is seen for ultrasound at 28 weeks' gestation for late prenatal care. The ultrasound reveals a grossly abnormal brain and cyclopia. Which of the following chromosomal anomalies is most strongly associated with the ultrasound findings?
   a. Down's syndrome
   b. Edwards' syndrome
   c. Patau's syndrome
   d. Triploidy
   e. Turner's syndrome

8. Which of following techniques is the correct method of nuchal translucency measurement?
   a. midsagittal plane, inside skin line to soft tissue of neck
   b. transverse plane, inside skin line to soft tissue of neck
   c. midsagittal plane, outside skin line to soft tissue of neck
   d. transverse plane, outside skin line to soft tissue of neck
   e. midsagittal plane, longitudinal measurement of lucent region

9. A 40-year-old woman is seen for an obstetric ultrasound at 24 weeks for size greater than dates. The sonographer identifies duodenal atresia and an absent middle phalanx of the fifth digit. Which of the following chromosomal anomalies is of primary concern?
   a. trisomy 13
   b. trisomy 18
   c. trisomy 21
   d. triploidy
   e. 45,X

10. Which of the following soft findings is most specific for Edwards' syndrome?
    a. choroid plexus cyst
    b. echogenic bowel
    c. echogenic intracardiac focus
    d. increased nuchal translucency
    e. pyelectasis

ACKNOWLEDGMENT

The authors thank Melissa Spagnuolo, Fetal Diagnostic Center of Orlando, for many of the images for this chapter.

REFERENCES

1. Spencer K, Liao AW, Ong CY et al: First trimester maternal serum placenta growth factor (PIGF) concentrations in pregnancies with fetal trisomy 21 or trisomy 18, *Prenat Diagn* 21:718-722, 2001.
2. Michailidis GD, Spencer K, Economides DL: The use of nuchal translucency measurement and second trimester biochemical markers in screening for Down's Syndrome, *Br J Obstet Gynaecol* 108:1047-1052, 2001.
3. Devieve F, Bouckaert A, Hubinont C et al: Multiple screening for Down's syndrome with the classic triple test, dimeric inhibin A and ultrasound, *Gynecol Obstet Invest* 49:221-226, 2000.
4. Himes P: Early pregnancy prenatal diagnostic testing: risks associated with chorionic villus sampling and early amniocentesis and screening options, *J Perinat Neonat Nurs* 13:1-13, 1999.
5. De Catte L, Liebaers I, Foulon W: Outcome of twin gestations after first trimester chorionic villus sampling, *Obstet Gynecol* 96:714-720, 2000.
6. Hagen-Ansert SA: *Textbook of diagnostic ultrasonography*, vol 1, ed 5, St Louis, 2001, Mosby.
7. Brambati B, Tului L, Guercilena S et al: Outcome of first-trimester chorionic villus sampling for genetic investigation in multiple pregnancy, *Ultrasound Obstet Gynecol* 17:209-216, 2001.
8. Callen P: *Ultrasonography in obstetrics and gynecology*, ed 4, Philadelphia, 2000, WB Saunders.
9. Leung WC et al: Role of amniotic fluid interphase fluorescence in situ hybridization (FISH) analysis in patient management, *Prenat Diagn* 21:327-332, 2001.
10. Pergament E, Chen PX, Thangavelu M et al: The clinical application of interphase FISH in prenatal diagnosis, *Prenat Diagn* 20:215-220, 2000.
11. Shulman LP et al: Fetal 'space-suit' hydrops in the first trimester: differentiating risk for chromosome abnormalities by delineating characteristics of nuchal translucency, *Prenat Diagn* 20:30-32, 2000.
12. Souter VL, Nyberg DA: Sonographic screening for fetal aneuploidy, *J Ultrasound Med* 20:775-790, 2001.
13. Souka AP, Krampl E, Bakalis S et al: Outcome of pregnancy in chromosomally normal fetuses with increased nuchal translucency in the first trimester, *Ultrasound Obstet Gynecol* 18:9-17, 2001.
14. de Graaf IM, Muller MA, van Zuylen-Vie AA et al: The influence of fetal position on nuchal translucency thickness, *Ultrasound Obstet Gynecol* 15:520-522, 2000.
15. Sullivan A, Giudice T, Vavelidis F et al: Choroid plexus cysts: is biochemical testing a valuable adjunct to targeted ultrasonography? *Am J Obstet Gynecol* 181:260-265, 1999.
16. Kubas C: Noninvasive means of identifying fetuses with possible Down syndrome: a review, *J Perinat Neonat Nurs* 13:27-46, 1999.
17. Huggon IC, Cook AC, Simpson JM et al: Isolated echogenic foci in the fetal heart as marker of chromosomal abnormality, *Ultrasound Obstet Gynecol* 17:11-16, 2001.
18. Prefumo F, Presti F, Mavrides E et al: Isolated echogenic foci in the fetal heart: do they increase the risk of trisomy 21 in a population previously screened by nuchal translucency? *Ultrasound Obstet Gynecol* 18:126-130, 2001.
19. Al-Kouatly HB, Chasen ST, Streltzoff J et al: The clinical significance of fetal echogenic bowel, *Am J Obstet Gynecol* 185:1035-1038, 2001.
20. Harrison KL, Martinez D, Mason G: The subjective assessment of echogenic fetal bowel, *Ultrasound Obstet Gynecol* 16:524-529, 2000.
21. Benacerraf BR: *Ultrasound of fetal syndromes*, Philadelphia, 1998, Churchill Livingstone.
22. Egan JF, Malakh L, Turner GW et al: Role of ultrasound for Down syndrome screening in advanced maternal age, *Am J Obstet Gynecol* 183:1028-1031, 2001.
23. DeVore GR: Second trimester ultrasonography may identify 77 to 97% of fetuses with trisomy 18, *J Ultrasound Med* 19:565-576, 2000.

Fetal Anomaly

CHARLOTTE HENNINGSEN

CLINICAL SCENARIO

■ A young woman is seen for an ultrasound for late prenatal care. The ultrasound reveals a single fetus in the late second trimester and the findings in Fig. 25-1. What are the most likely diagnosis and prognosis?

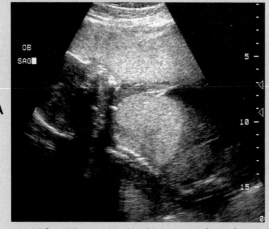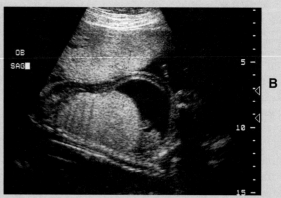

Fig. 25-1 Sagittal images of, **A,** fetal thorax and, **B,** abdomen reveal echogenic lesion in thorax with, **B,** fluid in abdomen with skin thickening.

OBJECTIVES

■ Describe anomalies that may be identified with prenatal ultrasound.

■ Identify the sonographic features that differentiate fetal anomalies.

■ List anomalies that may benefit from in utero treatment.

■ Identify anomalies that are incompatible with survival after birth.

■ List other methods of fetal evaluation used in the diagnosis of anomalies.

GLOSSARY OF TERMS

Aneuploidy: abnormal chromosomes

Aqueductal stenosis: congenital stenosis of the aqueduct of Sylvius (the part of the ventricular system that connects the third and fourth ventricles) that results in dilation of the lateral and third ventricles and is usually the result of an X-linked recessive pattern of inheritance

Arachnoid cysts: cysts located between the layers of the pia mater and arachnoid

Camptomelic dysplasia: a lethal skeletal dysplasia characterized by bent bones (camptomelia)

Cebocephaly: hypotelorism and a nose with single nostril

Choledochal cysts: cystic dilations of the biliary tree

Cyclopia: one orbit or the fusion of two orbits

Diastrophic dysplasia: an autosomal recessive short-limbed skeletal dysplasia with a characteristic fixed abducted thumb (hitchhiker thumb)

Ethmocephaly: cyclopia or hypotelorism with a proboscis or double proboscis

Heterozygous: inherited from both parents

Homozygous: inherited from one parent

Hydrops: a condition of fluid overload that can be diagnosed with the identification of skin edema plus fluid in one body cavity or fluid in two body cavities

Hypotelorism: closely spaced eyes

Polyhydramnios: an excessive accumulation of amniotic fluid

Proboscis: Fleshy, trunklike appendage

Rhizomelia: shortening of the proximal segment of the extremity

Thrombocytopenia–absent radius syndrome: syndrome characterized by thrombocytopenia and absent radii

Urachal cysts: persistence and distension of the embryologic allantois; midline in location; abuts the bladder

Volvulus: a twisting of the bowel that results in obstruction

X-linked: anomalies that are transmitted from the mother to the male fetus

---

Patients may be referred for an obstetric ultrasound for suspected fetal anomaly. With little additional information, the sonographer must carefully survey the fetus to identify and clarify the nature of the abnormality. Sonographers must be familiar with a variety of fetal anomalies. Proper documentation and subsequent diagnosis must be made for a meaningful discussion with the patient of pregnancy, treatment, and delivery options. This chapter explores many of the fetal anomalies that are identified with ultrasound (Table 25-1). Additional chapters in this text review renal anomalies (see Chapter 20), neural tube and abdominal wall anomalies (see Chapter 23), chromosomal anomalies (see Chapter 24), and fetal heart defects (see Chapter 26).

FETAL BRAIN

Hydrocephaly

Hydrocephalus is defined as a dilated ventricle with enlargement of the head and ventriculomegaly is a dilation of the ventricles without enlargement of the head, although these terms are sometimes used interchangeably. Hydrocephalus occurs in 0.5:1000 to 3:1000 live births and is associated with a high morbidity and mortality rate.[1] Hydrocephalus may be the result of a congenital anomaly or acquired, and when hydrocephalus leads to intracranial pressure, brain parenchyma may also be damaged. In addition, ventricular enlargement may result from compensation for atrophy or abnormal development of brain parenchyma.[2] The outcome is variable depending on the associated anomalies and the severity of the dilation.

The multiple causes of hydrocephalus include holoprosencephaly, spina bifida, encephalocele, Dandy-Walker malformation (DWM), **aqueductal stenosis, arachnoid cysts,** and agenesis of the corpus callosum (ACC). Hydrocephalus may be identified in fetuses affected by congenital infections, neoplasms, and musculoskeletal anomalies and may be identified as an isolated finding. Ventriculomegaly may also be associated with **aneuploidy.**

Sonographic Findings. The diagnosis of ventriculomegaly can be made when the atrium of the lateral ventricle exceeds 10 mm (Fig. 25-2) in the second and third trimesters of pregnancy.[3] When ventriculomegaly is identified, an evaluation of all fetal measurements can help to determine the degree of hydrocephalus present and whether fetal head enlargement is present. A thorough sonographic evaluation should also be performed in a search for associated anomalies.

Table 25-1	*Fetal Anomalies*
Diagnosis	**Sonographic Findings**
Hydrocephaly	Enlarged head; atrium of lateral ventricle > 10 mm
Holoprosencephaly	Single ventricle, fused thalami, absent cavum septum pellucidum and corpus callosum, absent falx; facial anomalies (clefts, hypotelorism, cyclopia, proboscis)
Hydranencephaly	Liquefaction of brain parenchyma; brain stem may be identified
Dandy-Walker malformation	Posterior fossa cyst with enlarged cisterna magna, splaying of cerebellar hemispheres with absent or dysplastic vermis; commonly associated with hydrocephalus
Agenesis of the corpus callosum	Absent cavum septum pellucidum, mild ventriculomegaly with dilated occipital horns; lateral displacement of lateral ventricles and superior displacement of third ventricle; dilated third ventricle
Cleft lip	Disruption of soft tissue of upper lip; bilateral cleft may appear to have premaxillary mass
Micrognathia	Recessed chin
Congenital diaphragmatic hernia	Abdominal contents, usually in stomach, in thorax; malposition of fetal heart; absence of intraabdominal stomach
Congenital cystic adenomatoid malformation	Type I: multiple large cysts; type II: visible cysts < 1 cm; type III: large echogenic mass in thorax
Pulmonary sequestration	Echogenic mass, may be triangular; separate blood supply from aorta
Pleural effusion	Fluid collection surrounding lungs; unilateral or bilateral
Duodenal atresia	Dilated stomach and proximal duodenum appearing as double bubble, polyhydramnios common
Bowel obstruction	Dilated loops of bowel proximal to obstruction
Meconium peritonitis	Calcifications on peritoneal surfaces; meconium pseudocyst; associated ascites or polyhydramnios may be identified
Ascites	Collection of fluid in fetal abdomen outlining organs and bowel
Abdominal cysts	Usually round, thin-walled anechoic structure; location and gender should be identified to identify origin
Sacrococcygeal teratoma	Heterogeneous or complex mass extending from fetal sacrum
Thanatophoric dysplasia	Significant micromelia, narrow thorax with protuberant abdomen, bowed limbs, macrocephaly with frontal bossing, trilobular skull may be identified
Achondrogenesis	Extreme micromelia, variable degrees of ossification of spine and calvaria, narrow thorax and ribs, rib fractures may be noted
Achondroplasia	Rhizomelia, trident hand, macrocephalus with frontal bossing, depressed nasal bridge
Short rib–polydactyl syndrome	Micromelia, narrow thorax, short ribs, polydactyly, cleft lip and palate may be identified
Osteogenesis imperfecta	Decreased ossification of bones, compressible calvaria, narrow ribs, short limbs, multiple fractures

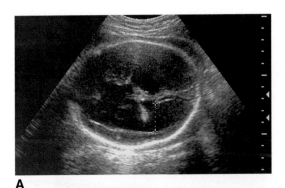

A

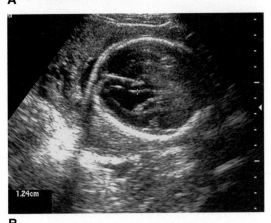

1.24cm

B

Fig. 25-2 A, Lateral ventricle of fetus measured 24 mm. Dandy-Walker malformation was also identified. **B,** Lateral ventricle measured 12 mm and was associated with Down's syndrome.

Holoprosencephaly

Holoprosencephaly encompasses a range of severity characterized by incomplete or lack of cleavage of the forebrain. The condition has been identified in 1:8000 second-trimester pregnancies, and many cases spontaneously abort in the first trimester.[4] The most severe form, alobar holoprosencephaly, presents with a complete failure of separation of the forebrain with subsequent fusion of the thalamus, a single ventricle, and cerebral hemispheres. Absence of the falx, corpus callosum, olfactory bulbs, and optic tracts is also noted. Semilobar holoprosencephaly is seen with partial cleavage of the forebrain and absence of the corpus callosum and olfactory bulbs. Identification of the mildest form, lobar holoprosencephaly, may be difficult because separation of the cerebrum will be evident although fusion of the lateral ventricles and absence of the corpus callosum may be noted. The outcome is variable depending on the severity, but the most severe forms of holoprosencephaly carry an extremely poor prognosis.[5]

Holoprosencephaly is associated with severe facial anomalies, including **cyclopia, ethmocephaly, cebocephaly,** and facial clefts. Holoprosencephaly is also associated with multiple chromosomal anomalies, most commonly trisomy 13. In addition, holoprosencephaly may be identified in many syndromes, including Edwards' syndrome (trisomy 18), Meckel's syndrome, Smith-Lemli-Opitz syndrome, and Hall-Pallister syndrome. Holoprosencephaly may also be transmitted through autosomal dominant, autosomal recessive, and **X-linked** modes. Also, several teratogenic effects have been linked to holoprosencephaly, including hyperglycemia (in diabetes) and alcohol.[4,5]

Sonographic Findings. Sonographic identification of holoprosencephaly is easier in its most severe form, and identification of a single ventricle (Fig. 25-3, *A*) surrounded by brain parenchyma is diagnostic. The thalamus appears fused, and the falx is absent as are the cavum septum pellucidum (CSP) and corpus callosum. In semilobar holoprosencephaly (Fig. 25-3, *B* and *C*), variable fusion may be identified and lobar holoprosencephaly may be difficult to distinguish from ACC, which should be suspected when the CSP is not identified. When enlargement of the ventricle is identified, holoprosencephaly may be difficult to differentiate from hydranencephalus or severe hydrocephalus, unless the characteristic facial anomalies are also identified.

When holoprosencephaly is identified, the face should be meticulously surveyed for the presence of associated anomalies, including (Fig 25-3, *C* to *E*) facial clefts, **hypotelorism,** a nose with a single nostril, a **proboscis,** and cyclopia. Other anomalies, such as a heart defect, polydactyly, or encephalocele, may suggest association with a chromosomal anomaly or syndrome.[5]

Hydranencephaly

Hydranencephaly is characterized by destruction of the brain parenchyma that may result from carotid artery occlusion, congenital infections, cocaine abuse, and some less common causes. Hydranencephaly is a rare anomaly, with a prevalence of less than 1:10,000 births.[6] The destruction to the brain usually occurs in the second trimester of pregnancy and may be preceded by a normal sonographic evaluation. The outcome of hydranencephaly is grave.

Sonographic Findings. The sonographic findings of hydranencephaly (Fig. 25-4) include liquefaction of the brain parenchyma with replacement by cerebrospinal fluid. The brainstem is intact and visible on

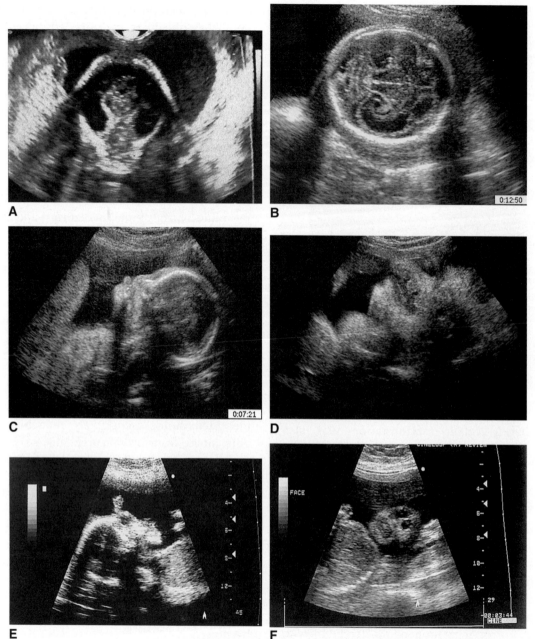

Fig. 25-3 **A,** Monoventricle associated with alobar holoprosencephaly is shown in fetal head. **B,** Semilobar holoprosencephaly was suspected in fetus with normal chromosomes. Anterior portion of brain was abnormal, and absent cavum septum pellucidum was noted. **C,** Abnormal profile and, **D,** bilateral cleft lip were also identified. Semilobar holoprosencephaly was confirmed at birth, and infant died within first few days of birth. Other facial anomalies may be identified in association with holoprosencephaly, including, **E,** proboscis and, **F,** hypotelorism.

ultrasound. The head may be normal or large in size. Hydranencephaly can be differentiated from severe hydrocephaly by a lack of surrounding brain parenchyma.

Dandy-Walker Malformation

Dandy-Walker malformation is characterized by absence or dysplasia of the cerebellar vermis and maldevelopment of the fourth ventricle with replacement by a posterior fossa cyst. A less severe form, referred to as the Dandy-Walker variant, may occur with dysplasia of the cerebellar vermis without enlargement of the posterior fossa. DWM is associated with numerous syndromes and chromosomal anomalies, including Meckel-Gruber syndrome, Neu Laxova syndrome, and short rib–

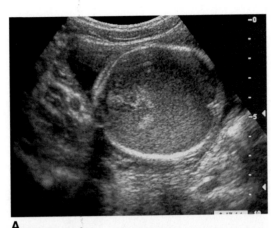

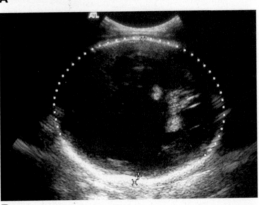

Fig. 25-4 Hydranencephaly. Young woman with poorly controlled diabetes was seen for ultrasound for late prenatal care. Fetal head was disproportionately large compared with abdominal circumference and femur length. **A,** Normal head anatomy was not seen, and homogeneous echogenic matter was identified swirling within calvaria. **B,** Follow-up examinations showed fetal head filled with anechoic fluid. Fetus died in utero near term.

polydactyly syndrome (SRPS). Chromosomal anomalies may be associated with as many as 55% of fetuses with DWM and include trisomy 13, trisomy 18, trisomy 21, and triploidy.[7] DWM has also been linked to the teratogenic effects of congenital infections and multiple intracranial anomalies, including ACC.

Sonographic Findings. The diagnosis of DWM can be made with the identification of a posterior fossa cyst, with a resultant enlarged cisterna magna, and splaying of the cerebellar hemispheres (Fig. 25-5) from the abnormal development of the cerebellar vermis. Hydrocephalus (see Fig. 25-2, *A*) frequently accompanies DWM. A thorough search for additional anomalies may assist in determination of whether DWM is isolated or associated with a chromosomal anomaly or syndrome.

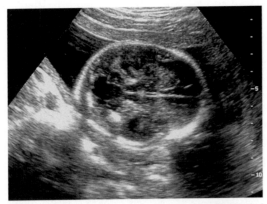

Fig. 25-5 Splaying of cerebellar hemispheres is identified in posterior fossa of fetus with Dandy-Walker malformation.

Agenesis of the Corpus Callosum

Agenesis of the corpus callosum is considered relatively common, although the condition may go undiagnosed. The corpus callosum connects the cerebral hemispheres and aids in learning and memory. ACC may be found in isolation but is often associated with other anomalies of the central nervous system, including holoprosencephaly, encephalocele, and DWM. A variety of chromosomal anomalies and syndromes may also be identified with ACC, including trisomies 13 and 18 and X-linked syndromes.[8] The outcome is variable depending on the association and severity of other anomalies, but ACC can be asymptomatic or carry a grave prognosis when severe anomalies are identified.[9]

Sonographic Findings. The diagnosis of ACC should be suspected when the CSP is absent (Fig. 25-6) because the corpus callosum develops with the CSP. In addition, colpocephaly may be identified and is defined as mild ventriculomegaly with dilation of the occipital horns, giving the ventricle a teardrop appearance. The lateral ventricles will also be displaced laterally, and the third ventricle may appear dilated and displaced superiorly. The sonographic examination should include a thorough search for additional anomalies that would suggest a more extensive CNS anomaly, aneuploidy, or syndrome.

FETAL FACE
Cleft Lip

Cleft lip or cleft palate is characterized by a defect in the upper lip or palate in the roof of the mouth. These anomalies comprise the most common congenital defects of the face, with occurrence in approximately 9:10,000 births.[10] Cleft palate is difficult to detect

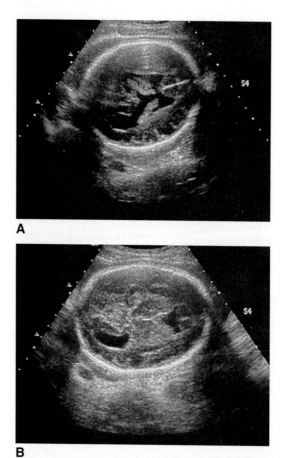

A

B

Fig. 25-6 **A,** Agenesis of corpus was diagnosed in fetus. Cavum septum pellucidum was also absent, and **(B)** occipital horns of lateral ventricles were dilated. (Courtesy Melissa Spagnuolo, Fetal Diagnostic Center of Orlando.)

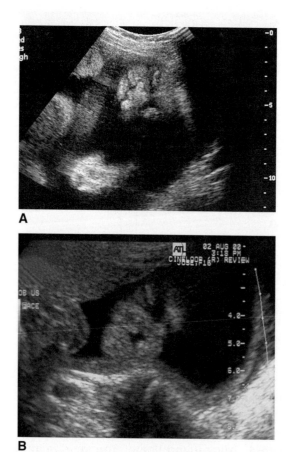

A

B

Fig. 25-7 Cleft lip may be unilateral; **A,** bilateral; or, **B,** median. Bilateral and median clefts are more frequently associated with other anomalies.

sonographically, especially in isolation. Cleft lip may be unilateral, bilateral, and median in location (Fig. 25-7). Unilateral clefts more commonly are left sided. Median clefts and bilateral clefts frequently have an associated cleft palate with an increased frequency of associated anomalies, including aneuploidy, skeletal anomalies, and syndromes.[8]

Sonographic Findings. A sonographic evaluation for a facial cleft includes imaging the soft tissue of the lips and nose in the coronal plane. A fetal profile may also show the cleft, especially bilateral clefts, which may appear as a premaxillary mass.

Micrognathia

Micrognathia is defined as a small or recessed chin. Micrognathia has been associated with aneuploidy, skeletal anomalies, and multiple syndromes. The most common anomaly associated with micrognathia is trisomy 18.[11] The outcome for fetuses with micrognathia is dependant on the associated anomalies.

Sonographic Findings. Micrognathia may be identified sonographically in the sagittal plane. A recessed chin (Fig. 25-8) may be identified in visualization of the fetal profile. Polyhydramnios may also be identified in association with the micrognathia.

FETAL THORAX

Congenital Diaphragmatic Hernia

Congenital diaphragmatic hernia (CDH) is a herniation of abdominal contents into the thorax through a defect in the diaphragm. The cause remains unknown, although genetic and teratogenic factors have been associated. This uncommon malformation is most commonly left sided and carries a high mortality rate of 73% to 86%.[12] Although associated anomalies influence the outcome, isolated defects carry a high morbidity and mortality because of respiratory complications from pulmonary hypoplasia.[13]

CDH has been associated with chromosomal anomalies. In addition, defects of the central nervous system and heart have been identified, as have defects of

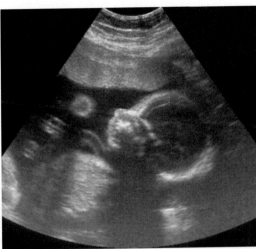

Fig. 25-8 Micrognathia. Recessed chin was identified in fetus with Edwards' syndrome.

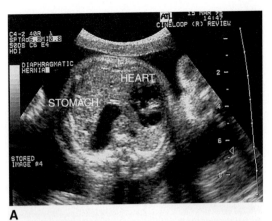

A

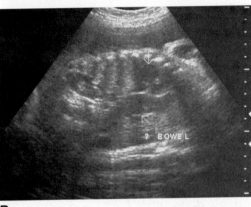

B

Fig. 25-9 **A,** Congenital diaphragmatic hernia most commonly presents with intrathoracic stomach and malpositioned heart as seen in fetus. **B,** Unusual presentation shows bowel extending from abdomen to thorax.

the lungs and genitourinary, skeletal, and gastrointestinal systems.[12] Sonographic examination and karyotyping assists in patient counseling, so that pregnancy options and surgical management, including prenatal surgery, can be discussed.

Sonographic Findings. Because left-sided defects more frequently occur, the most common sonographic finding is identification of the stomach above the diaphragm (Fig. 25-9, *A*). The intestines (Fig. 25-9, *B*) may also be identified in the thorax, and the heart will be malpositioned in the chest. Identification of the absence of an intraabdominal stomach is important to differentiate between CDH and cystic lung defects. Right-sided defects may show the liver and gallbladder within the thoracic cavity. **Polyhydramnios** and **hydrops** may also be identified in association with CDH. A thorough search for additional anomalies that may effect pregnancy management is imperative.

Congenital Cystic Adenomatoid Malformation

Congenital cystic adenomatoid malformation (CCAM) is a rare lung abnormality characterized by an overgrowth of terminal bronchopulmonary tissue. The three classifications are based on cyst size. Types I and II are macrocystic masses that consist of multiple large cysts and smaller cysts of less than 1 cm, respectively. Type III is a microcystic variety that appears as a large echogenic mass.[14] CCAM is usually unilateral and is without gender prevalence.

CCAM may be associated with hydrops, polyhydramnios, and pulmonary hypoplasia, all of which are associated with a poor outcome. Some lesions identified in the prenatal period may involute spon-

taneously, although they may become symptomatic after birth from infection or hemorrhage, and malignant transformation has also been reported.[14] Early diagnosis is important for pregnancy management, which may include prenatal interventions, such as fetal thoracentesis or cyst aspiration,[15] and in utero surgery in fetuses with hydrops, which has shown an improved outcome.[16] Delivery at a hospital with a neonatal intensive care unit should be arranged because newborns are frequently in respiratory distress and need support or surgery.

Sonographic Findings. The sonographic appearance (Fig. 25-10) of CCAM type I is one or more large cysts in the thorax; type II appears as multiple small cysts; and type III appears as a large echogenic mass.[17] Displacement of the fetal heart, polyhydramnios, and hydrops may also be identified. Ultrasound may be used to monitor for possible regression of the lesion.

Pulmonary Sequestration

Pulmonary sequestration is a rare abnormality characterized by a mass of lung tissue (Fig. 25-11) that does

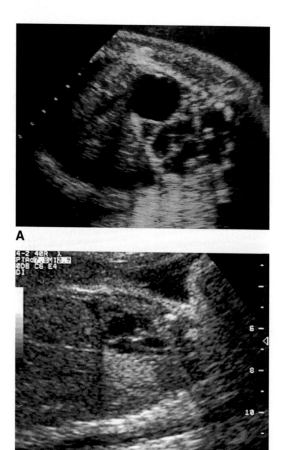

A

B

Fig. 25-10 Congenital cystic adenomatoid malformation may have, **A,** cystic appearance as in type I or, **B,** solid echogenic mass appearance as identified in fetus with type III.

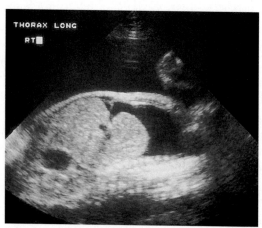

Fig. 25-11 Pulmonary sequestration was identified in fetus, in addition to large pulmonary embolus that surrounded mass of lung tissue.

not connect with the tracheobronchial tree and a separate blood supply that usually originates from the abdominal aorta.[18] Intralobar and extralobar varieties are seen, with intralobar pulmonary sequestration representing 75% of this anomaly. The extralobar variety may appear above or below the diaphragm.[14]

Although pulmonary sequestration may regress in utero and may be asymptomatic after birth, it has been associated with mediastinal shift, pleural effusion (PE), and hydrops. Polyhydramnios may also develop and initiate preterm labor. The outcome for pulmonary sequestration is variable. Fetuses may die in utero, and newborns may die of pulmonary hypoplasia or be completely asymptomatic and need respiratory support or surgery to resect the sequestered lung. In utero intervention to decrease polyhydramnios or drain pleural fluid may improve the outcome.[19]

Sonographic Findings. The sonographic appearance of pulmonary sequestration is an echogenic mass that may be triangular. Differentiation of this lesion from other echogenic thoracic lesions can be made with demonstration of the aberrant blood supply with color Doppler.[20] Serial ultrasound examinations may be used to monitor the fetus for lesion regression or the development of polyhydramnios, PE, or hydrops.

Pleural Effusion

Pleural effusion, also known as *hydrothorax,* is a rare entity characterized by an abnormal accumulation of fluid in the fetal thorax (see Fig. 25-11). PE may be unilateral or bilateral and isolated or a component of a generalized fluid overload (hydrops). PE may spontaneously resolve, lead to pulmonary hypoplasia, or progress to hydrops and fetal death.[21]

PE may be associated with other abnormalities of the thorax, including CCAM, pulmonary sequestration, CDH, and cardiac defects. PE may also be associated with trisomy 21, 45,X, cystic hygroma, and polyhydramnios.[14] Fetal thoracentesis may improve outcome in fetuses without associated anomalies that would preclude intervention and should be reserved for severe cases of PE.

Sonographic Findings. Sonographic diagnosis of PE can be made when fluid is identified in the fetal thorax surrounding lung tissue. A survey for associated findings provides the information necessary to explore pregnancy management and treatment options.

FETAL ABDOMEN

Duodenal Atresia

Duodenal atresia is characterized by stenosis, atresia, or development of webs that obstruct the distal duodenum.

The condition occurs in 2.5:100,000 to 10:100,000 live births and has been identified with increased frequency in twins and in the black population. An increased familial inheritance and a strong association with aneuploidy are also seen, most specifically trisomy 21, which has been identified in 35% of cases of duodenal atresia.[22]

Sonographic Findings. Sonographic evaluation of duodenal atresia reveals a dilated stomach and proximal duodenum that gives the characteristic double-bubble sign (Fig. 25-12). Polyhydramnios is commonly associated with duodenal atresia. This anomaly may not be evident until after 20 weeks' gestation. When duodenal atresia is identified, ultrasound may also be used for amniocentesis guidance for evaluation for chromosomal anomalies.

Esophageal Atresia

Esophageal atresia is the result of a congenital blockage of the esophagus and is identified in 1:2500 live births.[8] The condition may be associated with a fistula connecting the esophagus and trachea. Esophageal atresia may be associated with chromosomal anomalies, especially trisomies 21 and 18, and the VACTERL association. The outcome is dependent on the severity of associated abnormalities.

Sonographic Findings. Prenatal diagnosis of esophageal atresia is difficult. The most suggestive sonographic finding is an absent stomach from failure of amniotic fluid to pass from the esophagus to the stomach.[23] When a tracheoesophageal fistula is present, a normal or small stomach may be visualized. Atypically, sonography may show the fluid-filled esophagus coming to a blind end. Polyhydramnios (Fig 25-13) may also be identified because of the inability to effectively swallow.

Bowel Obstruction

Obstruction of fetal bowel may occur anywhere along the length of the small or large bowel. The more proximal the level of obstruction, the more likely polyhydramnios will be identified in association with this anomaly. Obstructions may occur with malrotation, atresia, **volvulus**, and peritoneal bands, and they may be isolated or associated with cystic fibrosis, ascites, meconium peritonitis, or other anomalies.[8]

Sonographic Findings. Obstructed bowel appears as dilated loops (Fig. 25-14) to the level of obstruction. Proximal obstructions are more likely to appear fluid filled. Dilated bowel may also be hypoechoic or hyperechoic, and peristalsis is noted on real time. Serial ultrasound examinations should be ordered to monitor

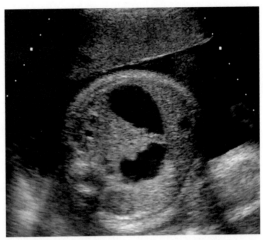

Fig. 25-12 Characteristic double-bubble sign is seen in fetus with duodenal atresia.

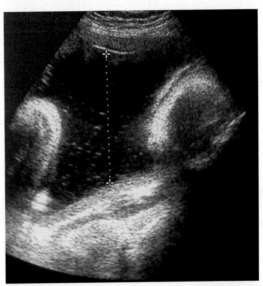

Fig. 25-13 Polyhydramnios was diagnosed in fetus with amniotic fluid index of 24 cm. Stomach bubble was not identified on multiple examinations. Amniocentesis confirmed trisomy 21. Esophageal atresia was suspected and confirmed at birth.

fetal well being. Changes in echogenicity and a lack of peristalsis may indicate that torsion of the bowel has occurred.[24]

Meconium Peritonitis

Meconium peritonitis may occur in fetuses with perforation of a bowel obstruction. This sterile chemical peritonitis may further result in an inflammatory reaction and formation of a meconium pseudocyst. Polyhydramnios may also be identified in fetuses with meconium peritonitis.

Sonographic Findings. Sonographic examination may reveal calcifications (Fig 25-15) in the fetal abdomen

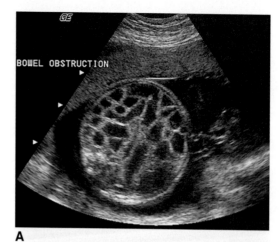

A

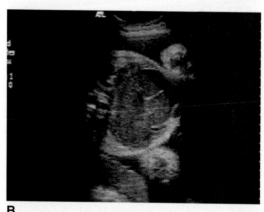

B

Fig. 25-14 **A,** Dilated loops of bowel are identified in fetus with bowel obstruction. **B,** Bowel obstruction was identified in fetus with later diagnosis of cystic fibrosis. (**A** Courtesy GE Medical Systems.)

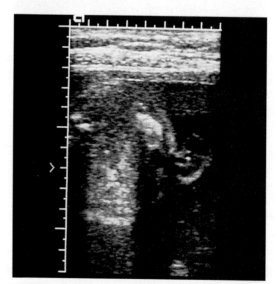

Fig. 25-15 Echogenic shadowing may be identified in fetuses with meconium peritonitis.

on the peritoneal surfaces and in the scrotum in male fetuses. Ascites are also identified in the abdomen, and polyhydramnios may be noted.

Ascites

Fetal ascites is the result of fluid collection in the fetal abdomen. The condition may be associated with bowel or bladder perforations or fetal hydrops. Fetal ascites has also been associated with congenital infections and fetal abdominal neoplasms.

Sonographic Findings. The sonographic evaluation of fetal ascites should show fluid outlining the abdominal organs and the fetal bowel (Fig. 25-16). The hypoechoic muscle adjacent to the fetal skin line should not be confused with fluid in the fetal abdomen.

Abdominal Cysts

Numerous cystic lesions within the fetal abdomen (Fig. 25-17) may be identified prenatally. The focus of the sonographic examination of a cystic lesion is identification

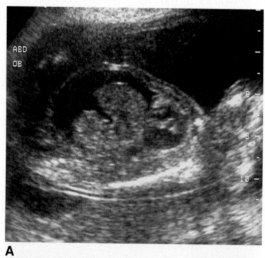

A

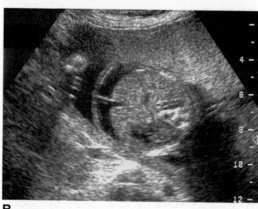

B

Fig. 25-16 **A** and **B,** Fluid can be identified surrounding fetal abdominal organs and bowel.

of the origin of the cyst and determination of the gender of the fetus because many cystic lesions identified in female fetuses are ovarian in origin. Serial sonographic examinations may also document resolution or a change in size or a change in echogenicity of these lesions. Cystic lesions that are located in the liver or right upper quadrant include **choledochal cysts,** hepatic cysts, and gallbladder duplication. **Urachal cysts** will be located between the bladder and umbilicus. Duplication cysts may be identified anywhere along the gastro-intestinal tract and may show the muscular layers of gut rather than a thin wall. Mesenteric cysts and renal cysts may also be identified, in addition to cystic lesions of other origins.

Sacrococcygeal Teratoma

Sacrococcygeal teratoma (SCT) occurs in 1:40,000 infants and is the most common congenital neoplasm, affecting females in 75% of cases.[25] This neoplasm arises from the three germ cell layers (the ectoderm, endoderm, and mesoderm) and is usually benign. SCTs are primarily external tumors, but they may have intrapelvic extension or arise entirely within the pelvis or abdomen. In addition, teratomas may arise anywhere in the fetus (Fig. 25-18), including the liver and brain.

The outcome for a fetus with SCT is generally poor because of the development of fetal hydrops, cardiac failure, anemia, tumor hemorrhage or rupture, and premature delivery from polyhydramnios.[25] Prenatal diagnosis provides for pregnancy options to be con-sidered, including termination, amniotic fluid reduction, and delivery with cesarean section. In utero invasive procedures have also been performed with some success. Infants can have successful resection of these tumors, although there is still an increase in neonatal morbidity and mortality.

Sonographic Findings. SCT will most commonly appear as a mass extending from the sacral region (Fig. 25-18, *B* to *D*) of the fetus. The tumor may vary greatly in size and echogenicity. Heterogeneous or complex tumors are frequently noted, and Doppler may show the increased vascularity of this mass. Evaluation of tumor size and identification of hydrops, urinary obstruction, and polyhydramnios should also be noted because these findings carry an increased fetal mortality rate.[26]

FETAL SKELETON

Skeletal dysplasias are a rare group of anomalies that involve abnormal development of bone and cartilage.

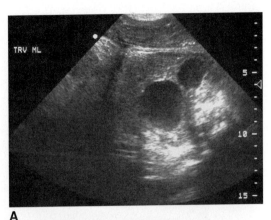

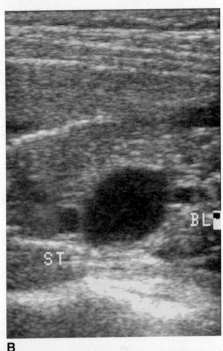

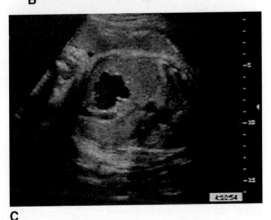

Fig. 25-17 Fetal abdominal cysts. **A,** Ovarian cyst was confirmed in female fetus with cystic lesion identified adjacent to bladder. **B,** Mesenteric cyst was confirmed in fetus after birth. **C,** Irregular cyst was identified in liver of fetus, and diagnosis of choledochal cyst was made after infant was delivered.

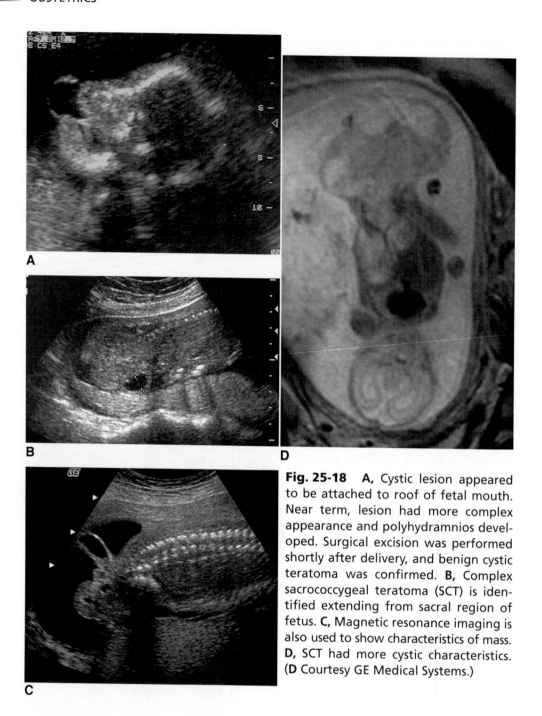

Fig. 25-18 **A,** Cystic lesion appeared to be attached to roof of fetal mouth. Near term, lesion had more complex appearance and polyhydramnios developed. Surgical excision was performed shortly after delivery, and benign cystic teratoma was confirmed. **B,** Complex sacrococcygeal teratoma (SCT) is identified extending from sacral region of fetus. **C,** Magnetic resonance imaging is also used to show characteristics of mass. **D,** SCT had more cystic characteristics. (**D** Courtesy GE Medical Systems.)

The occurrence rate is 2.3:10,000 to 7.6:10,000 births, and the most common of the skeletal dysplasias are thanatophoric dysplasia, achondrogenesis, achondroplasia, osteogenesis imperfecta (OI), and SRPS.[27] Fetal skeletal anomalies can be a challenge in accurate diagnosis because of the overlap of similar sonographic findings. Imaging protocol should be adjusted when a skeletal dysplasia is suspected to aid in the diagnosis and determination of chances for survival after birth. In addition to the sonographic evaluation, fetal radiographs, chromosomal analysis, and genetic testing may be used to assist in an accurate diagnosis.

The sonographic evaluation should include the imaging and measurement of all long bones because some skeletal dysplasia are associated with shortening or absence of a specific bone or segment of the extremities, as in **thrombocytopenia–absent radius (TAR) syndrome,** which presents with an absent radius.

Bones should also be evaluated for shape and for fractures. The hands and feet should be assessed for abnormal posturing and polydactyly, which may help in the diagnosis of certain dysplasias such as **diastrophic dysplasia**, which presents with a hitchhiker thumb, and SRPS. The fetal thorax should be analyzed for narrowing, associated with pulmonary hypoplasia, which is a feature of many of the lethal skeletal dysplasias. The absence or presence of other associated anomalies, such as facial clefts, hydrocephalus, and heart defects, may also lead to a specific diagnosis.

Thanatophoric Dysplasia

Thanatophoric dysplasia is the most common lethal skeletal dysplasia and occurs in 1:10,000 births.[8] It is usually a sporadic anomaly, although a 2% recurrence risk rate is seen.[28] The condition is divided into two types, types I and II, based on characteristic features. Both types of thanatophoric dysplasia have been linked with a mutation of the *FGFR3* gene. Infants born with thanatophoric dysplasia usually die shortly after birth of pulmonary hypoplasia and respiratory distress.

Type I thanatophoric dysplasia is the more common of the two types and is characterized by micromelia, curved femora, and a narrow thorax. Type II is characterized by micromelia, straight femora, a narrow thorax, and a cloverleaf skull.[29]

Sonographic Findings. The sonographic features of thanatophoric dysplasia (Fig. 25-19) include significant shortening of the extremities and a narrow thorax with a protuberant abdomen. Long bones may appear bowed with a "telephone receiver" appearance, and macrocephaly with frontal bossing may be evident. A trilobular appearance of the skull suggests type II, although this cloverleaf appearance may be identified in other anomalies, including homozygous achondroplasia and **camptomelic dysplasia.** Other anomalies that have been identified with thanatophoric dysplasia include holoprosencephaly, ACC, ventriculomegaly, and renal and heart defects.[30]

Achondrogenesis

Achondrogenesis is a lethal skeletal dysplasia caused by a defect in cartilage formation that leads to abnormal bone formation and hypomineralization of the bones. The condition occurs in 2.3:100,000 to 2.8:100,000 births and is usually transmitted in an autosomal recessive manner.[31] The two types of achondrogenesis are classified based on histologic and radiologic characteristics.

Type I achondrogenesis (Parenti-Fraccaro) is the more severe of the two types and is characterized by severe micromelia, a lack of ossification of the spine and calvaria, and fractured ribs. Type II achondrogenesis (Langer-Saldino) is the more common of the two types and is characterized by micromelia and variable ossification of the spine and calvaria.

Sonographic Findings. The sonographic findings (Fig. 25-20) associated with achondrogenesis include extreme shortening of the extremities. Variable degrees of ossification may be noted of the spine and calvaria. The thorax and ribs may be shortened, and the ribs may appear to have multiple fractures. Polyhydramnios and hydrops may also be identified in association with achondrogenesis.

Achondroplasia

Achondroplasia is the most common of the nonlethal skeletal dysplasias, occurring in 5:10,000 to 15:10,000 births.[8] This condition occurs from abnormal endochondral bone formation that results in **rhizomelia.** The phenotypic appearance also includes a large head with a prominent forehead, a depressed nasal bridge, and marked lumbar lordosis. Individuals with this skeletal dysplasia can have a normal life expectancy unless they have the uncommon severe complications of this disorder, including brain stem or cervical spinal cord compression, severe hydrocephalus, or spinal stenosis.

Achondroplasia is transmitted through an autosomal dominant mode, although most instances are the result of spontaneous mutation. There are **heterozygous** and **homozygous** forms of achondroplasia, and the homozygous form is rare and lethal.

Sonographic Findings. The sonographic findings of achondroplasia include shortening of the proximal segment of the extremities. An additional finding of the trident hand may be documented when the hand is extended and the fingers appear shortened and of similar lengths.[30] Macrocephalus with frontal bossing and a depressed nasal bridge may also be noted. The homozygous form of achondroplasia is indistinguishable from thanatophoric dysplasia.

Short Rib–Polydactyly Syndrome

Short rib–polydactyly syndrome (SRPS) is an autosomal recessive skeletal dysplasia characterized by the presence of short limbs and ribs and polydactyly. The narrow thorax associated with this syndrome is of a lethal nature because most infants die shortly after birth of

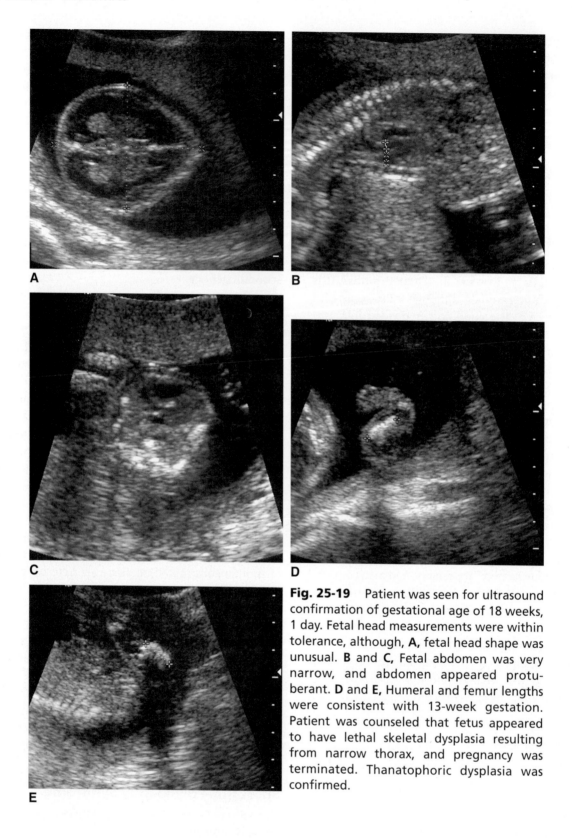

Fig. 25-19 Patient was seen for ultrasound confirmation of gestational age of 18 weeks, 1 day. Fetal head measurements were within tolerance, although, **A,** fetal head shape was unusual. **B** and **C,** Fetal abdomen was very narrow, and abdomen appeared protuberant. **D** and **E,** Humeral and femur lengths were consistent with 13-week gestation. Patient was counseled that fetus appeared to have lethal skeletal dysplasia resulting from narrow thorax, and pregnancy was terminated. Thanatophoric dysplasia was confirmed.

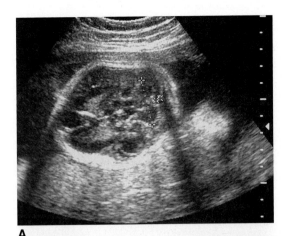

A

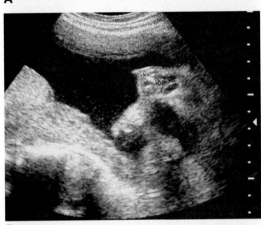

B

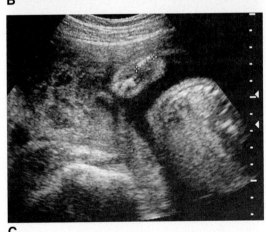

C

Fig. 25-20 Fetus was diagnosed with achondrogenesis at birth and died within hours. **A,** Fetal head was poorly ossified as shown by compression of calvaria with transducer pressure. At 24 weeks' gestation, **B,** femur and, **C,** humerus measured approximately 13 weeks.

pulmonary hypoplasia. The four types of SRPS may be classified based on radiologic and pathologic findings. Type I is also known as *Saldino-Noonan syndrome,* type II is also known as *Majewski syndrome,* type III is also known as *Verma-Naumoff syndrome,* and type IV is also known as *Beemer-Langer syndrome.*[32]

Sonographic Findings. The typical sonographic features of SRPS are micromelia, a narrow thorax with short ribs, and polydactyly (Fig. 25-21). Cleft lip and palate may also be identified, and numerous other anomalies have been identified in association with the various types.

Osteogenesis Imperfecta

Osteogenesis imperfecta (OI) is a rare disorder of connective tissue that leads to brittle bones (Fig. 25-22) and affects the teeth, ligaments, skin, and blue sclera. Four types of OI are seen, with types I and IV as the mildest forms transmitted through autosomal dominant modes of inheritance. Type III is a severe form transmitted through autosomal dominant or recessive modes.

Type II is the most severe and lethal form of OI and may be transmitted through autosomal dominant or recessive modes or the result of a spontaneous mutation.[8] Type II occurs in approximately 1:55,000 births[33] and is the most likely to be diagnosed prenatally. Infants with type II OI usually die shortly after birth of pulmonary complications.

Sonographic Findings. The sonographic features (Fig. 25-23) of OI type II include decreased ossification of the bones and multiple fractures. Hypomineralization of the bones may be identified with noting that the bones are decreased in echogenicity with decreased attenuation. The fetal head structures may be seen exquisitely well, and the reverberation artifact typically

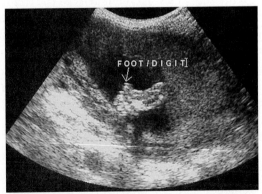

Fig. 25-21 Polydactyly coupled with narrow thorax and micromelia suggests short rib–polydactyly syndrome.

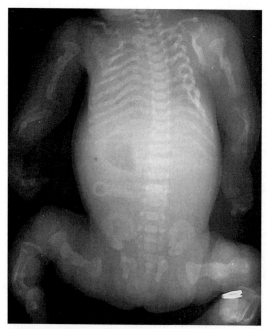

Fig. 25-22 Multiple fractures can be seen in post-mortem radiograph of newborn with osteogenesis imperfecta type II.

identified in the proximal hemisphere is absent. The calvaria may also be compressible with slight transducer pressure. The thorax appears narrow, and the limbs are shortened and may show marked deformities from the numerous fractures. Polyhydramnios may also be identified. OI type III may also be diagnosed prenatally, although sonographic findings will be less severe.

VACTERL ASSOCIATION

The VACTERL association is characterized by a group of anomalies that occur in concert and include *v*ertebral anomalies, *a*nal atresia, *c*ardiac defects, *t*racheo*e*sophageal fistula, *r*enal anomalies, and *l*imb defects. The condition usually occurs spontaneously and is of unknown etiology. The VATER association is a more narrow classification of anomalies that includes *v*ertebral anomalies, imperforate *a*nus, *t*racheo*e*sophageal fistula, and *r*adial and *r*enal dysplasias.[34] The diagnosis of these spectra of fetal anomalies can be made with the identification of three features of the association. Single umbilical artery and polyhydramnios may also be identified.

This association is considered nonlethal, although morbidity and mortality are affected by the severity of the anomalies and the presence of polyhydramnios, which may lead to premature labor and delivery. Most infants will need significant neonatal care and surgical treatment.[35] Accurate diagnosis with sonographic

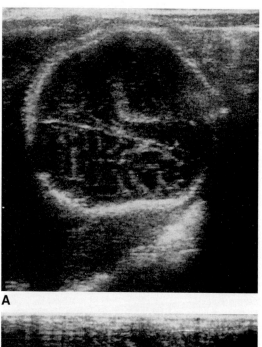

A

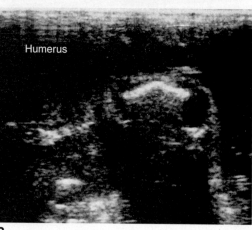

Humerus

B

Fig. 25-23 **A,** Poorly ossified calvaria and, **B,** shortened and fractured long bones are sonographic findings associated with osteogenesis imperfecta type II.

evaluation may assist in adequate planning for pregnancy management and delivery and treatment options.

Limb Anomalies

Limb abnormalities are numerous and may occur in isolation or as a feature of a chromosomal anomaly, skeletal dysplasia, or syndrome. When a limb anomaly is identified sonographically, a thorough evaluation for additional anomalies should ensue.

Talipes, also known as *clubfoot* (Fig. 25-24, *A*), involves abnormalities of the foot and ankle. The condition may be unilateral or bilateral, and a male prevalence is seen. Most cases are isolated and idiopathic in nature. Talipes may be associated with oligohydramnios and chromosomal anomalies, skeletal dysplasias, and other syndromes. It has also been identified in multiple

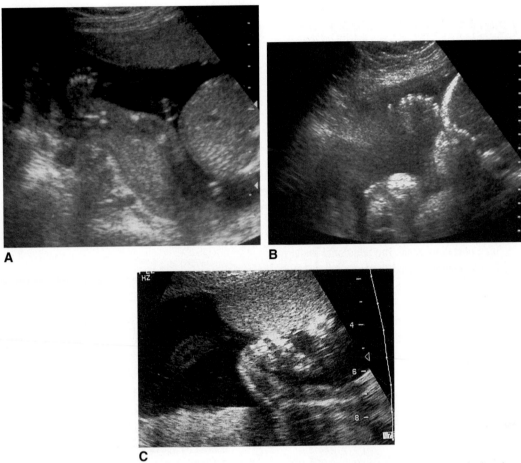

Fig. 25-24 Limb abnormalities may be isolated or part of syndrome, skeletal dysplasia, or chromosomal anomaly. **A,** Isolated clubfoot. **B,** Polydactyly was associated with trisomy 13. **C,** Clubhand deformity may be identified with absent radius.

gestations and with spina bifida and some teratogens.

Rocker bottom feet can be identified when the bottom of the foot is convex. This condition has been found in association with syndromes and chromosomal anomalies, especially trisomy 18.

Polydactyly (extra digits) may involve the hands (Fig. 25-24, *B*) or feet (see Fig. 25-21) and may be isolated or associated with syndromes or chromosomal anomalies. Abnormal posturing, including clenched hands or overlapping digits, may also be associated with chromosomal anomalies or syndromes. Absence of all or part of an extremity may be the result of an amputation associated with amniotic band syndrome. Fusion of extremities or digits may be associated with a variety of syndromes.

Absence or hypoplasia of the radius is termed a radial ray defect and has been associated with skeletal dysplasias, chromosomal anomalies, and syndromes. The hand will turn back toward the arm (Fig. 25-24, *C*), giving a characteristic clubhand appearance that may be identified sonographically.

SUMMARY

Obstetric sonography is challenging when a fetal anomaly is identified. An understanding of the many associated anomalies and completion of a thorough survey of the fetus are essential. Accurate diagnosis of an abnormality provides the patient and the physician with the information necessary to make decisions regarding pregnancy management, treatment, and delivery options.

CLINICAL SCENARIO—DIAGNOSIS

■ The echogenic lesion in the thorax is consistent with congenital cystic adenomatoid malformation type III. The diaphragm is inverted, and transverse imaging also revealed a mediastinal shift and malpositioning of the heart. The presence of ascites with skin edema indicated that hydrops was present. The fetus died in utero in the third trimester.

CASE STUDIES FOR DISCUSSION

1. A 17-year-old girl, G1 P0, is seen for ultrasound for size and dates for an uncertain last menstrual period. The sonographic evaluation shows a 28-week gestation and the findings in Fig. 25-25. The gender is identified as male, and the remainder of the examination is unremarkable. What is the most likely diagnosis?

2. A 20-year-old woman, G2 P1, is seen for ultrasound at the maternal fetal center at 30 ⁴/₇ weeks' gestation for evaluation of fetal hydrocephalus. The ventricles are enlarged, and the head measurements correspond with a 36-week gestation. Other measurements are consistent with the previously defined gestational age. The additional finding seen in Fig. 25-26 is identified, and the remainder of the examination is unremarkable. What is the most likely diagnosis?

3. A 42-year-old woman, G2 P0, is seen for ultrasound for advanced maternal age at 16 ³/₇ weeks' gestation. Amniocentesis reveals a 46,XX karyotype. The patient returns at 38 weeks' gestation because of a fetal abdominal mass (Fig. 25-27) identified in the obstetrician's office. What is the most likely diagnosis?

4. An ultrasound is performed for size and dates. A complete patient history is not possible because of a language barrier. The ultrasound shows the findings in Fig. 25-28. What is the most likely diagnosis?

5. A 32-year-old woman is seen for ultrasound for size and dates. The ultrasound reveals a 25-week fetus with the finding in Fig. 25-29. The remainder of the examination is unremarkable. What is the most likely diagnosis?

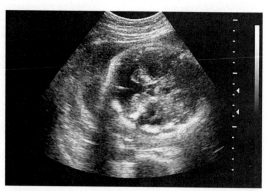

Fig. 25-26 Image of fetal head shows cerebellum and region of cisterna magna.

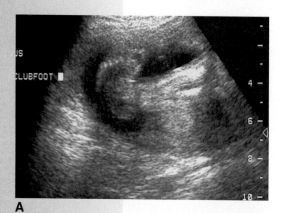

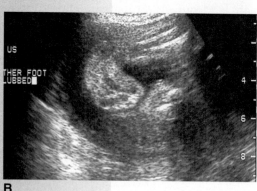

Fig. 25-25 Images of, **A**, right and, **B**, left lower legs and feet show abnormal posturing.

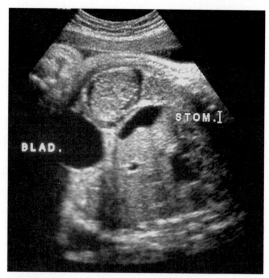

Fig. 25-27 Coronal view of fetal abdomen shows mass on left side of abdomen. Gender is female.

CASE STUDIES FOR DISCUSSION—cont'd

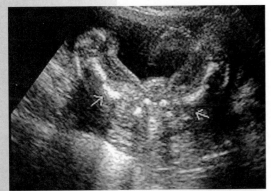

A

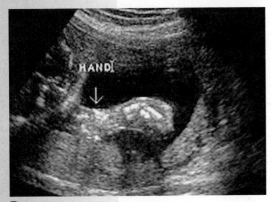

B

Fig. 25-28 Ultrasound images of, **A,** femora and, **B,** right arm show multiple fractures. Multiple fractures of ribs were also noted, and ribs were concave in appearance. Fetal head anatomy was well demonstrated, and calvaria compressed with minimal transducer pressure.

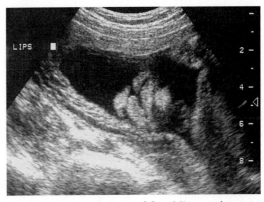

Fig. 25-29 Coronal view of fetal lips and nose.

STUDY QUESTIONS

1. A sonographic evaluation of a 27-week gestation reveals that the lateral ventricle measures 15 mm and the fetal head measurement is consistent with a 31-week gestation. The remainder of the examination is unremarkable. This is consistent with which of the following?
   a. colpocephaly
   b. holoprosencephaly
   c. hydranencephaly
   d. hydrocephaly
   e. ventriculomegaly

2. A 35-year-old woman is seen for a sonographic evaluation for advanced maternal age. The examination reveals polyhydramnios and absence of the stomach. This is most suggestive of which of the following anomalies?
   a. congenital diaphragmatic hernia
   b. cystic fibrosis
   c. duodenal atresia
   d. esophageal atresia
   e. jejunal atresia

3. Sonographic evaluation of a fetal head reveals cyclopia with a proboscis. Severe microcephaly is present, preventing adequate visualization of fetal head anatomy. On the basis of the findings that are evident, what is the most likely diagnosis?
   a. cebocephaly

b. Dandy-Walker malformation
c. holoprosencephaly
d. hydranencephaly
e. hydrocephaly

4. Which of the following describes the decreased length of the humerus or femur?
a. amelia
b. mesomelia
c. micromelia
d. phocomelia
e. rhizomelia

5. A 28-year-old woman is seen for obstetric ultrasound for size greater than dates. The ultrasound reveals polyhydramnios and the presence of two stomachs in the fetal abdomen. This is suggestive of which of the following anomalies?
a. bowel obstruction
b. congenital diaphragmatic hernia
c. duodenal atresia
d. esophageal atresia
e. tracheoesophageal fistula

6. A transverse image of a fetal thorax shows a cystic structure adjacent to a malpositioned fetal heart. A normally placed stomach is visualized in the fetal abdomen. This is most suggestive of which of the following anomalies?
a. congenital cystic adenomatoid malformation
b. congenital diaphragmatic hernia
c. esophageal atresia
d. pulmonary sequestration
e. tracheoesophageal fistula

7. A cystic lesion is identified in the abdomen of a female fetus. It appears to be in the region of the left lower quadrant and inferior to a normal stomach. This is most suggestive of which of the following?
a. duplication cyst
b. splenic cyst
c. mesenteric cyst
d. ovarian cyst
e. urachal cyst

8. A 30-year-old woman is seen for an ultrasound for late prenatal care. The ultrasound examination shows an approximately 28-week gestation. The femoral measurements are consistent with a 21-week gestation, and the humeral lengths are consistent with 22 weeks' gestation. The fetal head is trilobular in appearance, and the thorax is extremely small as compared with the abdominal circumference. This would be most consistent with which of the following?
a. achondrogenesis
b. achondroplasia
c. camptomelic dysplasia
d. osteogenesis imperfecta
e. thanatophoric dysplasia

9. Rocker bottom feet are identified in a fetus that has a heart defect. Which of the following is most likely?
a. diastrophic dysplasia
b. trisomy 13
c. trisomy 18
d. trisomy 21
e. VACTERL association

10. A sonographic evaluation reveals a fetus with a narrow thorax, micromelia, and polydactyly. This would be most suggestive of which of the following?
a. achondrogenesis
b. diastrophic dysplasia
c. osteogenesis imperfecta type II
d. short rib–polydactyly syndrome
e. thanatophoric dysplasia

REFERENCES

1. Durfee SM, Kim FM, Benson CB: Postnatal outcome of fetuses with the prenatal diagnosis of asymmetric hydrocephalus, *J Ultrasound Med* 20:263-268, 2001.
2. Bannister CM, Russell SA, Rimmer S et al: Prenatal ventriculomegaly and hydrocephalus, *Neurol Res* 22:37-42, 2000.
3. Benacerraf BR: Unilateral cerebral ventriculomegaly, is one better than two? *J Ultrasound Med* 20:179-181, 2001.
4. Bullen PJ, Rankin JM, Robson SC: Investigation of the epidemiology and prenatal diagnosis of holoprosencephaly in the North of England, *Am J Obstet Gynecol* 184:1256-1262, 2001.
5. Peebles DM: Holoprosencephaly, *Prenat Diagn* 18:477-480,1998.
6. Kurtz AB, Johnson PT: Case 7: hydranencephaly, *Radiology* 210:419-422, 1999.
7. Sherer DM, Shane H, Anyane-Yeboa K: First-trimester transvaginal ultrasonographic diagnosis of Dandy-Walker malformation, *Am J Perinatol* 18:373-377, 2001.
8. Hagen-Ansert SA: *Textbook of diagnostic ultrasonography*, vol 1, ed 5, St Louis, 2001, Mosby.
9. D'Ercole C et al: Prenatal diagnosis of fetal corpus callosum agenesis by ultrasonography and magnetic resonance imaging, *Prenat Diagn* 18:247-253, 1998.

10. Sohan K, Freer M, Mercer N et al: Prenatal detection of facial clefts, *Fetal Diagn Ther* 16:196-199, 2001.

11. Callen P: *Ultrasonography in obstetrics and gynecology*, ed 4, Philadelphia, WB Saunders, 2000.

12. Geary M: Management of congenital diaphragmatic hernia diagnosed prenatally: an update, *Prenat Diagn* 18:1155-1158, 1998.

13. Kim M-J, Cho JY: Prenatal ultrasonographic diagnosis of congenital diaphragmatic hernia at 11 weeks gestation, *J Diagn Med Sonogr* 17:286-289, 2001.

14. Hubbard AM, Crombleholme TM: Anomalies and malformations affecting the fetal/neonatal chest, *Semin Roentgenol* 33:117-125, 1998.

15. Marshall KW, Blane CE, Teitelbaum DH et al: Congenital cystic adenomatoid malformation: impact of prenatal diagnosis and changing strategies in the treatment of the asymptomatic patient, *AJR Am J Roentgenol* 175:1551-1554, 2000.

16. Mahle WT, Rychik J, Tian ZY et al: Echocardiographic evaluation of the fetus with congenital cystic adenomatoid malformation, *Ultrasound Obstet Gynecol* 16:620-624, 2000.

17. Ratner AN, Frisoli G: Congenital cystic adenomatoid malformation of the lung—type III, *J Diagn Med Sonogr* 15:249-251, 1999.

18. Nicolini U, Cerri V, Groli C et al: A new approach to prenatal treatment of extralobar pulmonary sequestration, *Prenat Diagn* 20:758-760, 2000.

19. Adzick NS, Harrison MR, Crombleholme TM et al: Fetal lung lesions: management and outcome, *Am J Obstet Gynecol* 179:884-889, 1998.

20. Lopoo JB, Goldstein RB, Lipshutz GS et al: Fetal pulmonary sequestration: a favorable congenital lung lesion, *Obstet Gynecol* 94:567-571, 1999.

21. Grisaru-Granovsky S, Seaward PG, Windrim R et al: Mid-trimester thoracoamniotic shunting for the treatment of fetal primary pleural effusions in a twin pregnancy, *Fetal Diagn Ther* 15:209-211, 2000.

22. Lawrence MJ, Ford WD, Furness ME et al: Congenital duodenal obstruction: early antenatal ultrasound diagnosis, *Pediatr Surg Int* 16:342-345, 2000.

23. Langer JC, Hussain H, Khan A et al: Prenatal diagnosis of esophageal atresia using sonography and magnetic resonance imaging, *J Pediatr Surg* 36:804-807, 2001.

24. Miyakoshi K, Tanaka M, Miyazaki T et al: Prenatal ultrasound diagnosis of small-bowel torsion, *Obstet Gynecol* 91:802-803, 1998.

25. Chisholm CA, Heider AL, Kuller JA et al: Prenatal diagnosis and perinatal management of fetal sacrococcygeal teratoma, *Am J Perinatol* 16:47-50, 1999.

26. Brace V, Grant SR, Brackley KJ et al: Prenatal diagnosis and outcome in sacrococcygeal teratomas: a review of cases between 1992 and 1998, *Prenat Diagn*, 20:51-55, 2000.

27. Gabrielli S, Falco P, Pilu G et al: Can transvaginal fetal biometry be considered a useful tool for early detection of skeletal dysplasias in high-risk patients? *Ultrasound Obstet Gynecol* 13:107-111, 1999.

28. Machado LE, Bonilla-Musoles F, Osborne NG: Thanatophoric dysplasia, *Ultrasound Obstet Gynecol* 18:85-86, 2001.

29. Chen CP, Chern SR, Shih JC et al: Prenatal diagnosis and genetic analysis of type I and type II thanatophoric dysplasia, *Prenat Diagn* 21:89-95, 2001.

30. Lemyre E, Azouz EM, Teebi AS et al: Achondroplasia, hypochondroplasia and thanatophoric dysplasia: review and update, *Can Assoc Radiol J*, 50:185-197, 1999.

31. Won HS, Yoo HK, Lee PR et al: A case of achondrogenesis type II associated with huge cystic hygroma: prenatal diagnosis by ultrasonography, *Ultrasound Obstet Gynecol* 14:288-290, 1999.

32. Golombeck K, Jacobs VR, von Kaisenberg C et al: Short-rib-polydactyly syndrome type III: comparison of ultrasound, radiology, and pathology findings, *Fetal Diagn Ther* 16:133-138, 2001.

33. Palmer TM, Rouse GA, Song A et al: Transparent bone and concave ribs, additional sonographic features of lethal osteogenesis imperfecta, *J Diagn Med Sonogr* 14:246-250, 1998.

34. Miller OF, Kolon TF: Prenatal diagnosis of VACTERL association, *J Urol* 166:2389-2391, 2001.

35. Tongsong T, Wanapirak C, Piyamongkol W et al: Prenatal sonographic diagnosis of VATER association, *J Clin Ultrasound* 27:378-384, 1999.

BIBLIOGRAPHY

Blaicher W, Prayer D, Kuhle S et al: Combined prenatal ultrasound and magnetic resonance imaging in two fetuses with suspected arachnoid cysts, *Ultrasound Obstet Gynecol* 18:166-168, 2001.

Hamada H, Watanabe H, Sugimoto M et al: Autosomal recessive hydrocephalus due to congenital stenosis of the aqueduct of sylvius, *Prenat Diagn*, 19:1067-1069, 1999.

Abnormal Fetal Echocardiography

SANDRA HAGEN-ANSERT

CLINICAL SCENARIO

■ A 39-year-old patient is seen at the obstetric service at 24 weeks of her third pregnancy. Her first child died shortly after birth of hypoplastic left heart syndrome. Her second child is 4 years old and is undergoing evaluation for a systolic ejection murmur. The patient has a history of a bicuspid aortic valve and underwent a balloon valvulotomy nearly 20 years ago. She was referred to the pediatric cardiology department for a fetal echocardiogram.

A complete fetal echocardiogram is performed. The aortic valve is thickened with reduced cusp excursion. The ascending aorta measures 2.3 mm, compared with the pulmonary artery measurement of 4.1 mm. The left ventricle is thicker and smaller than the right ventricle, measuring 6.7 mm with the right ventricular measurement of 8.0 mm. The velocity taken at the root of the aorta is increased and measures 2.0 m/sec.

What conclusions may be drawn from the fetal echocardiogram? What is the risk of congenital heart disease in this fetus?

OBJECTIVES

- Describe the echocardiographic appearance of premature atrial and ventricular contractions versus supraventricular tachycardia.
- List the various septal defects and their sonographic appearances.
- Differentiate between a complete and partial atrioventricular septal defect.
- List the echocardiographic findings in the tetralogy of Fallot.
- Describe the sonographic characteristics of hypoplastic left heart syndrome.
- Identify the risk factors associated with congenital heart disease.
- Describe the sonographic findings and Doppler characteristics in Ebstein's anomaly.
- Differentiate how the sonographer may distinguish transposition of the great arteries from truncus arteriosus.

GLOSSARY OF TERMS

Atrial fibrillation: occurs when the atrial rate is 400 to 700 beats per minute

Atrial flutter: occurs when the atrial rate is 240 to 400 beats per minute

Atrial septal defect: a hole in the septum that separates the right atrium filling chamber from the left atrium filling chamber

Atrioventricular block: blockage of the transmission of the electrical impulse from the atria to the ventricles

Atrioventricular node: areas of cardiac muscle that receive and conduct the electrical cardiac impulse

Atrioventricular septal defect: defect that occurs when the endocardial cushion fails to fuse in the center of the heart; may involve the atrioventricular valves as well

Bulbus cordis: primitive chamber of the heart that forms the right ventricle

Ebstein's anomaly: abnormal apical displacement of the septal leaflet of the tricuspid valve

Foramen ovale, or fossa ovalis: opening between the free edge of the septum secundum and the dorsal wall of the atrium

Hypoplastic left heart syndrome: underdevelopment of the left heart; may involve the mitral valve, aorta, and left ventricle

Inferior vena cava: venous return from the abdomen and lower extremities into the lateral wall of the right atrium

Left atrium: filling chamber of the heart

Left ventricle: pumping chamber of the heart

Mitral valve: atrioventricular valve between the left atrium and left ventricle

Premature atrial or ventricular contractions: cardiac arrhythmias that result from extra systoles and ectopic beats

Pulmonary artery: principal artery that carries blood from the right ventricle to the lungs

Pulmonary stenosis: thickening and narrowing of the pulmonary cusps

Pulmonary veins: the four pulmonary veins that bring blood from the lungs back into the posterior wall of the left atrium

Right atrium: filling chamber of the heart

Right ventricle: pumping chamber of the heart

Septum primum: first part of the atrial septum to grow from the dorsal wall of the primitive atrium and fuse with the endocardial cushion in the center of the heart

Septum secundum: second part of the atrial septum to grow to the right of the septum primum

Sinoatrial node: forms in the wall of the sinus venosus near its opening into the right atrium

Superior vena cava: venous return from the head and upper extremity into the posterior medial wall of the right atrium

Supraventricular tachyarrhythmias: abnormal cardiac rhythms of more than 200 beats per minute with a normal sinus conduction rate

Tetralogy of Fallot: membranous ventricular septal defect, overriding of the aorta, and pulmonary stenosis

Transposition of the great arteries: abnormal connection of the aorta to the right heart and of the pulmonary artery to the left heart

Tricuspid valve: atrioventricular valve found between the right atrium and the right ventricle

Truncus arteriosus: common arterial trunk in which both the pulmonary artery and the aorta arise

Ventricular septal defect: communication between the right and left ventricles

RISK FACTORS THAT INDICATE FETAL ECHOCARDIOGRAPHY

Specific risk factors indicate the fetus is at a higher than normal risk for congenital heart disease and warrant fetal echocardiography. These risk factors may be divided into the following three categories: fetal, maternal, and familial risk factors.

Fetal Risk Factors

Fetal risk factors include the presence of intrauterine growth retardation, cardiac arrhythmias, abnormal amniocentesis indicating a chromosomal anomaly, abnormal amniotic fluid collections, abnormal heart rate, or other anomalies as detected with the sonogram, such as hydrops fetalis.

Maternal Risk Factors

Maternal risk factors include the previous occurrence of congenital heart disease in siblings or parents; a maternal disease known to affect the fetus, such as diabetes mellitus or connective tissue disease (i.e., lupus erythematosus); or maternal use of drugs such as lithium or alcohol.

Familial Risk Factors

Familial risk factors include genetic syndromes or the presence of congenital heart disease in a previous sibling. The recurrence risk rate with a sibling with one of the most common cardiovascular abnormalities (**ventricular septal defect, atrial septal defect,** patent ductus arteriosus, **tetralogy of Fallot**) varies from 2.5% to 3%. Similar data with one parent with a congenital heart defect suggest that for the common defects listed, the recurrence risk rate ranges from 2.5% (atrial septal defect) to 4% (ventricular septal defect, patent ductus arteriosus, tetralogy of Fallot) (see Hagen-Ansert in bibliography, p. 389).

FETAL RHYTHM IRREGULARITIES
Fetal Cardiac Arrhythmias

The fetal heart undergoes multiple changes during the embryologic stages. One of these stages is the progression of the cardiac electrical system, which matures at the end of fetal life to cause a normal sinus rhythm in the cardiac cycle. The heart's pacemaker is the **sinoatrial (SA) node,** which fires 60 to 100 electrical impulses each minute. From the SA node, the electrical activity travels to the **atrioventricular (AV) node,** across the bundle of His to the ventricles, and down the right and left bundle branches, before being distributed to the rest of the cardiac muscle. This electrical activity precedes the ventricular contraction of the heart.

During this developmental stage, deceleration of the normal fetal heart rate from 150 beats per minute (bpm) to a bradycardia stage (<55 bpm), or even a pause of a few seconds, is not uncommon during the course of a fetal echocardiogram. This deceleration may occur if the fetus is lying on the umbilical cord or if the transducer pressure is too great. The fetus should be given a recovery time to bring the heart rate to a normal sinus rhythm, which is usually done with changing the position of the mother (i.e., rolling to her left side to release pressure from **inferior vena cava** compression) or with releasing the pressure from the transducer.

Normally, the fetal heart should have a baseline rate of 110 to 160 bpm. Some variability may be seen in rhythm and acceleration. Abnormal rate and rhythm may lead to fetal asphyxia, and thus, early recognition of "normal" from "abnormal" is critical. Short episodes of sinus bradycardia may be common in early pregnancy. However, if the bradycardia (<100 bpm) continues for several minutes, it is abnormal. Likewise, sinus tachycardia (>160 bpm) is common in later stages of pregnancy and may be associated with fetal movement.

This rate becomes abnormal when it exceeds 200 bpm or has frequent "dropped" beats (**premature ventricular contractions [PVCs]**).

The sonographer should evaluate the fetus for normal cardiac structure and signs of cardiac failure (enlarged **right ventricle,** hydrops, ascites, edema, pleural effusion, or pericardial effusion) and perform a simultaneous M-mode study through the atrial and ventricular cavities. Every ventricular contraction should be preceded by an atrial contraction.

Other changes in rhythm patterns seen during fetal development may result from **premature atrial contractions** (PACs) and PVCs, supraventricular tachycardia, tachycardia, or AV block.

Premature Atrial and Ventricular Contractions

Premature atrial and ventricular contractions arise from the electrical impulses generated outside the cardiac pacemaker (sinus node; Fig. 26-1). The sinus node is located along the lateral right atrial wall. Why these ectopic premature contractions develop in some patients is not clearly understood, and these contractions are rarely associated with structural heart disease. Some investigators have tried to link them to increased amounts of caffeine, alcohol, or smoking, but our patients with PACs do not have these associations. An increased redundancy of the flap of the **foramen ovale** has been noted in these patients. The flap is larger than seen in the normal fetus and appears to swing with a great excursion from the **left atrium** into the right atrial cavity, touching the right atrial node. The arrhythmia

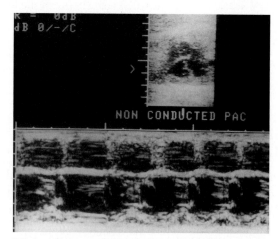

Fig. 26-1 Nonconducted premature atrial contractions. M-mode tracing is through atrium *(top)* and ventricle *(bottom)*. Note that atrial beats are continuous and ventricular strip shows skipped beat. Atrium has fired, but pulse is not conducted to ventricle.

usually regresses towards the end of pregnancy or soon after delivery.

The patient is usually referred for a fetal cardiac examination after an arrhythmia is heard on the routine obstetric examination with Doptone or auscultation. This technique provides information about the ventricular rate only. For adequate assessment of the fetal rhythm, the ventricular and atrial rates must be analyzed simultaneously.

The atrium and ventricle may have ectopic beats that give rise to complex echocardiographic patterns. The PACs may either be conducted to the ventricles or blocked, depending on the moment of the cardiac cycle in which they occur. Repeated PACs may lead to an increased or decreased ventricular rate.

A blocked PAC must be differentiated from an AV block. This distinction relies on the demonstration of an atrial contraction that appears prematurely. *PVCs* are ventricular contractions that are not preceded by atrial contractions.

The sonographer can help sort out the rhythm with M-mode and real-time ultrasound. For simultaneous recording of the atrial and ventricular rates, the four-chamber heart must be perpendicular to the transducer. The M-mode beam must dissect the ventricle and atria of the heart. Whether the right heart or left heart is more anterior does not matter. The best area for recording of atrial motion is usually just superior to the AV junction along the lateral wall of the atria. The atrial pattern appears to move with a box type of motion.

The ventricular rate is best recorded at the level of the AV valve and is seen to move as a smooth, uniform, well-defined pattern. If the sonographer cannot obtain adequate images from the four-chamber view, the parasternal short-axis view may be used. The M-mode beam should be directed through the right atrial wall and aortic cusps or the left atrial wall and aortic cusps. As the aorta moves in an anterior direction, the aortic cusps open in systole and close in diastole. Thus, the aortic leaflets may signify the ventricular systolic event, whereas the atrial wall signifies the atrial event. The M-mode should be expanded to its full extent for a clear view of the movement of the atrial and ventricular walls.

Changes in the AV valve patterns are also noted in patients with arrhythmias. Doppler of the AV valves determines whether regurgitation is present during the disturbance in rhythm. Patients with PACs and PVCs are assured that this development is a normal benign condition that results from the immaturity of the electrical conduction system of the heart. This pattern is not associated with other cardiac anomalies.

Supraventricular Tachyarrhythmias

Supraventricular tachyarrhythmias include abnormal rhythms of more than 200 bpm with a conduction rate of 1:1 (Fig. 26-2). These rhythm disturbances may be sinus and junctional tachycardia, paroxysmal atrial tachycardia, **atrial flutter,** or **atrial fibrillation.**

Supraventricular tachycardia occurs by automaticity or reentry mechanisms.

In cases of automatic induced tachyarrhythmias, an irritable ectopic focus discharges at a high frequency. The reentry mechanism consists of an electrical impulse reentering the atria, giving rise to repeated electrical activity. Reentry may occur at the level of the SA node, inside the atrium, at the AV node, and in the His-Purkinje system. Reentry may also occur along an anomalous AV connection, such as Kent's bundle in the Wolff-Parkinson-White (WPW) syndrome.

Supraventricular tachycardia is the most frequent arrhythmia caused by AV nodal reentry, occurring in one in 25,000 births. Maternal causes include viral infections and anticholinergic medications (e.g., atropine, prednisone, Benadryl), or hypoplasia of the SA tract

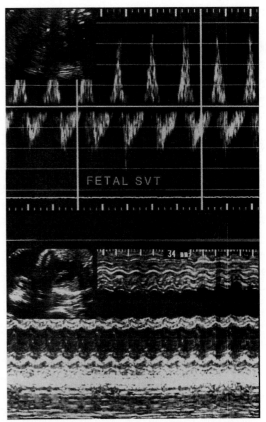

Fig. 26-2 Doppler and M-mode tracing of fetus in supraventricular tachycardia with heart rate of more than 200 beats per minute.

may trigger supraventricular tachycardia. Fetal causes for supraventricular tachycardia include hypoxia, anemia, or tachyarrhythmia.

The finding of supraventricular tachycardia in a fetus is an emergent situation. The fetus should undergo immediate scanning for assessment of signs of heart rate, ventricular and atrial size, amount of regurgitation, ventricular function, and presence of pericardial effusion and hydrops. With supraventricular tachycardia, the fetus has suboptimal filling of the ventricles, decreased cardiac output, and right ventricular volume overload develop, which lead to subsequent congestive heart failure.

The cardiac anomalies associated with supraventricular tachycardia are atrial septal defects, **mitral valve** disease, cardiac tumors, and WPW syndrome.

In atrial flutter, the atrial rate is recorded at 300 to 460 bpm, with a normal ventricular rate. Atrial fibrillation shows the atria to beat at more than 400 bpm, with a ventricular rate of 120 to 200 bpm.

Atrial flutter and fibrillation often alternate and are thought to result from a mechanism similar to that found in supraventricular tachycardia. Atrial flutter and fibrillation have been described in patients with WPW syndrome, cardiomyopathies, and thyrotoxicosis. The fetus with this arrhythmia is usually admitted into the hospital and medically treated with antiarrhythmic drugs to control the ventricular rate, with the goal of converting the rate into normal sinus rhythm. Fetal echocardiography may be clinically useful in monitoring recovery.

Atrioventricular Block

When the transmission of the electrical impulse from the atria to the ventricles is blocked, the condition is called an **atrioventricular** (AV) **block** (Fig. 26-3). Normally the atria fill in ventricular diastole and empty in ventricular systole. Just before ventricular systole occurs, the pressure in the atria is at its peak (this corresponds to the P wave on the electrocardiogram [ECG]). The QRS complex signifies the onset of ventricular systole, causing the pressure from the atria to open the AV valves so the **left ventricle** may fill. If this electrical process is blocked, the blood remains in the atria and does not cause the AV valves to open so blood can fill the ventricular cavities.

This condition may be attributed to immaturity of the conduction system, absence of connection to the AV node, or an abnormal anatomic position of the AV node. The fetus may have a first-degree, second-degree, or third-degree heart block.

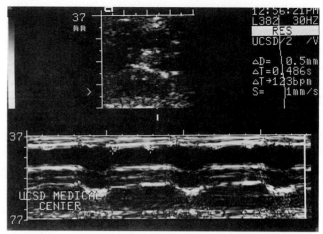

Fig. 26-3 M-mode tracing of fetus with 2:1 heart block rhythm. Atrial wall beats twice to aortic cusp opening.

Fetuses with a third-degree AV block have been found to have associated structural anomalies, including corrected transposition, atrioventricular septal defect (AVSD), univentricular heart, cardiac tumors, and cardiomyopathies. Patients with a connective tissue disorder, such as lupus erythematosus, have also been found to have heart block.

The first-degree and second-degree AV blocks are not associated with any significant hemodynamic disturbance.

A complete heart block may result in bradycardia, leading to decreased cardiac output and congestive heart failure during fetal life.

CONGENITAL HEART ANOMALIES

The most common type of congenital heart disease is ventricular septal defect (VSD), followed by atrial septal defects and **pulmonary stenosis**. Environmental factors may influence the development of congenital heart disease. Chromosomal abnormalities also have a high association with congenital heart disease (i.e., fetuses with trisomy 21 have a 50% incidence rate of congenital heart disease, specifically AVSDs).

Atrial Septal Defects

Atrial septal defects are usually not recognized during fetal life unless a large part of the intraatrial septum is missing. The development of the interatrial septum evolves in several stages; interruption of any of these stages could lead to the formation of an atrial septal defect. A natural communication exists between the right and left atria during fetal life. This communication (fossa ovalis) is covered by the flap of the foramen ovale and remains open in the fetal heart until after birth

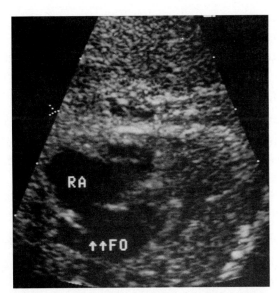

Fig. 26-4 Modified four-chamber view through atrial cavities shows flap of foramen ovale and opening into left atrium. In real-time imaging, flap may be shown to open and close with each cardiac contraction. Septum secundum is seen near base of heart, and septum primum is near center of heart (crux).

when the pressures change between the right and left heart to force the foramen to close completely (Fig. 26-4). Failure of the foramen to close may result in one type of atrial septal defect, the secundum defect.

The area of the foramen ovale is thinner in the fetus than in the surrounding atrial tissue; therefore, it is prone to signal dropout during sonographic evaluation, particularly in the apical four-chamber view when the transducer is parallel to the septum. Any break in the atrial septum in this view must be confirmed with the short-axis or perpendicular four-chamber view in which the septum is more perpendicular to the transducer. Because of beam-width artifacts, the edges of the defect may be slightly blunted and appear brighter than the remaining septum.

In utero, the natural flow is right to left across the foramen because the pressures are slightly higher on the right. A small reversal of flow may be present. The flap of the foramen should open into the left atrial cavity. The flap should not be so large as to touch the lateral wall of the atrium; when this redundancy of the foramen occurs, the SA node may become agitated in the **right atrium** and be the cause of fetal arrhythmias. The sonographer should sweep inferior to superior along the atrial septum to identify the three parts of the septum: the **primum septum** (near the center of the heart), the fossa ovalis (middle of the atrial septum), and the **septum secundum** (base of the heart, near the right upper pulmonary vein).

Secundum Atrial Septal Defect

Secundum atrial septal defect is the most common defect and occurs in the area of the fossa ovalis. Usually an absence of the foramen ovale flap is noted, with the fossa ovalis opening larger than normal.

Doppler tracings of the septal defect with the sample volume placed at the site of the defect show a right-to-left flow with a velocity of 20 to 30 cm/sec. The size of the normal foramen should measure at least 60% of the aortic diameter (i.e., if the aorta measures 4 mm, the foramen should be at least 2.4 mm). The flow patterns of the mitral and **tricuspid valves** are slightly increased with the increased shunt flow.

Sinus Venosus Septal Defect

The sinus venosus atrial septal defect is technically more difficult to visualize with echocardiogram. This defect lies in the superior portion of the atrial septum, close to the inflow pattern of the **superior vena cava,** and is best visualized with the four-chamber view. If signs of right ventricular volume overload are present, with no atrial septal defect obvious, then care should be taken to study the septum in search of a sinus venosus type of defect.

Partial anomalous pulmonary venous drainage of the right pulmonary vein is usually associated with this type of defect; thus, identification of the entry site of the **pulmonary veins** into the left atrial cavity is important. Color-flow mapping is useful in this type of problem because the sonographer can actually visualize the venous return to the left atrium and a flow pattern crossing into the right atrial cavity.

Ventricular Septal Defect

VSD is the most common congenital lesion of the heart, accounting for 30% of all structural heart defects. The septum is divided into two basic segments: the membranous and muscular areas. A number of sites exist in which VSDs may occur within the septum. Muscular defects occur lower in the septum, are usually very small, and may be multiple in number. Often the smaller defects close spontaneously shortly after birth and are difficult to image.

The prognosis is good for a patient with a single VSD. However, the association of other cardiac anomalies, such as tetralogy of Fallot, single ventricle, **transposition of the great arteries,** and endocardial cushion defect, is increased when a VSD is found.

Membranous Septal Defect

The (perimembranous) VSD may be classified as membranous, aneurysmal, or supracristal. The significant anatomic landmark is the crista supraventricularis ridge. The defect lies either above or below this ridge. Defects that lie above are supracristal. These defects are located just beneath the pulmonary orifice so that the pulmonary valve forms part of the superior margin of the interventricular communication. Defects that lie below the crista are infracristal and may be found in the membranous or muscular part of the septum. These are the most common defects.

The lesion may be partially covered by the tricuspid septal leaflet, and care must be taken for careful evaluation of this area with Doppler and color-flow tracings. The membranous defect is found just below the aortic leaflets; sometimes the aortic leaflet is sucked into this defect. The presence of an isolated VSD in utero usually does not change the hemodynamics of the fetus. Septal defects must be at least half the size of the aorta to be imaged. Defects smaller than 2 mm are not detected with fetal echocardiography. Malalignment of the anterior wall of the aorta with the septum is a sign that a septal defect may be present.

The sonographer must take care in the four-chamber view to carefully sweep the transducer posterior (to record the inlet part of the septum) to anterior (to record the outlet part of the septum).

VSDs may close with the formation of aneurysm tissue that is commonly found along the right side of the septal defect (Fig. 26-5).

Muscular Septal Defect

A less common infracristal defect is located in the muscular septum. These defects may be large or small, or they may be multiple fenestrated holes. The multiple defects are more difficult to repair, and their combi-

nation may have the same ventricular overload effect as a single large communication. Pressures between the right and left heart are different in utero, and therefore, a small defect will probably not show a flow velocity change.

Atrioventricular Septal Defect

Atrioventricular septal defect (AVSD) is also called *ostium primum atrial septal defect, AV canal malformation,* and *endocardial cushion defect.* These defects are subdivided into complete, incomplete, and partial forms. The defect occurs at the crux (center) of the heart.

Incomplete Atrioventricular Septal Defect

The failure of the endocardial cushion to fuse is termed *incomplete atrioventricular septal defect.* This condition results in a membranous VSD, an abnormal **tricuspid valve,** a primum atrial septal defect, and a cleft mitral valve (Fig. 26-6). A cleft mitral valve means that the anterior part of the leaflet is divided into two parts: medial and lateral. When the leaflet closes, blood leaks through this hole into the left atrial cavity. The leaflet is usually somewhat malformed, causing further regurgitation into the atrium.

In addition, there is a communication between the left ventricle and right atrium (left ventricular to right atrial shunt) because of the absent primum atrial septum and membranous interventricular septum. The VSD occurs just below the mitral ring and is continuous with the primum atrial septal defect.

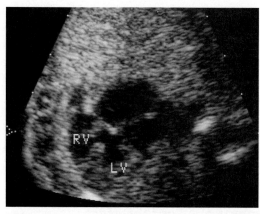

Fig. 26-5 Four-chamber view of heart with prominent membranous septal defect between right *(RV)* and left ventricles *(LV)*.

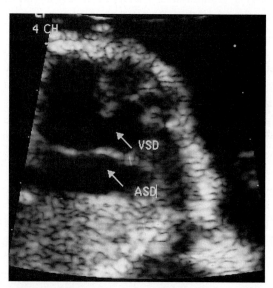

Fig. 26-6 Atrioventricular septal defect may have several characteristics. Patient has large atrial *(ASD)* and ventricular septal defects *(VSD)*.

Complete Atrioventricular Septal Defect

The endocardial defect may be further described into Rastelli types A, B, and C. Types A and B are characterized by insertion of the chordae from the cleft mitral and tricuspid valve into the crest of the ventricular septum or a right ventricular papillary muscle. Type C is the most primitive form and is called *complete AVSD*. This defect has a single, undivided, free-floating leaflet stretching across both ventricles.

The anterior and posterior leaflets are on both sides of the interventricular septum, which causes the valve to override or straddle the septum. This abnormality is more complex to repair because the defect is larger and the single AV valve is more difficult to clinically manage, depending on the amount of regurgitation.

Complete AVSDs are frequently associated with malpositions of the heart (mesocardia and dextrocardia) and AV block (caused by distortion of the conduction tissues). AVSDs are frequently associated with other cardiac defects, including truncoconal abnormalities, coarctation of the aorta, and pulmonary stenosis or atresia. Increased incidence rates of Down's syndrome (50% of babies with trisomy 21 have congenital heart disease) and asplenia and polysplenia syndromes also are seen.

Occasionally, complete absence of the interatrial septum is noted in the fetal four-chamber view. With color flow, the entire atria are completely filled throughout systole and diastole. This is termed *common atria*.

Partial Atrioventricular Septal Defect

A partial AVSD means that the fetus has only some of the previous findings, usually an absent primum atrial septum and a cleft mitral valve (Fig. 26-7). The ideal views for this anomaly are the long-axis, the short-axis (to search for abnormalities in the AV valves, such as presence of cleft), and the four-chamber views (to search for chordal attachment, overriding, or straddling of the valves).

The crux of the heart is carefully analyzed by sweeping the transducer anteroposteriorly to record the outlet and inlet portions of the membranous septum. Doppler and color flow are extremely useful in determination of the direction and degree of regurgitation present in the AV valves and the direction of shunt flow (increased right heart pressure causes a right ventricular to left atrial shunt in the fetus).

Tetralogy of Fallot

Tetralogy of Fallot is the most common form of cyanotic heart disease. The severity of the disease varies according to the degree of pulmonary stenosis present; the more stenosis, the greater the cyanosis. A mild form of pulmonary stenosis without any cyanosis after birth is possible.

Tetralogy of Fallot is characterized by the following:
1. High membranous ventricular septal defect
2. Large anteriorly displaced aorta, which overrides the septal defect (Fig. 26-8)
3. Pulmonary stenosis
4. Right ventricular hypertrophy (not seen in fetal life; occurs after birth when pulmonary stenosis causes increased pressures in the right ventricle).

A large septal defect with mild to moderate pulmonary stenosis is classified as acyanotic disease, whereas a large septal defect with severe pulmonary stenosis is considered cyanotic disease ("blue baby" at birth).

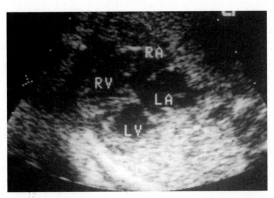

Fig. 26-7   Patient with atrioventricular septal defect with primum septal defect. Patient also had cleft mitral valve and regurgitation from left ventricle into right atrial cavity.

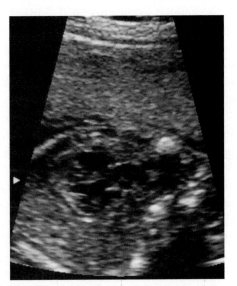

Fig. 26-8   Long-axis view of fetal heart in patient with tetralogy of Fallot shows membranous septal defect and overriding of aorta.

A number of other congenital cardiac malformations tend to occur in patients with pulmonary stenosis and VSD, including (1) right aortic arch, (2) persistent left superior vena cava, (3) anomalies of the **pulmonary artery** and its branches, (4) absence of the pulmonary valve (5) regurgitation of the aortic valve, and (6) variations in coronary arterial anatomy.

The demonstration of tetralogy of Fallot is distinguished on the parasternal long-axis view. The large aorta overrides the ventricular septum. If the override is greater than 50%, the condition is called *double-outlet right ventricle* (both great vessels arise from the right heart). A septal defect is present and may vary in size from small to large.

The short-axis view shows the small hypertrophied right ventricle (if significant pulmonary stenosis is present). The pulmonary artery is usually small, and the cusps may be thickened and domed or difficult to image well. A sample volume should be made in the high parasternal short-axis view to determine the turbulence of the right ventricular outflow tract and pulmonary valve stenosis.

Color flow is helpful in this condition for actual delineation of the abnormal high-velocity pattern and for directing the sample volume into the proper jet flow. If the VSD is large, increased flow is seen in the right heart (increased tricuspid velocity, right ventricular outflow tract velocity, and also increased pulmonic velocity).

Aortic Atresia or Hypoplastic Left Heart Syndrome

Hypoplastic left heart syndrome is characterized by a small, hypertrophied left ventricle with aortic or mitral dysplasia or atresia. This syndrome has been found to be an autosomal recessive condition. If a couple has had one child with hypoplastic left heart syndrome, the recurrence rate is 4%; if two births have been affected, the recurrence rate increases to 25%.

The cause of hypoplastic left heart syndrome is unknown and is thought to be decreased filling and perfusion of the left ventricle during embryologic development. When this closure occurs, the blood cannot cross the foramen to help the left ventricle grow. The real-time image shows a reduction in the size of the foramen ovale (the foramen should measure at least 0.6 multiplied by the diameter of the aortic root). Premature closure of the foramen would also show increased velocities across the interatrial septum (around 40 to 50 cm/sec).

The right ventricle supplies both the pulmonic and systemic circulations. The pulmonary venous return is diverted from the left atrium to the right atrium through the interatrial communication. Through the pulmonary artery and ductus arteriosus, the right ventricle supplies the descending aorta, along with retrograde flow to the aortic arch and the ascending aorta.

Overload on the right ventricle may lead to congestive heart failure in utero with the development of pericardial effusion and hydrops.

A fetus that has had a major disturbance in the development of the mitral valve or aortic valve would show dramatic changes in the development of the left ventricle (Fig. 26-9). The amount of hypoplasia would depend on when the left-sided atresia developed in the valvar area. If mitral atresia is the cause, the blood cannot fill the left ventricle to provide volume, and thus the aortic valve would become atretic as well, with concentric hypertrophy of the small left ventricular cavity. If the cause is aortic stenosis, the myocardium will show extreme hypertrophy from the increased pressure overload.

Ebstein's Anomaly

Ebstein's anomaly is an abnormal displacement of the septal leaflet of the tricuspid valve toward the apex of the right ventricle (Fig. 26-10). Tricuspid valvar tissue may adhere directly to the ventricular endocardium or may be closely attached to the ventricular wall by multiple, anomalous, short chordae tendineae. The portion of the right ventricle underlying the adherent tricuspid valvar tissue is thin and functions as a receiving chamber analogous to the right atrium and is referred to as the *atrialized chamber*.

The anterior leaflet of the tricuspid valve is the least affected of the three leaflets. The septal and posterior leaflets show the greatest deformity, and the posterior cusp may be rudimentary or entirely absent. The right atrium is usually massively dilated. Often the patients have an incompetent or fenestrated foramen ovale or a secundum atrial septal defect.

Sonographic evaluation shows apical displacement of the septal leaflet of the tricuspid valve with resultant insufficiency (as seen on the apical four-chamber view). The atrialized right ventricle is clearly visualized.

Doppler tracings are useful in recording the amount of insufficiency present from the abnormal tricuspid valve. The sample volume should be placed at the anulus of the tricuspid valve and then mapped through the atrialized right ventricle into the right atrial cavity to record the maximum jet of insufficiency. The earlier the regurgitation is seen, the poorer is the prognosis for the fetus.

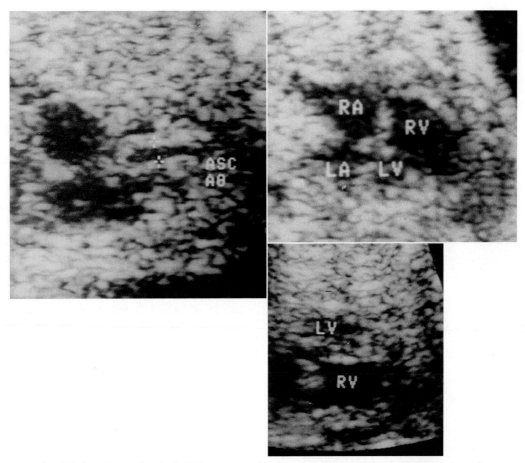

Fig. 26-9 Hypoplastic left heart syndrome shows small hypoplastic ascending aorta arising from thick hypoplastic left ventricle. *LA,* Left atrium; *LV,* left ventricle; *RA,* right atrium; *RV,* right ventricle.

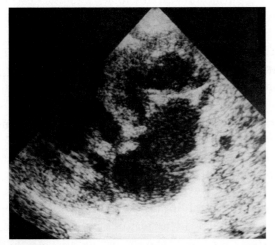

Fig. 26-10 Patient with Ebstein's anomaly with huge right atrialized chamber with apical displacement of septal leaflet of tricuspid valve.

Transposition of the Great Arteries

Transposition of the great arteries is an abnormal condition that exists when the aorta is connected to the right ventricle and the pulmonary artery is connected to the left ventricle. The AV valves are normally attached and related.

Transposition occurs because of an abnormal completion of the "loop" in embryonic development. The great vessels originate as a common truncus and undergo rotation and spiraling; if this development is interrupted, the great arteries do not complete their spiral and transposition occurs. Usually the aorta is anterior and to the right of the pulmonary artery (Fig. 26-11).

In the fetal heart, no hemodynamic compromise is seen in the fetus when the great arteries are transposed. The problems occur in the neonatal period with inadequate mixing of oxygenated and unoxygenated blood.

The short-axis view is the key view for imaging of the great arteries and their normal relationship. In the

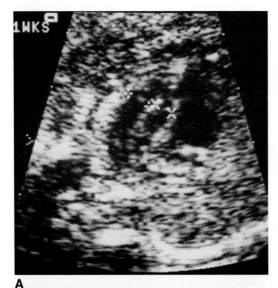

A

B

Fig. 26-11 **A,** Transportation of great arteries shows short-axis view of two great vessels side by side. **B,** Aorta is seen to arise from anterior ventricle.

normal fetus, the right ventricular outflow tract and pulmonary artery with its bifurcation should be seen anterior to the aorta in the parasternal short-axis view. In transposition, this relationship would not be present; it would be impossible to show the bifurcation of the pulmonary artery because the aorta would be the anterior vessel. Sometimes, the double circles of the great arteries can be seen in this view.

On the modified long-axis view, the normal criss-cross pattern obtained from a normal fetal echocardiogram occurs when the transducer is swept from the left ventricular outflow tract anterior and medial into the right ventricular outflow tract. In a fetus with trans-

position, this criss-cross sweep of the great arteries is not possible. The parallel great arteries are sometimes seen in this view because they both arise from the ventricles.

Other associated cardiac anomalies include atrial septal defects, anomalies of the AV valves, and underdevelopment of the right or left ventricles.

Corrected Transposition of the Great Arteries

Corrected transposition is a cardiac condition in which the right and left atria are connected to the morphologic left and right ventricles, respectively; and the great arteries are transposed. Therefore, these two defects essentially cancel each other out without hemodynamic consequences. Corrected transposition is associated with malpositions of the heart and sometimes with situs inversus.

A ventricular perimembranous septal defect may be present in half of the fetuses. The pulmonary artery may be seen to override the septal defect, with pulmonary stenosis in 50%.

Abnormalities of the AV valves, such as an Ebstein type of malformation and straddling of the tricuspid valve, may be present. AV heart block may also be recorded.

Truncus Arteriosus

Truncus arteriosus is a complex congenital heart lesion in which only one great artery arises from the base of the heart. From this single great artery arise the pulmonary trunk, the systemic arteries, and the coronary arteries.

This defect occurs in the early embryologic period when the conotruncus fails to separate into two great arteries. The conus corresponds to the middle third of the **bulbus cordis.**

This condition gives rise to the outflow tract of both ventricles and to the muscular portion of the ventricles located between the AV valves and the semilunar valves. The truncus is the distal part of the bulbus cordis. This structure rotates and divides into the two great semilunar valvar structures that represent the aortic and pulmonic leaflets. Failure of the bulbus to divide causes a single great artery with multiple cusps within.

Sonographic evaluation shows an abnormal, large, single great vessel arising from the ventricles. Usually an infundibular ventricular septal defect is present (Fig. 26-12; see Color Plate 18). Significant septal override is present. The truncal valve is usually dysplastic, thick, and domed. Multiple cusps are seen within the great artery. If truncal regurgitation is present, the prognosis is grim; the fetus usually has congestive heart failure, pericardial effusion, and hydrops develop.

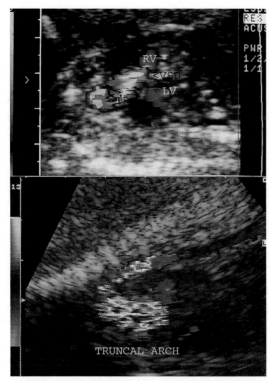

Fig. 26-12 Color Doppler imaging shows single large vessel arising from both ventricles. Multiple cusps within large vessel may be deformed and dysplastic, resulting in moderate to significant aortic insufficiency. *LV,* Left ventricle; *RV,* right ventricle; *TR,* tricuspid regurgitation; *VSD,* ventricular septal defect.

Truncus arteriosus may be difficult to separate from a severe tetralogy of Fallot with pulmonary atresia (small pulmonary artery and large aorta overriding septal defect). Associated anomalies include mitral atresia, atrial septal defect, univentricular heart, and aortic arch abnormalities. In the neonatal stage, the prognosis is poor for truncus arteriosus.

SUMMARY

Echocardiographic evaluation of a fetus with a suspected congenital heart problem has been a tremendous aid to the obstetrician and pediatric cardiologist in the management of the mother and fetus. For the mother of a child with congenital heart disease, a normal fetal echocardiogram in subsequent pregnancies is reassuring. On the other hand, a new diagnosis of congenital heart disease in utero may allow time for the pediatric cardiologist and surgeon to discuss possible options for the fetus after delivery. It also allows time to arrange the delivery in a medical center equipped to manage congenital heart problems.

CLINICAL SCENARIO—DIAGNOSIS

■ Once a mother has given birth to a child with congenital heart disease, the risk increases for subsequent pregnancies. In the case of left-sided heart disease, the risk is slightly greater with each subsequent pregnancy. Because the first child had hypoplastic left heart syndrome, the chance of the second child having left-sided heart disease increases to 4%. If the second child also has left-sided congenital heart disease, the third pregnancy risk factor increases to 25%. In addition, because the mother is known to have aortic valve disease, the risk further increases for each pregnancy.

This patient needs to be followed closely to evaluate for the presence of left-sided heart disease that may lead to hypoplastic left heart syndrome. This patient was seen at 24 weeks' gestation, but typically the initial sonographic evaluation may occur as early as 16 weeks to look for symmetry between the ventricular sizes. The fetus should again be scanned at 20 to 22 weeks for a detailed cardiac anatomy study. The last scan should be made at the beginning of the third trimester, at about 28 weeks. At that time, the ventricular growth pattern should be established, with the right ventricle being only slightly larger than the left. Any variation of more than 5 to 10 mm in growth pattern between the ventricles is suspicious for the development of hypoplastic left heart syndrome.

CASE STUDIES FOR DISCUSSION

1. A fetus is diagnosed with trisomy 21 after amniocentesis. Which heart abnormality is most specifically linked with trisomy 21, and what will the sonographer identify to make this diagnosis?
2. A four-chamber view of the heart shows a huge right atrial cavity. The tricuspid valve "does not look right." The right ventricle and pulmonary artery are seen. What abnormality do you expect, and what else should be evaluated?
3. A ventricular septal defect is seen in the outflow tract. The short-axis view shows asymmetry of the great vessels.

What do you expect to find, and what else should you look for?
4. Asymmetry of the four-chamber heart view is seen, with the left atria closest to the fetal aorta. The aortic arch is difficult to image. What is your differential consideration?
5. A sweep from the traditional four-chamber view to the anterior great vessels shows two great vessels that arise from the ventricles in parallel. What is the normal relationship of the great vessels, and what other areas should you view?

STUDY QUESTIONS

1. Premature atrial and ventricular contractions arise from electrical impulses generated outside the cardiac pacemaker (sinus node). In the presence of an atrial septum aneurysm, which arrhythmia is most likely to occur?
   a. left bundle branch block
   b. premature atrial contraction
   c. right bundle branch block
   d. premature ventricular contraction

2. What two areas of the heart must be observed with M-mode to record the irregular rhythm?
   a. right atrium, left atrium
   b. right atrium, left ventricle
   c. left atrium, pulmonary artery
   d. tricuspid valve, right ventricle

3. The three types of atrial septal defects that may occur in the fetus include all except:
   a. the secundum type, which occurs in the area of the foramen ovale
   b. the sinus venosus type, located in the most superior portion of the atrial septum and usually associated with partial anomalous pulmonary venous drainage
   c. the fossa type, located at the base of the heart
   d. the primum type, located just superior to the atrioventricular ring and usually associated with a cleft mitral valve leaflet

4. Which of the four findings in tetralogy of Fallot is not found in the fetus?

   a. high membranous ventricular septal defect
   b. large anteriorly displaced aorta, which overrides the septal defect
   c. pulmonary stenosis
   d. right ventricular hypertrophy

5. All of the following descriptors may relate to hypoplastic left heart syndrome except:
   a. tricuspid atresia
   b. hypertrophied left ventricle
   c. aortic atresia
   d. mitral atresia

6. How does supraventricular tachyarrhythmia differ from atrial fibrillation and atrial flutter? Which statement is false?
   a. supraventricular tachyarrhythmias include abnormal rhythms of more than 100 beats per minute with a conduction rate of 3:1
   b. in atrial flutter, the atrial rate is recorded at 300 to 460 beats per minute, with a normal ventricular rate
   c. atrial fibrillation shows the atria to beat at more than 400 beats per minute (bpm), with a ventricular rate of 120 to 200 bpm
   d. atrial flutter and fibrillation often alternate and are thought to result from a mechanism similar to that found in supraventricular tachycardia

7. The problems associated with a complete atrioventricular heart block include all except:
   a. bradycardia
   b. decreased cardiac output

c. increased cardiac output
d. congestive heart failure

8. Cardiac anomalies associated with transposition of the great arteries may include all except:
   a. anomalies of the atrioventricular valves
   b. hypoplasia of the ventricles
   c. atrial septal defect
   d. Ebstein's anomaly

9. Which statement is correct regarding truncus arteriosus?
   a. one great artery arises from the base of the heart
   b. the great arteries are reversed
   c. the aorta arises from the ductus arteriosus
   d. the pulmonary artery arises from the coronary sinus

10. Cyanosis, or "blue baby" after birth, most likely occurs in which congenital heart defect?
    a. atrial septal defect
    b. atrioventricular septal defect
    c. transposition of the great arteries with a patent foramen ovale
    d. tetralogy of Fallot with severe pulmonary stenosis

BIBLIOGRAPHY

Allan LD: *Manual of fetal echocardiography,* Lancaster, England, 1986, MTP Press Limited.

Fink BW: *Congenital heart disease,* ed 3, St Louis, 1991, Mosby.

Hagen-Ansert SL: Fetal echocardiography. In *Textbook of diagnostic ultrasonography,* vol II, Mosby, St Louis, 2001.

IV SUPERFICIAL STRUCTURES

27 Breast Mass

DANA SALMONS

CLINICAL SCENARIO

■ An 11-year-old black menstrual-age girl is seen in the emergency department with rapidly increasing breast size, with the left breast noticeably larger than the right. She is referred for an ultrasound the following day. According to the patient's mother, the girl wore a size 36A bra 2 months previously and now wears a size 36D on the right and a 36DD on the left. She went to her family physician 1 week previously for this condition and was told that this was part of the girl's normal breast development.

The day of the sonogram, the patient has no pain and is not febrile. The clinical breast examination is negative for discrete masses, but the breasts feel hard, similar to encapsulated breast implants, with a foamlike, spongy consistency. The skin and nipples are stretched taut, but the nipples are not displaced. The sonographic examination shows little to no normal-looking tissue. Homogeneous branching tissue is seen beneath both areolas with a positive Doppler signal. Ductal ectasia is noted bilaterally. Multiple lobular areas are seen with a lacy heterogeneous "Swiss cheese" appearance. The patient also undergoes a left breast magnetic resonance imaging examination that reveals a 13-cm neoplasm (Fig. 27-1, *A* and *B*). What is the most likely diagnosis?

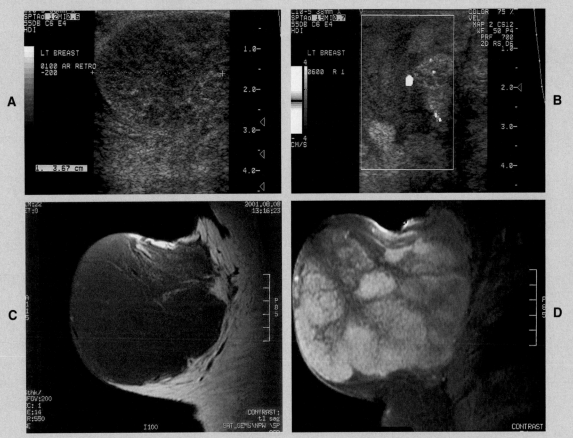

Fig. 27-1 **A**, Ultrasound of 11-year-old girl with bilateral breast enlargement. **B**, Color Doppler of lesion. **C** and **D**, magnetic resonance imaging of same case.

OBJECTIVES ■■■■■■■

■ Describe the sonographic appearance of common cystic masses of the breast.

■ Describe the sonographic appearance of the more common benign neoplasms of the breast.

■ Describe the sonographic appearance of the more common malignant neoplasms of the breast.

■ Describe the sonographic appearance of the augmented breast.

■ Describe the sonographic appearance of the inflamed breast.

■ Describe the sonographic appearance of the injured or postsurgical breast.

■ Describe the sonographic appearance of the male breast.

GLOSSARY OF TERMS ■■■■■■■

Antiradial: a plane of breast imaging for ultrasound perpendicular to a line radiating from the nipple (the hub) to the periphery of the breast like hands of a clock (90 degrees to radial)

Areola: the circular area of different pigmentation around the nipple of the breast

Asymptomatic: without symptoms

Axilla: the armpit

Breast: mammary gland, a compound alveolar gland consisting of 15 to 20 lobes of glandular tissue separated from each other by interlobular septa; each lobe is drained by a lactiferous duct that opens on the tip of the nipple; the mammary gland secretes milk used for nourishment of infants

Cooper's ligaments: support fibrous structures throughout the breast that partially sheathe the lobes shaping the breast; these ligaments affect the image of the glandular tissue on a mammogram

Cryptorchidism: failure of the testicles to descend into the scrotum

Cyst: a sac or pouch with a definite wall that contains fluid, semifluid, or solid material; when pertaining to the breast, a cyst is usually an abnormal structure resulting from obstruction of ducts

Eklund maneuver: a method for imaging augmented breasts that involves pulling the breast tissue away from the implant while displacing the implant posteriorly, excluding it from view and allowing for better visualization of the breast tissue

Fibroadenoma: a benign breast tumor composed of glandular and fibrous tissue

Granuloma: a tumor or growth that results when macrophages are unable to destroy a foreign body; when pertaining to breast implants, a granuloma is a glob of silicone with an associated inflammatory response

Gynecomastia: enlargement of the breast tissue in the male

Hormone replacement therapy: supplemental hormones used with postmenopausal women in preventing osteoporosis and providing cardiovascular benefits

Inspissated: thickened by evaporation or absorption of fluid; diminished fluidity

Intracapsular rupture: a breast implant rupture that extends outside the implant shell but not outside the fibrous capsule the body typically forms around the implant

Klinefelter's syndrome: a congenital endocrine condition of primary testicular failure that usually is not present before puberty; the classical form is associated with the presence of an extra X chromosome; the testes are small and firm; sterility, gynecomastia, abnormally long legs, and subnormal intelligence usually are present

Lymphoscintigraphy, or sentinel node mapping: scintillation scanning of lymph nodes after an injection of a radionuclide; the sentinel nodes are the first lymph nodes to absorb the radionuclide and these lymph nodes are surgically removed to determine whether cancer has metastasized to the lymphatic system

Mammary layer: the middle of the three layers of the breast

Palpable: able to be felt

Peau d'orange: French for *skin of an orange*; a dimpled skin condition that resembles an orange seen in lymphatic edemas and sometimes over an area of carcinoma of the breast

Radial: a plane of imaging the breast for ultrasound that radiates out from the nipple to the periphery of

GLOSSARY OF TERMS—cont'd

the breast like hands of a clock (90 degrees to antiradial)

Retroareolar: area beneath the nipple

Retromammary layer: the deepest of the three layers of the breast and the layer of the breast that is superficial to the pectoralis major muscle

Snowstorm sign: a sonographic sign of implant rupture that appears as echogenic noise or dirty shadowing with a similar sonographic appearance of bowel gas

Stepladder sign: a sonographic sign of implant rupture that appears as parallel echogenic lines within the interior of the implant

Subcutaneous layer: the most superficial of the three layers of the breast located just below the skin

Terminal ductal-lobular unit: each of hundreds of individual milk-producing glands within the breast and the terminal end of a lactiferous duct together form the terminal ductal-lobular unit, which is where almost all breast pathology is located

The two most common indications for **breast** ultrasound examinations are a **palpable** breast mass and the need for more information regarding a lesion seen with another method. Other indications for breast ultrasound include evaluation of dense breasts and areas of asymmetry not well visualized with mammography, evaluation of implant integrity, follow-up on either accidentally or surgically traumatized breasts, and serial sonogram evaluation of tumor size.[1] In addition, ultrasound guidance is often advantageous in invasive procedures such as **cyst** aspiration, abscess drainage, needle localization, **lymphoscintigraphy,** and core biopsy.

With the improvement in resolution of ultrasound imagery, there is a growing movement toward screening breast sonograms; however, sonography is not to be used as a replacement for mammography. Ultrasound cannot consistently detect microcalcifications that are often an indicator of breast cancer.[2]

BREAST

Ultrasound Scanning Planes

There are two accepted scanning systems of breast ultrasound. The preferred method uses **radial** and **antiradial** planes (Fig. 27-2, A). However, the breast may also be scanned in longitudinal and transverse planes.

Multiple ducts start at the nipple and radiate out towards the periphery of the breast parenchyma. With radial and antiradial scanning, ductal involvement of a mass is more readily seen.[2] With either method, scanning while turning on the lesion is important so that all aspects of the lesion are evaluated.

Breast Ultrasound Annotation

Documentation of the location within the breast that is being imaged is imperative. This proves that the area of interest was evaluated, and it facilitates relocation of any discovered pathology for follow-up.

The preferred method of annotation uses a quasigrid pattern. First, the breasts are viewed as a clock face. Directly above the nipple on either breast is 12:00. Right medial breast and left lateral breast are 3:00. Directly below the nipple bilaterally is 6:00. And right lateral breast and left medial breast are 9:00 (Fig. 27-2, B).

Next, the breast is divided into three equal concentric circles, with the center being the nipple. The first ring circles one third of the breast tissue, encompassing the area just outside the nipple, zone 1. The second ring is about two thirds of the breast surface from the nipple, zone 2. The final ring is to the breast periphery, zone 3 (Fig. 27-2, C).

Finally, depth of any pathology is documented. The breast is again divided into thirds from skin to the pectoralis major. Depth A is the most superficial third of the breast. Depth B is the middle layer. And depth C is the deepest third of the breast (Fig. 27-2, D).

The pathology in Fig. 27-2, E, would be labeled: RT BREAST, 5:00 1A rad (radial) or arad (antiradial); LT BREAST, 1:00 3B rad or arad.

Location of a Mass with Mammographic Images

With a search for a mass first seen via mammogram, isolation of the quadrant of interest is essential. An understanding of mammographic images is vital to correlation of sonographic findings.

The craniocaudal (CC) mammogram is used to discover whether a mass is in the medial or lateral portion of the breast. The CC mammogram is acquired with placement of the film inferior to the breast, and the radiograph beam is directed superiorly to inferiorly (Fig. 27-2, F).[3] The CC marker is placed just outside the

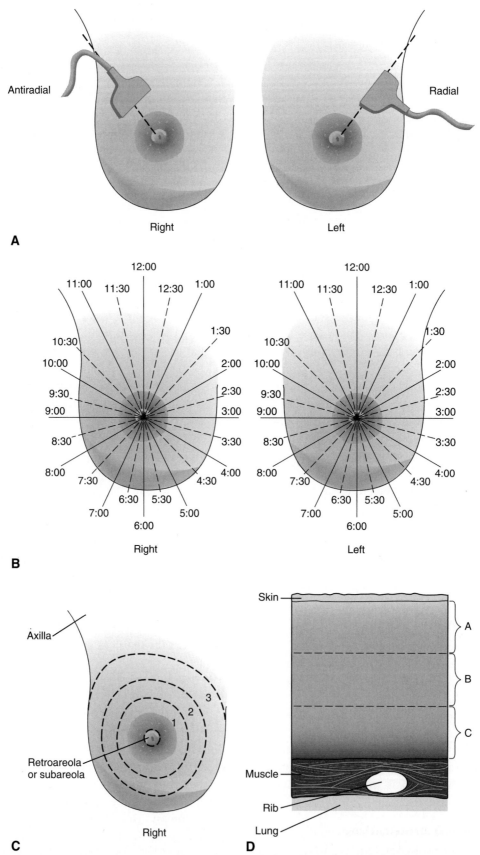

Fig. 27-2 **A,** Radial and antiradial scanning planes. **B,** Annotation uses clock face technique. **C,** Zones of breast are shown. **D,** Documentation of depth.

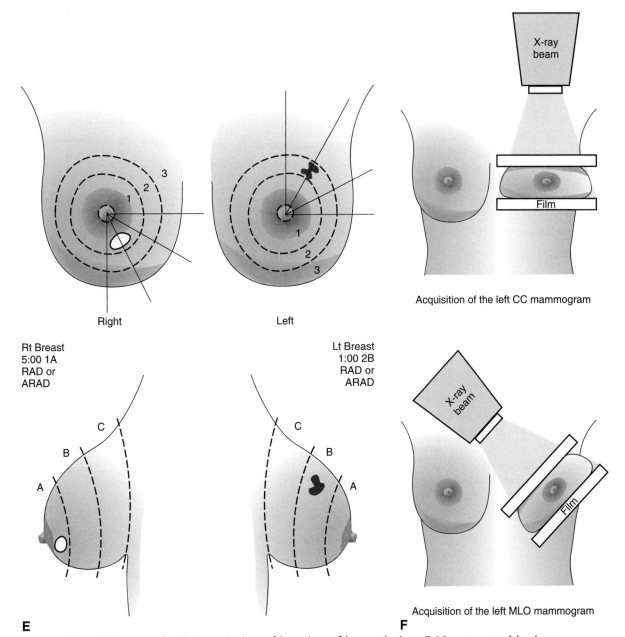

Right

Left

Rt Breast
5:00 1A
RAD or
ARAD

Lt Breast
1:00 2B
RAD or
ARAD

Acquisition of the left CC mammogram

Acquisition of the left MLO mammogram

E

F

Fig. 27-2, cont'd   **E,** Annotation of location of breast lesion. **F,** Mammographic views.

lateral breast border. If the mass is located between the nipple and the CC marker, the mass is in the lateral portion of the breast. If the mass is located between the nipple and the contralateral side of the CC marker, the mass is medial. Superior and inferior mass location is determined with the mediolateral oblique (MLO) mammogram. The MLO mammogram is acquired with placement of the film at an oblique angle that is lateral and slightly inferior to the breast. The radiograph beam is directed mediolaterally at the same obliquity as the film (see Fig. 27-2, *F*).[3] Because this is not a true mediolateral image, masses on the lateral breast will be slightly lower than that which appear in the image. Masses in the medial breast will be slightly higher.

Normal Sonographic Anatomy

Normal human breasts are two modified sweat glands on the upper anterior portion of the chest, lying anterior to the pectoralis major. The **areola** and nipple are centrally located on each breast. Each adult female breast has a conic formation with a "tail" that extends toward the associated **axilla** (Fig. 27-3).[4] The function is to

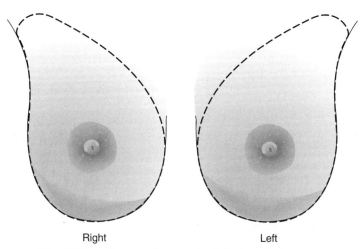

Right   Left

Fig. 27-3 Shape of normal adult female breasts.

produce and release milk during reproduction. The breasts are composed of fatty, glandular, and fibrous connective tissues, all with differing echogenicities. Proportions of these tissues vary from patient to patient and can also vary within the breast of the same patient. The normal sonographic appearance is therefore quite diverse.

The normal skin thickness overlying the breast is less than 2 mm.[5] Beneath the skin are three layers of mammary tissue. Starting superficially, the **subcutaneous layer** located just under the skin is mainly fat and, in the breast, is sonographically hypoechoic. The middle **mammary layer** contains the ducts, glands, and stroma of the breast and is relatively echogenic. The deep **retromammary layer** is also composed of hypoechoic

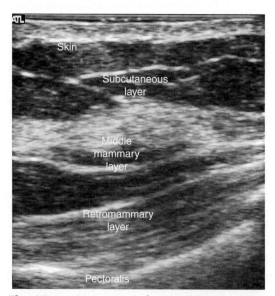

Fig. 27-4 Sonogram of normal breast tissue.

fat and is the portion of the breast that lies superficial to the pectoralis major. Traversing through these layers are **Cooper's ligaments** that are hyperechoic (Fig. 27-4).[6]

CYSTIC MASSES

Cysts are fluid-filled masses that form at the **terminal ductal-lobular unit** (TDLU) or from an obstructed duct and are the most common breast mass in women 40 to 50 years of age. They are frequent findings in perimenopausal women and often fluctuate with the menstrual cycle.[7,8]

Patients with cysts may have firm, smooth, mobile, palpable masses. Cysts are often painful and hard when they are full of fluid and the walls are stretched taut[8]; however, the patient may be **asymptomatic.** Cysts typically regress after menopause[2] but may persist or be new findings in postmenopausal women undergoing **hormone replacement therapy** (HRT). They may be singular or multiple, ranging in size from a few millimeters to multiple centimeters. Sonographically, they may further be classified as simple or complex.[1]

Aspiration of a cyst is generally done for one of three reasons: 1, the cyst is painful; 2, the cyst is radiographically or sonographically abnormal in appearance; or 3, the cyst obscures the diagnostic quality of a mammogram because of its size. Simple cysts do not become malignant and are usually left alone.[7]

Simple Cyst

Sonographic Findings. A simple cyst must have certain sonographic qualities to be considered simple. The mnemonic STAR may assist in identification of a

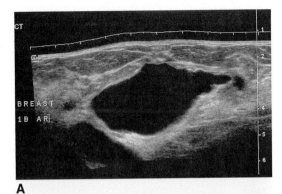

A

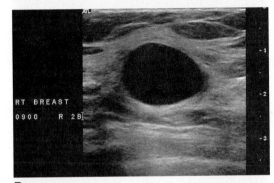

B

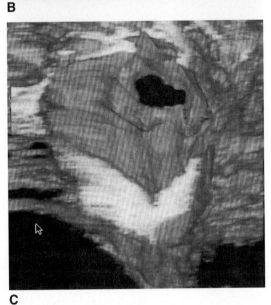

C

Fig. 27-5 Simple cysts measuring 5.6 cm seen in 50-year-old woman. **A,** Antiradial and, **B,** radial views show lesion. **C,** Three-dimensional image of same cyst shows smooth walls.

simple cyst. (Fig. 27-5, *A* and *B*). A simple cyst should be: *S, s*mooth and thin-walled; *T, t*hrough transmit; *A, a*nechoic; and *R, r*ound or oval.

Interior echoes within a cyst can be the result of improper gain or power settings or anterior reverberation artifact, or they may be real and therefore considered complex.[9]

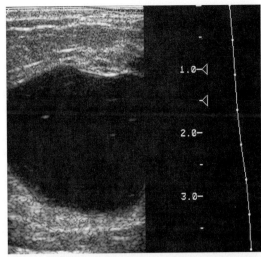

Fig. 27-6 Benign-appearing cyst with internal floating debris.

Newer ultrasound machines are better at depicting debris within cysts. This debris may be seen and yet not be considered worrisome for malignant disease. In these cases, some radiologists use the term benign-appearing instead of simple-appearing cyst (Fig. 27-6).

Complex Cyst

Complex cysts are cysts that do not meet the criteria of STAR, meaning they are cystic with a solid component.[9]

The reasons for a cyst to be classified as complex are multiple. Just as skin sloughs its cells, so do the cyst walls. This causes layering debris within the cyst. Cysts may also have internal echoes from infection, hemorrhage, mass, or abscess. Seromas may also be considered complex if they have septations and irregular walls.

Sonographic Findings. A cyst that deviates from STAR is considered complex. It may have thick, irregularly shaped walls or internal echoes or lack through transmission (Fig. 27-7).

Oil Cyst

Oil cysts are the liquefaction of injured fat, usually from trauma or surgery. Clinically, when palpable, they present as smooth masses. Galactoceles resolve to oil cysts because of their fatty milk properties.[10,11]

Sonographic Findings. Oil cysts are usually anechoic but can have hyperechoic internal echoes. They appear as round or oval and well-marginated masses (Fig. 27-8).

Galactocele

During pregnancy or lactation, a milky cyst may form from an obstruction of the lactiferous ducts. Galactoceles

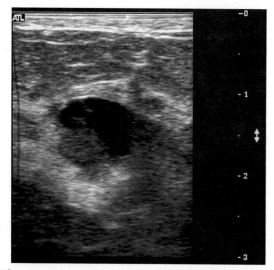

Fig. 27-7 Complex cyst in 48-year-old woman.

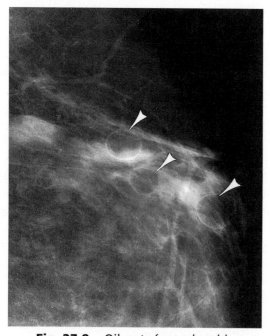

Fig. 27-8 Oil cysts *(arrowheads)*.

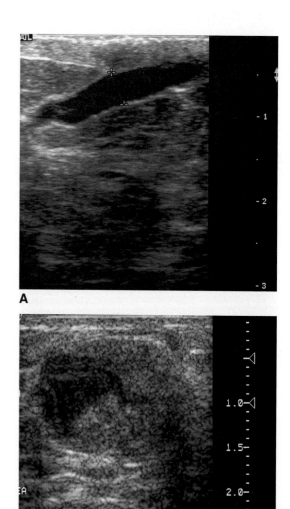

A

B

Fig. 27-9 **A,** Dilated lactiferous ducts. **B,** Galactocele in postpartum woman.

are considered rare, but when galactoceles are present, patients usually have periareolar palpable masses.[1,2,5] As expected, ductal ectasia may be present (Fig. 27-9, *A*). Abnormalities associated with galactoceles are mastitis and abscess.

Sonographic Findings. Galactoceles appear as well-marginated, round or oval masses. They typically contain echoes from fatty, milky material and can demonstrate fat-fluid levels. They resolve to an oil cyst because of their composition and usually change from a complex cyst to one with a more anechoic appearance. Limited

through transmission may be visualized. Doppler evaluation should be negative for internal blood flow (Fig. 27-9, *B*).[7]

Sebaceous Cyst

A sebaceous cyst is a retention cyst that occurs from the blockage of a sebaceous gland in the skin.[3,7,10] Sebaceous cysts can become infected, containing thick, white material on drainage. Patients usually have a small, superficial, smooth, mobile, palpable mass.

Sonographic Findings. A sebaceous cyst is a well-marginated mass that arises from the skin. The appearance may be variable from anechoic to echogenic with through transmission (Fig. 27-10).

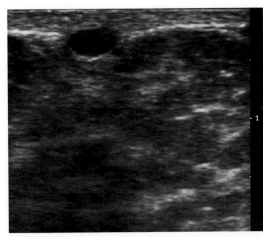

Fig. 27-10 Palpable area in 57-year-old woman that has been present for several years representing sebaceous or inclusion cyst.

BENIGN NEOPLASMS

When benign lesions are palpable clinically, they are usually discrete, mobile, and somewhat compressible masses. Several types of benign neoplasms that can occur in the breast are described.

Sonographic Findings

The general sonographic characteristics of benign breast lesions are smooth or macrolobulated masses with well-marginated borders. They are homogeneous, oval, and more wide than tall. They do not attenuate the ultrasound beam and thus have no posterior shadowing. They can, however, demonstrate through transmission. Benign neoplasms displace rather than infiltrate surrounding tissue. Doppler evaluation either is negative or shows some peripheral flow.

Fibroadenoma

Fibroadenoma is the most common benign mass in premenopausal women and is more common in black women. About 50% of all breast biopsies result in a fibroadenoma tissue diagnosis.[1,5,7,8,11] Fibroadenomas are estrogen stimulated and are frequently identified in women of reproductive age, usually between the ages of 15 and 35 years, with a mean age of 30 years.[8] Because they are hormonally stimulated, they can grow rapidly in pregnant women. Rarely are new fibroadenomas found in postmenopausal women with or without HRT. These masses, as with any new solid mass in a postmenopausal woman, should be considered highly suspicious for cancer, and tissue diagnosis is essential.

Fibroadenomas are composed of the normal tissues of the breast just in an abnormal formation; thus, they can have carcinoma within them. But the risk of cancer within a fibroadenoma is no greater than that of other breast tissue.[7]

Clinically, when palpable, the patient usually has a firm, rubbery, mobile mass. Fibroadenomas are more frequently found in the upper outer breast quadrants.[8] Bilateral masses are found in 9.9% of cases, and multiple masses are found in 10% to 16% of cases. If small and proven to be a fibroadenoma via core biopsy, they may be left within the breast and followed with serial sonograms. When fibroadenomas are large, surgical removal is usually recommended. Fibroadenoma variants consist of giant fibroadenomas and juvenile fibroadenomas. There is no standard measurement a fibroadenoma must reach before it is considered giant, but the term is usually reserved for those measuring 6 to 8 cm or greater.[7]

Juvenile fibroadenomas are found in adolescents and can have extremely rapid growth, to the point of deforming the breast and causing nipple displacement.[10] They may be multiple and bilateral. Sonographically, they are indistinct from other fibroadenomas. When large, these masses can concurrently be called juvenile and giant.[7]

Sonographic Findings. Fibroadenomas are smooth or macrolobulated masses that are more wide than tall. Usually they measure less than 3 cm.[2] These lesions displace rather than infiltrate surrounding tissue, making them well-marginated masses. They are typically homogeneous with low-level internal echoes but can show areas of cystic necrosis if they outgrow their blood supply. Through transmission may or may not be seen (Fig. 27-11, *A* and *B*). Peripheral vascularity may be visualized with Doppler. "Popcorn" calcifications can form, and sonographically these masses may completely attenuate the ultrasound beam, producing significant posterior shadowing.[7] An ultrasound examination may not be of assistance in these cases (Fig. 27-11, *C*).

Cystosarcoma Phylloides

Cystosarcoma phylloides are also called *phylloides tumors, proliferative fibroadenomas,* or *periductal stromal tumors.* The peak age for cystosarcoma phylloides is 30 to 40 years, roughly 10 years after the peak age for fibroadenomas. Cystosarcoma phylloides are rare but when seen are usually unilateral.[1,5,11] Approximately 10% of cystosarcoma phylloides are malignant and have the potential for metastases, usually to the lung. Malignant

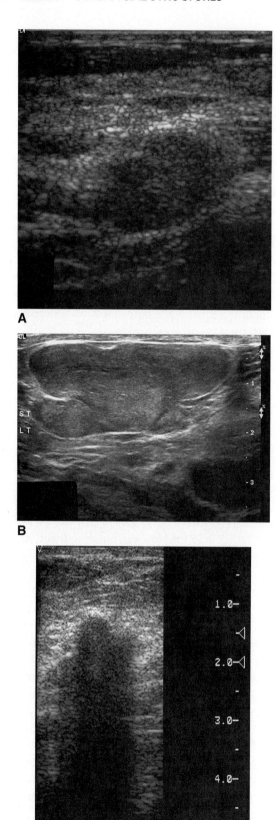

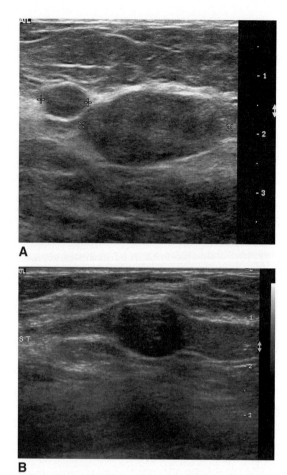

Fig. 27-12 A to D, Variable appearances of benign cystosarcoma phylloides are seen in images.

phylloides tumors tend to grow faster and larger than benign phylloides tumors. Unfortunately, ultrasound cannot differentiate between benign phylloides tumors, malignant phylloides tumors, or fibroadenomas.[1]

Sonographic Findings. The sonographic appearance is similar to that of fibroadenoma. Cystosarcoma phylloides show rapid growth on serial imaging examinations. They often contain cystic spaces from hemorrhage, necrosis, and mucinous fluid. Calcifications are atypical (Fig. 27-12).

Intraductal Papilloma

An intraductal papilloma is a proliferation of epithelial tissue within a duct or cyst that produces a mural nodule. Tumors are typically small and **retroareolar**. They are often undetectable but sometimes palpable. Intraductal papilloma is the most common cause of unilateral, spontaneous, bloody nipple discharge. This discharge can also be clear, serous, white, or dark green.[12] Patients are typically late in reproductive age or postmenopausal, between the ages of 30 and 55 years.[2,5,11]

Fig. 27-11 A, 1.5-cm palpable mass in 46-year-old woman with tissue diagnosis of fibroadenomas. B, 4.2-cm palpable mass in 51-year-old woman representing fibroadenoma. C, Calcified fibroadenoma in 75-year-old woman.

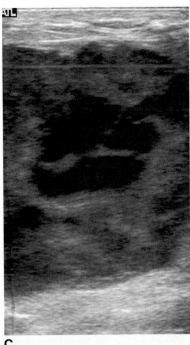

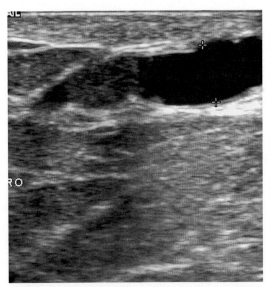

Fig. 27-13 Intraductal papilloma surgically removed from 32-year-old woman.

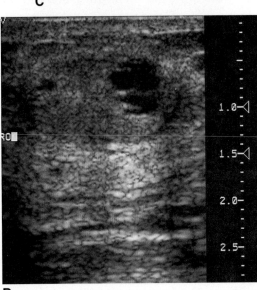

C

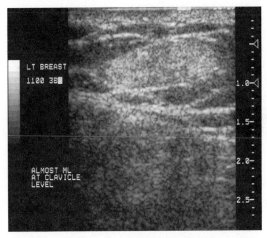

D

Fig. 27-12, cont'd.

Sonographic Findings. Unless some ductal ectasia is seen, intraductal papilloma is difficult to show and may result in a negative sonogram. Radial scanning to elongate ducts is essential. When visible, intraductal papilloma demonstrates a solid mass or solid tissue mural nodule within a duct or cyst. The nodule may be round, oval, or tubular following the contour of the duct or cyst (see also papillary carcinoma; Fig. 27-13).

Lipoma

Lipomas are not specific to the breast. Patients with lipomas are usually middle aged and older. Clinically,

Fig. 27-14 Lipoma. Incidental finding in 47-year-old woman.

the patient is either asymptomatic or has a soft, mobile, compressible, palpable mass. Lipomas are unilateral 97% of the time and are often incidental findings.[3,10]

Sonographic Findings. Lipomas can be hypoechoic or hyperechoic, but usually they are isoechoic to surrounding tissue.[3,10] They are discrete, and palpation during scanning may be necessary to locate these masses (Fig. 27-14). Calcifications may be present.[1,5,11]

BREAST CANCER

Breast cancer is not one disease. The several types of breast cancers have somewhat differing sonographic and clinical findings. Differing types of breast cancers can occur concurrently.

Clinically, most patients with breast cancer are either asymptomatic or have a hard, immobile mass. Pain is a rare indicator of breast cancer. In one study, only 7% of the women had pain as the only symptom.[13] More advanced malignant diseases with lymphatic and neurologic invasion are more painful. Patients may also have skin changes, such as discoloration, usually red[3]; edema with skin thickening; **peau d'orange** (Fig. 27-15); or inversion of the nipple. Nipple discharge is a common symptom but is rarely associated with breast cancer because it is found in only 3% to 11% of cases. The nipple discharge contains blood 70% to 85% of the time when concurrent with breast carcinoma. The chance of breast carcinoma with nipple discharge increases as the age of the patient increases.[13] Other skin changes include asymmetry and contour change, bulging, dimpling, or retraction.

Breast cancers metastasize to the lymph node, liver, lung, bone, and brain.

Sonographic Findings

Generally, malignant breast masses are hypoechoic and inhomogeneous. They often attenuate the ultrasound beam and cause posterior shadowing. Breast cancer usually infiltrates tissue rather than displacing it and has a tall rather than wide formation. These masses are generally speculated, and borders can be poorly marginated or microlobulated. In addition, microcalcifications may be present and may or may not be detectable with ultrasound. Neovascularity is necessary for a cancer to grow larger than a few millimeters.[14] Doppler evaluation typically shows an increase in blood flow in malignant masses.

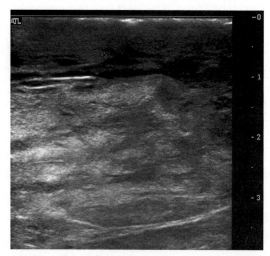

Fig. 27-15 Skin thickening seen on patient with invasive breast carcinoma.

Invasive Ductal Carcinoma

Invasive ductal carcinoma has many types of malignant diseases and comprises 70% to 80% of all breast cancers.[1] The peak age for this cancer is 50 years. With symptomatic disease, patients usually have a palpable mass. Focal breast tenderness and nipple discharge are possible symptoms. Depending on how advanced the lesion is, skin changes may also be noted.[10] Invasive ductal carcinoma originates in the lactiferous ducts of the breast.

Sonographic Findings. Invasive ductal carcinoma presents as a hypoechoic, spiculated mass with fingerlike extensions into dilated ducts. Sharp angulations may be identified with posterior shadowing and a tall rather than wide formation (Fig. 27-16, A to F).[10]

Invasive Lobular Carcinoma

Invasive lobular carcinoma comprises 8% to 15% of all breast cancers.[1] The peak age range is 55 to 70 years. It is credited with only 2% of breast cancers in women 35 years or younger[10] and with 11% of breast cancers in women over 75 years. Invasive lobular carcinoma is bilateral in 6% to 28% of cases and is often multicentric. Clinically, palpation of a discrete mass is rare with invasive lobular carcinoma because it is typically diffusely infiltrating. Patients may have an area of breast thickening and focal breast tenderness. The survival rate with early discovery is better than that with invasive ductal carcinoma.[7]

Microcalcifications are uncommon, and mammography has difficulty in showing these masses, resulting in a higher incidence rate of false-negative reports than with other invasive cancers. Even in retrospect, the mammogram can still look negative, which can explain why these masses are sometimes large when they are finally detected and already have lymph node involvement. There is often more underestimation than overestimation in size of these masses.[15-17]

Sonographic Findings. These masses are often spiculated, infiltrating, and rarely discrete, and demonstration of borders may be difficult. There may be hypoechoic areas with significant posterior shadowing,[7] but there may also be an area that simply appears distorted (Fig. 27-17, A to D).

Colloid Carcinoma

Colloid carcinoma is also known as *mucinous,* or *gelatinous, carcinoma* and comprises 2% of breast cancer. This disease is more prevalent in older women of ages 60 to 70 years. However, 1% of these cancers are found in women younger than 35 years and 7% occur in

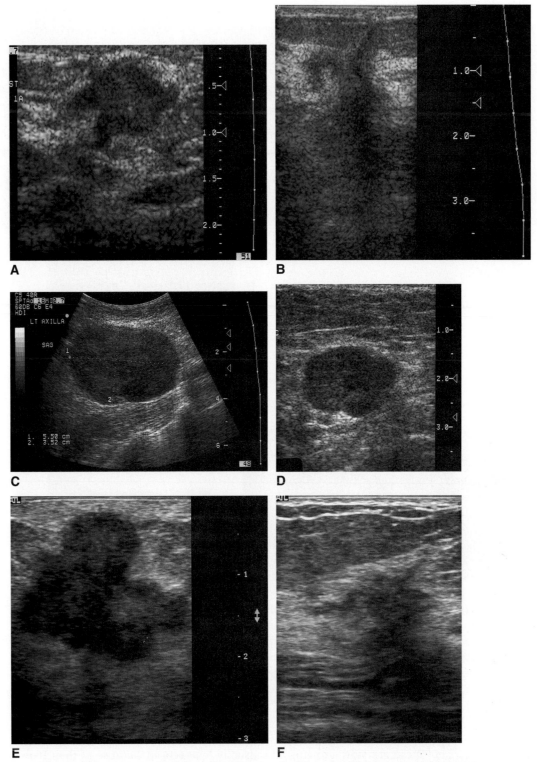

Fig. 27-16 **A,** Invasive ductal carcinoma in 54-year-old woman with metastases to two of four lymph nodes. **B,** Invasive ductal carcinoma in 44-year-old woman with no evidence of metastasis. **C,** Invasive ductal carcinoma in 75-year-old woman who is nonsurgical candidate. Mass measures 5.5 cm. **D,** Same patient as in Fig. 27-16, C, 12 months after chemotherapy. Mass now measures 2.3 cm. **E,** Invasive ductal carcinoma in 50-year-old woman with metastasis to one of seven lymph nodes. **F,** Invasive ductal and lobular carcinoma within same lesion.

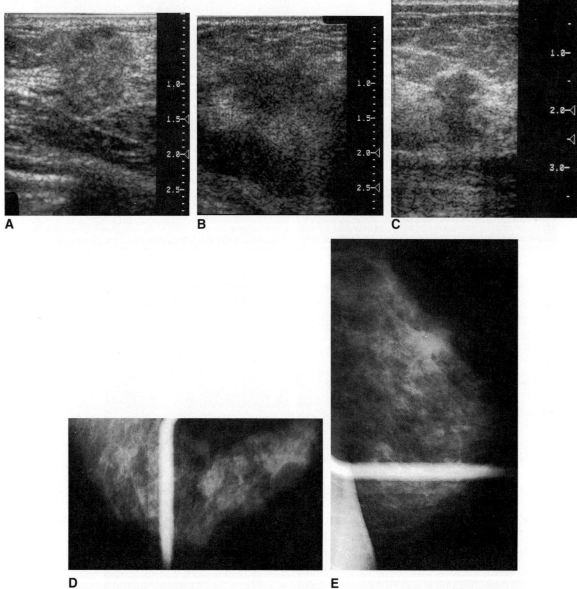

Fig. 27-17 **A,** Palpable mass that is pathologically proven to be invasive lobular carcinoma. **B,** Palpable masses bilaterally. Invasive lobular carcinoma was diagnosed in left breast, invasive ductal carcinoma in right. **C,** Invasive lobular carcinoma in 52-year-old woman; sonographically, mass measured 1.3 cm. Pathology documented lesion to be 4.5 cm. Mammograms of same patient in Fig. 27-17, *C,* document lesion in, **D,** craniocaudal and, **E,** mediolateral oblique views.

women older than 75 years. These are slow growing lesions with a fairly good prognosis.[1,5,7,10] Clinically, when palpable, these masses present as soft and discrete. This lesion does not typically produce skin or nipple changes.

   Sonographic Findings. These masses can appear somewhat benign. They may look well circumscribed, microlobulated, round or oval, and smooth. They are

usually hypoechoic. Because of their high cellular fluid content, sonographically they may show through transmission (Fig. 27-18).

Medullary Carcinoma

Medullary carcinoma accounts for 4% to 9% of all breast cancers. The peak age group is premenopausal. Medullary carcinoma represents 11% of breast cancers

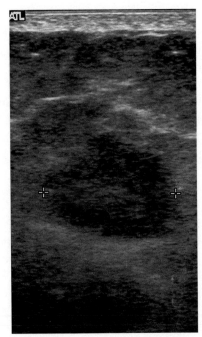

Fig. 27-18 Colloid carcinoma in 66-year-old woman with no metastasis.

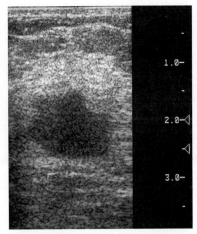

Fig. 27-19 Medullary carcinoma surgically removed from 39-year-old woman.

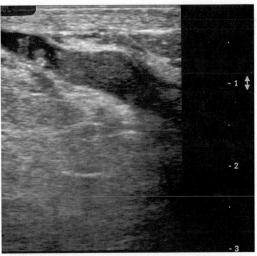

Fig. 27-20 Mural nodule seen within cyst pathologically proven to be papillary carcinoma.

in women younger than 35 years of age.[1,5,10] Although these are fast-growing cancers, the prognosis is good. Clinically, these present as discrete, mobile masses.

Sonographic Findings. These masses are usually hypoechoic, round, and well-marginated and appear misleadingly like fibroadenomas. Necrosis can produce a cystic component to this mass. Calcifications are atypical (Fig. 27-19).

Papillary Carcinoma

Papillary carcinoma represents 1% to 2% of breast cancers. It is more prevalent in older women, with the peak age of 63 to 67 years. These are slow-growing malignant diseases.[1,5,10] Clinically, patients have nipple discharge in 22% to 34% of cases. This discharge is typically bloody. When these masses are palpable, 90% are in the retroareolar area. Nipple and skin changes may be noted.

Sonographic Findings. Sonographically, these masses are as challenging to find as is their benign counterpart, intraductal papilloma, and they often cannot be differentiated from a papilloma. These are intraductal mural tissue masses. Microcalcifications may be present (Fig. 27-20).

METASTASES
Metastases to the Breast

Metastatic disease to the breast occurs in approximately 0.5% to 6.6% of cases and is considered uncommon.[18]

Diagnosis of the primary lesion is essential because treatment for metastatic breast cancer can be quite different from primary breast cancer. Mastectomy is not normally necessary.

Clinically, these are singular or multiple, round, palpable breast masses. They are hard but mobile and grow rapidly. They occur bilaterally in 8% to 25% of cases, with lymphadenopathy in 25% to 58% of cases.[18] Mammographically, these lesions are nonspiculated and discrete with slightly irregular margins. Usually there are no microcalcifications.

Primary cancers that metastasize to the breast are non-Hodgkin's lymphoma, melanoma, lung, ovarian, cervical, prostate, and bladder.[5]

Sonographic Findings. Sonographically, metastatic breast disease appears as a discrete solid breast mass. It

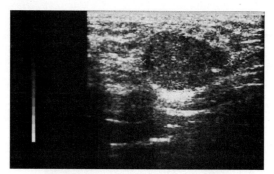

Fig. 27-21 Metastases to breast.

does not typically infiltrate surrounding tissue and can appear relatively indistinguishable from some well-marginated primary breast cancers (Fig. 27-21).[18]

AUGMENTATION

Approximately 2 million women in the United States have undergone breast augmentation for either cosmetic or reconstructive reasons.[19] In the augmented breast, the imaging role of ultrasound includes surveying for breast tissue abnormalities and implant integrity. The tissue abnormalities may or may not be implant related.

The most successful methods in identification of implant rupture are magnetic resonance imaging (MRI) and ultrasound. Because of the expense of MRI, the patient typically has an ultrasound first, and if the examination is unequivocal, they proceed to MRI. MRI is also the best way to evaluate the area around the chest wall.[19] Mammographically, implants can still obscure a reported 35% to 40% of breast tissue, even with the use of the **Eklund maneuver**.[11] Nevertheless, mammography is still important for these patients to assess the breast tissue for abnormalities, unless all breast tissue was removed before reconstruction.

Currently, in the United States, augmentation prostheses are placed in either the subglandular or the subpectoral position. Some countries inject silicone directly into the tissue, resulting in a difficult and confusing ultrasound because of **granuloma** formation (Fig. 27-22, A).[19]

Complications of implants in addition to rupture include hematoma, abscess, implant displacement, and autoimmune disease.

Clinically, a patient with suspected implant rupture has a palpable mass, pain or burning, a contour change, increase or decrease of breast fullness, or a compromised autoimmune system.[2]

Sonographic Findings

There are several types of implants with varying sonographic findings. The following is a description of double-lumen silicone implants.

Sonographically, implants should be anechoic internally with three echogenic rings surrounding the implant. From inner to outer, these rings are: the inner surface of the implant shell, the outer surface of the implant shell, and the body's reactive fibrous capsule (Fig. 27-22, B and C).

The sonographic signs for implant rupture are the **stepladder sign** and the **snowstorm sign**. The stepladder sign is parallel echogenic lines within the interior of the implant and indicates an **intracapsular rupture**. The stepladder sign correlates with the linguine sign on MRI. The snowstorm sign is described as echogenic noise with dirty shadowing similar to the appearance of bowel gas.[2,5] These sonographic signs may be noted concurrently (Fig. 27-22, D).

INFLAMMATION
Mastitis

Mastitis is inflammation of the breast. Mastitis can happen at any age, but most cases occur during lactation, usually in the second or third postpartum week,[20] and are usually caused by a bacterial infection.[2,7] Mastitis can begin with a crack on the nipple or a skin wound[2] and may lead to abscess formation.[10] It may also be caused by a foreign body, parasite, or disease or be the result of an infected cyst.[2] Clinically, patients have warm, red, swollen, and tender breasts. They may be febrile. There may be associated purulent discharge or a clogged lactiferous duct.[2] Compression during mammography may be difficult because of the patient's skin edema and pain.[7] Antibiotics may resolve mastitis.

One percent of breast cancers are inflammatory carcinoma, which can have a similar patient presentation as mastitis. Differentiation between these two conditions is essential.

Sonographic Findings. The ultrasound evaluation of mastitis may be normal or may reveal diffuse edema with an increase in tissue echogenicity. Skin thickening measuring greater than 2 mm[5] and **inspissated** material within dilated ducts can sometimes be seen.[2] Visualization of reactive lymph nodes is possible (Fig. 27-23, A to D).

Abscess

An abscess is a localized area of pus and can form anywhere in the body. Within the breast, it is usually found

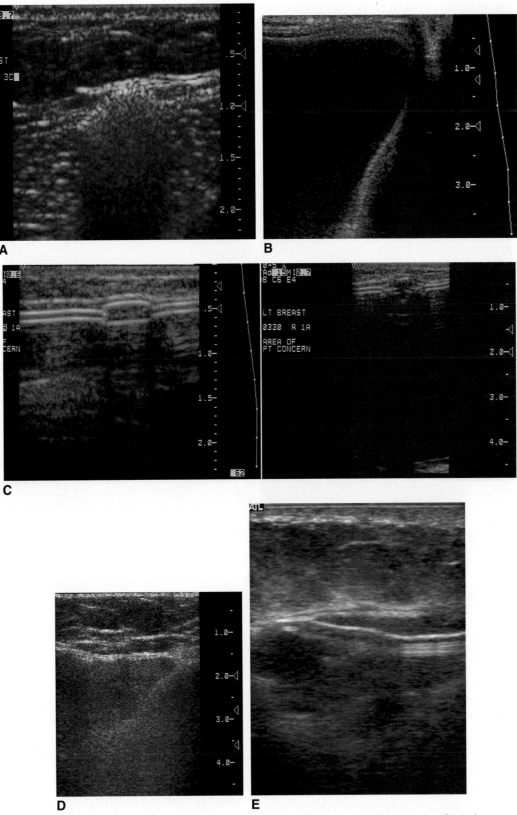

Fig. 27-22 **A,** Palpable granuloma in 58-year-old woman with history of implant rupture and removal. **B,** Normal-looking breast implant. **C,** Palpable area in 26-year-old woman with breast implants proved to be normal valve on implant. Implants with both, **D,** snowstorm sign and, **E,** stepladder sign, indicating implant rupture.

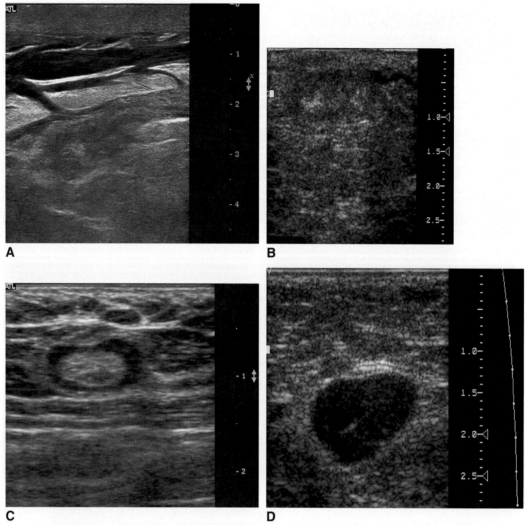

Fig. 27-23 **A,** Woman at 13 days postpartum with signs of mastitis. **B,** Inspissated material seen within duct of 35-year-old nursing woman. Patient was seen with palpable lump and had decreased milk flow from this breast. **C,** Normal appearance of lymph node, reniform in shape with echogenic fatty hilum. **D,** Abnormal-appearing lymph node pathologically proven to be benign reactive process.

retroareolar.[2] Abscesses form in a small percentage of patients from mastitis,[11] usually in lactating or weaning women.[5,20] It can also be a byproduct of an infected cyst. Clinically, the patient usually has a palpable lump and tender, enlarged lymph nodes, in addition to symptoms of mastitis.[5] Drainage or surgical removal may be necessary.[2]

Sonographic Findings. An abscess is usually a complex mass with irregular thick walls. Debris levels and septations are common.[2,5] Edema, skin thickening, and reactive lymph nodes are also common findings (see Figs. 27-15 and 27-23, *C* and *D*). As the abscess ages, the walls become more discrete (Fig. 27-24).[5]

HEMATOMA

Breast hematomas typically form after an accidental or surgical trauma. Clinically, these patients often have a painful palpable mass. Depending on the age of the hematoma, skin bruising and edema may also be noted.[5] A seroma is similar to a hematoma only if it contains serous fluid. The term *seroma* is usually used for a postsurgical fluid cavity.

Sonographic Findings

Depending on the age and amount of blood within the fluid, a hematoma may appear as an anechoic and well-marginated mass or as complex with thick walls and

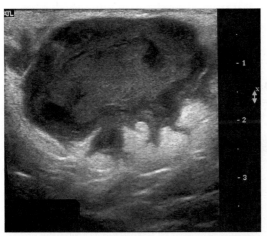

Fig. 27-24   Palpable abscess in woman at 39 weeks' gestation.

layering debris.[5,6] Hematomas can decrease in size with age. Sonographically, they may regress and show no abnormality or they may become a scar with some tissue distortion.[7] Associated edema can look like a general area of increased echogenicity. Sonographically, a hematoma and a seroma may be indistinguishable (Fig. 27-25, *A* to *D*).

MALE BREAST DISEASES
Gynecomastia

All breast anomalies found in the female breast can also be found in the male breast with reduced incidence.[1,10] The most common male breast anomaly is **gyneco-mastia**, which is enlargement from benign ductal and stromal proliferation.[7] It typically occurs at three age periods: transiently at birth; again at puberty, declining in the late teens; and at adulthood, between 50 and 80 years old.[20] Gynecomastia may be idiopathic but has been associated with estrogen excess, androgen deficiency, increased age, **Klinefelter's syndrome,** testicular failure, renal failure, cirrhosis, AIDS, and certain drugs, including marijuana, digitalis, heroin, and steroids.[10] Gynecomastia can regress on its own, but treatment depends on the cause.[20] Clinically, it will present as unilateral or bilateral breast enlargement with a tender or nontender retroareolar mass.

Sonographic Findings. Gynecomastia will present sonographically as normal-appearing fibroglandular breast tissue with a triangular-shaped pattern.[2] Occasionally the ducts may also be appreciated (Fig. 27-26, *A* to *E*).

Male Breast Cancer

Male breast cancer is rare, representing 0.5% to 1% of all breast cancers.[2,10] It usually occurs later than in women, with a mean age of 59 years. The most common form, representing 85% of occurrences, is invasive ductal carcinoma.[7] Male breast cancer has been associated with Klinefelter's syndrome, family history, testicular injury, **cryptorchidism,** and advancing age.[2] Clinically, breast cancer is usually palpated in the retroareolar region and will feel similar to breast cancers in women. Bloody nipple discharge is seen in 14% of men with breast cancer and is a stronger indicator of breast carcinoma in males than in that of females.[2,7]

Sonographic Findings. Sonographically, male breast cancers will look the same as female breast cancers (Fig. 27-27, *A* and *B*).

SUMMARY

Ultrasonography is an essential diagnostic tool used to better define the characteristics of a mass by quantifying its size, shape, and location. Ultrasonography is dynamic, making it uniquely qualified for invasive procedures and examinations involving the breast. Further, patient comfort is not usually compromised in the process. Performance of an ultrasound can help reduce the number of unwarranted surgeries. Tables 27-1 to 27-3 are summaries of the pathologies of the breast.

CLINICAL SCENARIO—DIAGNOSIS

■ The patient was sent to a breast surgeon and was diagnosed with bilateral juvenile fibroadenomas. The fibroadenomas in this case are sonographically atypical. Fibroadenomas are usually discrete masses. The patient underwent bilateral breast reductions.

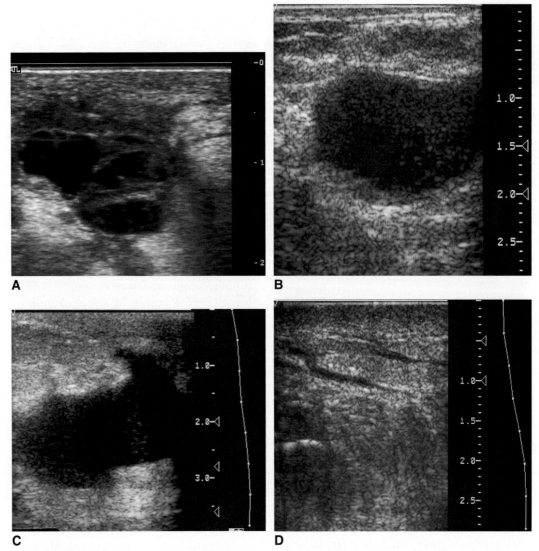

Fig. 27-25 Hematoma/seroma. **A,** Hematoma/seroma in 2-week postlumpectomy sight. **B,** Decreasing hematoma on serial sonograms in patient with history of automobile accident. **C,** Five-year-old seroma in patient with history of lumpectomy and radiation therapy. **D,** Edema in patient 8 days after needle core biopsy.

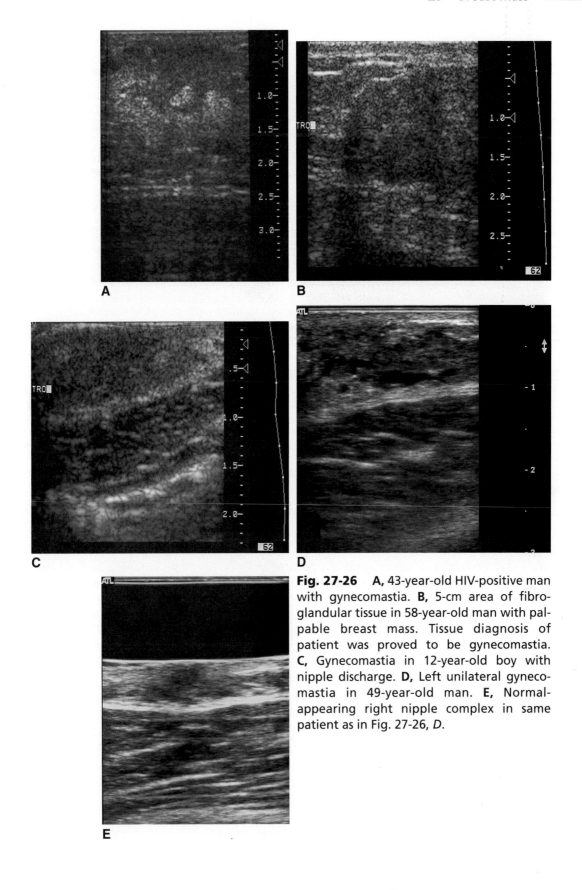

Fig. 27-26 **A,** 43-year-old HIV-positive man with gynecomastia. **B,** 5-cm area of fibroglandular tissue in 58-year-old man with palpable breast mass. Tissue diagnosis of patient was proved to be gynecomastia. **C,** Gynecomastia in 12-year-old boy with nipple discharge. **D,** Left unilateral gynecomastia in 49-year-old man. **E,** Normal-appearing right nipple complex in same patient as in Fig. 27-26, *D.*

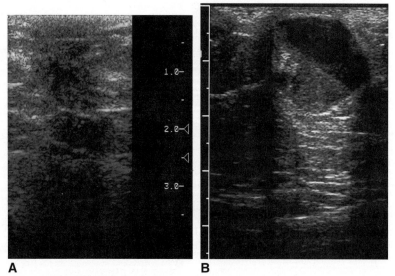

A   **B**

Fig. 27-27 **A,** Invasive ductal breast cancer in man with palpable abnormality. **B,** Papillary carcinoma in 55-year-old man.

Table 27-1	*Cysts of Breast*	
Pathology	**Symptoms**	**Sonographic Findings**
Simple cyst	Asymptomatic, tender, palpable mass	Round or oval, anechoic, thin-walled, through transmission
Complex cyst	Asymptomatic, tender, palpable mass	Irregular or thick-walled, hypoechoic, may lack through transmission
Oil cyst	Usually result of surgical or accidental trauma; smooth, palpable mass; asymptomatic	Usually anechoic, may have hyperechoic internal echoes
Galactocele	Pregnancy or lactating; usually periareolar; palpable mass; associated with mastitis and abscess	Anechoic, complex, fat-fluid level, may have through transmission
Sebaceous cyst	Smooth, superficial, palpable mass	Anechoic to echogenic, through transmission

Table 27-2	*Benign Neoplasms of Breast*	
Pathology	**Symptoms**	**Sonographic Findings**
Fibroadenoma	Firm, rubbery, mobile mass; asymptomatic	Smooth, macrolobulated, usually homogeneous, hypoechoic, wide rather than tall
Cystosarcoma phylloides	Palpable, firm, mobile, rapidly enlarging mass	Similar to fibroadenoma, often contains cystic spaces
Papilloma	Nipple discharge; retroareolar when palpable; asymptomatic	Small solid mass within cyst or dilated duct
Lipoma	Soft, mobile, compressible mass; asymptomatic	Usually isoechoic

Table 27-3	Carcinoma of Breast	
Pathology	Symptoms	Sonographic Findings
Invasive ductal carcinoma	Hard, fixed, palpable mass; skin changes; asymptomatic	Hypoechoic, spiculated mass, posterior shadowing, tall rather than wide
Invasive lobular carcinoma	Breast thickening; usually not palpable; asymptomatic	Areas of distortion with heavy posterior shadowing, indiscrete borders
Colloid or mucinous carcinoma	Soft mass; skin changes are atypical; asymptomatic	Hypoechoic, microlobulated, well-defined mass, may have through transmission
Medullary carcinoma	Discrete, mobile, rapidly enlarging mass	Hypoechoic round mass
Papillary carcinoma	Nipple discharge; retroareolar; palpable mass; asymptomatic	Cystic or intraductal solid mass
Metastatic carcinoma	Hard, round, mobile, rapidly enlarging mass or masses	Hypoechoic discrete mass or masses
Inflammatory carcinoma	Mastitis	Diffuse increase in tissue echogenicity, skin thickening

CASE STUDIES FOR DISCUSSION

1. A 25-year-old woman with a history of nipple piercing is seen for a diagnostic mammogram and breast sonogram. She has periareolar pain with intermittent focal skin eruption and drainage for the past 12 months. The nipple ring has been removed for some time. She had been on seven different antibiotics with no change in the lesion. Clinically, the skin appears intact. Ultrasound examination reveals a 1-cm hypoechoic area 0.5 cm below the skin with a tract running to the skin surface (Fig. 27-28, A and B). What is the most likely diagnosis?

2. A 34-year-old woman 38 days postpartum is seen for a breast sonogram with a palpable mass for 5 weeks. She is still breast-feeding her baby. The ultrasound revels a 2-cm oval complex mass (Fig. 27-29). What is the most likely diagnosis?

3. A 52-year-old woman is seen for a diagnostic mammogram and sonogram of a palpable breast lump. A sonogram 2 years previously showed a palpable cyst in the area. One year previously, the patient had a non–ultrasound-guided breast biopsy of this palpable nodule that was negative for

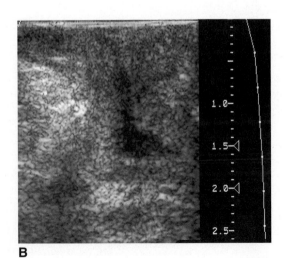

A   **B**

Fig. 27-28 **A,** Initial sonogram shows hypoechoic region. **B,** At 2.5 weeks later.

CASE STUDIES FOR DISCUSSION—cont'd

malignancy. The current mammogram notes a possible distortion in this region. Sonographically, the palpable area corresponds to a small cyst located within an area of dense fibroglandular tissue. Adjacent to this area is an $8 \times 5 \times 6$-mm hypoechoic irregularly shaped mass with angular margins (Fig. 27-30). What is the most likely diagnosis?

4. A 52-year-old woman is seen for a diagnostic mammogram and sonogram to rule out breast mass. She has a history of numerous bilateral benign breast biopsies. She has a 5-cm circular brown skin discoloration medial and including the right areola. According to the patient, it has been present for more than 6 months and was initially red. Her physician sent her to a dermatologist, and she was told that the area was a result of her hormone levels. Two masses are shown better sonographically than mammographically. One lesion is at 12:00 and measures 3 cm. It has irregular margins with posterior shadowing and is hypoechoic to the surrounding tissue (Fig. 27-31, *A*). The other lesion is at 8:00 and measures 1 cm. It is also hypoechoic with posterior shadowing (Fig. 27-31, *B*). What is the most likely diagnosis?

5. A 43-year-old man is seen for a diagnostic mammogram and sonogram for breast hypertrophy. The patient is on antidepressant medications. Clinically, a small lump is felt under the left nipple. According to the patient, this mass has been present and unchanged for about 10 years. Sonographically, there is a 1.4-cm hypoechoic poorly marginated mass with posterior shadowing (Fig. 27-32). What is the most likely diagnosis?

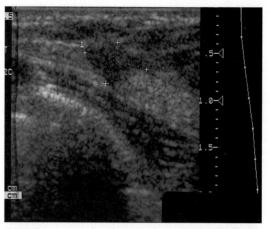

Fig. 27-30   Irregular, hypoechoic lesion is shown.

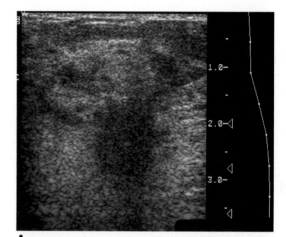

A

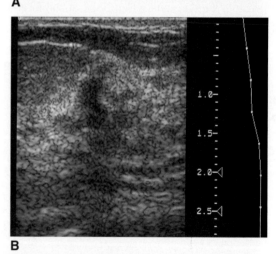

B

Fig. 27-31   **A,** 12:00 lesion measures 3 cm and appears irregular and hypoechoic with posterior shadowing. **B,** 08:00 lesion measures 1 cm and is also hypoechoic with posterior shadowing.

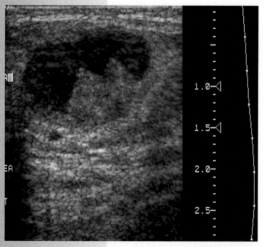

Fig. 27-29   Oval, complex mass is identified in image.

CASE STUDIES FOR DISCUSSION—cont'd

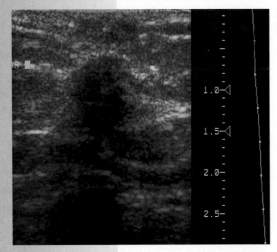

Fig. 27-32   Poorly marginated mass with posterior shadowing is shown.

STUDY QUESTIONS

1. An oval structure that shadows is identified posterior to the mammary and muscle tissues. What does it most likely represent?
   a. cyst
   b. fibroadenoma
   c. abscess
   d. breast cancer
   e. rib

2. A 30-year-old woman who recently started taking contraceptives has a palpable breast mass that is firm and mobile and rapidly increasing in size. The sonogram shows a hypoechoic, macrolobulated mass without posterior attenuation. Doppler shows peripheral blood flow. This most likely represents which of the following?
   a. cyst
   b. fibroadenoma
   c. abscess
   d. breast cancer
   e. rib

3. Primary cancers that metastasize to the breast include:
   a. brain
   b. prostate
   c. liver
   d. kidney
   e. bone

4. A 50-year-old man with a history of immuno-suppressant drug therapy for HIV has a tender palpable breast mass. Sonographic findings include retroareolar fibroglandular tissue. What is the likely diagnosis?
   a. metastatic disease
   b. lymphadenopathy
   c. gynecomastia
   d. breast cancer
   e. cyst

5. Which of the following structures that may be identified during a breast sonogram is the least echogenic?
   a. calcification
   b. Cooper's ligaments
   c. glandular tissue
   d. ribs
   e. subcutaneous fat

6. A 75-year-old woman is seen with unilateral bloody nipple discharge and a palpable retroareolar mass. Her nipple is inverted and has been for the last few years. Sonographically, there is an enlarged duct containing a mural nodule. What do these findings suggest?
   a. intraductal papilloma
   b. colloid carcinoma
   c. invasive lobular carcinoma
   d. papillary carcinoma
   e. medullary carcinoma

7. A spiculated heterogeneous mass with posterior attenuation and positive internal Doppler flow is seen in a woman of any age. What is the most likely diagnosis?

  a. invasive ductal carcinoma

  b. invasive lobular carcinoma

  c. lipoma

  d. hematoma

  e. cyst

8. A woman is seen for a breast ultrasound for evaluation of an area that is discrete and hard within her breast. She has a history of a lumpectomy 6 months previously. The sonographic evaluation reveals a smooth-walled anechoic area containing septae. What is the most likely diagnosis?

  a. breast cancer

  b. seroma

  c. lymph node

  d. papilloma

  e. metastases

9. A women with a history of breast implant removal for rupture has an abnormal mammogram. On the breast sonogram, a discrete hypoechoic area is shown with posterior dirty shadowing. What is the most likely diagnosis?

  a. fibroadenoma

  b. invasive ductal carcinoma

  c. lobular carcinoma

  d. granuloma

  e. lymph node

10. A 3-mm bean-shaped structure is identified within the breast and has an echogenic center and hypoechoic rim. The remainder of the evaluation is unremarkable. What is the likely diagnosis?

  a. lymph node

  b. hematoma

  c. simple cyst

  d. complex cyst

  e. seroma

REFERENCES

1. Sohn C, Blohmer JU, Hamper UM: *Breast ultrasound: a systematic approach to technique and image interpretation,* New York, 1999, Tieme.

2. Carr-Hoefer C, Grube JA: *National certification examination review: breast ultrasound,* Dallas, 2001, Society of Diagnostic Medical Sonography.

3. Andolina VF, Lille SL, Willison KM: *Mammographic imaging: a practical guide,* Philadelphia, 1992, Lippincott Williams & Wilkins.

4. Monda LA: Differentiation of breast calcifications, *Radiol Technol* 72:532-554, 2001.

5. Carr-Hoefer C: Breast sonography. In Kawamura DM: *Abdomen and superficial structures,* ed 2, Philadelphia, 1997, Lippincott.

6. Hagen-Ansert SL: *Textbook of diagnostic ultrasonography,* vol 1, ed 5, St Louis, 2001, Mosby.

7. Bassett LW, Jackson VP, Jahan R et al: *Diagnosis of diseases of the breast,* Philadelphia, 1997, WB Saunders.

8. Pruthi S: Detection and evaluation of a palpable breast mass, *Mayo Clinic Proc* 76:641-648, 2001.

9. Rapp C: Sonography of the breast. Official proceedings of the SDMS 17th Annual Conference, Dallas, 2000, 57-67.

10. Cardenosa G: *Breast imaging companion,* Philadelphia, 1997, Lippincott-Raven.

11. Lanfranchi ME: *Breast ultrasound,* Madrid, 2000, Marban.

12. Morrow M: The evaluation of common breast problems, *Am Fam Physician* 61:2371-2378, 2000.

13. Scott S, Morrow M: Breast cancer: making the diagnosis, *Surg Clin North Am* 79:991-1003, 1999.

14. Moon WK, Im JG, Noh DY et al: Nonpalpable breast lesions: evaluation with power Doppler US and a microbubble contrast agent: initial experience, *Radiology* 217:240-245, 2000.

15. Helvie MA, Paramagul C, Oberman HA et al: Invasive lobular carcinoma: imaging features and clinical detection, *Invest Radiol* 28:202-207, 1993.

16. Krecke KN, Gisvold JJ: Invasive lobular carcinoma of the breast: mammographic findings and extent of disease at diagnosis in 184 patients, *Am J Radiol* 161:957-960, 1993.

17. Le Gal M, Ollivier L, Asselain B et al: Mammographic features of 455 invasive lobular carcinomas, *Radiology* 185:705-708, 1992.

18. Yang WT, Kwan WH, Chow LT, et al: Unusual sonographic appearance with color Doppler imaging of bilateral breast metastases I a patient with alveolar rhabdomyosarcoma of an extremity, *J Ultrasound Med* 15:531-533, 1996.

19. Kimbro M: A sound alternative: for imaging the woman with augmented breast, *Advance* 14:36-37, 2001.

20. Thomas CL: *Taber's cyclopedic medical dictionary,* ed 18, Philadelphia, 1997, Davis.

28 Scrotal Mass

KIMBERLY WATTS

CLINICAL SCENARIO

■ A 30-year-old medical student in his first year of residency is seen in the sonography department with swelling in the right scrotum. The patient appears to be in excellent health and has no additional symptoms. Sonographic evaluation of the scrotum identifies a solid, slightly hypoechoic-appearing mass (Fig. 28-1) within the right testicle. Discuss possible causes for the sonographic appearance noted.

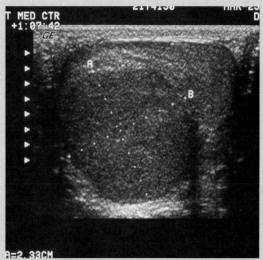

Fig. 28-1 Large fairly homogeneous mass is identified. (Courtesy Cindy Rapp, Radiology Imaging Associates, Greenwood Village, Colorado.)

OBJECTIVES

■ Describe the sonographic appearance of the normal scrotum.
■ Describe the sonographic appearance of benign pathology of the scrotum.
■ Describe the sonographic appearance of the more common malignant pathologies of the scrotum.

■ Identify the clinical symptoms of benign processes in the scrotum.
■ Identify the clinical symptoms of malignant processes in the scrotum.

GLOSSARY OF TERMS ■■■■■

Abscess: a localized collection of pus

Appendix testis: small oval structure located under the head of the epididymis

Chlamydia: microorganisms that cause a wide variety of diseases, including urethritis

Choriocarcinoma: an extremely rare, very malignant neoplasm

Cryptorchidism: testicles that do not descend into the scrotal sac

Epidermoid: pertaining to the epidermis of the skin

Epididymis: a small, oblong body resting on and beside the posterior surface of the testes and consisting of a convoluted tube 13 to 20 feet in length

Epididymitis: inflammation of the epididymis

Epididymoorchitis: inflammation of the epididymis and corresponding testis

Human chorionic gonadotropin: hormone secreted by the placenta

Hematoma: a swelling or mass of blood confined to an organ, tissue, or space

Hematocele: extratesticular hematoma

Hernia: the protrusion of part or all of an organ through the wall that normally contains it

Hydrocele: the accumulation of serous fluid in the tunica vaginalis testis

Incarcerated: imprisoned, confined, restricted

Inguinal canal: the canal carrying the spermatic cord

Lymphoma: growth of new tissue in the lymphatic system

Mediastinum testis: the thickened portion of the tunica albuginea on the posterior surface of the testis

Microlithiasis: calcifications within the seminiferous tubules

Omentum: a double fold of peritoneum

Orchiectomy: surgical excision of the testicle

Orchitis: inflammation of the testis

Scrotum: the double pouch of the male that contains the testicles and part of the spermatic cord

Seminomas: germ cell tumors of the testis

Sperm: the mature male sex or germ cell formed within the seminiferous tubules of the testes

Spermatocele: retention cyst that involves the seminiferous tubules containing sperm

Teratomas: congenital tumors that contain embryonic elements of all three primary germ cell layers

Testicle: male gonad; one of two reproductive organs located in the scrotum

Tunica albuginea: white, fibrous capsule that surrounds the testicle

Tunica vaginalis: serous membrane that surrounds the front and sides of the testicle

Torsion: twisting of the spermatic cord

Varicocele: a group of dilated veins caused by venous return obstruction

Vas deferens: the excretory duct of the testis; transports sperm from each testis to the prostatic urethra

---

Sonography is the imaging method of choice for examination of the **scrotum.** When a scrotal mass is discovered clinically, an ultrasound is usually ordered for identification of the location and sonographic characteristics of the scrotal mass. Not only are neoplasms of the **testicle** easily seen with ultrasound, but other conditions of the scrotum can also be identified, such as fluid collections and infectious processes. Along with clinical findings, sonography can provide valuable information in diagnosis and treatment planning of abnormal conditions of the scrotum.

SCROTUM
Normal Sonographic Appearance

The scrotum is a pouch of skin that extends from the abdomen. Several structures are contained within the scrotum (Fig. 28-2). These structures are the **epididymis,** the proximal portion of the ductus deferens, and the testicles.[1] The epididymis is a tightly coiled tube located posterior and superior to the testicle.[1,2] The three parts to the epididymis are the head, body, and tail.

Sonographic Findings. The normal epididymis has an echogenicity that is the same as or greater than the testicle.[1] The ductus deferens is a continuation of the epididymis and part of the spermatic cord. The testicles are paired structures located within the scrotum. Each testicle is ovoid in shape, homogeneous, and mildly echogenic (Fig. 28-3).[3] Each testicle is approximately $5 \times 3 \times 2$ cm in size.[4] Each testicle is covered by a fibrous tissue termed the *tunica albuginea.*[4] The posterior surface of the tunica albuginea enters the testicular tissue and forms the **mediastinum testis.**[4] The mediastinum testis runs through the testicle in a craniocaudal direction.[2]

This line can be of variable thickness and echogenicity.[2] The **tunica vaginalis** lines the **hydrocele** sac.[5] A small amount of fluid also surrounds each testicle and allows the testicle to move freely within the scrotal sac.[5]

EXTRATESTICULAR MASS

Unlike intratesticular masses, which are almost always malignant, extratesticular masses tend to be benign. An extratesticular lesion is more likely to be the result of inflammation, trauma, or a benign lesion.[6] Extratesticular masses include hydrocele, **varicocele, spermatocele,** scrotal **hernia, abscess, hematoma,** and **epididymitis.**

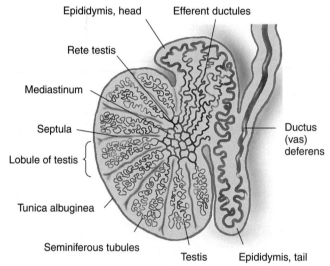

Fig. 28-2 Anatomy of testis and epididymis.

Epididymis, head
Efferent ductules
Rete testis
Mediastinum
Septula
Lobule of testis
Tunica albuginea
Seminiferous tubules
Testis
Epididymis, tail
Ductus (vas) deferens

Sonographic Findings

Extratesticular masses may be anechoic, hypoechoic, hyperechoic, or a combination of echogenicities.

Hydrocele

A hydrocele is an abnormal collection of serous fluid in the potential space between the two layers of the tunica vaginalis.[2] Hydroceles may be unilateral or bilateral and occur in children and adults. Hydroceles are also common in male newborns.[2,3,7,8] Acquired hydroceles can have many causes, including trauma, infection, infarction, **torsion,** and testicular neoplasms.[3,7]

Sonographic Findings. Hydroceles appear as a fluid collection anterolateral to the testis (Fig. 28-4). In chronic hydroceles, echoes may be seen within the fluid surrounded by a thick scrotal wall.[7,8] An acute hydrocele transilluminates light and has a thin scrotal wall.

CYSTS OF THE SCROTUM

Cysts of the scrotum include simple, epididymal, **epidermoid,** tunica albuginea, and intratesticular cysts.

Simple Cysts

Simple cysts of the testicle occur in men 40 years of age or older and are usually an incidental finding because they are not palpable.[9] The size of the simple cysts can range from 2 mm to 2 cm.[9] These cysts are usually found in the upper pole of the testicle.[8]

Sonographic Findings. Simple cysts of the testicle have characteristics that are seen in other simple cysts (Fig. 28-5): smooth walls, anechoic centers, and through

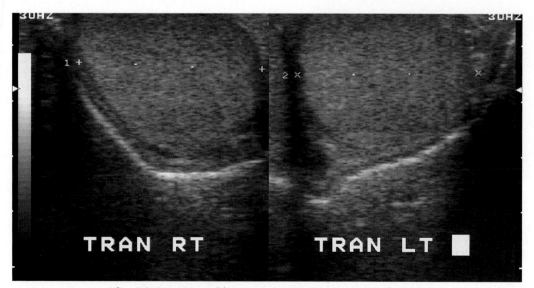

Fig. 28-3 Normal homogeneous appearance of testes.

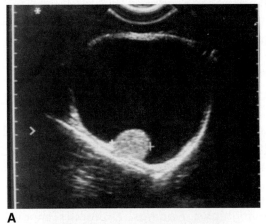

A

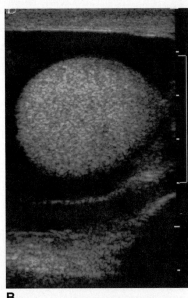

B

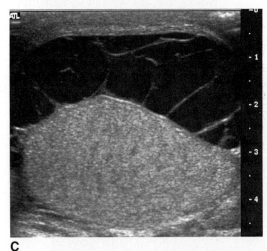

C

Fig. 28-4 **A,** 66-year-old man is seen with enlarged left hemiscrotum. Large hydrocele is shown. **B,** Hydrocele is shown in 43-year-old man. **C,** Complex hydrocele was from infection. (Courtesy Cindy Rapp, Radiology Imaging Associates, Greenwood Village, Colorado.)

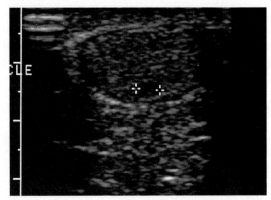

Fig. 28-5 Small simple cyst is noted within testicle.

transmission.[9] The cyst must be located completely within the testicular parenchyma.[10]

Epididymal Cysts

Epididymal cysts are cysts that can occur anywhere in the epididymis.[7] They are uncommon and result from cystic dilation of the epididymal tubules. These cysts contain clear serous fluid.[2]

Sonographic Findings. Epididymal cysts (Fig. 28-6) have the same sonographic characteristics of other cysts. The cyst is located within the epididymis.

Epidermoid Cysts

Epidermoid cysts account for 1% to 2% of testicular neoplasms.[8,11] They are more common in men 20 to 40 years of age[8] and are benign.[11]

Sonographic Findings. An epidermoid cyst (Fig. 28-7) presents as a well-defined, round or oval mass with echogenic walls within the testis.[7,10] The cysts may contain calcifications,[7,8] and acoustic enhancement may not be present.[12]

Tunica Albuginea Cysts

Tunica albuginea cysts are typically seen in men 50 to 60 years of age.[8] They are found anterior and lateral to the testicle at the testicular surface[8] and range in size from 2 mm to 5 mm.[8,9]

Sonographic Findings. These cysts appear as well-defined anechoic areas with posterior enhancement.[7]

Varicocele

A varicocele is a group of dilated veins caused by incompetent valves in the internal spermatic veins. Varicoceles are typically larger on the left because the left testicular vein is longer and enters the left renal vein at a right angle.[13] Most varicoceles are extratesticular and rarely intratesticular.[13] Varicoceles generally occur

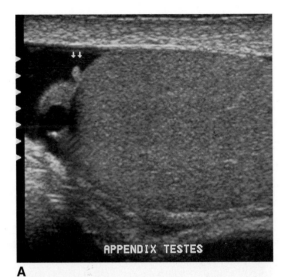

APPENDIX TESTES

A

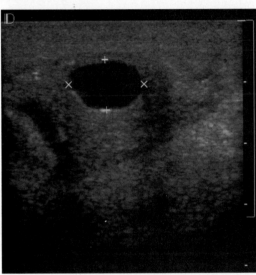

B

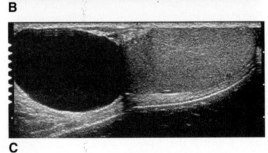

C

Fig. 28-6 **A,** Small epididymal cyst is shown. Note appendix testis *(arrows).* **B,** Clinically palpable small mass was identified as epididymal cyst. **C,** Large epididymal cyst displaced testis inferiorly. (**A** and **C,** Courtesy Cindy Rapp, Radiology Imaging Associates, Greenwood Village, Colorado.)

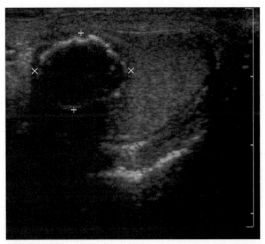

Fig. 28-7 Intratesticular lesion was found to be epidermoid cyst.

in 10% to 15% of men. Varicoceles are divided into two categories: primary and secondary.[2] Primary varicoceles are more common in younger men between 15 and 25 years of age.[2,7] They are the most common correctable cause of infertility, occurring in 21% to 39% of men with infertility.[7] Secondary varicoceles are caused by compression of the spermatic vein by tumor, hydronephrosis, muscle strain, hepatomegaly, and splenomegaly.[2,7]

Sonographic Findings. Varicoceles (Fig. 28-8; see Color Plate 19) appear as dilated tubular structures greater than 2 mm in the inferior aspect of the scrotum. Color Doppler is useful in the diagnosis of a varicocele, with an accuracy rate of 98%. Increased flow is identified within the prominent veins when the patient performs the Valsalva's maneuver or the patient is scanned standing upright.

Spermatocele

A spermatocele is a retention cyst located along the course of the **vas deferens** or more commonly in the head of the epididymis. Spermatoceles may be single or multiple, unilateral or bilateral.[3,8] Spermatoceles range in size from 0.2 cm to 9 cm. The fluid found in a spermatocele is thick and creamy and contains nonviable **sperm.**[2]

Sonographic Findings. Typically located superiorly (Fig. 28-9), a spermatocele appears as a round or oval predominantly anechoic mass.[2] Spermatoceles may reposition the testicle anteriorly. Spermatoceles are of little clinical significance.[3]

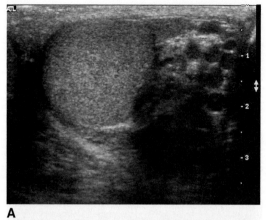

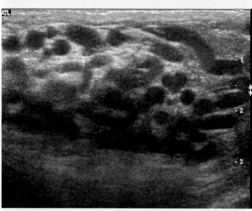

B

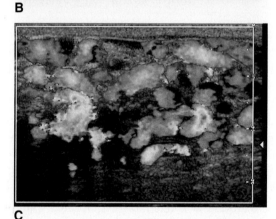

C

Fig. 28-8 **A,** Transverse and, **B,** longitudinal images show dilated tubular structures. **C,** Color Doppler confirms vascular nature of varicoceles. (Courtesy Cindy Rapp, Radiology Imaging Associates, Greenwood Village, Colorado.)

Scrotal Hernia

Scrotal hernias are inguinal hernias that enter the scrotum.[7] These hernias may contain small bowel, colon, or **omentum.**[8] Bowel is able to enter the scrotum because the processus vaginalis, which connects the abdomen and scrotum in the fetus, persists after birth.[3,7] The two types of inguinal hernias are external or

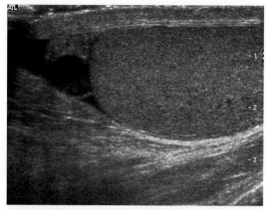

Fig. 28-9 Spermatocele is identified superior to testis. (Courtesy Cindy Rapp, Radiology Imaging Associates, Greenwood Village, Colorado.)

indirect and internal or direct. External or indirect inguinal hernias are the most common. The patient has a swollen scrotum that contains a firm, palpable mass.[8] **Incarcerated** hernias are hernias that are no longer able to move between the abdomen and scrotum. The bowel is "trapped" within the scrotum, causing the blood supply of the herniated bowel to be obstructed. If emergency surgery is not performed, the bowel becomes gangrenous.[7]

Sonographic Findings. Sonographic scans reveal a scrotal mass with both echogenic and anechoic areas.[8] Shadowing from air may also be identified within the scrotum. If peristaltic motion (Fig. 28-10) is identified, the diagnosis of scrotal hernia is confirmed.[3,8]

CALCIFICATIONS

Calcifications that occur in the scrotum include scrotal pearls and **microlithiasis.**

Scrotal Pearls

Scrotal pearls are free-floating calcifications within the scrotum or along the tunica. They can be caused by epididymitis torsion, torsion of the **appendix testis,** inflammation, or a chronic hydrocele.[8]

Sonographic Findings. Scrotal pearls appear highly echogenic and may shadow.

Microlithiasis

Testicular microlithiasis occurs as a result of calcifications in the seminiferous tubules.[8] The condition is rare[14] but has been seen in patients with infertility, **cryptorchidism,** torsion, Klinefelter's syndrome, male pseudohermaphroditism, intratubular germ cell neo-

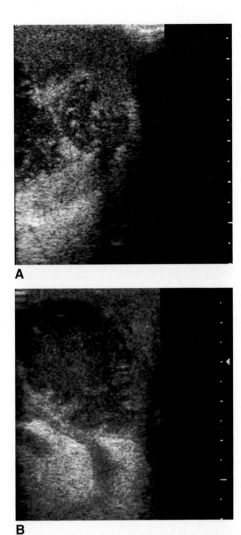

A

B

Fig. 28-10 Mass is identified within scrotum, separate from testes. **A,** Longitudinal and, **B,** transverse images show mass in which peristalsis was identified in real time, for diagnosis of scrotal hernia.

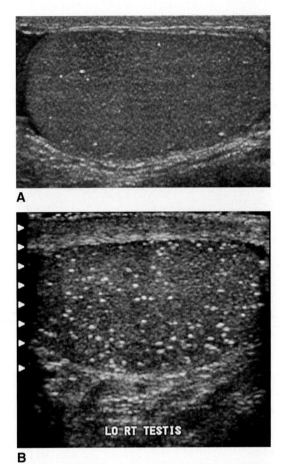

A

LO RT TESTIS

B

Fig. 28-11 Examples of, **A,** mild microlithiasis and, **B,** severe microlithiasis. (Courtesy Cindy Rapp, Radiology Imaging Associates, Greenwood Village, Colorado.)

plasia, and granulomatous disease.[7] Microlithiasis was once considered completely benign but has been linked to the presence or development of testicular neoplasm in 40% of cases where it is identified.[7,8]

Sonographic Findings. Testicular microlithiasis (Fig. 28-11) appears as small, echogenic foci within the testes that do not shadow.[7] It is common to see microlithiasis bilaterally.[7]

Epididymitis

Epididymitis accounts for 75% to 80% of acute inflammatory disease of the scrotum.[7,8] Swelling and sonographic epididymal abnormalities, skin thickening, and hydrocele are more suggestive of an infectious process than of tumor.[15] Patients have pain for at least 2 days and may have a discharge.[8] The most frequent cause of epididymitis is a bacterial infection.[7,8] This infection is usually from an urinary tract infection. In younger men, the most common cause of epididymitis is **chlamydia**.[8] It is usually a unilateral condition but may be bilateral.[7,8] If epididymitis is not successfully treated, **epididymoorchitis** develops.

Sonographic Findings. The epididymis is thickened and enlarged (Fig. 28-12) with a decrease in echogenicity compared with a normal epididymis. If the infection becomes chronic, the epididymis is thickened and focally echogenic and may have calcifications.[3]

Orchitis

Orchitis is defined as inflammation of the testis. The entire testicle or an isolated focal area may be involved.[3] The condition may be bacterial or viral in origin.[16] Bacterial orchitis is usually a secondary infection from epididymitis and may be a manifestation of a sexually transmitted disease, such as gonorrhea or chlamydia.

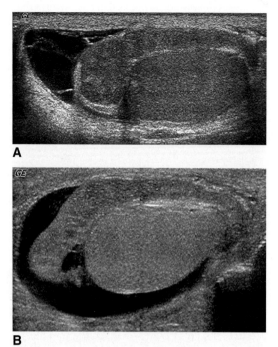

A

B

Fig. 28-12 Epididymitis is identified in images with, **A,** enlarged epididymis and loculated fluid and with, **B,** simple hydrocele.

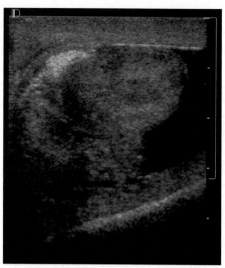

Fig. 28-13 Epididymoorchitis was diagnosed in 85-year-old man with history of recurrent urinary tract infections.

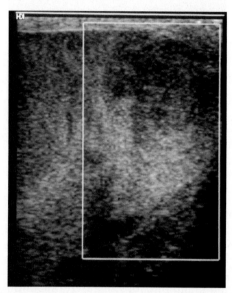

Fig. 28-14 Irregular hypoechoic region within testis was diagnosed as abscess in patient with severe epididymoorchitis. (Courtesy Cindy Rapp, Radiology Imaging Associates, Greenwood Village, Colorado.)

Viral causes of orchitis include mumps, influenza, and tonsillitis.[8,16] Approximately 20% of prepubertal patients with mumps have orchitis develop.[16] Orchitis develops in 15% to 25% of men with mumps after puberty. Isolated orchitis is typically caused by a virus.[16] Patients with orchitis may have pain, fever, nausea, and vomiting.[2] If the disease is left untreated, areas of necrosis or abscess may develop.[17]

Sonographic Findings. In the acute phase of orchitis, the testis or focal areas of the testis appear less echogenic (Fig. 28-13) than a normal testicle.[3] Increased blood flow from hyperemia may be identified, and a reactive hydrocele may be present.[2] In the chronic phase, the testicle appears atrophied with degeneration of the tubules. The scrotal wall may be thickened with acute or chronic orchitis.[2] In 60% of patients with orchitis, unilateral testicular atrophy occurs.[16]

Testicular Abscess

A testicular abscess is a localized and encapsulated area of infection.[18] This condition is a rare occurrence and usually follows epididymoorchitis.[2,8] Other causes of testicular abscess include torsion, smallpox, scarlet fever, appendicitis, and mumps.[2,8] Diabetes mellitus and tuberculosis may also be predisposing factors for testicular abscess.[2] Clinically, the patient has a swollen, painful scrotum.[7]

Sonographic Findings. A testicular abscess appears complex and irregular (Fig. 28-14) with increased blood flow evident with color Doppler around the periphery of the abscess and absent flow within the abscess.

INTRATESTICULAR MASS

An intratesticular mass is malignant until proven otherwise.[6] Determination by the sonographer of whether the mass is intratesticular or extratesticular in location is important.[19] Scrotal sonography approaches 100% accuracy in distinguishing an intratesticular mass from an extratesticular mass.[6] In addition, sonography is extremely accurate in determination of the exact location of a scrotal mass, but it is less accurate in distinguishing whether an intratesticular mass is malignant or benign.[19]

Sonographic Findings

Most intratesticular malignant masses are hypoechoic when compared with the normal testicular tissue. Almost all benign intratesticular masses are echogenic.[20]

Seminoma

Most scrotal neoplasms are of primary germ cell origin.[7] Included in this category are **seminomas, teratomas,** embryonal cell carcinoma, and **choriocarcinoma.**[7] The most common type of testicular neoplasm is the seminoma. Seminomas constitute 40% to 50% of primary testicular tumors.[8] They tend to occur in men between 35 and 39 years of age,[8] which is a slightly older age group from other testicular malignant diseases. Seminomas are also the most common malignant disease associated with undescended testes.[2] Fortunately seminomas are not aggressive tumors and are radiosensitive. Compared with other testicular malignant diseases, seminomas have the best prognosis.[8]

Sonographic Findings. Seminomas present as a solid, hypoechoic mass (Fig. 28-15) that is homogeneous,[8] although occasionally scattered echogenic areas may be identified.[7] Seminomas are usually unilateral[7] and may be very small (2 to 3 mm) in size.[3] Seminomas may also almost completely replace normal testicular parenchyma.

Embryonal Cell Carcinoma

Embryonal cell carcinoma typically occurs in men between 25 and 35 years of age.[7] It is the second most common type of testicular neoplasm and accounts for 25% of primary testicular neoplasms.[8] Metastasis can occur through the blood stream and lymph nodes.[8] Elevated serum alpha fetoprotein and **human chorionic gonadotropin** (hCG) levels are detectable in 70% of cases of embryonal cell carcinoma.[21]

Sonographic Findings. Embryonal cell tumors (Fig. 28-16; see Color Plate 20) usually present as a hypoechoic mass in the testicle[8] but may have areas of increased echogenicity.[3] These tumors are aggressive and may distort the normal contour of the testicle when invasion of the tunica albuginea occurs.[7,8]

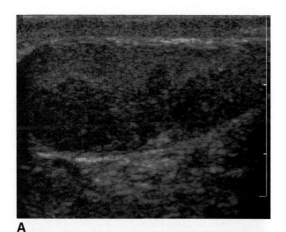

A

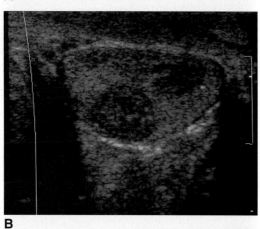

B

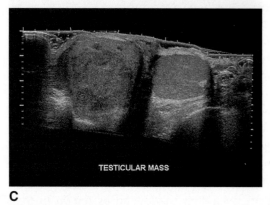

TESTICULAR MASS

C

Fig. 28-15 This 35-year-old man was seen with history of left **orchiectomy** for testicular cancer 5 years previously. Right testis is imaged in, **A,** longitudinal and, **B,** transverse views, revealing hypoechoic lesions that were diagnosed as recurrent seminoma. **C,** Side-by-side comparison in image of seminoma shows significant size tumors may obtain. (Courtesy GE Medical Systems.)

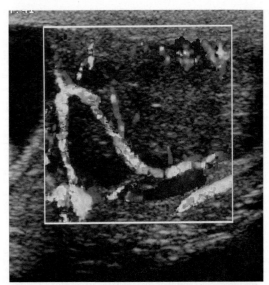

Fig. 28-16 Color Doppler outlines example of embryonal cell carcinoma. (Courtesy Cindy Rapp, Radiology Imaging Associates, Greenwood Village, Colorado.)

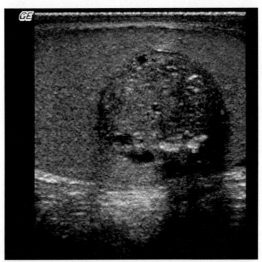

Fig. 28-17 Teratomas may demonstrate mixed echogenicity, including shadowing as shown in testicular tumor. (Courtesy GE Medical Systems.)

Teratoma

Teratomas account for 5% to 10% of scrotal tumors and are generally seen in men between 25 and 35 years of age.[7,8] Teratomas may contain hair, bone, and teeth.[7,8]

If testicular teratomas are left untreated, they generally metastasize within 5 years.[8]

Sonographic Findings. Teratomas are usually well differentiated[17] and, depending on which tissue components they contain, may be hyperechoic, hypoechoic, or complex and demonstrate shadowing (Fig. 28-17).[7]

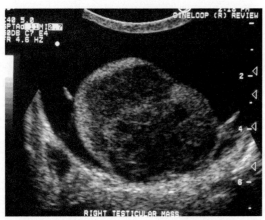

Fig. 28-18 Heterogeneous intratesticular mass is shown in addition to hydrocele. Pathology report revealed choriocarcinoma. (Courtesy Cindy Rapp, Radiology Imaging Associates, Greenwood Village, Colorado.)

Choriocarcinoma

Choriocarcinomas account for a small percentage of testicular tumors (<3%)[7] and are the rarest form of germ cell tumors.[17] They are almost always part of a mixed tumor,[17] with elements of embryonal cell carcinoma, seminoma, and teratoma.[7,8] The most common age group is 20 to 30 years of age. Choriocarcinomas respond poorly to radiation and chemotherapy, resulting in a high mortality rate.[22] On clinical examination, these tumors may be too small to be palpable. Elevated levels of hCG are found in 100% of men with choriocarcinomas.[7] However, an important note is that 60% of men with any type of testicular neoplasm have elevated hCG levels.[7]

Sonographic Findings. Choriocarcinomas (Fig. 28-18) usually present as a small mass with mixed echogenicity from hemorrhage, necrosis, and calcifications.[7,8]

Lymphoma

Lymphoma accounts for approximately 5% of testicular neoplasms, with 2.5% of patients with lymphoma having testicular lymphoma.[7,8] The peak age for the occurrence of testicular lymphoma is 60 years of age,[7,8] which makes lymphoma the most common testicular mass in this age group.[20] Testicular lymphoma is usually unilateral but may be bilateral.[17]

Sonographic Findings. Testicular lymphoma may appear hypoechoic and enlarged with anechoic masses.[8] Lymphoma usually presents as a diffuse mass (Fig. 28-19) but occasionally may be focal.[20]

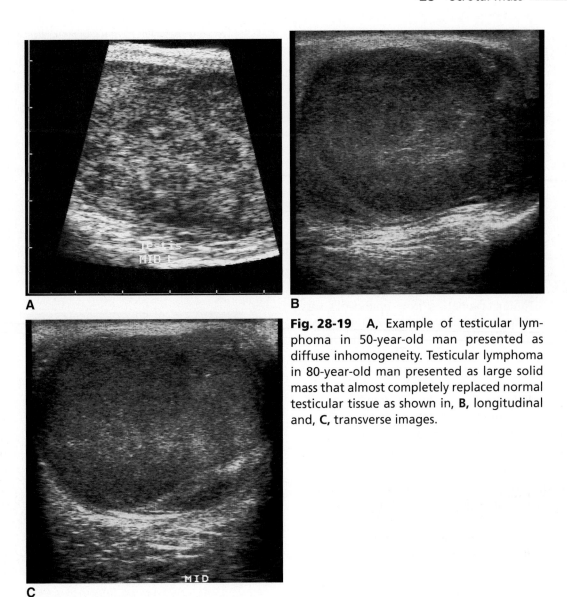

A

B

Fig. 28-19   **A,** Example of testicular lymphoma in 50-year-old man presented as diffuse inhomogeneity. Testicular lymphoma in 80-year-old man presented as large solid mass that almost completely replaced normal testicular tissue as shown in, **B,** longitudinal and, **C,** transverse images.

C

Leydig's Cell Tumors

Leydig's cell tumors are also called *interstitial cell tumors*[7] and occur in men between the ages of 20 and 50 years.[20] These tumors account for 1% to 3% of testicular neoplasms.[20] They are usually considered benign, but 10% of these tumors are malignant, which makes them the most common non–germ cell tumor of the testis.[7] They may produce excessive amounts of estrogen and testosterone, causing virilization or feminization.[17] Determination of whether such tumors are benign or malignant with pathologic examination alone is often difficult. Metastatic lesions may reveal the presence of a malignant Leydig's cell tumor.[23] Patients normally have painless enlargement of the testicle or a palpable mass. Fifteen percent of patients have breast enlargement.[20]

Sonographic Findings. Leydig's cell tumors appear as a solid intratesticular mass and are usually hypoechoic.[7]

They may contain focal areas of hemorrhage and necrosis within the tumor, creating cystic areas identified in 25% of Leydig's cell tumors.

Adenomatoid Tumor

Adenomatoid tumors are benign and more commonly found in the epididymis (Fig. 28-20).[24] Most scrotal adenomatoid tumors are less than 2 cm in size and attach to the surface of the epididymis.[24] The mean age for scrotal adenomatoid tumors is 36 years of age.[24] Testicular adenomatoid tumors are rare benign tumors.[7] They typically attach to the tunica albuginea of the testicle.[25] These tumors may be discovered by the patient or physician as a painless testicular nodule.[24] Adenomatoid tumors identified within the testicle may have the same sonographic findings as malignant neoplasms. Because benign neoplasms within the

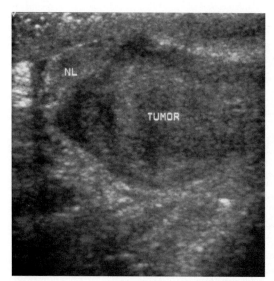

Fig. 28-20 Tumor originating from epididymis was determined to be malignant. (Courtesy Cindy Rapp, Radiology Imaging Associates, Greenwood Village, Colorado.)

testicle are extremely rare, any intratesticular mass should be treated initially as a malignant disease.[25]

Sonographic Findings. Adenomatoid tumors most commonly appear as a small solid mass with echogenicity ranging from hypoechoic to hyperechoic.[7]

TESTICULAR TRAUMA

Trauma to the testicle is uncommon because of the location and mobility of the testicles within the scrotal sac.[4] Testicular trauma may result in blood being released into the scrotum. Hematomas and testicular rupture are conditions that may be caused by trauma.[26] Examples include sports injuries, motor vehicle accidents, and straddle injuries.[4] Testicular trauma (Fig. 28-21) usually occurs in men ages 15 to 40 years.[5] The three categories of trauma are blunt, penetrating, and degloving.[5] Blunt trauma results from a kick or a baseball injury. Penetrating trauma is caused by a gunshot or stab wound. Degloving trauma results in the scrotal skin being sheared off, such as entrapment in heavy machinery.[5] Sonography has the potential to show the cause of scrotal swelling after trauma. The swelling may be from an actual testicular injury or a scrotal hematoma surrounding a normal testicle.[26]

Sonographic Findings

Because the age of a hemorrhage determines the sonographic pattern, hypoechoic or hyperechoic areas may be present within the scrotum. A long-term sequela of

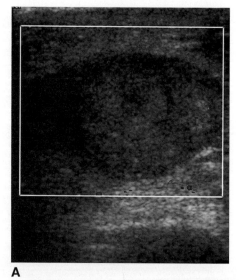

A

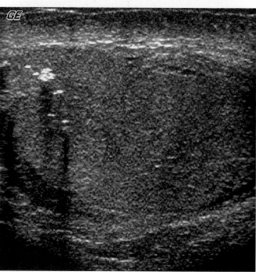

B

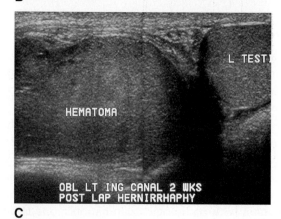

C

Fig. 28-21 Types of trauma to scrotum. **A,** Testicular hematoma resulting from motorcycle straddle injury. **B,** Gunshot wound to testis. **C,** Large hematoma status after surgery. (**B,** Courtesy GE Medical Systems. **C,** Courtesy Cindy Rapp, Radiology Imaging Associates, Greenwood Village, Colorado.)

scrotal trauma may be testicular atrophy, which is apparent clinically and sonographically.[26]

Testicular Rupture

In rupture of the testicle, the tunica albuginea is ripped or torn by trauma.[5,7] Blunt scrotal trauma is the most common cause of testicular rupture.[8] Blunt trauma usually involves either a sports injury or a kick to the groin.[5] Most testicular ruptures occur in males 16 to 20 years of age.[4] Testicular rupture is a rare occurrence[7] but is considered a urologic emergency.[4] If surgery is performed within 72 hours of the injury, 90% of testicles can be salvaged.[7,8,17] The unrepaired testicle may lose the ability to produce sperm and hormones. In addition, the patient may have chronic scrotal pain and may have scrotal gangrene develop.[7] Clinical examination shows a scrotum tender to the touch with scrotal edema. The testicles may be hard to palpate because of the edema.[4]

Sonographic Findings. A ruptured testicle has an irregular outline with anechoic and hyperechoic areas within the testicle (Fig. 28-22).[7,8] A fracture line is rarely seen.[17] Color Doppler may indicate absent or decreased intratesticular blood flow. In 33% of patients with testicular rupture, a **hematocele** is present.[7,8]

Testicular Torsion

Testicular torsion is a twisting of the spermatic cord. This twisting results in the loss of blood supply to the testis and blocks the venous drainage of blood from the testicle.[2,7,8] The two types of testicular torsion are intravaginal and extravaginal.[7] Extravaginal torsion is rare and is seen most frequently in newborns.[2,7] Intravaginal torsion typically involves adolescents and occasionally adults.[2] Unilateral torsion occurs in young males, with a peak incidence at 14 years of age.[27] Bilateral torsion accounts for approximately 2% of testicular torsion.[27]

Intravaginal testicular torsion occurs when the testicle is suspended within the tunica vaginalis by a long stalk of spermatic cord. Extravaginal testicular torsion is the twisting of the testicle at its covering at the level of the external ring.[7] Patients with testicular torsion have sudden severe testicular pain during rest or sleep. Fifty percent of patients have nausea and vomiting. The affected testicle sits higher and horizontal in the scrotum.[7] The left testicle is more often affected than is the right.[28]

The timing of the diagnosis is critical to the prognosis. If surgery occurs within 6 hours of the onset of symptoms, 80% to 100% of torsed testicles are saved.

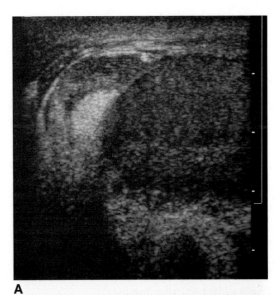

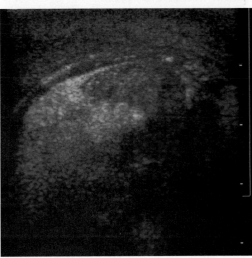

A

B

Fig. 28-22   Testicular rupture of right testis was diagnosed in 26-year-old who had been hit in scrotum with baseball. **A,** Longitudinal and, **B,** transverse images.

Surgery occurring between 6 and 12 hours of the onset of symptoms almost always results in the loss of the testicle.[7] The appearance of the torsed testicle changes over time. The following three phases of torsion have been identified: 1, acute (within 24 hours); 2, subacute (24 hours to 10 days); and 3, chronic (>10 days).[7,8]

Sonographic Findings. In the acute phase, the epididymis and testis enlarge and the testis appears hypoechoic[2] and inhomogeneous.[27] Decreased blood flow to the testis is noted with the Doppler evaluation. After 24 hours, absent blood flow (Fig. 28-23; see Color Plate 21) to the testis is seen. In chronic torsion, the testis atrophies with the epididymis remaining enlarged and hyperechoic.[8]

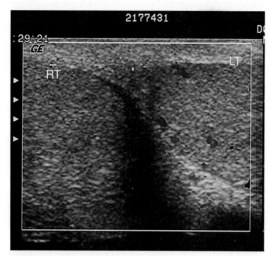

Fig. 28-23 Lack of blood flow is shown in right testis in patient with testicular torsion.

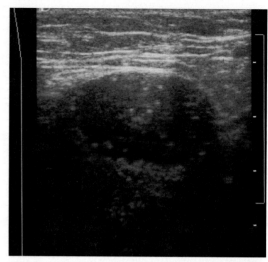

Fig. 28-24 Undescended left testicle was identified in inguinal canal of 72-year-old man. Microlithiasis was also noted.

Cryptorchidism

In the normal fetus, the testicles descend into the scrotal sac at approximately 36 weeks' gestation. If the testes fail to descend into the scrotum, cryptorchidism results. The several causes of cryptorchidism include a narrow **inguinal canal**, a short spermatic cord, fibrosis, or adhesions.[8] Several conditions are associated with cryptorchidism, including infertility, cancer, and scrotal hernia. Infertility results from the testis being exposed to higher temperatures within the body.[7]

An undescended testicle has a 35 to 48 times higher risk of cancer than does a testicle within the scrotal sac.[7,8] Scrotal hernia results because of failure of the processus vaginalis to close as the testicle never descends through this opening.[7] Cryptorchidism is bilateral in 10% of cases. Undescended testicles can be located in the inguinal canal (80%) or the peritoneal cavity (20%).[7] Intraabdominal testicles may be located as high as the renal pedicle.[17]

Sonographic Findings. An undescended testicle is identified as a soft tissue mass in the inguinal canal (Fig. 28-24) or peritoneal cavity. The undescended testicle is typically smaller than a normally located testicle and may be mobile on palpation. The echo texture of an undescended testicle is homogeneous and hypoechoic.[7] For surgical correction of cryptorchidism in infants and young children, the undescended testicles are placed in the scrotal sac.[8] Surgery within the second year of life is recommended.[29] Undescended testicles in pubertal and adult males to the age of 32 years are removed.[8] After 32 years of age, no treatment is recommended.[8]

SUMMARY

Sonography plays a major role in the diagnosis of scrotal masses. The sonographer must be familiar with normal echo patterns of scrotal structures and abnormal echo patterns (Table 28-1). Sonography is sensitive in distinguishing extratesticular from intratesticular masses. This distinction is valuable in diagnosis of scrotal masses. Infectious processes are usually extratesticular, and most intratesticular masses are malignant. Clinicians agree that ultrasound is the preferred method for imaging the scrotum.

CLINICAL SCENARIO—DIAGNOSIS

■ The finding that the mass is intratesticular is highly suggestive of carcinoma of the right testicle because masses within the testicle are usually malignant. Because the patient is 30 years old and the identified mass is intratesticular and hypoechoic, this mass would most likely be a seminoma, although other neoplasms cannot be definitively ruled out with ultrasound. The pathology confirmed the mass to be a seminoma.

Table 28-1	*Pathology of Scrotum*	
Pathology	**Symptoms**	**Sonographic Findings**
Simple cyst	Usually asymptomatic	Round or oval, anechoic, thin-walled, posterior enhancement
Abscess	Scrotal pain, fever, nausea and vomiting	Round or oval lesion with irregular wall; hypoechoic, anechoic, or mixed; with or without enhancement
Infarct	Testicular pain	Normal echo pattern or wedge-shaped, hypoechoic lesion; may be round with variable echogenicity
Hydrocele	Asymptomatic or scrotal enlargement	Fluid collection anterolateral to testis
Varicocele	Prominent scrotal vessels with standing	Increased blood flow in prominent veins, usually on left
Spermatocele	Painless scrotal mass	Round or oval lesion predominately anechoic
Hernia	Swollen scrotum with firm palpable mass	Scrotal mass with echogenic and anechoic areas; peristaltic motion may be identified
Epididymitis	Scrotal pain and possible discharge	Thick, enlarged epididymis with decreased echogenicity
Orchitis	Pain, fever, nausea and vomiting	Decreased echogenicity; possible hydrocele; in advanced stages, testicular atrophy occurs
Cryptorchidism	Asymptomatic or palpable mass in pelvis or lower abdomen	Homogeneous, hypoechoic mobile mass in inguinal canal or peritoneal cavity
Torsion	Sudden severe testicular pain, nausea and vomiting	Initially, enlargement of hypoechoic testicle with greatly diminished or absent blood flow; later, testicular atrophy of hyperechoic testicle with no blood flow
Seminoma	Palpable testicular mass	Solid, hypoechoic, homogeneous neoplasm
Embryonal cell carcinoma	Palpable testicular mass	Hypoechoic neoplasm that may have echogenic areas
Teratoma	Palpable testicular mass	Hyperechoic, hypoechoic, or complex well-differentiated mass; shadowing
Choriocarcinoma	Elevated hCG level with or without palpable mass	Small mass with mixed echogenicity
Lymphoma	Enlarged testicles with or without palpable mass	Hypoechoic enlarged testicles with possible anechoic masses
Leydig's cell tumor	Painless testicular enlargement	Solid hypoechoic intratesticular mass
Adenomatoid tumor	Painless testicular nodule	Small, solid, hypoechoic or hyperechoic
Rupture	Scrotal edema; painful to touch	Irregular testicular outline with hypoechoic or hyperechoic areas; absent or decreased blood flow

CASE STUDIES FOR DISCUSSION ▬▬▬▬▬▬▬

1. A 59-year-old man is seen in the sonography department with enlargement of the right testicle. He has had general malaise for the past month but only last week noticed the irregularity in his testicle. Sonography reveals the findings in Fig. 28-25. What is the most likely diagnosis?

2. A 15-year-old boy is hit in the scrotum by a "line drive" during a high school baseball game. He enters the sonography department the following day with a swollen and bruised right testicle. The results of the sonographic evaluation are shown in Fig. 28-26. What is the most likely diagnosis?

3. A 19-year-old man is seen in the emergency department with an onset of severe scrotal pain from no apparent cause.

The sonographic examination reveals a slightly enlarged left testicle when compared with the right testicle. Color Doppler of the left testis is shown in Fig. 28-27, *A*, and the Doppler evaluation of the right testis is shown in Fig. 28-27, *B*. The left epididymis is shown in Fig. 28-27, *C*. What is the most likely diagnosis?

4. A 40-year-old man is seen in the sonography department with some swelling and pain in the left hemiscrotum of 5 days' duration. The ultrasound reveals the findings in Fig. 28-28 (see Color Plate 22). The right hemiscrotum is unremarkable. What is the most likely diagnosis?

5. A 71-year-old man is seen with swelling and what appears to be a mass in the left scrotum. On further questioning,

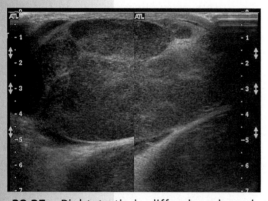

Fig. 28-25 Right testis is diffusely enlarged and inhomogeneous. (Courtesy Cindy Rapp, Radiology Imaging Associates, Greenwood Village, Colorado.)

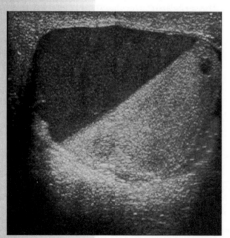

Fig. 28-26 Sonographic evaluation of right testicle after sports injury. (Courtesy Cindy Rapp, Radiology Imaging Associates, Greenwood Village, Colorado.)

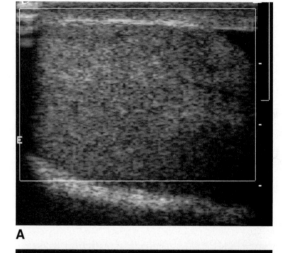

A

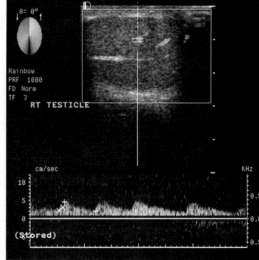

B

Fig. 28-27 **A,** Color Doppler evaluation of left testis, and, **B,** Doppler evaluation of right testis in young man with acute scrotal pain.

CASE STUDIES FOR DISCUSSION—cont'd

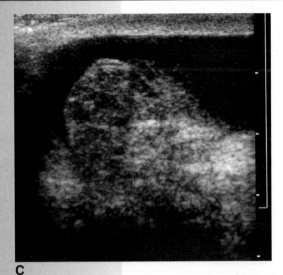

C

Fig. 28-27, cont'd   C, Epididymis is also shown.

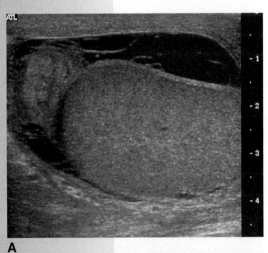

A

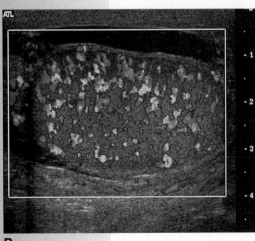

B

Fig. 28-28   A, Sonographic evaluation of left hemiscrotum is shown in addition to, **B,** Color Doppler evaluation. (Courtesy Cindy Rapp, Radiology Imaging Associates, Greenwood Village, Colorado.)

the patient reveals that he has had intermittent pain for several weeks in his lower abdomen. Ultrasound examination reveals both hypoechoic and hyperechoic structures (Fig. 28-29) with a "ladder" appearance. Peristalsis is associated with these structures in the left scrotum. What is the most likely diagnosis?

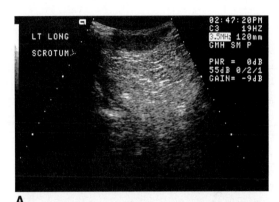

A

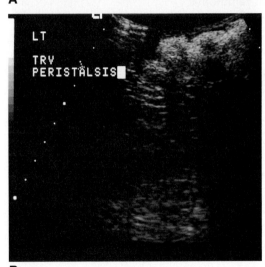

B

Fig. 28-29   A, Longitudinal and, **B,** transverse images of scrotum.

STUDY QUESTIONS

1. A 10-year-old boy is seen for a scrotal ultrasound. On clinical examination, no testicles were palpated within the scrotal sac. A homogeneous ovoid mass is identified within the left inguinal canal. This mass probably represents:
   a. testicular rupture
   b. lymphoma
   c. spermatocele
   d. cryptorchidism
   e. metastasis

2. A 52-year-old man is seen with pain and enlargement of the scrotum. An ultrasound evaluation is ordered by the attending physician and reveals a small hydrocele on the left with a swollen heterogeneous-appearing left testicle and left epididymis. Increased blood flow is also identified on color Doppler examination. This is suggestive of:
   a. testicular torsion
   b. epididymoorchitis
   c. epididymitis
   d. seminoma
   e. scrotal hernia

3. A 22-year-old man is awakened with a sudden onset of scrotal pain. On examination in the emergency department, a scrotal ultrasound is ordered. The sonogram reveals slight enlargement of the right testicle and a small hydrocele. On color Doppler examination, no blood flow can be shown. What do these findings suggest?
   a. epididymitis
   b. orchitis
   c. embryonal cell tumor
   d. testicular torsion
   e. varicocele

4. A 43-year-old male is seen with a grossly enlarged scrotum. Sonographic examination reveals bilateral large hydroceles. In addition, a hypoechoic area in the head of the right epididymis is identified. This hypoechoic area probably represents:
   a. varicocele
   b. spermatocele
   c. focal epididymitis
   d. cryptorchidism
   e. teratoma

5. A 35-year-old man is seen for sonographic examination of the scrotum for palpable mass in the right hemiscrotum. The sonogram reveals multiple punctate foci and a large area of decreased echogenicity in the right testis. These findings are suggestive of:
   a. testicular carcinoma with microlithiasis
   b. orchitis with microlithiasis
   c. torsion with hydrocele
   d. varicocele with microlithiasis
   e. hematoma with clotted blood

6. A 40-year-old man undergoes evaluation for infertility. His physician orders an ultrasound for further evaluation. During the ultrasound examination, an area of dilated vessels is identified in the left scrotum. Some of these vessels measure 1.5 mm to 2.0 mm. These vessels are suggestive of:
   a. spermatocele
   b. abscess
   c. hydrocele
   d. epididymal cyst
   e. varicocele

7. A 26-year-old male construction worker is seen in the emergency department after falling onto a metal pipe from a ladder. He currently has pain and swelling of the scrotum. An ultrasound is ordered. During the sonogram, increased echogenicity of the right testicle is noted. In addition, hypervascularity of the right testicle is noted on color Doppler examination. An area of echogenic material is seen in the upper margin of the right testicle. These findings are suggestive of:
   a. testicular torsion
   b. scrotal hernia
   c. testicular rupture
   d. seminoma
   e. hydrocele

8. A 28-year-old undergoes clinical evaluation for a palpable mass in the left testicle. An ultrasound examination is ordered for further evaluation. The sonogram reveals a solid hypoechoic mass within the left testicle. A small amount of fluid also surrounds the left testicle. These findings are suggestive of:
   a. scrotal hernia
   b. epididymitis
   c. seminoma
   d. epididymal cyst
   e. teratoma

9. A 61-year-old man is seen with intermittent pain and swelling of the right scrotum. He also has pain in the area of the right inguinal canal. A sonogram is ordered for further evaluation. On sonographic examination, an abnormal area is seen in the right scrotum containing tubular-appearing structures that show peristalsis. These sonographic findings are consistent with:
   a. varicocele
   b. epididymal cyst
   c. orchitis
   d. scrotal hernia
   e. scrotal abscess

10. A 2-week-old male is seen with an enlarged scrotum. During the clinical examination, the swollen scrotum transilluminates light coming from a flashlight. Sonographically, anechoic fluid surrounds both testicles. The scrotal wall appears to be thin. These sonographic findings are suggestive of:
   a. an acute hydrocele
   b. a chronic hydrocele
   c. cryptorchidism
   d. hematocele
   e. scrotal hernia

ACKNOWLEDGMENT

The author thanks Cindy Rapp, BS, RDMS, FSDMS, FAIUM, sonographer practitioner, Radiology Imaging Associates, Greenwood Village, Colorado, for providing many of the images in this chapter.

REFERENCES

1. Curry RA, Tempkin BB: *Ultrasonography: an introduction to normal structure and functional anatomy,* Philadelphia, 1995, WB Saunders.
2. Krebs CA, Giyanani VL, Eisenberg RL: *Ultrasound atlas of disease processes,* Norwalk, Conn, 1993, Appleton & Lange.
3. Saunders RC: *Clinical sonography,* ed 3, Philadelphia, 1998, Lippincott Williams & Wilkins.
4. Dogra VS: *Testicle, trauma,* www.emedicine.com/radio/topic682.htm, retrieved August 12, 2003.
5. Chow JM: *Testicular trauma,* www.emedicine.com/med/byname/testicular-trauma.htm, retrieved August 12, 2003.
6. Rosser CJ, Scharling E, Salmon J et al: *Scrotal leiomyoma,* www.duj.com/Article/Rosser3.html, retrieved September 11, 2003.
7. Kawamura DM: *Abdomen and superficial structures,* ed 2, Philadelphia and New York, 1997, Lippincott.
8. Gill KA: *Abdominal ultrasound,* Philadelphia, 2001, WB Saunders.
9. Dogra VS, Gottlieb RH, Rubens DJ et al: Benign intratesticular cystic lesions: US features, *Radiographics* 21:S273-S281, 2001.
10. Ririe K, Bowman K, Townsend R: Intratesticular spermatocele in occurrence with seminiferous tubular ectasia, *J Diagn Med Sonogr* 14:203-206, 1998.
11. Langer JE, Ramcharin P, Siegelman ES et al: Epidermoid cysts of the testicle: sonographic and MR imaging features, *AJR Am J Roentgenol* 173:1295-1299, 1999.
12. Garcia CJ, Zuniga S, Rosenberg H et al: Simple intratesticular cysts in children: preoperative sonographic diagnosis and histological correlation, *Pediatr Radiol* 29:851-855, 1999.
13. Mehta AL, Dogra VS: Intratesticular varicocele, *J Clin Ultrasound* 26:49-51, 1998.
14. Aizenstein RI, DiDomenico D, Wilbur AC et al: Testicular microlithiasis: association with male infertility, *J Clin Ultrasound* 26:195-198, 1998.
15. Muttarak M, Peh WC, Lojanapiwat B et al: Tuberculous epididymitis and epididymo-orchitis: sonographic appearances, *AJR Am J Roentgenol* 176:1459-1466, 2001.
16. Mycyk M: *Orchitis,* www.emedicine.com/emerg/byname/orchitis.htm, retrieved August 12, 2003.
17. Machin JA: *Scrotal ultrasound: recent advances including color Doppler,* www.com/phys_art1.html, retrieved September 11, 2003.
18. Chung SE, Frush DP, Fordham LA: Sonographic appearances of extratesticular fluid and fluid-containing scrotal masses in infants and children: clues to diagnosis, *AJR Am J Roentgenol* 173:741-745,1999.
19. Chin SC, Wu CJ, Chen A et al: Segmental hemorrhagic infarction of testis associated with epididymitis, *J Clin Ultrasound* 26:326-328, 1998.
20. Rose DI, Laing FC: Malignant Leydig cell adenoma of the testicle, *Brigham RAD,* April 1997, http://brighamrad.harvard.edu/Cases/bwh/hcache/224/full.html, retrieved September 9, 2003.
21. Yamase H: *Embryonal carcinoma,* http://uchc.edu/Code/786.htm, retrieved September 11, 2003.
22. Davis JW: *Testicular choriocarcinoma,* www.eMedicine.com/med/byname/testicular-choriocarcinoma.htm, retrieved August 12, 2003.
23. Anderson MS, Brogi E, Biller BM: Occult Leydig cell tumor in a patient with gynecomastia, *Endocr Pract* 7:267-271, 2001.
24. Yamase H: *Adenomatoid tumor,* http://radiology.uchc.edu/Code/805.htm, retrieved September 11, 2003.
25. Adler HL, Haddad JL, Wheeler TM et al: *Intratesticular adenomatoid tumor radiographically mimicking a primary testicular malignancy,* http://www.duj.com/Article/Kim/Kim.html, retrieved August 12, 2003.

26. Cross JJL, Berman LH, Elliott PG et al: Scrotal trauma: a cause of testicular atrophy, *Clin Radiol* 54:317-320, 1999.

27. Washowich TL: Synchronous bilateral testicular torsion in an adult, *J Ultrasound Med* 20:933-935, 2001.

28. Tamkin G: Evaluating acute scrotal pain, *Emerg Med* May:20-35, 2000.

29. Riebel T, Herrmann C, Wit J et al: Ultrasonographic late results after surgically treated cryptorchidism, *Pediatr Radiol* 30:151-155, 2000.

BIBLIOGRAPHY

Anthony CP, Kolthoff NJ: *Textbook of anatomy and physiology,* ed 8, St Louis, 1971, Mosby.

Blaivas M, Sierzenski P: Emergency ultrasonography in the evaluation of the acute scrotum, *Acad Emerg Med* 8:85-89, 2001.

Henderson SO: *Torsion of the appendices and epididymis,* www.emedicine.com/emerg/byname/torsion-of-the-appendices-and-epididymis.htm, retrieved August 12, 2003.

Rose DI, Laing FC: *Malignant Leydig cell adenoma of the testicle,* http://brighamrad.harvard.edu/Cases/bwh/hcache/224/full.html, retrieved August 12, 2003.

Swischuk LE: Swollen and painful left testicle, *Pediatr Emerg Care* 16:287-289, 2000.

Thomas CL: *Taber's cyclopedic medical dictionary,* Philadelphia, 1981, FA Davis.

29 Neck Mass

KATHRYN M. KUNTZ

CLINICAL SCENARIO

■ A 23-year-old man is referred to the ultrasound department for evaluation of a palpable neck mass. The left-sided mass was incidentally noted by the patient during shaving. The patient is in good general health and has no significant medical history; laboratory blood test evaluation results are normal. The mass is not tender and does not appear to have grown over the last year. A high-resolution neck ultrasound reveals not only the palpable left-sided thyroid nodule but also three other right-sided thyroid nodules. The predominate nodule is 1.5 cm and solid, and the sonographer notes tiny flecks of nonshadowing calcifications. The other three nodules are all less than 0.5 cm and also solid and lack the calcifications detected in the large predominate nodule. Also noted are numerous visible lymph nodes bilaterally along the carotid-jugular chain. The patient is concerned about thyroid cancer. Because the mass was already known, how is the diagnosis of carcinoma confirmed or discounted? What significance do the incidental nodules and the presence of enlarged lymph nodes have?

OBJECTIVES

- Name the most common neck masses encountered on sonographic examinations.
- List the risk factors associated with the development of neck masses.
- Describe the sonographic appearances of the most commonly seen neck masses.
- Recognize sonographic features that suggest a thyroid nodule is benign or malignant.
- List the risk factors, laboratory values, and sonographic features of parathyroid adenoma.
- Describe the less common cystic neck pathologies that can be diagnosed with ultrasound.

GLOSSARY OF TERMS

Adenomas: benign thyroid neoplasms

Adenopathy: enlargement of lymph nodes

Anaplastic thyroid cancer: a rare carcinoma of the thyroid

Branchial cleft cysts: congenital cystic mass in the lateral neck

Capillary lymphangioma: cystic neck mass caused by malformations of the cervical thoracic lymphatic system

Cavernous lymphangioma: cystic neck mass caused by malformations of the cervical thoracic lymphatic system

Cystic hygroma: cystic neck mass caused by malformations of the cervical thoracic lymphatic system

Fine-needle aspiration: usually performed with a 23- to 27-gauge needle

Follicular cancer: a malignant mass in the thyroid

Goiter: enlargement of the thyroid gland that can be focal or diffuse; nodules may be present

Graves' disease: an autoimmune disorder of diffuse toxic goiter characterized by bulging eyes

Hashimoto's disease: the most common form of thyroiditis

Hyperparathyroidism: disorder associated with elevated serum calcium levels, usually caused by a benign parathyroid adenoma

Hyperplastic nodules: thyroid nodules that form as the result of tissue degeneration

Hyperthyroidism: the oversecretion of thyroid hormones

Hypophosphatasia: low phosphatase level that can be seen with hyperparathyroidism

Isthmus: thin band of thyroid tissue that connects the right and left lobes

Longus colli muscles: wedge-shaped muscle posterior to the thyroid lobes

Medullary thyroid cancer: an uncommon thyroid cancer

Microcalcifications: tiny echogenic foci within a nodule that may or may not shadow

Papillary thyroid cancer: the most common form of thyroid cancer

Parathyroid hormone: a hormone that is secreted by parathyroid glands, which regulate serum calcium levels

Parathyroid hyperplasia: enlargement of multiple parathyroid glands

Primary hyperparathyroidism: oversecretion of parathyroid hormone, usually from a parathyroid adenoma

Psammoma bodies: fine, punctate, internal calcifications seen in papillary thyroid cancer nodules

Secondary hyperparathyroidism: enlargement of parathyroid glands in patients with renal failure or vitamin D deficiency

Serum calcium: laboratory value that is elevated with hyperparathyroidism

Sternocleidomastoid muscles: large muscles anterolateral to the thyroid

Strap muscles: sternohyoid and sternothyroid muscles that lie anterior to the thyroid

Thyroid inferno: increase in color Doppler vascular flow in the thyroid

High-frequency ultrasonography has been acknowledged as an important screening and diagnostic imaging method for the evaluation of the thyroid and parathyroid glands of the neck. The advantages of ultrasonography over other imaging methods include its high degree of accuracy, ready availability, fast examination time, and low cost. Ultrasound requires no patient preparation, and no ionizing radiation is used. The performance of interventional procedures with ultrasonographic guidance, including **fine-needle aspiration** (FNA) of thyroid nodules and alcohol ablation of parathyroid **adenomas,** is an important application of ultrasonography. In addition to thyroid and parathyroid disease, other less common congenital, cystic, and solid neck masses and lymph node diseases should be considered by any practitioner of ultrasound.[1]

THYROID GLAND

Normal Sonographic Anatomy

The thyroid gland is part of the endocrine system, which helps the body to maintain a normal metabolism. The thyroid consists of paired right and left lobes in the lower anterior neck. The lobes are joined at the midline by a thin bridge of thyroid tissue called the *isthmus,* which is draped over the anterior aspect of the trachea at the junction of the middle and lower thirds of the gland (Fig. 29-1). A midline pyramidal lobe that arises from

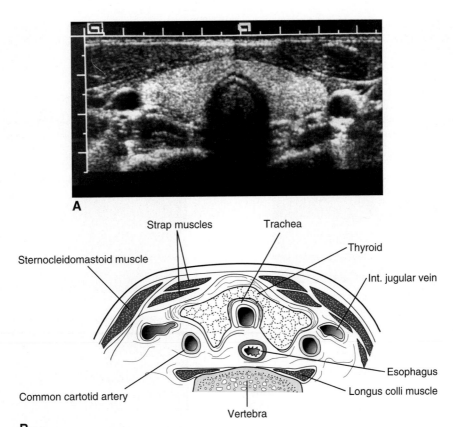

A

Strap muscles   Trachea

Sternocleidomastoid muscle   Thyroid

                                                    Int. jugular vein

                                                    Esophagus
                                                    Longus colli muscle

Common cartotid artery

                 Vertebra

B

Fig. 29-1   A, Transverse image of thyroid anatomy with, **B,** accompanying line drawing.

the isthmus and tapers superiorly, anterior to the thyroid cartilage, is seen in some patients. Anterior to the thyroid surface are the **strap muscles** of the neck, the sternohyoid and sternothyroid. The large **sternocleidomastoid muscles** are located anterolaterally. Laterally is the carotid sheath, which contains the common carotid artery and the jugular vein. The wedge-shaped **longus colli muscles** are located posteriorly. In the midline, the shadowing gas-filled trachea generally hides the esophagus, but the esophagus may be seen protruding slightly laterally and can be confused with a parathyroid adenoma with imaging in the transverse plane only.[2]

The normal thyroid has a fine homogeneous echotexture that is more echogenic than the adjacent muscles. In its periphery, the gland's echotexture is interrupted by vascular structures. Color-flow Doppler imaging of the normal thyroid shows minimal flow signal, which usually is located near the poles of the gland.[1]

Diffuse Disease

Goiter is the most common cause of diffuse thyroid hyperplasia with gland enlargement. Goiter is caused by

inadequate iodine ingestion but is not a significant problem in the United States. The most commonly encountered diffuse thyroid diseases in the United States are **Hashimoto's disease** (chronic thyroiditis) and **Graves' disease** (diffuse toxic goiter). Although these are distinctly different conditions, the ultrasound findings are relatively nonspecific. Visualization of a thyroid isthmus thicker than a few millimeters suggests a diffusely enlarged gland. A sonogram that reveals involvement of the entire gland can alert the physician to consider diffuse rather than focal disease.[2]

Graves' disease is an autoimmune disorder characterized by thyrotoxicosis and is the most frequent cause of **hyperthyroidism.**[1] Graves' disease usually produces a diffusely hypoechoic thyroid texture, with accompanying contour lobulation but without palpable nodules.[3,4] A characteristic increase in color-flow Doppler in the thyroid is present on examination, both in systole and diastole, leading to the term *thyroid inferno,* coined by Ralls and colleagues (Fig. 29-2; see Color Plate 23).[5]

Hashimoto's disease is the most common form of thyroiditis. The typical clinical presentation is a painless, diffusely enlarged gland in a young or middle-aged woman. No normal parenchyma is identified. The

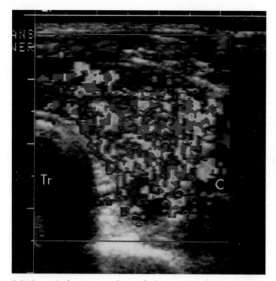

Fig. 29-2 Color Doppler of thyroid inferno seen with Graves' disease.

sonographic appearance is hypoechoic compared with a normal thyroid, with a coarse but overall homogeneous thyroid echotexture. Also seen are multiple ill-defined hypoechoic areas separated by thickened fibrous strands (Fig. 29-3). Discrete thyroid nodules are less common. Color-flow Doppler imaging usually demonstrates increased vascularity. In the final stages of the disease, a fibrotic gland may be seen that is small, ill defined, and heterogeneous. Because of the increased risk for malignant disease associated with Hashimoto's disease, follow-up examinations are recommended.[1]

Thyroid Mass

Nodular thyroid disease is the lesion of the thyroid gland most commonly encountered with ultrasound. Nodular thyroid disease is a common disorder. Between 4% and 7% of the adult population in the United States is estimated to have thyroid nodules, which can be detected with palpation. Twenty-seven percent to 41% have nodules visible with ultrasound, and 50% have nodules discovered at autopsy.[6-9] Thyroid cancer, however, is rare. The annual detection rate of clinically significant thyroid cancer is only 0.005%. Therefore, most nodules that the sonographer encounters are benign and not clinically significant. In the patient who is referred or has a palpable thyroid nodule, the challenge is to distinguish the few significant malignant nodules from the many benign ones and thus to identify those patients for whom surgery is indicated.

Benign Nodules

Sonographic Findings. Benign nodules either are hyperplastic (involution of underlying thyroid tissue)

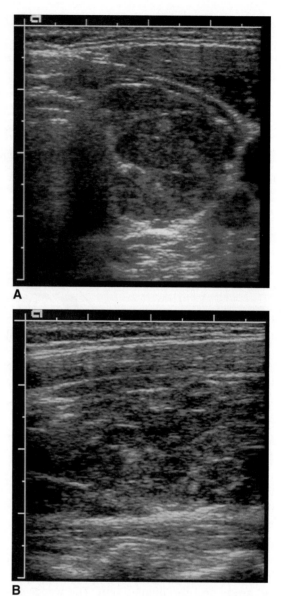

Fig. 29-3 **A**, Transverse and, **B**, longitudinal images of Hashimoto's disease.

or are adenomas, also called *follicular adenomas.* Adenomas are true thyroid nodules but are actually less common than **hyperplastic nodules.**[1] Sonographically, palpable thyroid nodules can be seen with a high degree of accuracy. However, the differentiation of benign from malignant nodules on the basis of ultrasound appearance is challenging. The sonographic findings with thyroid nodules can be thought of as a group of several features, each of which may aid in prediction of the benign or malignant nature of a given nodule.[10,11] Features that suggest a benign nodule include nodules that are mostly cystic. These cystic nodules almost always contain debris (Fig. 29-4). Less common types of a benign nodule are those that are hyperechoic relative to the adjacent thyroid parenchyma and

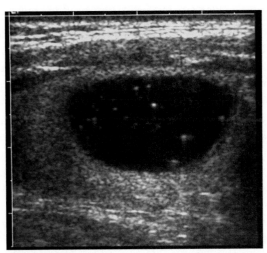

Fig. 29-4 Ultrasound image of cystic follicular adenoma.

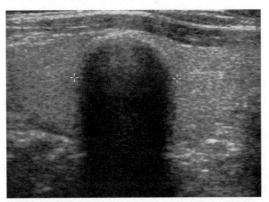

Fig. 29-5 Longitudinal image of eggshell calcification in benign nodule.

nodules that have peripheral eggshell-type calcification (Fig. 29-5).

Color Doppler, spectral Doppler, and power Doppler all have been applied to the evaluation of thyroid nodules.[10,12-14] The presence of increased flow in the nodule's periphery, or rim vascularity, may help in the initial decision of a subtle thyroid mass. However, the characterization of thyroid nodules based on Doppler findings is not definitive. For example, benign hyperplastic nodules show minimal or no flow within the nodule itself and low-velocity flow around the periphery of the nodule. Adenomas, on the other hand, show more intralesional and perilesional flow than hyperplastic nodules. However, this is true for some carcinomas as well.[15] In addition, some investigators report no correlation between pathologic findings and the presence or amount of blood flow detected with Doppler.[16] In one study, color Doppler flow patterns were believed to depend more on the size of the lesion than on the histologic type. The larger nodules, regardless of histology, had more flow than did the smaller nodules.[17]

Malignant Nodules

Sonographic Findings. Most thyroid cancer appears solid and hypoechoic. A wide, irregular halo surrounding the nodule and fine punctate internal calcifications known as *psammoma bodies* are also features commonly seen with **papillary thyroid cancer** (Fig. 29-6).[1] A study of approximately 300 patients showed that the combination of a hypoechoic solid nodule with **microcalcifications** had a 70% positive predictive value for malignant disease.[11] In addition, as discussed previously, some investigators believe that the marked

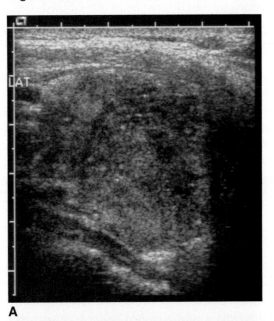

A

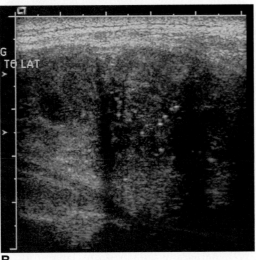

B

Fig. 29-6 A, Transverse and, B, longitudinal images of psammoma bodies in papillary thyroid cancer.

hypervascularity of many papillary carcinomas can assist in the diagnosis of these malignant diseases.[15] Papillary carcinomas are the most common of thyroid cancers; other types of cancers include **anaplastic, follicular,** and **medullary** cancers.

Fine-Needle Aspiration

Because a precise definition of the nature of a thyroid nodule on the basis of its sonographic features is difficult, in many practices, FNA is the primary method of evaluation of a palpable thyroid nodule. This procedure obtains thyroid follicular epithelial cells and minute tissue fragments for cytologic evaluation. FNA is relatively inexpensive and minimally invasive and provides more direct information than other diagnostic techniques.[18-21] In most cases, thyroid nodule FNA is performed by the clinician as an office-based outpatient procedure. It is considered a safe low-risk procedure. In one study of more than 6000 thyroid FNA procedures, only one patient had a significant complication of a neck hematoma that necessitated surgery.[19] Ultrasound guidance is used if the nodule is too poorly palpable to be accurately biopsied as an office-based procedure. When ultrasound-guided FNA and palpation are used, the typical results that can be expected are that approximately 5% of thyroid nodules will be positive for malignant disease, 10% will be suspicious for malignant disease, 70% will be negative, and 15% will be nondiagnostic.[19]

PARATHYROID GLAND

Primary hyperparathyroidism was once considered to be a rare endocrine disorder but is now recognized as a common disease. The prevalence of primary hyperparathyroidism in the United States is estimated to be 100 to 200 per 100,000 population. Women have this disease two to three times more frequently than do men, and the condition is particularly common in postmenopausal women. The parathyroid glands are the calcium-sensing organs in the body. They produce parathormone (PTH) and monitor the **serum calcium.**[22] Laboratory values that can raise suspicion for hyperparathyroidism include increased serum levels of calcium and **parathyroid hormone, hypophosphatasia,** and increased renal excretion of calcium. Nephrocalcinosis or recurrent renal stones may hint at the underlying disorder if found on ultrasound examination. Sonography is used for the preoperative localization of enlarged parathyroid glands in patients with suspected primary hyperparathyroidism from laboratory values. Primary hyperparathyroidism is caused by a single para-

thyroid adenoma in 80% to 90% of cases, by multiple gland enlargement in 10% to 20% of cases, and by parathyroid carcinoma in less than 1% of cases. Parathyroid carcinoma is rare. It is seen in less than 1% of patients with hyperparathyroidism. Malignant tumors tend to be more inhomogeneous in echotexture than do typical parathyroid adenomas, but no sonographic means of differentiating benign from malignant parathyroid disease exists.[23]

The term *secondary hyperparathyroidism* is used to describe parathyroid glands that show compensatory enlargement and hypersecretion in patients with renal failure or vitamin D deficiency. In secondary hyperparathyroidism, usually all parathyroid glands are affected.[1,22]

Normal Sonographic Anatomy

There are four paired parathyroid glands, two superior and two inferior, located in close proximity to the thyroid gland. Normal parathyroid glands, which typically measure $5.0 \times 3.0 \times 1.0$ mm in size, are similar in echogenicity to the adjacent thyroid and surrounding tissues and are difficult to visualize sonographically.

Sonographic Findings. Occasionally, normal glands are visualized in young adults. The typical parathyroid adenoma is sonographically seen as an oval solid mass of homogenous low-level echogenicity that usually measures slightly more than 1 cm in length (Fig. 29-7). However, the shape, echogenicity, internal architecture, and size can vary.

Parathyroid Adenoma

Color Doppler and power Doppler imaging of a parathyroid adenoma may show a hypervascular pattern or a peripheral vascular arc that can aid in the differentiation from hyperplastic regional lymph nodes, which have hilar flow.[24,25] Superior parathyroid adenomas are located adjacent to the posterior aspect of the mid portion of the thyroid. The location of inferior thyroid adenomas is more variable, but they usually lie in close proximity to the caudal tip of the lower pole of the thyroid. Most of these inferior adenomas are adjacent to the posterior thyroid aspect or in the soft tissues 1 to 2 cm inferior to the thyroid. Most superior and inferior adenomas are found in these typical locations, adjacent to the thyroid. One percent to 3% of adenomas are ectopic. Ectopic glands can be a cause of failure for sonographic location of the adenoma and lead to failed operations. The four most common locations for ectopic parathyroid glands are mediastinal, retrotracheal, intrathyroid, and carotid sheath/undescended.

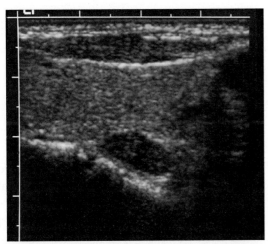

Fig. 29-7 Ultrasound image of a parathyroid adenoma.

Hyperparathyroidism and Hyperplasia

The sensitivity of sonographic parathyroid localization in primary hyperparathyroidism is between 70% and 85%.[26-29] Of the patients with hyperparathyroidism, approximately 10% have hyperplasia, the enlargement of multiple glands. The cause of **parathyroid hyperplasia** is not well understood. Although the hyperplasia involves all four glands, the glands are not involved equally and the enlargement is always asymmetric.[1]

Potential pitfalls in interpretation of parathyroid examinations include normal cervical structures, such as veins adjacent to the thyroid, the esophagus, and the longus colli muscles of the neck, which can simulate parathyroid adenomas and produce false-positive results during neck sonography. Besides these normal structures, pathologies such as thyroid nodules and cervical lymph nodes can also cause false-positive results.

LYMPH NODES

During the course of a neck ultrasound examination, normal, inflammatory, and malignant lymph nodes are readily identified with high-frequency techniques. **Adenopathy** describes enlarged nodes, and documentation of the size, shape, and internal architecture can be used to help differentiate benign from malignant lymph nodes.[30,31]

Normal Sonographic Anatomy

Enlarged benign inflammatory nodes occur commonly in the neck. Differentiation of these nodes from malignant nodes in patients with a known cervical malignant disease, such as thyroid cancer, can be difficult. Most

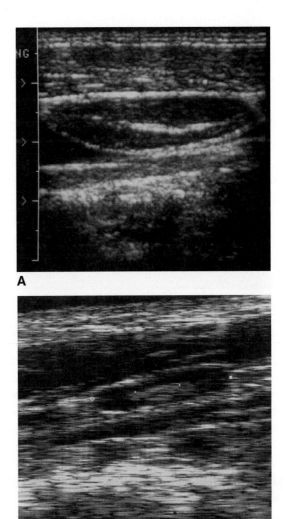

Fig. 29-8 **A** and **B**, Ultrasound images of normal cervical lymph node.

normal and inflammatory cervical lymph nodes have a flattened oblong oval shape, with their greatest dimension in the longitudinal axis (Fig. 29-8). This is presumably from compression by the adjacent longitudinally oriented tissue planes in the neck. Most normal nodes measure only a few millimeters in size.

Sonographic Findings. Sonographically visualized nodes are important features in evaluation for the distinction between benign and malignant or inflammatory nodes. In the neck, lymph node shape is probably the best method for this differentiation. It has been suggested that cervical lymph nodes with a short-to-long ratio of greater than 0.5 cm show a much higher prevalence of malignant disease than those with a ratio of less than 0.5 cm.[32] The more rounded the shape of the lymph node, the more likely it is to be malignant

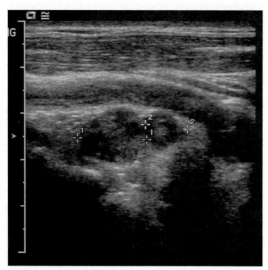

Fig. 29-9 Ultrasound image of abnormal cervical lymph node (malignant).

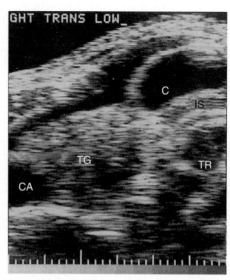

Fig. 29-10 Transverse image of neck shows thyroglossal duct cyst.

(Fig. 29-9). Care must be taken not to transfer these principles to other regions of the body; for example, the breast and axilla do have normal rounded lymph node appearances because surrounding tissue planes do not constrict the nodes. Malignant nodes often have an abnormal heterogeneous internal architecture. Microcalcifications, similar to those seen in primary malignant papillary thyroid nodule, are often seen in malignant nodes as well.

Color Doppler sonography may also demonstrate abnormal flow patterns in malignant cervical lymph nodes when compared with benign nodes. These differences can be subtle and are unlikely to be definitive.[33]

Because of the considerable overlap in the size and appearance of benign and malignant lymph nodes, percutaneous aspiration/biopsy of nodes suspicious for malignant disease can be performed.[34,35]

OTHER NECK MASSES

Other cystic neck masses may possibly develop from malformations in the cervical thoracic lymphatic system because of the complex embryology of the neck region. Some of these masses are **cystic hygroma, cavernous lymphangioma,** and simple **capillary lymphangioma.**[1] Thyroglossal duct cysts are congenital anomalies that form anterior in the midline of the neck (Fig. 29-10).[22] They are the most common, clinically significant congenital anomaly. The cyst can occur anywhere along the course of the duct from the base of the tongue to the

pyramidal lobe of the thyroid gland.[1] **Branchial cleft cysts** are usually located lateral to the thyroid gland along the anterior border of the sternocleidomastoid muscle. Most are located near the angle of the mandible, but they can occur at almost any level in the neck.[1,22]

Sonographic Findings

Cystic hygromas are most often seen as large cystic masses on the lateral aspect of the neck. They can be multiseptated and multiloculated. Cystic hygroma is differentiated from cavernous lymphangioma, capillary lymphangioma, and other lymphatic malformations based only on the size of its lymphatic spaces.

Thyroglossal duct cysts are oval or spherical masses, located in the midline of the neck and rarely larger than 2 to 3 cm.[22] These masses, along with cavernous lymphangioma and simple capillary lymphangioma, usually have echolucent cystic internal components and a thin rim; however, they can become infected, significantly changing their sonographic characteristics.[1]

SUMMARY

The ability of high-resolution ultrasound to detect small nonpalpable thyroid nodules is unsurpassed by any other imaging method. In one U.S. study, 1000 consecutive patients underwent neck sonography. Forty-one percent had sonographically visible nodules, of which only 8% were clinically palpable.[15] A high prevalence of thyroid nodules has also been detected in autopsy studies. However, the prevalence of thyroid malignant disease for these nodules was between only 2% and 4%. Of this small number of thyroid cancers, most have been proven to be tiny, incidentally discovered, occult papillary cancers.[17] Because most papillary carcinomas are slow growing and remain curable if and when they become clinically apparent at approximately 1.0 cm to 1.5 cm in size, aggressive pursuit of all of the small nodules that are detected with high-frequency ultrasound is considered impractical and imprudent. The pathologic conditions discussed in this chapter are listed in Table 29-1.

CLINICAL SCENARIO—DIAGNOSIS

■ The patient is a young man, in whom a thyroid nodule is more likely to be malignant. The mass is slow growing and painless, both also indicative of a malignant nodule. The sonographic appearance of the palpable nodule is solid and hypoechoic with microcalcification versus rim or wall calcification, also pointing toward a papillary thyroid cancer. That the patient also has several other nonpalpable masses and cervical lymph nodes visible with high-frequency sonographic techniques is not unique. This patient would likely undergo fine-needle aspiration to confirm the diagnosis of papillary thyroid cancer with subsequent thyroidectomy and cervical exploration.

Table 29-1	Pathology of Thyroid, Parathyroid, and Neck	
Pathology	**Symptoms**	**Sonographic Findings**
Adenoma	Usually asymptomatic; possibly palpable	Well-marginated, mostly cystic with internal debris
Adenopathy (cervical)	Variable dependent on cause; possibly palpable	Loss of normal flattened elongated oval lymph node shape with increase in AP dimension
Anaplastic thyroid cancer	Painful rapid enlargement of nodule; may mimic thyroiditis	Inhomogeneous hypoechoic invasive solid mass
Branchial cleft cyst	Painless mass on lateral neck; if infected, may be tender and painful	Noninfected: thin uniform wall surrounding homogeneous usually fluid filled core; infected: wall can become thick and internal fluid may be echogenic
Cystic hygroma	Painless, soft, semifirm mass in posterior neck	Usually multiloculated homogeneous cystic masses
Follicular cancer	Slow-growing nodule	Often isoechoic to normal adjacent thyroid
Goiter	Enlargement of thyroid	Nonspecific
Graves' disease	Symptoms associated with hyperthyroidism	Diffuse hypoechoic thyroid texture
Hashimoto's disease (chronic lymphocytic thyroiditis)	Painless, diffusely enlarging gland	Ill-defined hypoechoic areas separated by thickened fibrous strands; course but overall homogeneous thyroid echotexture
Parathyroid adenoma/ parathyroid hyperplasia	Increased levels of serum calcium and parathyroid hormone; hypophosphatasia; increased renal excretion of calcium; nephrocalcinosis and renal stones	Single or multiple oval homogeneous low-echogenicity solid masses; if minimally enlarged, may not be detected with ultrasound

Continued

Table 29-1	*Pathology of Thyroid, Parathyroid, and Neck—cont'd*	
Pathology	Symptoms	Sonographic Findings
Medullary thyroid cancer	Possible palpable nodule; increased calcitonin level	Discreet tumor in one lobe or numerous nodules involving both lobes; possible focal hemorrhage, necrosis, coarse calcification, and reactive fibrosis in tumor
Papillary thyroid cancer	Possible palpable mass	Variable, but almost always mass of low echogenicity; often multicentric; internal microcalcifications are common and specific finding

CASE STUDIES FOR DISCUSSION

1. A postmenopausal woman is referred for neck ultrasound for evaluation of a palpable left neck nodule. The nodule is painless and noted at the time of a routine physical examination. Ultrasound examination reveals a 1.5-cm mostly cystic nodule correlating with the palpable mass. What is the most likely diagnosis?

2. A 50-year-old woman is seen with several solid nodules incidentally noted at the time of carotid artery ultrasound. During the medical history, the clinician learns that the patient underwent neck radiation as a child for an enlarged thymus. What is the most likely diagnosis?

3. A 45-year-old woman is referred for ultrasound of a palpable neck nodule that is tender and swollen. High-resolution ultrasound reveals a rounded hypoechoic lymph node that contains microcalcifications and measures 1.2 cm in length and 1.5 cm in anteroposterior dimension that correlates with the palpable lesion. Also noted is a mostly solid thyroid nodule on the same side of the neck. What is the most likely diagnosis?

4. A 55-year-old woman is referred to the ultrasound department for evaluation of primary hyperparathyroidism. The neck ultrasound reveals an oblong hypoechoic mass adjacent to the posterior aspect of the lower third of the left thyroid lobe. What is the most likely diagnosis?

5. A 19-year-old woman ultrasound student is seen with an incidental mostly cystic thyroid nodule noted at the time of a practice scanning session. The mass is solitary and has some rim calcification. What is the most likely diagnosis?

STUDY QUESTIONS

1. A patient is seen for neck ultrasound 2 years after surgery for papillary thyroid cancer. The sonogram reveals bilateral multiple masses, presumable lymph nodes, along the carotid-jugular areas. Of note is one mass that is hypoechoic and rounded in shape. The shape and location of this mass make it most suggestive of:
   a. parathyroid adenoma
   b. thyroid adenoma
   c. malignant lymph node
   d. benign lymph node
   e. obstructed salivary duct

2. An oval solid homogeneous mass located adjacent to the posterior aspect of the midportion of the thyroid is discovered in a postmenopausal woman. The sonographic features of the mass, along with the patient gender and age, make it suspicious for:
   a. parathyroid adenoma
   b. ectopic thyroid nodule
   c. thymus gland
   d. thyroid isthmus
   e. papillary thyroid cancer

3. A patient with no significant medical history is seen with a palpable nodule in the left lobe of the thyroid. On ultrasound examination, the nodule is found to be mostly cystic but to contain debris. The features of this mass make it more likely to be:
   a. parathyroid adenoma
   b. papillary cancer

c. benign thyroid nodule
d. inflammatory lymph node
e. malignant lymph node

4. A 50-year-old patient who has undergone previous neck irradiation in his adolescence is seen with normal physical examination results. The referring physician has sent the patient for neck ultrasound because of a high-risk history. The sonogram reveals a hypoechoic solid nodule with microcalcifications. The most likely diagnosis for this mass is:
   a. parathyroid adenoma
   b. malignant thyroid nodule
   c. benign thyroid adenoma
   d. inflammatory lymph node
   e. malignant lymph node

5. A 25-year-old patient with an otherwise normal neck ultrasound has multiple bilateral masses adjacent to the carotid arteries and jugular veins. The masses are flattened, oblong, and oval shaped, with their greatest dimension in the longitudinal axis. The most likely diagnosis for these masses is:
   a. parathyroid adenomas
   b. thyroid adenomas
   c. benign lymph nodes
   d. malignant lymph nodes
   e. cystic hygroma

6. A postmenopausal woman is referred for neck ultrasound for evaluation of the parathyroid glands because of elevated parathyroid hormone and serum calcium levels. The sonogram reveals enlargement of all four glands, although the enlargement is asymmetric. This finding is indicative of:
   a. parathyroid adenoma
   b. parathyroid hyperplasia
   c. benign lymph nodes
   d. benign lymph node
   e. cystic hygroma

7. A patient with clinical hyperthyroidism is referred for sonogram for evaluation of an enlarged thyroid. The sonogram reveals a diffusely hypoechoic thyroid texture and lobulated contour. No discreet nodules are seen, but color-flow Doppler in the thyroid reveals dramatic flow in both systole and diastole. These findings are suggestive of:
   a. Graves' disease
   b. papillary cancer
   c. benign thyroid nodule

d. inflammatory lymph node
e. malignant lymph node

8. A middle-aged woman with a painless diffusely enlarged thyroid gland is referred for neck sonography. The sonogram reveals a hypoechoic but overall coarse homogeneous thyroid echotexture when compared with a normal thyroid. Also seen are multiple ill-defined hypoechoic areas separated by thickened fibrous strands. This is the appearance of:
   a. Graves' disease
   b. Hashimoto's disease
   c. goiter
   d. papillary cancer
   e. medullary cancer

9. A young child is referred to the ultrasound department for evaluation of a midline neck mass that the parents report has been present since birth. The sonogram reveals a cyst that appears adjacent to the base of the tongue. This mass should represent:
   a. cystic hygroma
   b. thyroglossal duct cyst
   c. branchial cleft cyst
   d. sternocleidomastoid muscle cyst
   e. the normal longus colli muscle

10. During a carotid artery ultrasound, the sonographer notes a 1.0-cm nodule in the left lobe of the thyroid. This mass contains fine punctate calcifications. Further examination reveals a 1.5-cm hypoechoic mass outside the thyroid gland but adjacent to the carotid artery. This mass also contains microcalcifications. Which of the following findings should the sonographer suggest to the interpreting physician?
    a. papillary thyroid cancer with regional lymph node involvement
    b. parathyroid hyperplasia with ectopic glands
    c. multinodular goiter
    d. incidental thyroid nodule and probable branchial cleft cyst with debris
    e. simultaneous thyroid and parathyroid adenomas

REFERENCES

1. McGahan JP: *Diagnostic ultrasound: a logical approach,* Philadelphia, 1998, Lippincott-Raven.
2. Reading CC: Thyroid, parathyroid and cervical nodes. In Rifkin MD, editor: *Syllabus: special course-ultrasound,* Oak Brooke, Ill, 1991, RSNA.

3. James EM, Charboneau JW, Hay ID: The thyroid. In Rumack CM, Wilson SR, Charboneau JW, editors: *Diagnostic ultrasound*, vol 1, St Louis, 1991, Mosby Year Book.

4. Kerr L: High resolution thyroid ultrasound: the value of color Doppler, *Ultrasound Q* 12:21, 1994.

5. Ralls PW, Mayekawa DS, Lee KP et al: Color-flow Doppler sonography in Graves' disease: "thyroid inferno," *AJR Am J Roentgenol* 150:781, 1988.

6. Ezzat S, Sarti DA, Cain DR et al: Thyroid incidentalomas: prevalence by palpation and ultrasonography, *Arch Intern Med* 154:1838-1840, 1994.

7. Brander A, Viikinkoski P, Nickels J et al: Thyroid gland: US screening in a random adult population, *Radiology* 181:683-687, 1991.

8. Mortenson JD, Woolner LB, Bennett WA: Gross and microscopic findings in clinically normal thyroid glands, *J Clin Endocrinol Metab* 12:1270-1280, 1955.

9. Hay ID, Reading CC, Charboneau JW: High-resolution real-time ultrasonography and unsuspected micronodular thyroid disease, *Lancet* 1:916, 1984.

10. Solbiati L, Cioffi V, Ballarati E: Ultrasonography of the neck, *Radiol Clin North Am* 30:941-954, 1992.

11. Takashima S, Fukuda H, Nomura N et al: Thyroid nodules: re-evaluation with ultrasound, *J Clin Ultrasound* 23:179-184, 1995.

12. Barreda R, Kaude JV, Fagein M et al: Hypervascularity of nontoxic goiter as shown by color-coded Doppler sonography, *AJR Am J Roentgenol* 156:199, 1991.

13. Kerr L: High resolution thyroid ultrasound: the value of color Doppler, *Ultrasound Q* 12:21-43, 1994.

14. Argalia G, D'Ambrosio F, Lucarelli F et al: Doppler thyroid nodule characterization, *Radiol Med (Torino)* 89:651-657, 1995.

15. Solbiati L, Livraghi T, Bellarati E et al: Thyroid gland. In Solbiati L, Rizzatto G, editors: *Ultrasound of superficial structures*, New York, 1995, Churchill Livingstone.

16. Clark KJ, Cronan JJ, Scola FH: Color Doppler sonography: anatomic and physiologic assessment of the thyroid, *J Clin Ultrasound* 23:215-223, 1995.

17. Shimamoto K, Endo T, Ishigaki T et al: Thyroid nodules: evaluation with color Doppler ultrasonography, *J Ultrasound Med* 12:673-678, 1993.

18. Gharib H, Goellner JR: Fine-needle aspiration biopsy of the thyroid: an appraisal, *Ann Intern Med* 118:282-289, 1993.

19. Goellner JR, Grant CS et al: Fine-needle aspiration of the thyroid: 1980 to 1986, *Acta Cytol* 31:587-590, 1987.

20. Yokozawa T, Miyauchi A, Kuma K et al: Accurate and simple method of diagnosing thyroid nodules by the modified technique of ultrasound-guided fine-needle aspiration biopsy, *Thyroid* 5:141-149, 1995.

21. Sanchez RB, van Sonnenberg E, D'Agostino HB et al: Ultrasound guided biopsy of nonpalpable and difficult to palpate thyroid masses, *J Am Coll Surg* 178:33-36, 1994.

22. Hagan-Ansert SL: *Textbook of diagnostic ultrasonography*, vol 1, ed 5, St Louis, 2001, Mosby.

23. Edmonson GR, Charboneau JW, James EM et al: Parathyroid carcinoma: high frequency sonographic features, *Radiology* 161:65, 1986.

24. Wolf RJ, Cronan JJ, Monchik JM: Color Doppler sonography: an adjunctive technique in assessment of parathyroid adenomas, *J Ultrasound Med* 13:303-308, 1994.

25. Gooding GA, Clark OH: Use of color Doppler imaging in the distinction between thyroid and parathyroid lesions, *Am J Surg* 164:51-56, 1992.

26. Hopkins CR, Reading CC: Thyroid and parathyroid imaging, *Semin Ultrasound CT MR* 16:279-295, 1995.

27. Buchwach KA, Mangum WB, Hahn FW Jr: Preoperative localization of parathyroid adenomas, *Laryngoscope* 97:13-15, 1987.

28. Attie JN, Khan A, Rumancik WM et al: Preoperative localization of parathyroid adenomas, *Am J Surg* 156:323-326, 1988.

29. Kohri K, Ishikawa Y, Kodama M et al: Comparison of imaging methods for localization of parathyroid tumors, *Am J Surg* 164:140-145, 1992.

30. Evans RM, Ahuja A, Metreweli C: The linear echogenic hilus in cervical lymphadenopathy: a sign of benignity or malignancy? *Clin Radiol* 47:262-264, 1993.

31. Vasallo P, Wernecke K, Roos N et al: Differentiation of benign from malignant superficial lymphadenopathy: the role of high-resolution ultrasound, *Radiology* 183:215-220, 1992.

32. Thnosu N, Onodo S, Isono K: Ultrasonographic evaluation of cervical lymph node metastasis in esophageal cancer with special reference to the relationship between the short to long axis ratio (S/L) and the cancer content, *J Ultrasound Med* 17:101-107, 1989.

33. Chang DG, Yang PC, Yu CJ et al: Differentiation of benign and malignant cervical lymph nodes with color Doppler sonography, *AJR Am J Roentgenol* 162:956-960, 1994.

34. Chang DG, Yang PC, Yu CJ et al: Ultrasonography and ultrasonographically guided fine-needle aspiration biopsy of impalpable cervical lymph nodes in patients with non-small cell lung cancer, *Cancer* 70:1111-1114, 1991.

35. Van Overhagen H, Lameris, JS, Berger MY et al: Supraclavicular lymph node metastasis in carcinoma of the esophagus and gastroesophageal junction: assessment with CT, US and US-guided fine-needle aspiration biopsy, *Radiology* 179:155-158, 1991.

30 Elevated Prostate Specific Antigen

ROBERT MAGNER and GARY E. CLAGETT

CLINICAL SCENARIO

■ A 56-year-old man is seen at the ultrasound department for an examination of his prostate. The patient is apprehensive because his uncle and father both have a history of prostate cancer. Within the past 2 months, he has had lethargy and lower back pain, which precipitated a visit to his doctor. His physician did a complete physical examination that included a digital rectal examination. This examination revealed a nodule posterior on the prostate.

Laboratory analysis revealed a free prostate specific antigen value of 12.

An endorectal ultrasound is performed to evaluate the nodule and shows a small hypoechoic mass with slight bulging of the posterior aspect of the capsule. The margins are poorly defined. What is the possible diagnosis for this lesion?

OBJECTIVES

■ Describe the normal sonographic appearance of the prostate.

■ Describe the sonographic appearance of benign prostatic hypertrophy.

■ Describe the sonographic appearance of prostatic inflammation and cysts.

■ List clinical symptoms associated with prostate cancer.

■ Describe the role prostate specific antigen plays in the detection of prostate cancer and its limitations.

An ultrasound of the prostate can be ordered for many reasons, including **benign** and **malignant** processes. The prostate is a small organ, yet diseases of this organ may be debilitating or lethal in some cases. Prostate **cancer** has become the most common cancer affecting North American men. Prostate cancer is the most commonly diagnosed form of cancer, other than skin cancer, among men in the United States and is second only to lung cancer as a cause of cancer-related death. The American Cancer Society estimated that 198,100 new cases of prostate cancer would be diagnosed and that 31,500 men would die of the disease in 2001.

Age, race, ethnicity, and family history are factors that affect the risk for prostate cancer. About 80% of all men with clinically diagnosed prostate cancer are 65 years or older. Because prostate cancer usually occurs at an age when conditions such as heart disease and stroke cause death, many men die with prostate cancer rather than of it. Fewer than 10% of men with prostate cancer die of the disease within 5 years of diagnosis.[1]

In most cases, the patient is a asymptomatic and may undergo a routine physical examination that reveals a **nodule** or elevated prostate specific antigen (PSA) value. Fortunately, there are tests that aid in the early detection of abnormalities of the prostate. Ultrasound is ideal for evaluation of pathologic processes of the prostate and may identify the cause of elevated PSA levels.

PROSTATE
Normal Sonographic Anatomy

The prostate is located behind the inferior arch of the pubic symphysis and in front of the rectal ampulla. The gland is shaped like an inverted pyramid. Normal prostatic parenchyma should appear homogeneous. The gland is basically divided into three zones: the transitional, central, and peripheral zones (Figs. 30-1 and 30-2). The peripheral zone comprises about 70% of the normal gland volume. In young men, this zone is isoechoic compared with the central zone and the transitional zone and is poorly seen. When the transitional zone becomes hypoechoic because of the changes of benign prostatic hypertrophy (BPH), the peripheral zone appears relatively hyperechoic and is more easily recognized.[2] Table 30-1 lists the components of a typical sonographic evaluation of the prostate.

Prostate Specific Antigen

Because prostate cancer is a huge public health burden and because most prostate cancer is asymptomatic, the current wide availability of PSA testing is fortunate.

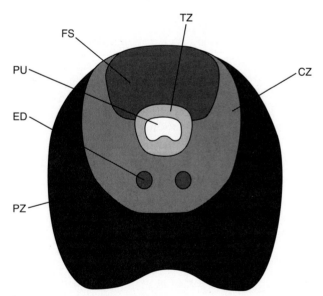

Fig. 30-1 Prostate zonal anatomy. *CZ,* Central zone; *ED,* ejaculatory ducts; *FS,* fibromuscular stroma; *PU,* periurethral glandular region; *PZ,* peripheral zone; *TZ,* transition zone.

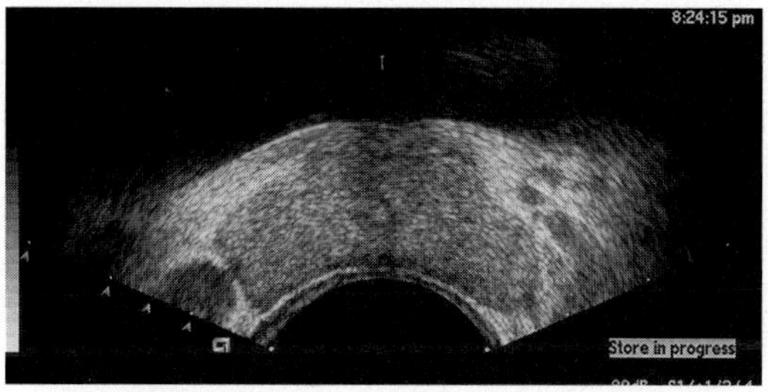

Fig. 30-2 Normal prostate.

Table 30-1	*Sonographic Evaluation of Prostate*

Imaging of prostate in two planes (sagittal and coronal)

Evaluation of gland for size, echogenicity, and symmetry

Evaluation of periprostatic fat and vessels for asymmetry

Examination of seminal vesicles in two planes for size, shape, position, symmetry, and echogenicity

Evaluation of vas deferens

Survey of perirectal space with attention to rectal wall and lumen

Screening with the digital rectal examination (DRE) and PSA is the best method for detection of prostate cancer while it is asymptomatic and at an organ-confined stage.

Prostate specific antigen is a protein produced by the cells of the prostate gland. The PSA test measures the level of PSA in the blood. The normal range for total PSA is 0.0 to 4.0 ng/ml (nanograms per millimeter of tissue).

Level of PSA has been shown to be one of the most useful tumor markers and is considered the most valuable tool available for the diagnosis of early curable organ-confined prostate cancer. Since PSA testing has become available, it has been shown to be twice as accurate as the DRE and superior to transrectal ultrasound (TRUS). Still, a normal PSA level does not exclude prostate cancer.

The PSA level can be elevated for a number of reasons, including inflammatory changes such as acute bacterial prostatitis, urinary tract infection (UTI), chronic prostatitis, and acute urinary retention. Prostate enlargement is by far the most common reason for increased PSA levels. An enlarged prostate from BPH is often the reason for elevated PSA levels. This condition, which is common as men get older (>50 years of age), is a benign enlargement of the prostate gland. BPH is not considered a precancerous state. The increase in serum PSA levels with gland volume explains most of the age-related increases in PSA. The net effect is that the bigger the prostate, the higher the PSA level.

The goal of PSA testing is identification of early cancers. On a volume per volume basis, prostate cancer contributes 10 times the amount of PSA to the serum as does benign prostate tissue. Serum PSA levels are often high in patients with prostate cancer. PSA level increases with tumor volume and stage. This increase is not the result of increased production of PSA; rather it is the result of increased diffusion (leaking) of PSA into the serum. Thus, the more aggressive the tumor, the more disruption of prostatic architecture and the higher the PSA.

As noted previously, a normal PSA level is 0.0 to 4.0 ng/ml. A PSA level of 4 to 10 ng/ml is considered slightly elevated, levels between 10 and 20 ng/ml are moderately elevated, and levels greater than 20 ng/ml are highly elevated. The higher the PSA level, the more likely cancer is present.

Several methods of evaluation of PSA are being researched to distinguish between cancerous and benign conditions and between slow-growing and fast-growing cancers. These methods are: volume-corrected PSA, PSA velocity, age-adjusted PSA, and free and attached PSA.

Volume-Corrected Prostate Specific Antigen. This PSA level is calculated during a TRUS, with the volume of the gland determined with sonography and then "corrected" with a formula. The volume-corrected PSA (volume-corrected PSA = prostate length [cm] × width [cm] × AP [cm] × 0.523 × 0.12 PSA density [PSAD]) considers the relationship of the PSA level to the size of the prostate. In other words, an elevated PSA level in a small gland may be suspicious, whereas an elevated PSA in a larger gland would be considered less suspicious.

The PSAD must also be derived to calculate the volume-corrected PSA. A PSAD of 0.1 or less is considered normal, a PSAD of 0.10 to 0.15 is intermediate, and a PSAD of higher than 0.15 is considered high (PSAD = serum PSA/prostate volume).

Prostate Specific Antigen Velocity. The PSA velocity is based on changes of PSA levels over time. A sharp rise in PSA level (>20% per year) is worrisome for malignant disease. Three PSA levels are recommended to established a PSA velocity.

Age-Adjusted Prostate Specific Antigen. Age is an important factor in determination of the meaning of increasing PSA levels. Some experts use age-adjusted PSA levels, which define a different PSA level for each 10-year age group, suggesting that men younger than 50 years of age should have a PSA of less than 2.5 ng/ml and that PSA levels up 6.5 ng/ml would be considered normal for men of age 70 years. Opinions on the accuracy of age-adjusted PSA levels vary.

Free and Attached Prostate Specific Antigen. Prostate specific antigen circulates in the blood in two forms: free or attached to a protein molecule. In benign prostate conditions, more free PSA is seen, and cancer produces more of the attached form.

Although PSA is an excellent screening tool, it still lacks sufficient sensitivity and specificity to consider it the "perfect" tumor marker. Nonetheless, screening with PSA increases the cancer detection rate by 75% over DRE alone and almost doubles the percentage in detection of tumors that are organ confined.[3] Because effective treatments exist for organ-confined disease, early treatment is believed to decrease mortality.

Benign Prostatic Hypertrophy

As a man ages, the prostate enlarges; this condition is BPH. The gland continues to grow throughout a man's life. As the prostate enlarges, the surrounding **capsule** stops it from expanding, causing the gland to press against the urethra like a clamp on a garden hose. The bladder wall subsequently becomes thicker and irritable, contracting even when it contains small amounts of urine and leading to frequent urination. As the bladder wall weakens, it loses the ability to empty itself and urine remains behind. Narrowing of the urethra and partial emptying of the bladder cause many of the problems associated with BPH. Symptoms of BPH include a hesitant or weak stream of urine, leaking/dribbling, and increased urinary frequency, particularly at night (nocturia). BPH rarely causes symptoms before age 40 years and is present in 50% of men over 50 years of age and in 95% of men over 70 years of age.[2] Nonmalignant enlargement of the prostate develops almost exclusively in the transitional zone.

Sonographic Findings. The most common appearance for BPH is enlargement of the gland with hyperechoic or hypoechoic areas or cystic regions, whereas **hyperplasia** of the **stroma** tends to be hypoechoic (Fig. 30-3). Nodules can compress both the central zone and the peripheral zone but do not infiltrate beyond the confines of the gland.[2]

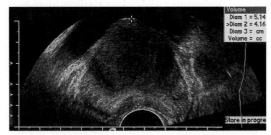

Fig. 30-3 Benign prostatic hypertrophy (hypoechoic) is identified in patient.

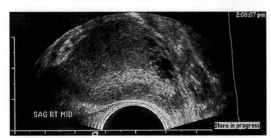

Fig. 30-4 Irregular hypoechoic lesion was confirmed to be abscess.

Inflammation

Infection of the prostate can spread as the result of a bladder or urethral infection. Symptoms of prostatitis are chills, fever, urinary urgency, and frequency. The patient may also have a urethral discharge and pain in the perineal region. During an acute phase of prostatitis, the gland remains normal in size. In severe forms, the gland becomes enlarged with extensive areas of hypoechogenic tissue.

Sonographic Findings. Prostatitis is seen with hypoechoic areas within the prostate, and reactive dilation of the periprostatic vessels may also be identified. In patients who are elderly or immunosuppressed, an abscess (Fig. 30-4) may form. This may appear as a cystic region with irregular borders.[4]

Cysts

Cystic changes can be seen in the prostate gland and usually appear as simple cysts. Ejaculatory duct dilation should not be confused with cystic changes seen in necrotic hyperplastic nodules. Ductal dilation, although rounded when viewed on axial or sagittal images, should appear tubular with perpendicular rotation of the transducer. Cysts that are caused by degeneration usually appear round.

Sonographic Findings. Cysts in the prostate should meet the same sonographic criteria for any simple cyst

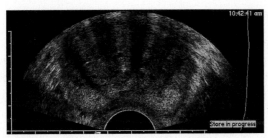

Fig. 30-5 Multiple small cysts are seen within enlarged prostate.

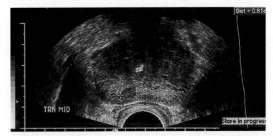

Fig. 30-7 Small hypoechoic lesion was confirmed to be prostate cancer.

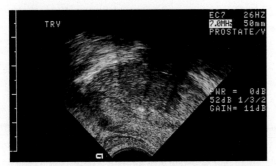

Fig. 30-6 Prostatic calcifications are identified in patient.

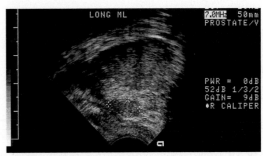

Fig. 30-8 Prostate cancer may cause contour abnormality as noted in image.

and be anechoic and smooth-walled with good through transmission (Fig. 30-5).

Calcifications

Prostatic calcifications are indicative of a benign process. If no acoustic attenuation is present, then these bright areas may not represent calcifications but may represent corpora amylacea. Corpora amylacea is a precursor of calcific formation.[5]

Sonographic Findings. Calcifications should appear as echogenic foci with acoustic shadowing (Fig. 30-6).

Prostate Cancer

Prostate cancer is particularly prevalent in western countries such as the United States. An increased incidence rate of prostate cancer is seen with increased age. Prostate cancer is an uncommon malignant disease in young men, particularly in those under 50 years. Some autopsy studies have shown that as many as 30% to 40% of all men over 60 years of age have prostate cancer.[5]

Sonographic Findings. Prostate cancer presents as an irregularly deformed area. Prostate cancers generally appear hypoechoic in relation to adjacent tissues. They may be anechoic, with irregular borders and no through transmission or hypoechoic (Fig. 30-7). Most early cancers that are detected with ultrasound are in the peripheral zone. Some prostatic cancers appear isoechoic to adjacent tissues, although asymmetry and increased Doppler flow may assist in defining these **lesions.** Tumor extension into the capsule, periprostatic lymph nodes, seminal vesicles, or surrounding tissues may be shown sonographically. If lymph nodes are detected, tumor extension should be suspected.

Most early cancers detected are located in the peripheral zone of the prostate and may be identified at only a few millimeters in size. Some lesions are quite subtle in appearance, and comparison of the echogenicity of prostate tissues is imperative.

As lesions increase in size, the echogenicity may change. Isoechoic lesions may be identified with a capsular bulge or distortion (Fig. 30-8).

The normal seminal vesicles tend to be moderate in echogenicity. Involvement of cancer can be suspected with asymmetry between the two. The seminal vesicles are normally fluid-filled structures. With tumor infiltration, this can change to a more solid composition. The criteria for determination of subtle seminal vesicle involvement is the obliteration of the "nipple" sign. Asymmetric erosion of the "nipple" has been determined to be a relatively reliable sign of tumor infiltration. This is not a consistent finding, and thus its absence may be inconclusive (Figs. 30-9 and 30-10).[5]

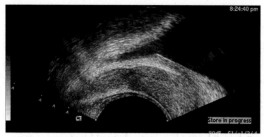

Fig. 30-9 Normal appearance of seminal vesicles.

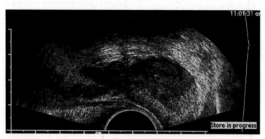

Fig. 30-10 Abnormal appearance of seminal vesicles from invasion of prostate cancer.

SUMMARY

Ultrasound is a valuable tool in evaluation of the prostate when combined with DRE and biochemical testing. Early treatment of prostate diseases may prevent debilitation to the patient. Sonography may effectively evaluate the prostate for benign and malignant neoplasms, cysts, inflammatory processes, and benign enlargement of the gland. An understanding of the symptoms and sonographic characteristics of diseases of the prostate is important.

Table 30-2 is a synopsis of the pathology of the prostate.

CLINICAL SCENARIO—DIAGNOSIS

■ Clinically the patient is seen with lethargy and lower back pain, which do not fit the clinical picture of BPH. The sonographic examination shows a hypoechoic mass with bulging of the capsule. This finding, coupled with the PSA value of 12, points to a malignant process. A biopsy of the prostate confirms the diagnosis of prostate cancer.

Table 30-2	*Pathology of Prostate*	
Pathology	**Symptoms**	**Sonographic Findings**
Prostate cancer	Usually asymptomatic; may have variety of urinary symptoms	Irregularly deformed area; generally hypoechoic
Benign prostatic hypertrophy	Hesitant or weak stream of urine, leaking/ dribbling, and increased urinary frequency, particularly at night	Enlargement of gland with hyperechoic or hypoechoic areas or cystic regions
Cysts	Usually asymptomatic	Anechoic, good posterior borders, and through transmission
Prostatitis	Chills, fever, urinary urgency and frequency	Enlargement of gland with hypoechoic areas and dilation of periprostatic vessels
Calcifications	Usually asymptomatic	Echogenic focus with posterior shadowing

---

CASE STUDIES FOR DISCUSSION

1. A 67-year-old man in generally good health has had difficulty in urination for the past 6 months. One morning he awakes in extreme discomfort unable to urinate. What is the most likely diagnosis?
2. A patient is referred to an urologist for enlargement of the prostate found during a physical examination. The digital rectal examination reveals a hard mass in the posterior/lateral aspect. The PSA value is 6.0. What is the most likely diagnosis?
3. A 70-year-old man is seen for ultrasound for evaluation of the prostate. The prostate measures 5.2 × 4.1 × 3.9 cm. What is the volume-corrected PSA?
4. A 25-year-old man has a history of dysuria and pain in the perineal region. A prostate ultrasound is performed. The gland measures 3 × 2 × 1 cm. The sonogram report notes identification of periprostatic vessels. The PSA value for this patient is 0.6. What is the most likely diagnosis?
5. An elderly man is referred to the clinic for the evaluation of his prostate. He has had some variation in urination stream, which is notably weak at times. He has been taking a prescribed medication for a cardiac condition. The PSA value is 2.1. He does have a significant history of prostatitis. The sonogram reports numerous calcific densities on the right. Immediately posterior to these calcifications is a cystic mass measuring 3 × 3 × 2 mm. What would be the most likely diagnosis?

STUDY QUESTIONS

1. A young man has a sonogram of the prostate for evaluation of dysuria and perineal pain. His white blood count is markedly elevated, and on physical examination, the prostate is boggy and the patient has extreme discomfort. The sonogram shows a cystic area with irregularly shaped border, and color Doppler shows hyperemia at the periphery of the lesion. What is the most likely diagnosis?
   a. abscess
   b. benign prostatic hypertrophy
   c. cancer of the prostate
   d. corpora amylacea
   e. ejaculatory duct cyst

2. An 87-year-old man without symptoms is seen by his physician for a routine physical examination. The physical examination results are unremarkable; however, the PSA level is markedly elevated. A sonogram of the prostate reveals a lateral solid mass. What is the most likely diagnosis?
   a. prostatitis
   b. ejaculatory duct cyst
   c. prostate cancer
   d. benign prostatic hypertrophy
   e. fibromuscular stroma

3. A 51-year-old man tells his provider that he has had difficulty in commencing urination and increased frequency in urination. The doctor performs a digital rectal examination and notes some enlargement of the prostate with no discrete nodules. The PSA value is 4.2, and the sonogram shows an enlarged prostate of 4.2 × 3.1 × 3.3 cm. What is the most likely diagnosis?
   a. prostate cancer
   b. benign prostatic hypertrophy
   c. abscess
   d. normal examination
   e. chronic prostatitis

4. A 30-year-old man has a computed tomographic scan of the abdomen/pelvis for abdominal pain. An incidental note is made of a mass in the prostate. All laboratory test results are normal, including PSA. Further evaluation of the prostate with endorectal sonography reveals an anechoic mass with sharp posterior borders and through transmission. On the sagittal orientation, the mass elongates. What is the most likely diagnosis?
   a. ejaculatory duct cyst
   b. prostate cancer
   c. benign prostatic hypertrophy
   d. corpora amylacea
   e. TURP defect

5. An elderly man is seen by his provider because he has not been feeling well for the past 3 months. He has had fatigue, increased urinary frequency, and a significant weight loss. A digital rectal examination reveals a lateral hard nodule. Ultrasound is performed and shows a large hypoechoic mass extending into

the bladder. The seminal vesicles are asymmetric with loss of the "nipple" sign on the side of the mass. What is the most likely diagnosis?

a. prostate cancer
b. advanced prostate cancer
c. benign prostatic hypertrophy
d. degenerative cystic nodule
e. seminal vessel cyst

6. A 45-year-old man reports to the emergency department with a recent history of painful urination radiating to the testicle. A rectal examination reveals some tenderness, and the emergency department provider orders a testicular and prostate ultrasound. The prostate ultrasound notes a homogeneous gland. The PSA levels are reported as normal. This would be consistent with which of the following?

a. normal examination
b. benign prostatic hypertrophy
c. chronic prostatitis
d. urinary tract infection
e. abscess

7. A 70-year-old man reports to his provider that he has had difficulty in urinating and an increase in frequency. A prostate ultrasound is ordered and reports an enlarged gland with several cystic regions in the left portion of the gland. What would be the most likely diagnosis?

a. normal examination
b. benign prostatic hypertrophy
c. prostate cancer
d. ejaculatory duct cyst
e. Gleason stage II mass

8. An elderly man receives results from his provider that his PSA is significantly elevated. What is the most common reason for his PSA results?

a. prostate cancer
b. prostatitis
c. prostate infection
d. benign prostatic hypertrophy
e. atrophic prostatic hypertrophy

9. A patient has a serum PSA value of 3.6. The measurements of this patient's prostate on endorectal sonography are as follows: anteroposterior, 3.4 cm; transverse, 5.2 cm; and longitudinal, 4.8 cm. What is the volume of this patient's prostate? What is the volume-corrected PSA for this patient?

10. Is the serum PSA value of the patient in question 9 appropriate for the size of the prostate?

ACKNOWLEDGMENTS
To my mother, Sheila Magner, who has left me with wonderful memories and whose support and encouragement guided me to where I am today. Last but not least to my family Sue, Anthony, Julie, and Daniel, for their love and support.

REFERENCES
1. Division of Cancer Prevention and Control (DCPC): http://www.cdc.gov/cancer/prostate/prostate.htm, retrieved September 11, 2003.
2. McGahan J, Goldberg B: *Diagnostic ultrasound: a logical approach*, Philadelphia, 1998, Lippincott-Raven.
3. Altruis Biomedical Network: http://www.E-prostate.net, retrieved August 12, 2003.
4. Prostatitis 2000: http://www.prostatitis2000.org/eng/metodiche1.htm, retrieved August 12, 2003.
5. Rifken MD: *Ultrasound of the prostate*, New York, 1988, Raven Press.

V   MISCELLANEOUS

31

Hip Dysplasia

CHARLOTTE HENNINGSEN

CLINICAL SCENARIO

■ A 4-week-old female infant is seen for a hip ultrasound to rule out hip dysplasia from a history of a breech presentation in utero. The ultrasound of the left hip reveals the finding in Fig. 31-1. What is the diagnosis and what is the possible treatment, if any, for this infant?

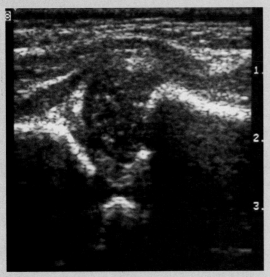

Fig. 31-1 Coronal/neutral view of hip shows relationship of femoral head to acetabulum.

OBJECTIVES

■ Identify the normal anatomy of infant hips.
■ List the risk factors associated with infant hip dysplasia.
■ Describe the clinical maneuvers used in evaluation for hip dysplasia.
■ Describe the sonographic protocol for imaging of infant hips.
■ Differentiate hip laxity, subluxation, and dislocation.

GLOSSARY OF TERMS

Abduction: the act of moving an extremity away from the body

Adduction: the act of moving an extremity towards the body

Oligohydramnios: a decreased amount of amniotic fluid that may restrict fetal movement

Primigravida: first pregnancy

Teratologic: caused by a congenital or developmental anomaly

Torticollis: a condition in which the head tilts to one side because of abnormal contraction of the muscles

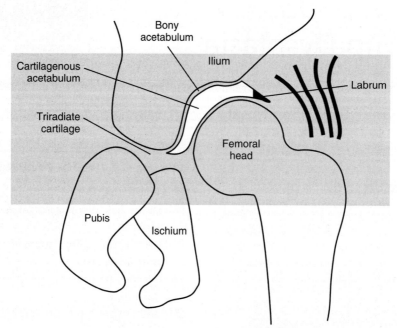

Fig. 31-2 Normal hip anatomy.

Every newborn examination includes an evaluation of the infant's hips for assessment for developmental dysplasia of the hip (DDH). This chapter explores the risk factors for DDH and the clinical examination that may be used to identify DDH. The various modes of testing, including ultrasonography, are examined, in addition to the types of treatment available on the basis of the severity of the disease. The sonographic evaluation of infant hips also includes a review of normal hip anatomy and imaging protocol for evaluation of DDH.

ANATOMY OF THE HIP

The hip forms from the embryonic mesoderm and is comprised of the femoral head and the acetabulum. The femoral head is cartilaginous at birth and begins to ossify between 2 and 8 months, with ossification occurring earlier in females.[1] The acetabulum is comprised of cartilage and bone. The bony acetabulum (Fig. 31-2) consists of the ilium, the ischium, and the pubis, which is joined by a growth plate known as the triradiate cartilage. The cartilaginous labrum is located at the acetabular rim and extends over the superolateral aspect of the femoral head.

At birth, the hip has a large cartilaginous component and the femoral head is more shallow in its relationship to the acetabulum. The hip its therefore subject to molding, especially in the first 6 weeks of life.[1] The normal development of the hip is contingent on the femur having adequate contact with the acetabulum without an abnormal amount of stress. When the femoral head is subluxed or dislocated for a significant amount of time, the acetabulum becomes increasingly dysplastic, the femoral head becomes deformed, and the supporting ligaments also deform.

The purpose of early treatment of abnormal hips is to position the hip so that the femoral head and acetabulum can develop normally, avoiding possible surgery and disability. Clinical evaluation and identification of risk factors can be used to identify those infants at risk for development of hip dysplasia. Ultrasound evaluation can be used to further define those infants who will benefit from treatment and to follow their progress. Screening for hip dysplasia is usually reserved for those infants with an abnormal clinical examination or for those infants with identified risk factors to avoid overtreatment of infants with physiologic laxity.

DEVELOPMENTAL DYSPLASIA OF THE HIP

Developmental dysplasia of the hip describes a spectrum of abnormalities that involve an abnormal relationship of the femoral head to the acetabulum, which includes mild instability, subluxation, and frank dislocation. DDH has also been referred to as congenital hip dysplasia, although this is a misnomer because hip dysplasia may develop after birth. The overall incidence rate of DDH is 0.6:1000 newborns, but significant geographic variability exists.[1]

Hip instability is associated with joint laxity and may be identified in newborns affected by maternal hormones. This laxity often resolves within the first few weeks of birth and necessitates no treatment. Subluxation of the hip refers to a femoral head that is shallow in location, allowing it to glide within the confines of the acetabulum. Hip dislocation is defined as a femoral head that is located outside of the acetabulum and may be reducible or irreducible. Hip dislocation can also be associated with congenital neurologic or musculoskeletal anomalies, including spina bifida, arthrogryposis, and numerous syndromes, and is referred to as *teratologic hips.*

Risk Factors

Many of the risk factors associated with DDH are related to the inability of the fetus or newborn to move freely. These conditions include pregnancies affected by **oligohydramnios** (including serious renal anomalies), breech presentation, first pregnancy **(primigravida)**, and high birth weight. Other factors include infants who are swaddled, infants born in the cold seasons of the year, female infants, and infants with **torticollis.** Laplanders and American Indians have an increased incidence rate of DDH. The left hip is affected more commonly than is the right, and DDH is bilateral in 20% of cases.[2] Family history is also an important factor in identification of those infants at risk for development of DDH. Conversely, infants at decreased risk for development of DDH include the black population and infants who are carried on the waist with the legs flexed and abducted.

Clinical Evaluation

Evaluation for hip dysplasia is part of every newborn examination. The accuracy of the evaluation is affected by the experience of the physician; and infants in whom hip dysplasia does not develop until after birth may have normal examination results. Clinical findings associated with DDH include asymmetric skin folds of the thighs and one knee appearing lower than the other when the hips and knees are flexed. The subluxed or dislocated hip appears shorter (known as the *Galeazzi* or *Allis' sign*).

Clinical maneuvers can also be used to detect hip instability and dislocation, but performance of these maneuvers may be difficult if the infant is not relaxed. The two maneuvers are performed with the infant's hips and knees flexed, and one hip should be examined at a time. The Ortolani maneuver (Fig. 31-3) involves **abduction** of the thigh while the hip is gently pulled anteriorly. If the hip is dislocated, the hip may relocate

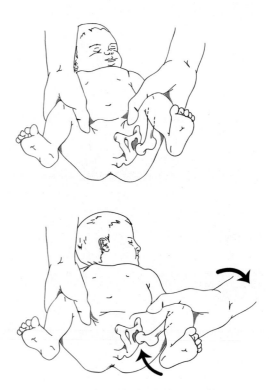

Fig. 31-3 Ortolani maneuver.

into the acetabulum with a palpable (and possibly audible) "clunk." The Barlow maneuver (Fig. 31-4) is performed with **adduction** of the hip with a gentle posterior push in an effort to solicit subluxation or dislocation in an abnormal hip.[3] These maneuvers are similar to those performed in a dynamic ultrasound evaluation.

SONOGRAPHIC EVALUATION OF INFANT HIPS

The technique for imaging the infant hip was initially described by Graf who used a static approach. Harcke developed a dynamic approach to sonographic imaging. The two approaches were combined to develop a minimum standard examination.[4] Imaging protocol should incorporate two orthogonal views with one view that includes stress views, which typically include the coronal/neutral or coronal/flexion view and the transverse flexion view. The transverse/neutral view and measurements are considered optional, and anterior views have also been described. Particular attention should be taken to image each view in the correct plane and with the appropriate anatomy identified because a minimal shift in the image may lead to an inaccurate diagnosis. This chapter defines the images for the minimum standard examination and describes normal and abnormal findings.

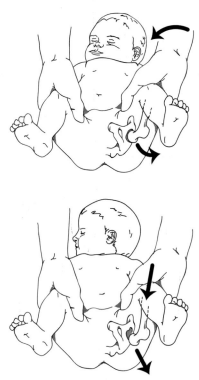

Fig. 31-4 Barlow maneuver.

Infant hips may be examined sonographically during the first year of life or until the ossification of the femoral head prevents adequate visualization. A linear transducer is preferred to avoid distortion and to cover a broader field of view. The highest frequency transducer should be used, and a 7.5-MHz transducer is recommended for infants from birth to 3 months of age, although 10-MHz transducers may be used in premature infants.

A successful examination requires that the infant be relaxed for accurate stress maneuvers. Infants should be imaged in a warm environment with distracters such as toys, pacifiers, or bottles. A parent should be available and visible to the infant to assist in maintaining a relaxed environment. The infant should be placed in a supine, slightly oblique or lateral decubitus position to accommodate the lateral and posterolateral position of the transducer. Bolsters should be used as needed to stabilize the infant's position. Harcke and Grissom[5] suggest that the ultrasound professional scan the left hip with the right hand while maneuvering the hip with the left hand and scan the right hip with the left hand while performing stress maneuvers with the right hand. Because two hands are needed to adequately image and maneuver the hip, sonographic evaluation is often a joint effort between the sonographer and radiologist. The second person may assist in maneuvering the hip or producing the images, depending on institutional protocol. A foot switch may also be used to acquire the images during stress maneuvers.

Coronal/Neutral View

The coronal/neutral view of the hip is obtained with placement of the transducer in a coronal plane at the lateral aspect of the hip. The hip is maintained in a physiologic neutral position with approximately 15 to 20 degrees of flexion. The ultrasound image should demonstrate the midportion of the acetabulum, with the ilium appearing as a straight line parallel to the transducer. The junction of the ilium and triradiate cartilage should be clearly identified, and the cartilaginous tip of the labrum should be visualized. The femoral metaphysis is also seen in this plane, which differentiates this view from the coronal/flexion view. A normal hip (Fig. 31-5, *A*) shows the hypoechoic femoral head resting against the acetabulum. An abnormal hip (Fig. 31-5, *B*) migrates laterally and superiorly.

In this view, the alpha angle (Fig. 31-5, *C*) may be obtained with measurement of a line along the lateral aspect of the ilium with respect to the slope of the acetabulum. According to the Graf classification, a normal hip would have an alpha angle of 60 degrees or more (type I). A type II hip (50 to 60 degrees) would reflect a physiologic immaturity in infants less than 3 months of age and would require follow-up but no treatment. If a type II hip is identified in an infant of more than 3 months of age, then treatment would be necessary. A type III hip describes subluxation with a shallow acetabulum and an alpha angle of more than 50 degrees, and a type IV hip is a dislocated hip that lacks contact between the acetabulum and the femoral head.[1,3,4,6] With the minimum standard examination, measurements are optional; however, they do provide a quantitative baseline for follow-up purposes.

In this view, a more subjective assessment method may be used with noting how deep the femoral head is located within the acetabulum. A normal hip shows at least 50% of femoral head coverage by the acetabulum. This can be assessed by drawing a line across the ilium through the femoral head and identifying whether 50% of the femoral head is below the line. On the basis of the amount of femoral head coverage, the hip can be classified as sitting deep, intermediate, or shallow. A visual assessment of the acetabulum and any irregularities should also be described. The acetabulum becomes progressively deformed when hip dysplasia is present, and fibrofatty tissue develops (appearing as a soft tissue echoes) between the femoral head, thus preventing reduction of the hip.[4]

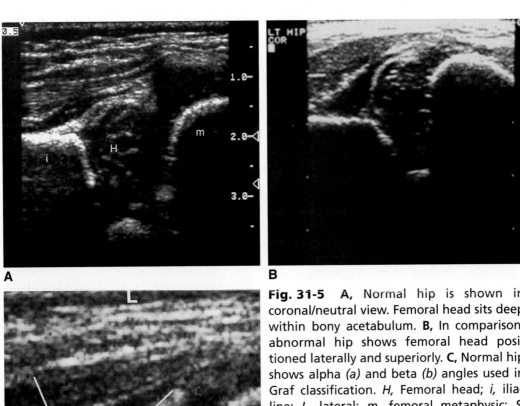

Fig. 31-5 **A,** Normal hip is shown in coronal/neutral view. Femoral head sits deep within bony acetabulum. **B,** In comparison, abnormal hip shows femoral head positioned laterally and superiorly. **C,** Normal hip shows alpha *(a)* and beta *(b)* angles used in Graf classification. *H,* Femoral head; *i,* iliac line; *L,* lateral; *m,* femoral metaphysic; *S,* superior.

Coronal/Flexion View

The coronal/flexion view is also imaged from the coronal plane, although the hip is flexed at a 90-degree angle. The sonographic appearance is similar to the coronal/neutral view, with the exception of visualization of the bony metaphysis. The lateral margin of the ilium should appear as a straight line, and the femoral head should be identified resting within the acetabulum (Fig. 31-6). As in the coronal/neutral view, the cartilaginous tip of the labrum is visualized. In this view, stress maneuvers can be performed for assessment of instability of the hip. The stress maneuvers performed are similar to the Ortolani and Barlow maneuvers to test for the reduction of a dislocated hip or to identify whether or not the hip can be dislocated. The infant must be relaxed for accurate assessment of instability. Gentle guiding of the hip, moving of the hip from a neutral to flexed position, and abducting and adducting while administering a gentle push/pull are also important. The sonographer should observe and document the absence or presence of any instability identified in real time. Notation of whether or not a dislocated hip will reduce is also important. The acetabulum should again be evaluated for any evidence of dysplasia.[5]

Transverse/Flexion View

The transverse/flexion view is obtained with the infant's hip flexed at a 90-degree angle. The transducer is rotated

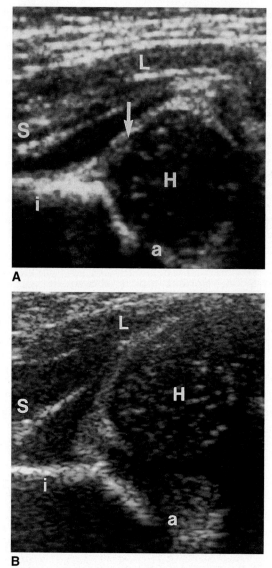

Fig. 31-6 **A,** Normal coronal/flexion view is identified with femoral head resting against acetabulum. **B,** Dislocated hip shows soft tissue echoes in acetabulum that may prevent hip from being reduced without surgical intervention. *a,* Acetabulum; *H,* femoral head; *i,* iliac line; *L,* lateral; *S,* superior; *arrow,* labrum.

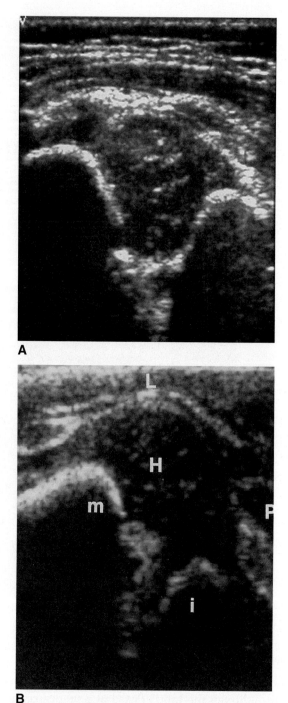

Fig. 31-7 **A,** Normal transverse/flexion view shows U-shaped configuration that is not present in, **B,** dislocated hip. *H,* Femoral head; *i,* ischium; *m,* femoral metaphysic; *L,* lateral; *P,* posterior.

90 degrees from a coronal to a transverse plane and should be positioned slightly posterolaterally over the hip. The infant may need to be slightly oblique to accommodate the transducer position. The ultrasound image shows the femoral head and metaphysis, which is identified anterior to the femoral head; and the ischium is identified posterior to the femoral head. The normal hip appears to have a U-shaped configuration (Fig. 31-7, *A*) as the metaphysis and ischium surround the femoral head. An abnormal hip (Fig. 31-7, *B*) lacks this

appearance as the femoral head shifts laterally with subluxation and posterolaterally with dislocation. Stress maneuvers should be used as described in the coronal/flexion view to assess for instability and the ability to reduce a dislocated hip.[4]

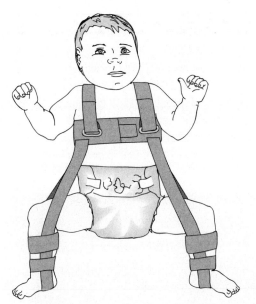

Fig. 31-8 Pavlik harness is often used in treatment of hip dysplasia.

TREATMENT

Treatment of abnormal hips may vary depending on the age at diagnosis and the severity of hip dysplasia. Some degree of laxity may be identified in the newborn period and resolve without intervention, although follow-up is necessary to ensure resolution of a subluxation. The triple diaper technique has also been used to prevent adduction without evidence of improvement when compared with infants without treatment within the first 3 weeks of life.[2] Treatment for hip dysplasia is indicated for infants with subluxation beyond 3 weeks of life and for infants with hip dislocation.

The Pavlik harness (Fig. 31-8) is the most common device used in the treatment of hip dysplasia; it prevents adduction of the hips and is used for infants with hip subluxations and reducible dislocations. The typical treatment period is 3 months, during which time the infant may be monitored regularly with radiography or ultrasound and adjustments to the harness may be made as necessary. When treatment is followed with ultrasound, the Pavlik harness should initially be left in place. As the infant is weaned from the harness, the sonographer may be directed to perform the ultrasound examination without the harness. Infants who do not have successful treatment with the Pavlik harness and those infants with irreducible dislocations may require an abduction brace, casting, or operative reduction.[2]

SUMMARY

Early diagnosis and treatment of hip dysplasia can reduce infant morbidity. Risk factors or abnormal clinical examination results can be used to identify those infants who will achieve the greatest benefit from ultrasound screening. Sonography is an important tool in the diagnosis, especially in those infants at risk with normal clinical examination results. A thorough knowledge of imaging technique is necessary to ensure reliability and reproducibility. This is of particular importance when ultrasound is used to follow the effectiveness of treatment.

CLINICAL SCENARIO—DIAGNOSIS

■ The femoral head is located in a shallow position within the acetabulum but is not completely dislocated. With proper patient compliance and follow-up for necessary adjustments, this infant may have successful treatment with a Pavlik harness.

CASE STUDIES FOR DISCUSSION

1. A family practice resident examines a newborn in the first day of life. The hips feel unstable, and an ultrasound is ordered. The ultrasound reveals a Graf type II hip with an alpha angle of 54 degrees. What is the appropriate treatment for this infant?

2. An infant is seen with a positive Allis' sign on the left side. Clinical examination is limited because of the fussy nature of the infant at the time of the appointment. An ultrasound is ordered to rule out hip dysplasia. The sonographer identifies a normal right hip and a dislocated left hip. As the sonographer performs stress maneuvers, the hip remains persistently out of the acetabulum. What are the treatment options for this infant?

3. A 5-week-old infant is referred for ultrasound to rule out hip dysplasia because of a positive family history. Ultrasound reveals the finding in Fig. 31-9. What is the diagnosis and treatment plan?

4. A sonographer presents the hip ultrasound image in Fig. 31-10 to the radiologist. The radiologist asks the sonographer to repeat the view. Can you explain why?

5. A mother brings her 6-week-old child in for a 2-week follow-up after placement of the Pavlik harness. Should the sonographer image the infant in or out of the harness?

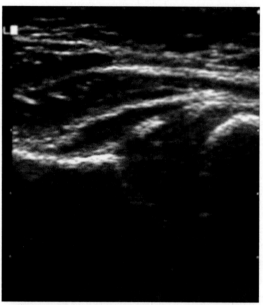

Fig. 31-10   Coronal/neutral view of hip.

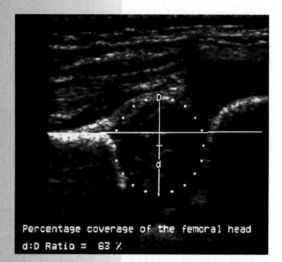

Fig. 31-9   Coronal/neutral view identifies percentage of femoral head contained within acetabulum.

STUDY QUESTIONS

1. Which of the following describes the type of hip abnormality in which the femoral head sits in a shallow position in the acetabulum, freely gliding as the hip is manipulated?
   a. dislocation
   b. dysplasia
   c. laxity
   d. subluxation
   e. teratologic

2. Which of the following views is taken at the lateral aspect of the infant with the transducer oriented parallel to the long axis of the body with the hip in a relaxed position?
   a. coronal/flexion view
   b. coronal/neutral view
   c. sagittal/neutral view
   d. transverse/flexion view
   e. transverse/neutral view

3. The risk factors for developmental dysplasia of the hip include which of the following?
   a. breech position, warm climate, congenital torticollis
   b. American Indian, family history, male gender
   c. black population, female gender, primigravida
   d. high birth weight, spina bifida, cold season
   e. Laplander, multigravida, oligohydramnios

4. The bony acetabulum consists of which of the following?
   a. femoral head, ilium, labrum
   b. ilium, ischium, pubis
   c. ischium, metaphysis, pubis
   d. metaphysis, labrum, femoral head
   e. pubis, labrum, ilium

5. Which of the following maneuvers is performed to reduce a dislocated hip?
   a. Allis' maneuver
   b. Barlow maneuver
   c. Graf maneuver
   d. Harcke maneuver
   e. Ortolani maneuver

6. Which of the following views are combined with stress maneuvers for evaluation of hip stability?
   a. anterior/neutral, coronal/neutral
   b. coronal/flexion, transverse/flexion
   c. coronal/flexion, coronal/neutral
   d. transverse/flexion, transverse/neutral
   e. transverse/flexion, anterior/flexion

7. Which of the following Graf classifications would include newborns with physiologic laxity?
   a. type 0
   b. type I
   c. type II
   d. type III
   e. type IV

8. A newborn infant, 2 weeks of age, is seen for hip ultrasound with a history of a "click" on clinical examination. The alpha angle measures 60 degrees on the right and 62 degrees on the left. This would be consistent with which of the following?
   a. right hip, type II; left hip, type I
   b. right hip, type I; left hip, type I
   c. right hip, shallow; left hip, deep
   d. right hip, type II; left hip, type II
   e. right hip, type III, left hip, type II

9. Which of the following views normally has a U shape?
   a. anterior/neutral
   b. coronal/neutral
   c. coronal/flexion
   d. transverse/neutral
   e. transverse/flexion

10. Which of the following would meet the criteria of the minimum standard examination?
    a. coronal/neutral view with stress maneuvers; coronal/flexion view
    b. coronal/flexion view with stress maneuvers; coronal/neutral view
    c. coronal/neutral view with alpha angle; transverse/flexion view
    d. transverse/flexion view with stress maneuvers; transverse neutral view
    e. coronal/neutral view with alpha angle; coronal/flexion view

REFERENCES

1. Gerscovich EO: Infant hip in developmental dysplasia: facts to consider for a successful diagnostic ultrasound examination, *Appl Radiol* March:18-25, 1999.
2. Guille JT, Pizzutillo PD, MacEwen GD: Developmental dsyplasia of the hip from birth to six months, *J Am Acad Orthop Surg* 8:232-242, 2000.
3. French LM, Dietz FR: Screening for developmental dysplasia of the hip, *Am Fam Physician* 60:177-184, 1999.
4. Rumack CM, Wilson SR, Charboneau JM: *Diagnostic ultrasound*, vol 2, ed 2, St Louis, 1998, Mosby.
5. Harcke HT, Grissom LE: Pediatric hip sonography, *Radiol Clin North Am* 37:787-796, 1999.
6. Weintroub S, Grill F: Ultrasonography in developmental dysplasia of the hip, *J Bone Joint Surg* 82A:1004-1018, 2000.

32

Neonatal Neurosonography

CHARLOTTE HENNINGSEN

CLINICAL SCENARIO

■ A woman delivers twins at 24 weeks' gestation. One of the twins dies at the time of birth. The other twin is placed in the neonatal intensive care unit, and laboratory test results reveal a falling hematocrit level. At 2 weeks of age, a neonatal head ultrasound is performed at bedside. The ultrasound reveals the findings in Fig. 32-1, *A*. A second examination is performed 1 week later and shows the changes noted in Fig. 32-1, *B* and *C*. What is the diagnosis and what is the prognosis for this infant?

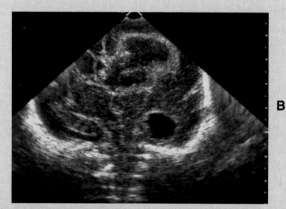

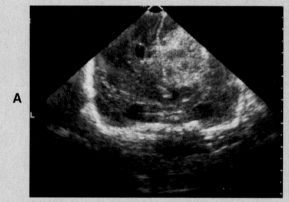

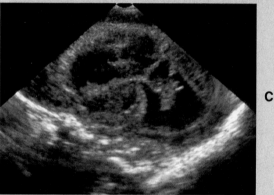

Fig. 32-1 Female infant born at 24 weeks' gestation. **A,** Coronal image was taken at 14 days. Second ultrasound was performed 1 week later. **B,** Coronal and, **C,** sagittal images show pertinent information.

OBJECTIVES

■ List the images that should routinely be taken in evaluation of a neonatal brain.

■ Differentiate the sonographic findings of intraventricular hemorrhage and periventricular leukomalacia.

■ Identify congenital anomalies seen in the neonatal brain.

■ Recognize the normal sonographic anatomy of the neonatal spine.

■ Define the sonographic criteria of a tethered cord.

GLOSSARY OF TERMS

Achondroplasia: the most common, nonlethal dwarfism

Aqueductal stenosis: a stricture of the aqueduct of Sylvius; the lateral and third ventricles are dilated

Asphyxia: severe hypoxia

Brainstem: includes midbrain, pons, and medulla oblongata

Caudothalamic notch, or caudothalamic groove: the region at which the thalamus and caudate nucleus join; the most common location of germinal matrix hemorrhage

Cebocephaly: hypotelorism (closely spaced eyes) and a normally placed nose with a single nostril

Cerebral palsy: a spectrum of disorders that occurs with brain dysfunction at the time of birth or in the neonatal period; can include spasticity, diplegia, hemiplegia (paralysis of half of the body), quadriplegia, seizure disorder, and varying degrees of mental retardation; decreased sight, vision, and impaired speech may also occur

Conus medullaris: the caudal end of the spinal cord

Cutaneous: relating to the skin

Cyclopia: one orbit or the fusion of two orbits

Diplegia: paralysis of both sides of the body

Ethmocephaly: cyclopia or hypotelorism with a proboscis (fleshy, trunklike appendage) or double proboscis

Forebrain, or prosencephalon: the part of the brain that includes the cerebral hemispheres and thalamus

Hematocrit: a measure of blood volume that specifically relates to the percentage of red blood cells; decreases with significant hemorrhage

Hypoxia: decreased oxygen

Interhemispheric fissure, or falx cerebri: separates the cerebral hemispheres

Quadriplegia: paralysis that includes the upper and lower extremities and the trunk

Spina bifida aperta: open (non–skin-covered lesions) neural tube defects, such as myelomeningocele and meningocele

Spina bifida occulta: closed (skin-covered lesions) neural tube defects, such as spinal lipoma and tethered cord

Ventriculomegaly: enlargement of the ventricles in the brain

Neonatal neurosonography is an effective diagnostic imaging method because of portability, low cost, non-invasiveness, and lack of radiation. Sonography of the neonate is often performed for findings noted in an abnormal obstetric ultrasound, for an infant born prematurely, or for abnormal physical examination results. Imaging of the neonatal head may confirm a congenital anomaly or be used to look for changes associated with **hypoxia** or **asphyxia** related to a premature or difficult delivery. Infants may not have been imaged in utero and at the time of delivery may show an abnormal behavior or appearance that precipitates a search for abnormal brain anatomy. Physical examination of a newborn may also reveal findings suggestive of **spina bifida occulta,** leading to sonographic evaluation for tethered cord. This chapter covers the most common neonatal brain and spine abnormalities encountered by sonographers. In addition, limited congenital abnormalities of the central nervous system are explored. Additional anomalies of the head and spine as identified in the fetus are found in Chapters 23 and 25.

NEONATAL HEAD
Imaging Technique

Neonatal imaging of the brain is an important aspect of the evaluation of infants at risk for diseases and anomalies. It is often performed on infants who are premature or critically ill. With a neonatal head ultrasound, care should be taken to maintain body temperature with warm gel, no unnecessary exposure, and minimization of scanning time. Efforts to minimize stress on the infant are imposed by maintaining a quiet, dark atmosphere; and care should be taken against disruption of that environment. Many infants have immunosuppression, so proper transducer disinfection and hand washing between infants are imperative for prevention of the spread of infection.

The neonatal imaging technique should include the selection of the highest frequency possible without sacrifice of adequate penetration. Transducers of 7.5 to 10 MHz are typically selected for premature infants, and 5-MHz transducers are usually adequate for infants with larger heads. In addition, transducers designed with a small transducer footprint are especially useful with imaging through small fontanelles. Most commonly, neonatal brain imaging is accomplished through the anterior fontanelle in the coronal, sagittal, and parasagittal planes. Parasagittal views are lateral to the midline (true sagittal) plane but are referred to as sagittal images in this chapter. Alternate views may be obtained with imaging through the posterior fontanelle for anatomy and pathology in the posterior and inferior aspects of the head. Axial views of the brain may be used with imaging through the mastoid.

Six standard coronal views exist for imaging from the anterior to the posterior aspect of the brain. Anterior coronal images should be taken (Fig. 32-2, A) at the level of the frontal lobes, anterior to the frontal horns of the lateral ventricle, and (Fig. 32-2, B) at the level of the frontal horns, caudate nucleus, cavum septum pellucidum (CSP), and corpus callosum. Midcoronal images include (Fig. 32-2, C) the lateral ventricles, third ventricle, CSP, and corpus callosum and (Fig. 32-2, D) should be slightly angled posterior to include the choroids plexus at the posterior aspects of the lateral ventricle and the roof of the third ventricle. The tentorium and cisterna magna are also noted in the midcoronal views. Posterior coronal images of the head include the (Fig. 32-2, E) glomus of the choroids in the trigone region of the lateral ventricles and (Fig. 32-2, F) posterior to the ventricles, including the occipital lobes of the brain.

Five standard sagittal views exist for imaging midline structures and the right and left lateral brain. A midline image (Fig. 32-3, A) of the brain includes the corpus callosum, CSP, third and fourth ventricles, and cerebellar vermis. Lateral views of right and left sides of the brain should include the **caudothalamic notch** (Fig. 32-3, B) and lateral ventricle (Fig. 32-3, C), showing the frontal, temporal, and occipital horns; and a steeply angled view of the brain (Fig. 32-3, D), including the sylvian fissure.

INTRACRANIAL HEMORRHAGE

Intracranial hemorrhage may be seen in premature and full-term infants and may be the sequela of an ischemic or hypoxic event, trauma, infarction, vascular malformation, or bleeding disorder. Subependymal hemorrhage is a common event in premature infants, and when the hemorrhage extends into the ventricle and brain parenchyma, devastating neurologic effects may result. Ultrasound imaging is frequently used in infants at increased risk for development of an intracranial hemorrhage with screening of low–birth weight (<1500 g) or premature (<30 weeks gestational age) infants.[1]

Approximately 80% of hemorrhages occur within the first 3 days of life, and screening for hemorrhage is usually performed at 1 week of age.[2]

The most common location of the origin of intracranial hemorrhage is in the germinal matrix, in the subependymal region, at the head of the caudate nucleus. This embryonic structure contains a fragile network of vessels that are prone to rupture with changes in pressure. The germinal matrix is greatest in size between 24 and 32 weeks' gestation and progressively decreases in size with only a small amount present at term, which explains why the risk for hemorrhage is greatest in preterm infants.

The severity of intracranial hemorrhage may be classified by the extent and location of the hemorrhage and the presence of ventricular enlargement. A hemorrhage that is subependymal (Fig. 32-4, A) without **ventriculomegaly** is classified as grade I. A grade II hemorrhage is defined by extension into the ventricle (Fig. 32-4, B, C, and D) without ventriculomegaly. An intraventricular hemorrhage with ventriculomegaly (Fig. 32-5) is classified as grade III, and a grade IV hemorrhage (Fig. 32-6) is defined as a hemorrhage that extends into the brain parenchyma with or without associated ventriculomegaly.

The prognosis of intracranial hemorrhage is variable depending on the extent of the bleed and includes an increase in morbidity and mortality. Grade I and grade II hemorrhages may spontaneously regress without evidence of long-term effects. Infants with grade III and IV hemorrhages are more likely to have neurologic effects, which range from developmental delays and behavioral problems to spastic motor deficits that may be accompanied by intellectual deficits.

Treatment for intracranial hemorrhage primarily focuses on controlling hydrocephalus to decrease neurologic deficits. Medical management may be used to decrease production of cerebral spinal fluid (CSF). Lumbar puncture can be used to drain excess CSF, and percutaneous ventricular punctures may be performed. Long-term treatment usually involves the placement of a ventricular shunt for drainage of CSF into the peritoneal cavity.[3] Although this treatment is considered effective, it is not without complications, such as increased infections and shunt blockage.

Sonographic Findings

Sonographic imaging for hemorrhage should identify the absence or presence of hemorrhage, ventricular enlargement, and parenchymal extension. Most commonly, a small, echogenic hemorrhage is identified in the region

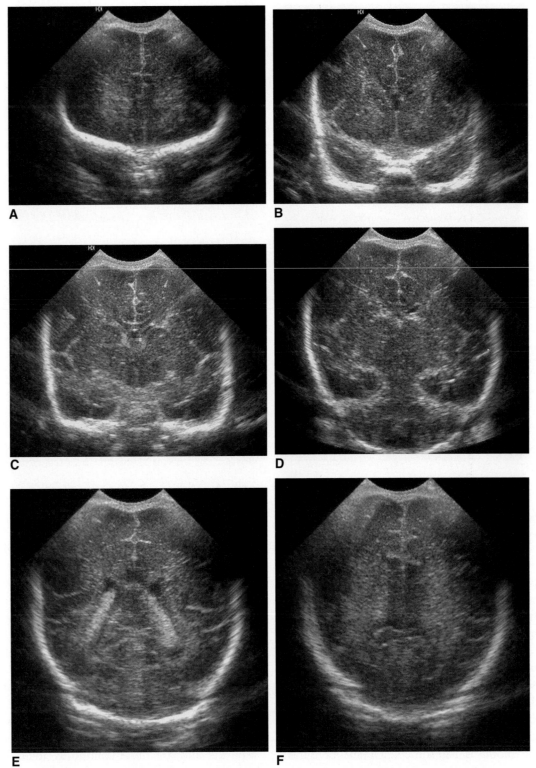

Fig. 32-2 Coronal views of neonatal head. **A** and **B,** Anterior coronal. **C** and **D,** Midcoronal. **E** and **F,** Posterior coronal. (Courtesy Douglas Dumas, Florida Hospital, Orlando, Florida.)

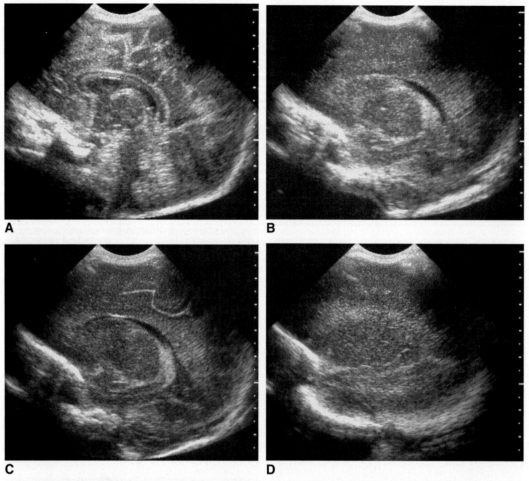

Fig. 32-3 Sagittal views of neonatal head. **A,** Midline. **B** and **C,** Lateral. **D,** Steeply angled. (Courtesy Douglas Dumas, Florida Hospital, Orlando, Florida.)

of the caudate nucleus. These subependymal hemorrhages are similar in echogenicity to the choroid plexus, and the coronal view shows asymmetry between normal choroid plexus and a hemorrhage in this region. In the sagittal plane, a small contour abnormality may be noted as the echogenic clot pushes against the ventricular wall. An intraventricular hemorrhage can be diagnosed with evidence of the echogenic hemorrhage within the ventricular cavity. When the hemorrhage extends into the parenchyma, the highly echogenic hemorrhage is identified extending from the ventricle to the adjacent white matter. The echogenicity of blood decreases over time. As the blood is reabsorbed, a cystic cavity is identified extending from the ventricle to the parenchyma and is known as a *porencephalic cyst.*[4]

PERIVENTRICULAR LEUKOMALACIA

Periventricular leukomalacia (PVL) defines white matter necrosis that may be diffuse or focal and is most

commonly identified at the external angles of the lateral ventricles. PVL is the result of ischemia to the vulnerable arterial border zones, also referred to as *watershed areas.* These areas are especially susceptible to changes in blood flow pressure in the premature infant because of lack of maturation of these zones.

Numerous risk factors contribute to the development of PVL. The perinatal risks include multiple gestations, chorioamnionitis, premature rupture of membranes, intrauterine growth restriction, congenital infections, and maternal hemorrhage. The postnatal risks usually relate to factors associated with hypotension and asphyxia and are most commonly identified in premature infants.[5,6]

The outcome for infants with PVL is variable depending on the severity and extent of white matter necrosis, although significantly increased morbidity and mortality are seen. **Cerebral palsy** is a prevalent sequela in infants with PVL. Infants are usually afflicted with major long-term neurologic deficits, including spastic

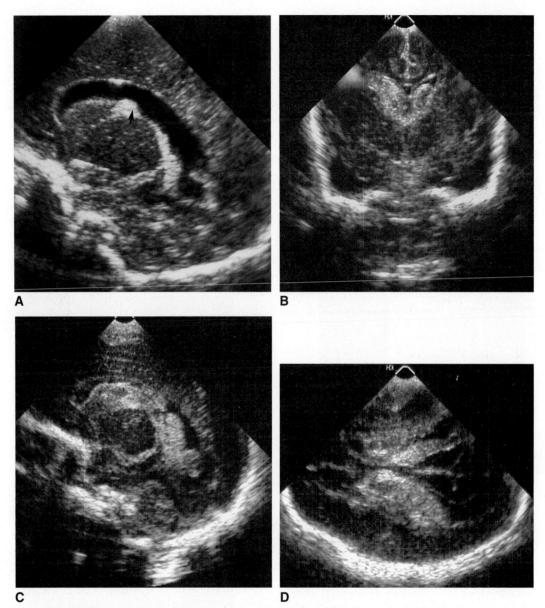

Fig. 32-4   Intracranial hemorrhage. **A,** Grade I bleed. Grade II bleed shown in, **B,** coronal, **C,** sagittal, and, **D,** axial planes.

diplegia, quadriplegia, seizure disorder, visual impairment, and mental retardation.

Sonographic Findings

The diagnosis of PVL may be initially inconclusive as the sonographic examination may reveal an increase in echogenicity in the periventricular parenchyma. This finding may be evident for the first few weeks of life and then may resolve. The more severe form of PVL progresses to the development of cystic lesions (Fig. 32-7) within the areas of increased echogenicity in approximately 2 to 3 weeks. These findings resolve within a few months with resultant brain atrophy and subsequent ventriculomegaly.[4,6]

CEREBRAL EDEMA

Cerebral edema (Fig. 32-8) may occur in full-term infants with significant anoxic or hypoxic events. Sonographic evaluation of the neonatal brain initially demonstrates diffuse increased echogenicity. The ventricles appear compressed, and the choroid plexus may blend with the increased echogenicity of the cerebellar hemispheres. The brain has a smooth, homogeneous appearance with a loss of differentiation of the sulci from the increased echogenicity. Within a couple of weeks, ventricular enlargement occurs from atrophy of the brain parenchyma and cystic changes may or may not be demonstrated.[1]

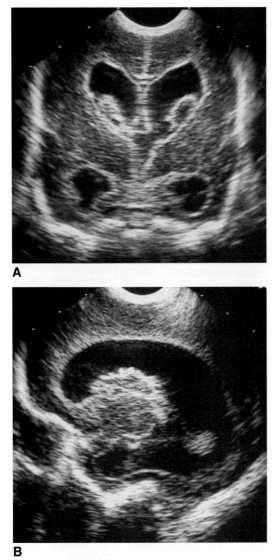

B

Fig. 32-5 Grade III hemorrhage with significant ventricular enlargement identified in, **A,** coronal and, **B,** sagittal planes.

HYDROCEPHALUS

Hydrocephalus is defined as enlargement of the ventricles with enlargement of the infant's head. Hydrocephalus may occur from obstruction of CSF, an overproduction of CSF, or abnormal absorption of CSF. Numerous congenital anomalies can contribute to the development of hydrocephalus, including, but not limited to, spina bifida, **aqueductal stenosis,** Dandy-Walker malformation (DWM), Arnold-Chiari malformation, congenital infections (Fig. 32-9), hemorrhage, and **achondroplasia.** Sonographic evaluation should include identification of the lateral, third, and fourth ventricles to show the level

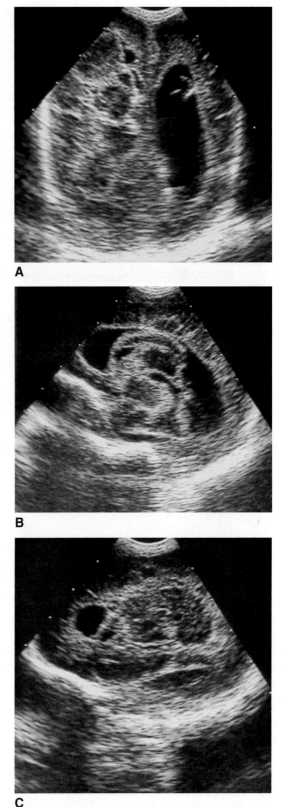

C

Fig. 32-6 Grade IV hemorrhage in infant born at 28 weeks' gestational age. **A,** Posterior coronal view. **B,** Sagittal view of right ventricle. **C,** Steeply angled sagittal view of brain.

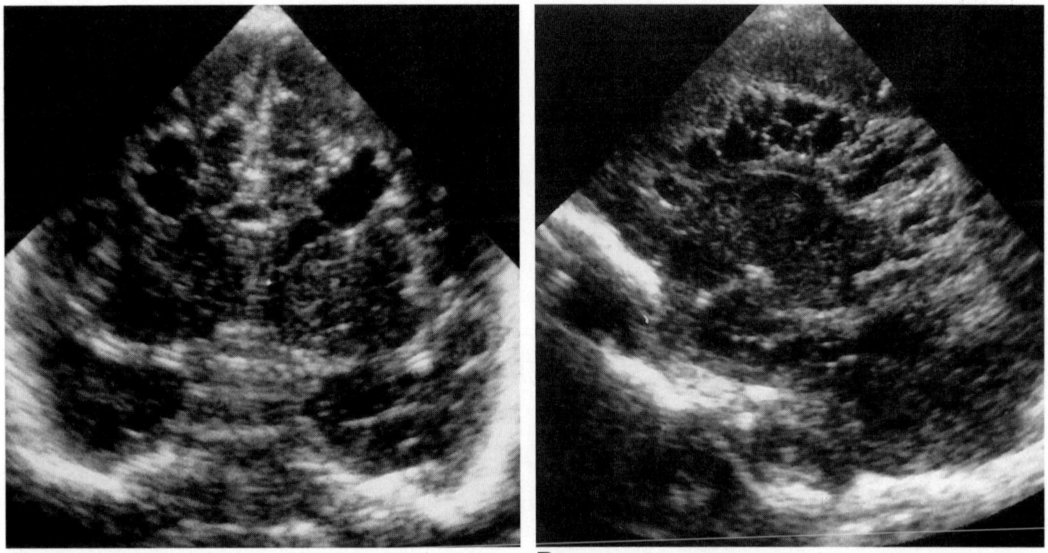

Fig. 32-7   Periventricular leukomalacia progresses to significant cavitation of brain parenchyma as shown in, **A,** coronal and, **B,** sagittal views of premature infant.

of obstruction and the identification of associated central nervous system anomalies if present. Serial ultrasound examinations may be used to follow progression or response to shunt placement (Fig. 32-9, *D, E,* and *F*).

CONGENITAL MALFORMATIONS

Chiari II Malformation

Chiari II malformation, also known as *Arnold-Chiari malformation,* represents the downward displacement of the cerebellum and **brainstem** in association with spina bifida (Fig. 32-10). The cisterna magna is obliterated, and the fourth ventricle and medulla are displaced into the cervical canal. Hydrocephalus is commonly associated.

Sonographic Findings. Sagittal and coronal views of the neonatal head show the absence of the cisterna magna and the downward displacement of the cerebellum. The fourth ventricle is also displaced, and the ventricles are increased in size, especially the lateral ventricles. The septum pellucidum also is absent.[4]

Agenesis of the Corpus Callosum

Agenesis of the corpus callosum (ACC) is considered relatively common, although the condition may go undiagnosed. The corpus callosum connects the cerebral hemispheres and aids in learning and memory. The corpus callosum may be completely absent or partially formed. ACC may be found in isolation but is often associated with other anomalies of the central nervous system, including holoprosencephaly (Fig. 32-11), encephalocele, and DWM. A variety of chromosomal anomalies and syndromes may also be identified with ACC, including trisomies 13 and 18 and X-linked syndromes.[4] The outcome is variable depending on the association and severity of other anomalies, but ACC can be asymptomatic or carry a grave prognosis when severe anomalies are identified.[7]

Sonographic Findings. The diagnosis of ACC may be made with notation of its absence on coronal and sagittal images of the head. In addition, colpocephaly may be identified, which is defined as mild ventriculomegaly with dilation of the occipital horns, giving the ventricle a teardrop appearance. The lateral ventricles are widely displaced laterally, and the third ventricle may appear dilated and displaced superiorly. The cingulate gyri, which are relatively parallel to the corpus callosum, radiate in a sunburst pattern. The CSP is usually absent as well.

Dandy-Walker Malformation

Dandy-Walker malformation is characterized by absence or dysplasia of the cerebellar vermis and maldevelopment of the fourth ventricle with replacement by a posterior fossa cyst. A less severe form, referred to as the *Dandy-*

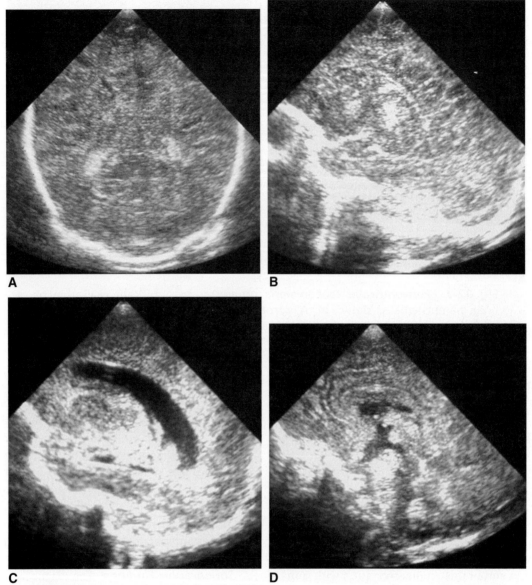

Fig. 32-8 Cerebral edema. Term infant was seen for neonatal head ultrasound after difficult delivery that resulted in severe hypoxia. Cerebral edema was evident as shown in, **A,** coronal and, **B,** sagittal views. Three weeks later, brain atrophy with ventricular enlargement was noted as shown in, **C** and **D,** sagittal views. **C,** Amount of ventricular enlargement in stark contrast to, **B,** slitlike ventricle. Infant was subsequently removed from life support and died.

Walker variant, may occur with dysplasia of the cerebellar vermis without enlargement of the posterior fossa. DWM is associated with numerous structural abnormalities, syndromes, and chromosomal anomalies. Chromosomal anomalies may be associated with up to 55% of fetuses with DWM and include trisomy 13, trisomy 18, trisomy 21, and triploidy.[8] DWM has also been linked to the teratogenic effects of congenital infections and multiple intracranial anomalies, including ACC.

The prognosis for infants born with DWM is variable depending on associated abnormalities and the absence or presence of an abnormal karyotype. Overall, the prognosis is considered poor, with high morbidity and mortality rates. Patients may have severe mental and physical disabilities, although infants with Dandy-Walker variant may function normally.[9]

Sonographic Findings. The diagnosis of DWM (Fig. 32-12) can be made with the identification of a posterior fossa cyst, with a resultant enlarged cisterna

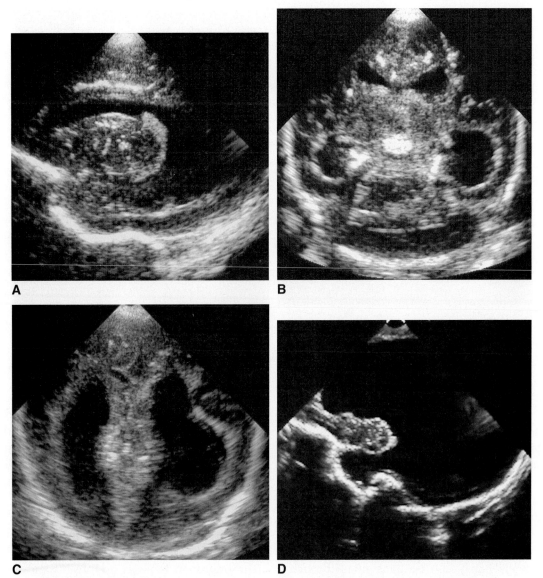

Fig. 32-9 Enlarged ventricles are noted in premature infant affected by congenital infection cytomegalovirus (CMV). **A,** Sagittal and, **B** and **C,** coronal images show ventricles and calcifications that are also identified in association with CMV. **D,** Greatly enlarged ventricles were identified in infant with spina bifida as noted in sagittal image. *Continued*

magna, and splaying of the cerebellar hemispheres from the abnormal development of the cerebellar vermis. Hydrocephalus frequently accompanies DWM. Sonographic imaging through the posterior fontanelle is useful in characterization of the cerebellar abnormality.

Holoprosencephaly

Holoprosencephaly encompasses a range of severity characterized by an incomplete or a lack of cleavage of the **forebrain.** The condition has been identified in 1:8000 second trimester pregnancies, and many cases spontaneously abort in the first trimester.[10] The most

severe form, alobar holoprosencephaly (Fig. 32-13, *A*), is seen with a complete failure of separation of the forebrain with subsequent fusion of the thalamus, a single ventricle, and cerebral hemispheres. Absences of the falx, corpus callosum, olfactory bulbs, and optic tracts also are noted. Semilobar holoprosencephaly (see Fig. 32-11 and Fig. 32-13, *B*) is seen with partial cleavage of the forebrain and absences of the corpus callosum and olfactory bulbs. The mildest form, lobar holoprosencephaly, is seen with a falx and **interhemispheric fissure,** although a small amount of the anterior brain parenchyma is fused. Fusion of the lateral ventricles and

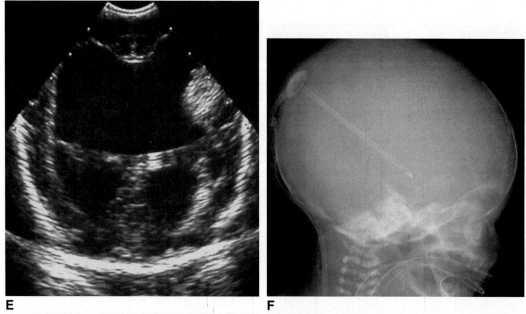

Fig. 32-9, cont'd **E,** One day after shunt placement, decrease was seen in ventricular size. Shunt was identified crossing lateral ventricles. Echogenic regions in parenchyma represent hemorrhage. **F,** Radiograph demonstrates shunt.

absence of the corpus callosum may be noted. The outcome is variable depending on the severity, but the most severe forms of holoprosencephaly carry an extremely poor prognosis.[11]

Holoprosencephaly is associated with severe facial anomalies, including **cyclopia, ethmocephaly, cebocephaly,** and facial clefts. Holoprosencephaly is also associated with many syndromes and multiple chromosomal anomalies, most commonly trisomy 13. Holoprosencephaly may also be transmitted through autosomal dominant, autosomal recessive, and X-linked modes. Several teratogenic effects have also been linked to holoprosencephaly, including hyperglycemia (in diabetes) and alcohol.[10,11]

Sonographic Findings. Sonographic identification of holoprosencephaly is easier in its most severe form. Identification of a single ventricle surrounded by brain parenchyma is diagnostic. The thalamus appears fused, and the falx is absent as are the CSP and corpus callosum. In semilobar holoprosencephaly and lobar holoprosencephaly, variable fusion may be identified and ACC and absence of the CSP are noted.

Hydranencephaly

Hydranencephaly is characterized by destruction of the brain parenchyma, which may result from carotid artery occlusion, congenital infections, cocaine abuse, and some less common causes. Hydranencephaly is usually isolated and sporadic. It is a rare anomaly, with a prevalence of less than 1:10,000 births.[12] The destruction to the brain usually occurs in the second trimester.

The outcome of hydranencephaly is grave. Death usually occurs shortly after birth, although survival for several months has been reported.[13]

Sonographic Findings. The sonographic findings of hydranencephaly include liquefaction of the brain parenchyma with replacement with CSF (Fig. 32-14). The brainstem is intact and visible on ultrasound. A portion of the falx and an atrophic thalami may be identified, and the head may be normal or large in size.

Schizencephaly

Schizencephaly is a rare disorder that results from a destructive assault in utero that leads to clefts in the cerebral cortex from the midline to the calvaria. The clefts may be open or closed and unilateral or bilateral. The clefts are lined with abnormal gray matter, although that is not distinguished sonographically. Absence of the corpus callosum and CSP are frequently seen.

The outcome for infants born with schizencephaly is variable. Close-lip clefts carry a better prognosis, as do unilateral clefts. Patients may have seizures and blindness and motor and mental deficits.[4]

Sonographic Findings. Sonographic evaluation of schizencephaly reveals an open cleft (Fig. 32-15) filled with fluid extending from the midline to the calvaria.

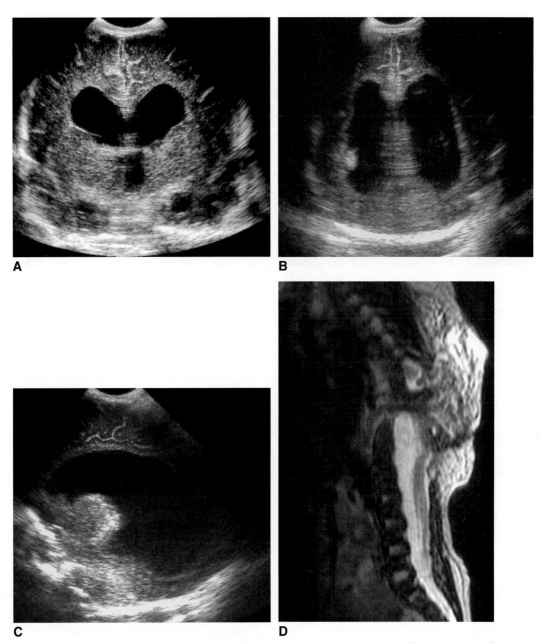

Fig. 32-10 Infant was delivered by cesarean section at 39 weeks' gestation for thoracic spina bifida. Chiari's malformation, type II, was identified. Enlarged ventricles can be appreciated in, **A,** anterior and, **B,** posterior coronal views and, **C,** lateral sagittal view of head. **D,** Magnetic resonance imaging shows spinal defect.

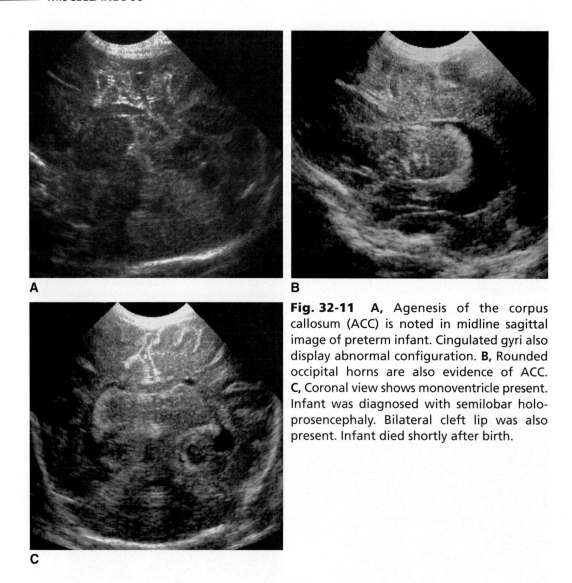

Fig. 32-11 **A,** Agenesis of the corpus callosum (ACC) is noted in midline sagittal image of preterm infant. Cingulated gyri also display abnormal configuration. **B,** Rounded occipital horns are also evidence of ACC. **C,** Coronal view shows monoventricle present. Infant was diagnosed with semilobar holoprosencephaly. Bilateral cleft lip was also present. Infant died shortly after birth.

Ventricular enlargement and absences of the corpus callosum and CSP may be present.

INFANT SPINE

An ultrasound of the neonatal spine may be ordered when the initial clinical examination reveals a dimple, hemangioma, tuft of hair, or other cutaneous lesion on an infant's back because these are associated with spinal dysraphism, which may be associated with tethering of the spinal cord. Spinal dysraphism encompasses disorders involving absent or incomplete closure of the neural tube. A range of severity exists from mild spina bifida occulta to severe **spina bifida aperta.** Ultrasound may be used in imaging the range of these disorders, with the most severe anomalies imaged in the perinatal period and the less severe usually evaluated in the neonatal period.

The sonographic evaluation is usually performed with the infant in the prone position with the spine flexed. This may be accomplished by extending the infant over a bolster or pillow. A high-frequency, linear transducer is preferred because of the larger transducer footprint needed to adequately visualize multiple vertebra along the longitudinal axis. The infant is scanned in longitudinal and transverse planes over the area of the spine.

The purpose of neonatal spine imaging is identification of the level of the **conus medullaris,** which should be located between the first (L1) and second (L2) lumbar vertebrae.[14] Sonography can be used in documentation of the level of the conus (Fig. 32-16) by counting the vertebrae. The most caudal rib is identified at the level of the 12th thoracic vertebra, which may be identified by scanning lateral to the vertebra. Because variants may occur (such as a missing or extra rib), identification of the vertebra should be confirmed also

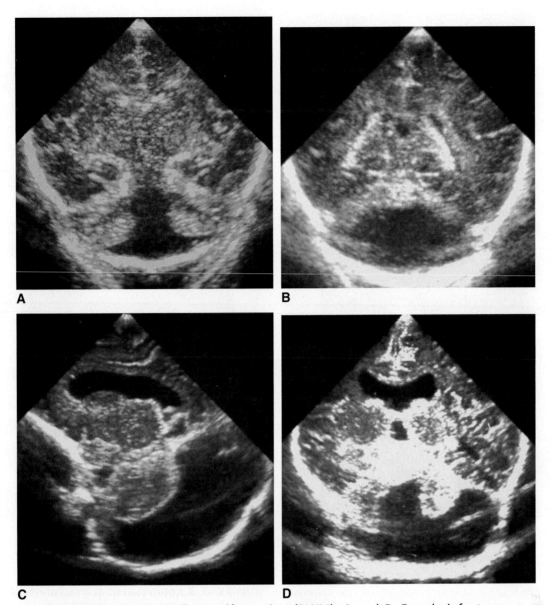

Fig. 32-12 Dandy-Walker malformation (DWM). **A** and **B,** Female infant was born at 37 weeks' gestation, and neonatal head ultrasound was ordered. Mother of the infant had no prenatal care. Sonographic evaluation showed posterior fossa cyst and splaying of cerebellar hemispheres as noted in coronal images. No hydrocephalus was identified. **C** and **D,** Hydrocephalus was identified in infant with DWM. **C,** Lateral sagittal and, **D,** coronal views show large posterior fossa cyst and accompanying ventricular enlargement.

by counting the sacral elements that follow the fifth lumbar vertebra. When the conus is identified at the same level when counting from the caudal and cephalic aspects of the lumbar vertebra, confidence exists in the identification of the level. For confirmation of the level of the conus or identification of the level with equivocal or difficult examinations, a radiopaque marker can be placed at the level of the conus with ultrasound guidance and a radiograph can confirm the level.

For identification of the level of the conus, an understanding of normal spinal anatomy is imperative. The normal spinal cord in the longitudinal plane is visualized between the vertebral bodies as an elongated hypoechoic structure surrounded by anechoic CSF. The cord contains one or two echogenic linear structures, known as the *central echo complex.* The spinal cord tapers at the caudal end, resembling the end of a carrot. Surrounding and distal to the conus, the echogenic

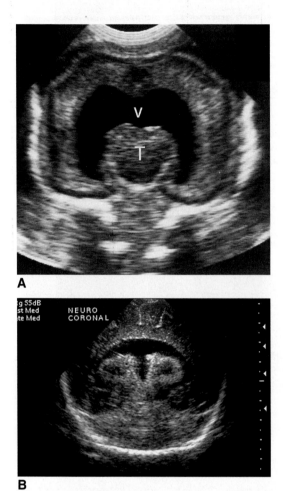

Fig. 32-13 **A,** Alobar holoprosencephaly is identified in image demonstrating single ventricle. **B,** Variable fusion identified in semilobar holoprosencephaly is seen in image.

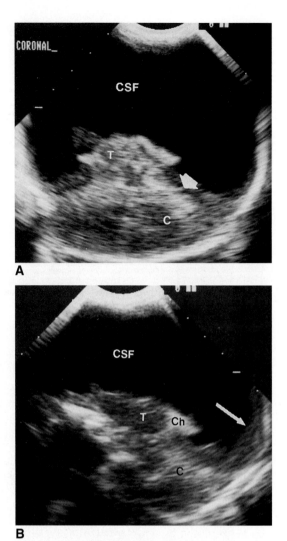

Fig. 32-14 Hydranencephaly is seen with replacement of cerebral hemispheres, although structures of posterior fossa appear normal as shown in, **A,** ultrasound and, **B,** computed tomographic images.

cauda equina is visualized. A normal spine also demonstrates pulsations of the nerve roots of the cauda equina. The coccyx is usually not ossified in the neonate, and the caudal end of the sac that encloses the spinal cord (the thecal sac) is usually located at the level of the second sacral element. The transverse cord in the lumbar region appears rounded, and the central echo complex appears as echogenic dots.[1]

TETHERED CORD

A tethered cord is defined as a fixed spinal cord that is positioned in an abnormal caudal position. A tethered cord may be suspected when cutaneous markers are identified on visual inspection of the infant, including skin tags, dimples, tufts of hair, hemangiomas, and raised skin lesions.[15] As the infant grows, increasing tension is placed on the cord, leading to increasing neurologic dysfunction, although the infant may be asymptomatic until ambulation occurs. Symptoms associated with tethering of the cord include bladder and bowel incontinence, leg weakness and atrophy, abnormal gait, abnormal posturing of the lower extremities, and sensory loss.[15] Early treatment can prevent the development of neurologic dysfunction.

Sonographic Findings

Sonographic evaluation of a tethered cord reveals the conus abnormally caudal in location (Fig. 32-17). The nerve roots of the cauda equina lack the pulsation

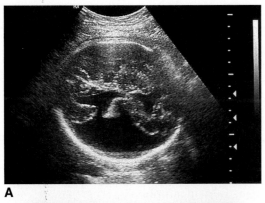

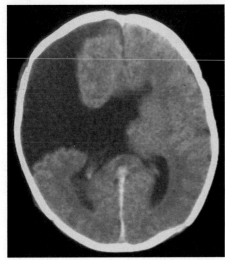

Fig. 32-15 **A,** Large cleft in brain parenchyma is identified on obstetric ultrasound and is consistent with schizencephaly. **B,** Confirmation with computed tomography was made after infant was born.

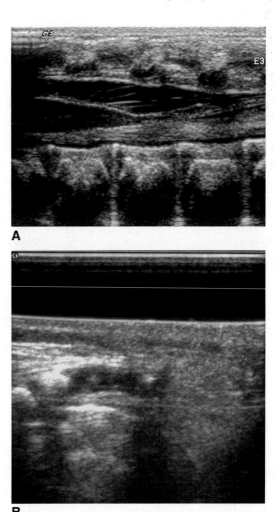

Fig. 32-16 **A,** Normal neonatal spine is shown. **B,** One-day-old infant was seen with dimple after newborn examination. Conus was identified between L1 and L2. Stand-off pad was used to image over region of dimple to look for sinus tract, which was not seen. (**A** Courtesy GE Medical Systems.)

identified in a normal spinal cord. If a **cutaneous** dimple is present, a stand-off pad or thick glob of gel should be used to determine whether the dimple is part of a sinus tract extending from the skin to the spinal cord.

SUMMARY

Ultrasound is an effective diagnostic imaging method for assessment of anomalies of the central nervous system in the neonate. Ultrasound evaluation of the neonatal head and spine is frequently used to analyze abnormalities. An understanding of the normal anatomy and most common pathologies (Table 32-1) assists the healthcare team with an accurate diagnosis so that appropriate treatment can be provided.

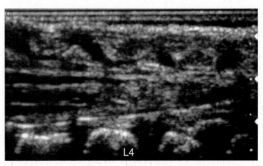

Fig. 32-17 Tethered cord was diagnosed in infant seen for ultrasound with dimple and skin tag. Conus was identified at L4.

Table 32-1	*Pathology of Neonatal Head*
Diagnosis	**Sonographic Findings**
Hemorrhage	Grade I: echogenic subependymal bleed; grade II: blood within ventricle; grade III: blood within ventricle with ventricular enlargement; grade IV: intraventricular blood extending to parenchyma
Periventricular leukomalacia	Increased echogenicity in periventricular parenchyma that becomes cystic over time
Cerebral edema	Increased echogenicity of cerebral hemispheres, slitlike ventricles; ventricular enlargement as brain atrophies
Hydrocephaly	Enlarged ventricles with enlarged head
Chiari II malformation	Absence of cisterna magna, inferiorly displaced cerebellum, enlarged ventricles
Agenesis of the corpus callosum	Absent corpus callosum and cavum septum pellucidum (CSP), mild ventriculomegaly with dilated occipital horns; lateral displacement of lateral ventricles and superior displacement of third ventricle; dilated third ventricle; cingulated gyri radiate in sunburst pattern
Dandy-Walker malformation	Posterior fossa cyst with enlarged cisterna magna, splaying of cerebellar hemispheres with absent or dysplastic vermis; commonly associated with hydrocephalus
Holoprosencephaly	Single ventricle, fused thalami, absent CSP and corpus callosum, absent falx; variable fusion with less severe forms
Hydranencephaly	Liquefaction of brain parenchyma; brain stem may be identified
Schizencephaly	Cleft in brain parenchyma from midline to calvaria

CLINICAL SCENARIO—DIAGNOSIS

■ The echogenic region identified in the anterior coronal view of the head suggests an intraventricular hemorrhage that extends into the parenchyma, which would classify this hemorrhage as a grade IV bleed. The follow-up shows the change in echogenicity as the hemorrhage begins to resolve.

This will leave a large porencephalic cyst in the left cerebral hemisphere and is consistent with a poor prognosis, which may include death. If this infant survives, she will probably have long-term neurologic deficits and may need shunt placement.

CASE STUDIES FOR DISCUSSION

1. A neonatal head ultrasound is ordered on an 8-day-old female infant for a premature delivery at 30 weeks' gestation. The infant is otherwise asymptomatic. The findings are revealed in Fig. 32-18. What is the most likely diagnosis?

2. A 4-day-old male infant with a history of a small dimple is seen in the radiology department for a spinal ultrasound to rule out tethered cord. The ultrasound reveals the finding in Fig. 32-19. What is the diagnosis?

3. A young woman is seen for an ultrasound at 34 weeks' gestation for late prenatal care. The abdominal circumference and femur length are consistent with the gestational age; however, the fetal head (Fig. 32-20, *A*) measures greater than 42 weeks. The patient is counseled regarding the severity of the fetal head anomaly. A cesarean section is scheduled at 38 weeks' gestation for the large size of the

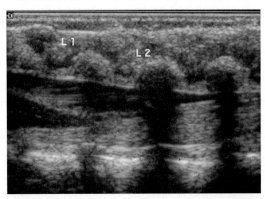

Fig. 32-19 Four-day-old male seen for ultrasound of spine.

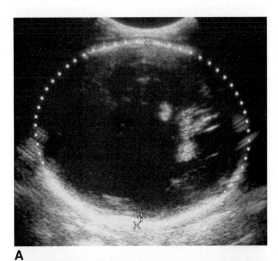

A

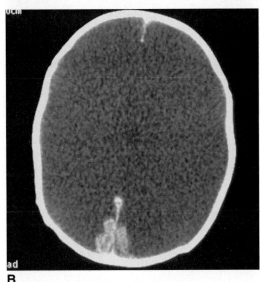

B

Fig. 32-20 **A,** Prenatal ultrasound of fetal head. **B,** Postnatal computed tomographic scan of infant brain.

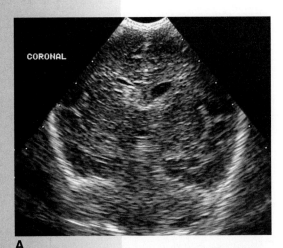

A

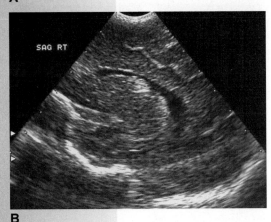

B

Fig. 32-18 **A,** Coronal and, **B,** sagittal images are shown in 8-day-old female. Left lateral sagittal view was within normal limits.

head. A T-incision is necessary to deliver the baby's head. A computed tomographic scan of the brain (Fig. 32-20, *B*) is performed the same day. What is the most likely diagnosis and prognosis for this infant?

4. An ultrasound is performed in the neonatal intensive care unit on a premature infant. The results are shown in Fig. 32-21. What is the most likely diagnosis?

5. A 6-week-old male infant born at 29 weeks' gestation is seen for a neonatal head ultrasound. The ultrasound examination reveals the findings in Fig. 32-22. What is the most likely diagnosis?

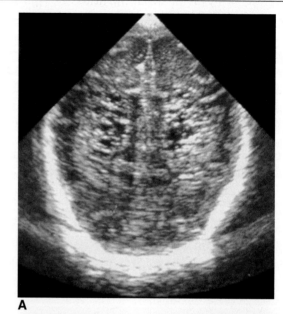

A

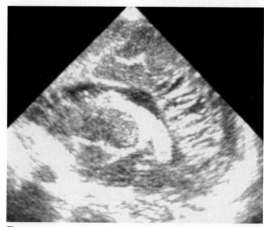

B

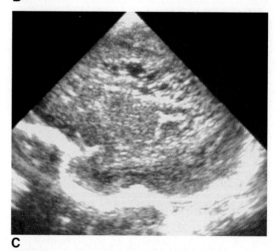

C

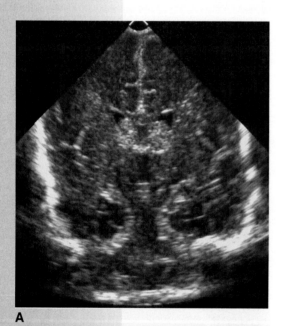

A

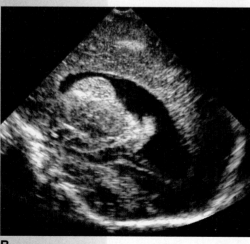

B

Fig. 32-21 **A,** Coronal and, **B,** left sagittal views of head are shown. Right and left ventricles were fairly symmetric.

Fig. 32-22 Representative images show, **A,** posterior coronal view and, **B,** right and, **C,** left lateral views in sagittal plane.

STUDY QUESTIONS

1. An infant is delivered via cesarean section and transported to the neonatal intensive care unit for severe enlargement of the head. Neonatal ultrasound of the brain reveals greatly enlarged ventricles. Examination of the posterior fossa reveals a large cystic structure and splaying of the cerebellar hemispheres. This would be consistent with which of the following anomalies?
   a. Dandy-Walker malformation
   b. Dandy-Walker variant
   c. holoprosencephaly
   d. hydranencephaly
   e. hydrocephalus

2. A neonatal head ultrasound is performed on a premature infant born at 27 weeks' gestation. The examination reveals an asymmetric echogenic bulge in the region of the caudothalamic notch that pushes into the ventricle on the right side. The ventricle appears normal in size, although an area of increased echogenicity is also identified in the occipital horn. What is the most likely diagnosis?
   a. grade I hemorrhage
   b. grade II hemorrhage
   c. grade III hemorrhage
   d. grade IV hemorrhage
   e. periventricular leukomalacia

3. An infant is born with a myelomeningocele and an enlarged head. The ultrasound reveals enlarged ventricles. Imaging through the posterior fontanelle shows an abnormally shaped cerebellum that appears to be pulled posteriorly and inferiorly. A cisterna magna is not identified. Which of the following most accurately defines the findings in the head?
   a. agenesis of the corpus callosum
   b. Chiari II malformation
   c. Dandy-Walker malformation
   d. hydranencephaly
   e. hydrocephaly

4. A woman is seen in the emergency department at 41 weeks' gestation and in advanced labor. The labor is difficult and prolonged because of the large size of the infant. Hypoxia is suspected, and a neonatal head ultrasound is ordered. The ultrasound reveals a diffusely echogenic brain with slitlike ventricles. This would be consistent with which of the following?
   a. cerebral edema
   b. hydrocephalus

   c. intraventricular hemorrhage
   d. periventricular leukomalacia
   e. porencephaly

5. A woman without history of prenatal care is seen in labor in the emergency department. The infant is delivered, and physical examination reveals a median cleft lip and hypotelorism. A neonatal head ultrasound is ordered. What will the sonogram reveal?
   a. holoprosencephaly
   b. hydranencephaly
   c. hydrocephaly
   d. porencephaly
   e. schizencephaly

6. A newborn is seen with a tuft of hair on the lower back on neonatal physical examination. An ultrasound is ordered and reveals the conus medullaris at the level of L4. What is the most accurate diagnosis?
   a. normal examination
   b. meningomyelocele
   c. spinal dysraphism
   d. spinal bifida aperta
   e. tethered cord

7. A premature infant born at 28 weeks' gestation undergoes scanning at 4 weeks of age to rule out brain pathology. The ultrasound reveals symmetric regions of increased echogenicity that contain multiple cystic spaces. The ventricles are enlarged but do not connect with the cystic regions. This would be consistent with which of the following diagnoses?
   a. cerebral edema
   b. hydrocephaly
   c. periventricular leukomalacia
   d. porencephaly
   e. schizencephaly

8. Which of the following defines a grade I hemorrhage?
   a. a subependymal hemorrhage without extension into the ventricle with ventriculomegaly
   b. a subependymal hemorrhage without extension into the ventricle without ventriculomegaly
   c. a subependymal hemorrhage with extension into the ventricle with ventriculomegaly
   d. a subependymal hemorrhage with extension into the ventricle without ventriculomegaly
   e. a subependymal hemorrhage with extension into the ventricle and adjacent brain parenchyma

9. A newborn with a history of an abnormal head ultrasound in utero is seen for an ultrasound examination of the head. The sonographic examination reveals widely spaced lateral ventricles and a widely spaced interhemispheric fissure. The occipital horns are dilated. Based on these findings, what is a likely diagnosis?
   a. agenesis of the corpus callosum
   b. holoprosencephaly
   c. hydrocephaly
   d. porencephaly
   e. schizencephaly

10. Which of the following is defined as a cleft in the brain extending from the midline to the calvaria?
    a. holoprosencephaly
    b. hydranencephaly
    c. hydrocephaly
    d. porencephaly
    e. schizencephaly

REFERENCES

1. Rumack CM: *Diagnostic ultrasound,* ed 2, St Louis, 1998, Mosby.
2. Furlow B: Neonatal imaging, *Radiol Technol* 72:577-597, 2001.
3. Whitelaw A: Intraventricular haemorrhage and posthaemorrhagic hydrocephalus: pathogenesis, prevention and future interventions, *Semin Neonatol* 6:135-146, 2001.
4. Hagen-Ansert SL: *Textbook of diagnostic ultrasound,* ed 5, St Louis, 2001, Mosby.
5. Resch B et al: Risk factors and determinants of neurodevelopmental outcome in cystic periventricular leucomalacia, *Eur J Pediatr* 159:663-670, 2000.
6. Perlman JM: White matter injury in the preterm infant: an important determination of abnormal neurodevelopment outcome, *Early Hum Dev* 53:99-120, 1998.
7. D'Ercole C et al: Prenatal diagnosis of fetal corpus callosum agenesis by ultrasonography and magnetic resonance imaging, *Prenat Diagn* 18:247-253, 1998.
8. Sherer DM, Shane H, Anyane-Yeboa K: First-trimester transvaginal ultrasonographic diagnosis of Dandy-Walker malformation, *Am J Perinatol* 18:373-377, 2001.
9. Ecker JL, Shipp TD, Bromley B et al: The sonographic diagnosis of Dandy-Walker and Dandy-Walker variant: associated findings and outcomes, *Prenat Diagn* 20:328-332, 2000.
10. Bullen PJ, Rankin JM, Robson SC: Investigation of the epidemiology and prenatal diagnosis of holoprosencephaly in the North of England, *Am J Obstet Gynecol* 184:1256-1262, 2001.
11. Peebles DM: Holoprosencephaly, *Prenat Diagn* 18:477-480, 1998.
12. Kurtz AB, Johnson PT: Case 7: hydranencephaly, *Radiology* 210:419-422, 1999.
13. Herman TE, Siegel MJ: Special imaging casebook, *J Perinatol* 4:274-275, 2000.
14. Unsinn KM, Geley T, Freund MC et al: US of the spinal cord in newborns: spectrum of normal findings, variants, congenital anomalies, and acquired diseases, *Radiographics* 20:923-938, 2000.
15. Kriss VM, Desai NS: Occult spinal dysraphism in neonates: assessment of high-risk cutaneous stigmata on sonography, *AJR Am J Roentgenol* 171:1687-1692, 1998.

BIBLIOGRAPHY

Anderson KN, Anderson LE, Glanze WD: *Mosby's medical, nursing, & allied health dictionary,* ed 5, St Louis, 1998, Mosby.

Peneff C, Swearengin R: National certification examination review, Neurosonology, SDMS, Dallas, 2001.

Ramey J: Evaluation of periventricular-intraventricular hemorrhage in premature infants using cranial ultrasounds, *Neonatal Network* 17:65-72, 1998.

Tegeler CH, Babikian VL, Gomez CR: *Neurosonology,* St Louis, 1996, Mosby-Year Book, Inc.

Volpe JJ: Brain injury in the premature infant: overview of clinical aspects, neuropathology, and pathogenesis, *Semin Pediatr Neurol* 5:135-151, 1998.

33

Carotid Artery Disease

LISA MULLEE

CLINICAL SCENARIO

■ A man in his early 30s is seen in the emergency department via ambulance after a motor vehicle accident. He is found to have left hemiplegia, hemianopia, and dysphasia. After consultation with family members, the patient is noted to have been in excellent physical health and very active before the accident.

A carotid ultrasound is performed, and a thin line is noted bilaterally in the carotid arteries. Doppler analysis shows a high-resistance waveform with decreased velocities in the right internal carotid artery. What do these findings suggest?

OBJECTIVES

■ Identify risk factors associated with disease of the carotid or vertebral arteries.

■ Identify signs and symptoms associated with abnormalities of the carotid or vertebral arteries.

■ Recognize the sonographic appearances of normal and abnormal carotid arteries.

■ Differentiate Doppler findings from normal to hemodynamically significant lesions.

■ Distinguish rare forms of cerebrovascular disease/accidents.

GLOSSARY OF TERMS

Amaurosis fugax: transient blindness described as a shade being pulled over the eye

Aphasia: impaired ability or absence of ability to communicate, particularly by speaking

Carotid bruit: a systolic murmur heard in the neck produced by blood flow in the carotid arteries

Cerebrovascular accident: permanent neurologic deficit

Endarterectomy: surgical removal of plaque or diseased structure to the endothelial or media layer of the vessel wall

Hemianopia: loss of vision in one or both eyes that affects half of the visual field

Hemiplegia: paralysis of half of the body

Transient ischemic attack: temporary neurologic deficit, with symptoms lasting a few minutes to several hours but never more than 24 hours

Stroke, also known as *cerebrovascular accident,* is the third leading cause of death in the United States, preceded only by heart disease and cancer. Each year, about 500,000 people have a first stroke and an additional 100,000 have a recurrent stroke. On average, someone in the United States has a stroke every 53 seconds; and every 3.1 minutes, someone dies of a stroke. Approximately 83% of all strokes are the result of ischemia, and the additional 17% are hemorrhagic.[1]

Carotid ultrasound has proved to be a useful and cost-effective method of evaluation of the cervical carotid and vertebral arteries. With early detection and intervention in patients with more than 70% blockage, the relative risk for stroke has been reduced by approximately 65%.[2] Knowledge of risk factors, signs, symptoms, and presentation of impending stroke are key factors. Disease of the carotids affects the ipsilateral side of the head and the contralateral side of body.

Risk factors for stroke include hypertension, cigarette smoking, heart disease, diabetes, and history of **transient ischemic attack** (TIA). Some of the more common warning signs of stroke are unilateral weakness or numbness of the face, arm, or leg; difficulty speaking; loss of vision, particularly in one eye; and a **bruit** heard by a physician. Additional generalized symptoms may include dizziness, syncope, headache, or confusion.

NORMAL ANATOMY

The aortic root leaves the left ventricle with the left and right coronary arteries immediately branching off near the aortic cusp. The innominate, or brachiocephalic, is the first major branch off the aortic arch. The innominate splits into the right subclavian and right common carotid artery. The right common carotid then bifurcates into the right internal carotid artery (ICA) and external carotid artery (ECA). The right vertebral artery branches off the right subclavian and travels cephalad until it joins the left vertebral artery to form the basilar artery. The left common carotid is the next branch directly off the aortic arch. It also bifurcates into the ICA and ECA. The third branch off the arch is the left subclavian artery, which supplies blood to the left arm. The left vertebral artery branches off the left subclavian and combines with the right vertebral to form the basilar artery, which provides blood for the posterior circulation of the brain (Fig. 33-1).

SONOGRAPHIC IMAGING TECHNIQUES

A typical carotid ultrasound begins with a focused history obtained from the patient or chart. Some laboratory protocols then require bilateral arm blood pressures; others may only require blood pressures if

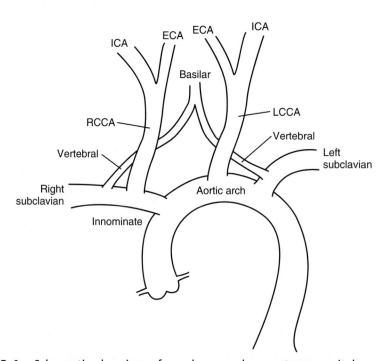

Fig. 33-1 Schematic drawing of cerebrovascular anatomy as it branches off aortic arch. *ECA,* External carotid artery; *ICA,* internal carotid artery; *LCCA,* left common carotid artery; *RCCA,* right common carotid artery.

retrograde flow is seen in one of the vertebral arteries. The patient is placed in a supine position with the head turned away from the side being scanned. Although consistency is the only necessary factor, most sonographers begin the examination on the right side. A 7-MHz linear transducer is most frequently used, but a 5- or 10-MHz transducer may be preferred, depending on the size of the patient.

The examination begins with grayscale interrogation from a transverse plane. The transducer is usually placed in an anterolateral position near the supraclavicular notch and moved cephalad to the angle of the mandible (Fig. 33-2). During scanning in the transverse plane, notation of the orientation of the ICA and ECA as they split just past the bulb (Fig. 33-3) is helpful. The location and amount of plaque should also be noted when present. Area measurements for determination of the percent of stenosis are taken from this plane.

Longitudinal views then are obtained, again with a start at the proximal common carotid artery near the clavicle (Fig. 33-4). The widening of the artery at the bifurcation is identified as the carotid bulb (Fig. 33-5), seen at the more cephalad portion of the vessel. The artery then splits into the ICA and ECA (Fig. 33-6). Again, plaque characterization should take place. Diameter measurements of a stenotic lesion should also be taken in this view.

The ICA is typically the larger vessel when compared with the ECA. In most patients, the ICA is posterior and lateral to the ECA and very rarely has branches off the vessel seen in the neck. The ECA, on the other hand, may be identified by the superior thyroid artery branching off in the cervical area. The vertebral arteries originate from the subclavian artery and are imaged

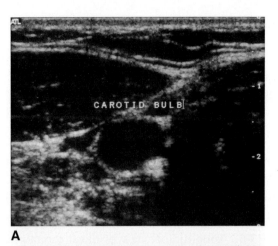

A

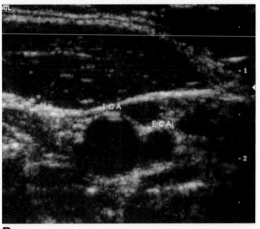

B

Fig. 33-3 Transverse views of, **A,** carotid bulb just before bifurcation of internal carotid artery (ICA) and external carotid artery (ECA) and, **B,** ICA and ECA just past carotid bulb.

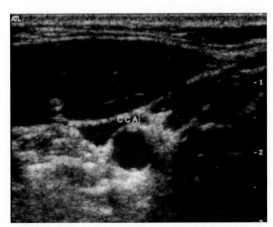

Fig. 33-2 Transverse view of proximal common carotid artery.

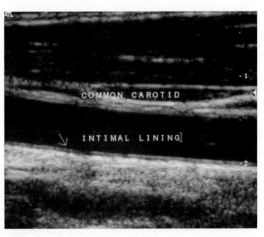

Fig. 33-4 Longitudinal view of common carotid artery low on neck.

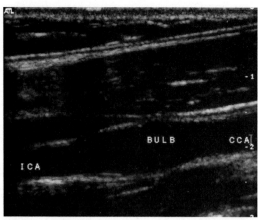

Fig. 33-5 Longitudinal view of distal common bulb and proximal internal carotid artery. Note widening of artery at area of bulb.

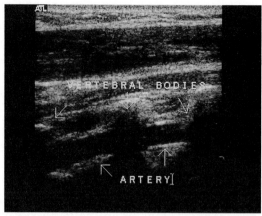

Fig. 33-7 Posterolateral angle shows vertebral processes with vertebral artery running through vertebral bodies.

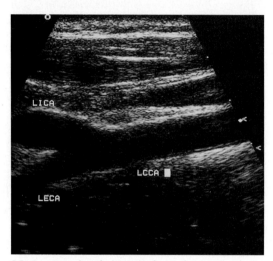

Fig. 33-6 Proximal internal and external carotid arteries seen from longitudinal view.

with posterolaterally directing the sound beam until the vertebral bodies are identified. The vertebral artery is seen running between the vertebral processes (Fig. 33-7). Color and spectral Doppler are instrumental in visualization of the vertebral artery.

DOPPLER IMAGING: SPECTRAL ANALYSIS

Doppler spectral analysis is valuable in determination of the hemodynamic significance of a stenotic lesion. The common carotid artery, the ICA, and the ECA all have distinct flow characteristics that can be evaluated with peak systolic velocities (PSVs), diastolic velocities, or velocity ratios.

The ICA receives approximately 80% of the blood supplied by the common carotid artery and is needed to supply an adequate amount of blood to the brain. Therefore, the Doppler spectral waveform has a low-resistance appearance, demonstrating antegrade flow in diastole (Fig. 33-8).

The ECA supplies blood to the facial musculature and demonstrates a high-resistance Doppler waveform. The ECA waveform shows a sharp systolic rise and a sharp diastolic fall with a brief diastolic flow reversal. The ECA can be distinguished from the ICA with a temporal tap, which can be accomplished by locating the superficial temporal artery near the ipsilateral ear and providing quick sequential taps. This can be seen on the ECA spectral waveform during diastole (Fig. 33-9).

The common carotid artery has flow characteristics of both the ICA and the ECA. Like the ICA, it has antegrade flow during diastole (Fig. 33-10).

COLOR DOPPLER

Color Doppler imaging is very helpful in quickly distinguishing between laminar and turbulent flow. The cervical arteries are typically displayed in shades of red that represent antegrade flow. With laminar flow, the lighter color shades are seen in the center of the vessel, showing the highest velocity flows. Turbulent flow is easily identified by the mixture of color shades that represent blood flow traveling at higher speeds and variable directions.

Color Doppler in the common carotid artery and ICA shows a continuous flow pattern that indicates flow throughout the cardiac cycle. The ECA has diminished

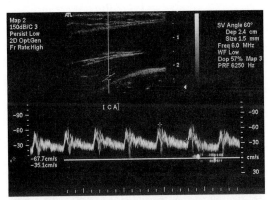

Fig. 33-8 Doppler flow seen in normal internal carotid artery. Note antegrade flow seen in diastole.

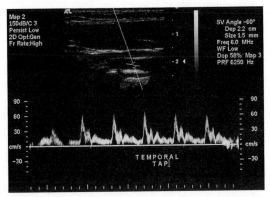

Fig. 33-9 Doppler flow seen in normal external carotid artery (ECA). Diastolic pulsations seen during temporal tap confirm ECA flow.

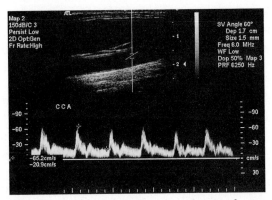

Fig. 33-10 Normal Doppler waveform of common carotid artery shows characteristics of both internal and external carotid arteries.

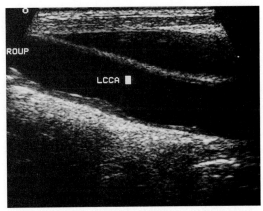

Fig. 33-11 Minimal homogeneous plaque seen in lining wall of common carotid artery.

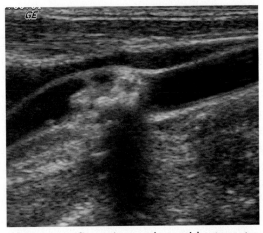

Fig. 33-12 Significant internal carotid artery stenosis shows complex heterogeneous plaque with area of intraplaque hemorrhage. (Courtesy GE Medical Systems.)

diastolic flow that can be described with color as having a "blinking" appearance.

CAROTID ARTERY STENOSIS

A carotid ultrasound examination consists of grayscale imaging, Doppler, and color-flow analysis, with each one providing support in determination of the percent of stenosis. Direct imaging of the vessel allows evaluation and characterization of plaque. For example, a homogeneous layer along the intimal lining with smooth borders may indicate a minimal stenosis, sometimes referred to as a fatty streak (Fig. 33-11). A more complex plaque may show echogenic areas made up of calcium mixed with soft echoes, reflective of collagen and fibrous tissue. Sonolucent areas seen within a complex plaque would indicate areas of intraplaque hemorrhage (Fig. 33-12). Calcific plaque can easily be

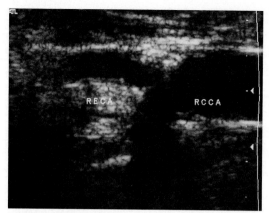

Fig. 33-13 Calcified plaque in carotid bulb shows acoustic shadowing.

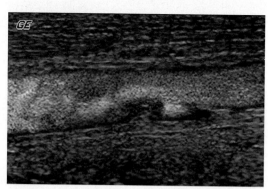

Fig. 33-14 Area of ulceration seen in common carotid artery. (Courtesy GE Medical Systems.)

identified with distal acoustic shadowing (Fig. 33-13). Shadowing from a calcific plaque can make determination of vessel patency difficult with sonographic imaging techniques.

Plaque texture should be described as homogeneous or heterogeneous, and borders should be described as smooth or irregular. Careful attention should be given to irregular borders to evaluate for areas of ulceration (Fig. 33-14). Ulcer craters allow for thrombus formation and embolic possibilities.

Depending on department protocol, area or diameter measurements may be taken for determination of percent stenosis. Area measurements are taken from a transverse plane with tracing the residual and original lumens and calculating the percent stenosis. Diameter measurements are usually taken from a sagittal plane, again with measuring the residual and original lumens (Fig. 33-15). Diameter reductions of greater than 50% and area reductions of greater than 70% are considered significant enough to cause an increase in flow velocities.

Color-flow Doppler should be used to interrogate the common, internal, and external carotid vessels. Areas of flow disturbance can easily be identified with color Doppler, with aliasing representing the highest velocity shifts, which aids in quick identification of stenosis and determination of placement of the Doppler sample volume.

Doppler spectral analysis helps in quantification of a stenotic lesion. Doppler measurements should be taken in a sagittal view, with the sample volume placed in the area of the greatest color Doppler shift. For accurate spectral information, a Doppler angle between 45 and 60 degrees should be used. Department protocols should be established and followed for consistency and reproducibility.

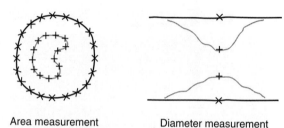

Area measurement   Diameter measurement

Fig. 33-15 Schematic drawing shows difference between area and diameter measurements.

Spectral waveforms should be obtained in the common carotid artery, bulb, proximal and distal ICA, and ECA. PSVs and end diastolic velocities (EDVs) of common and ICAs should be taken. PSVs should be obtained in the ECA and vertebral vessels (Fig. 33-16). Systolic ratios can also be obtained with dividing the PSVs of a stenotic ICA by the PSVs of a normal common carotid artery. End diastolic ratios can also be useful in prediction of stenoses greater than 80%. The velocity ranges in Table 33-1 are used in our laboratory and correlate well with our quality assurance (QA) data. Department-specific protocols and QA data should be established for each laboratory.

When performed correctly, Doppler spectral analysis is accurate in determination of stenosis within the ICA. Soft plaque or thrombus may be difficult to see with imaging techniques alone; therefore, Doppler plays a vital role in evaluation for blockage.

The most common treatment for hemodynamically significant lesions is carotid **endarterectomy**. In multiple clinical trials, including the North American Symptomatic Carotid Endarterectomy Trial (NASCET) and the European Carotid Surgery Trial (ECST), the benefit of carotid endarterectomy has been established in patients with at least 70% stenosis.[2] Vascular

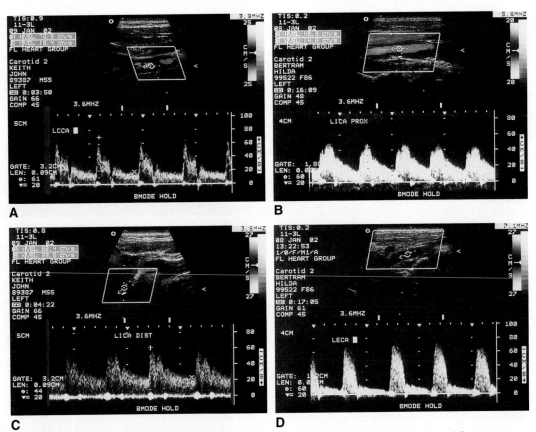

Fig. 33-16 Spectral Doppler waveforms taken in, **A,** common carotid artery, **B,** proximal internal carotid artery (ICA), **C,** distal ICA, and, **D,** external carotid artery. Peak systolic and end diastolic measurements are seen in common carotid artery and proximal and distal ICA.

Table 33-1	*Carotid Artery Stenosis*			
Percent Stenosis	**Peak Systolic Velocity (cm/sec)**	**End Diastolic Velocities (cm/sec)**	**Systolic Velocity Ratio (ICA/CCA)**	**Diastolic Velocity Ratio (ICA/CCA)**
<49%	<140	<100	<1.8	<2.6
50% to 79%	>140	<100	>1.8	>2.6
80% to 99%	>140	>100	>3.7	>5.5
100%	Absent	Absent	Absent	Absent

CCA, Common carotid artery; *ICA,* internal carotid artery.

surgeons may also use ultrasound to evaluate the vessel and flow within the vessel before closing the neck. This is believed to help reduce potential problems that may arise after the endarterectomy.

CAROTID ARTERY OCCLUSION

Carotid artery occlusion can be suspected when echogenic material appears to totally fill the vessel lumen (Fig. 33-17). Absence of color and Doppler flow are also indicators of occlusion. Doppler within the common carotid artery has a thumping or "drum-beat" sound in systole. The ipsilateral ECA may take on an internal flow pattern as it tries to compensate for the occlusion. The ECA can be identified with a temporal tap. ICAs that are chronically occluded appear reduced in size.

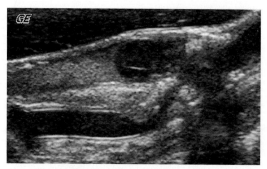

Fig. 33-17 Completely occluded internal carotid artery. (Courtesy GE Medical Systems.)

SUBCLAVIAN STEAL

Subclavian steal syndrome (SSS) is a result of stenosis or occlusion proximal to the vertebral artery. The pressure in the arm drops from decreased blood flow, resulting in reversal of flow in the ipsilateral vertebral artery.

Subclavian steal syndrome is found in males more frequently than in females and usually affects individuals of more than 50 years of age. SSS is commonly asymptomatic and found incidentally during a carotid ultrasound examination. Symptomatic patients may have arm pain with exercise or at rest. Signs of vertebrobasilar ischemia may include ataxia, vertigo, or bilateral visual disturbances.

Subclavian steal syndrome can be diagnosed with reversed flow in the vertebral artery, which is usually proven with color-flow Doppler and confirmed with spectral Doppler. For proven flow reversal in the vertebral artery, antegrade flow should be demonstrated in the common carotid artery. A difference in bilateral blood pressures of greater than 20 mm Hg is also an indication of SSS.

CAROTID DISSECTION

Carotid artery dissection should be considered a possible cause in patients less than 40 years of age with symptoms associated with a stroke. Carotid dissection is seen slightly more often in males than in females. The morbidity from a carotid dissection varies in severity from transient ischemic neurologic deficit to death. A 75% mortality rate is associated with dissections that extend intracranially.[3]

Some predisposing factors associated with carotid artery dissection may include Marfan syndrome, fibromuscular dysplasia, syphilis, or atherosclerosis, or the condition may be familial. With patients with a

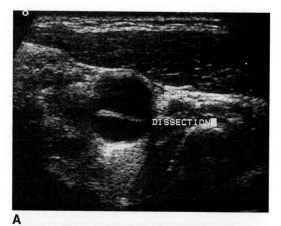

A

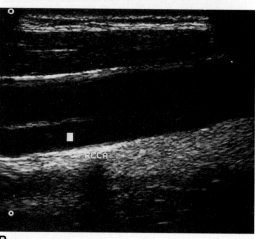

B

Fig. 33-18 Carotid artery dissection seen in, **A,** transverse and, **B,** sagittal views. Note intimal flap that creates double lumen. (Courtesy Erin Simard, Florida Heart Group, Orlando, Florida.)

neurologic deficit with sustained injury or trauma, carotid dissection should be considered. Chiropractic manipulation, blunt trauma, and injury from seat belts in motor vehicle accidents have all been associated with carotid artery dissection.

Dissection of the cervical carotid arteries can be diagnosed when an intimal flap creates a double lumen (Fig. 33-18). The formation of thrombus may be visualized within the false lumen. The vessels should be carefully interrogated in an attempt to determine the extent of the dissection.

Doppler analysis is helpful in identification of a stenosis or occlusion caused by the false lumen. A dissected ICA may have an appearance of a high-resistance waveform with a decreased velocity (Fig. 33-19). With color Doppler, red and blue may be seen within the lumen in a transverse view.

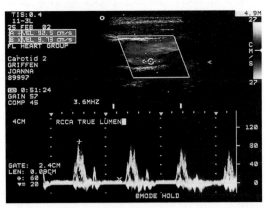

Fig. 33-19 Doppler waveform seen in presence of carotid dissection. Although it is internal carotid artery waveform, it has appearance of high-resistance flow with little to no diastolic flow noted. (Courtesy Erin Simard, Florida Heart Group, Orlando, Florida.)

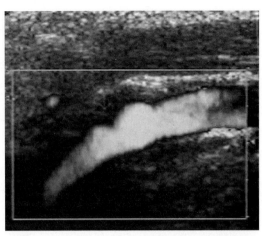

Fig. 33-20 Internal carotid artery from patient with fibromuscular dysplasia. Note peapod appearance of artery. (Courtesy Doug Marcum, Orlando Ultrasound Associates, Inc., Orlando, Florida.)

FIBROMUSCULAR DYSPLASIA

Fibromuscular dysplasia is a noninflammatory disease of unknown cause that has been found to affect several members of the same family, implying a hereditary factor. Fibromuscular dysplasia can involve both systemic and cervicocerebral vessels, with the most common being the renal arteries and ICAs. Fibromuscular dysplasia is seen more often in females and is typically diagnosed between the ages of 30 and 50 years. Individuals may go without diagnosis until the development of hypertension from affected renal arteries or symptoms of TIA or stroke from affected ICAs.

Sonographic evaluation of the ICA reveals expanded and narrowed areas of the arterial lumen often described as having a "string-of-beads" or a "peapod" appearance (Fig. 33-20; see Color Plate 24). The distal portion of the ICA is usually affected. The expanded areas provide an environment for blood to swirl and have a pooling effect that allows for clot formation. Smaller clots may then travel, causing TIAs. The narrowed segments of fibromuscular dysplasia may have varying degrees of stenosis and must be interrogated carefully, particularly with Doppler. Because fibromuscular dysplasia commonly involves the distal ICA, angiogram follow-up is necessary for further evaluation and diagnosis.

Patients with fibromuscular dysplasia affecting the ICAs are typically placed on antiplatelet and anticoagulation therapy to prevent thrombus formation or are given a carotid endarterectomy to revascularize stenosed segments.[4] Because of the nonatherosclerotic nature of fibromuscular dysplasia, carotid stent grafting has become an additional treatment option for patients with this condition. Carotid artery stenting is a relatively new procedure and needs additional clinical trials to determine long-term benefit and complications.

SUMMARY

Carotid ultrasound is a safe and cost-effective method for evaluation of vessels that supply blood to the brain. In the hands of a skilled and knowledgeable sonographer, carotid ultrasound has been accurate in determination of disease of the carotid or vertebral arteries. Early detection and prevention of impending stroke has the potential for saving millions of dollars in healthcare and rehabilitation costs.

CLINICAL SCENARIO—DIAGNOSIS

■ The thin line seen bilaterally on carotid ultrasound is actually an intimal flap from bilateral carotid dissections. During the accident, the vehicle flipped several times. The trauma from a three-point restraint seat belt is believed to have contributed to the bilateral dissections. The dissection on the left seems to be contained to the common carotid, and the right originated in the common and extended into the right ICA and proves to be the most significant.

This young man has had to relearn to be self sufficient. Five years after the accident, he walks with a limp from the hemiplegia and has little to no use of his left arm. As part of his personal rehabilitation, he spends many volunteer hours traveling and assisting children who are disabled.

CASE STUDIES FOR DISCUSSION

1. A carotid ultrasound is performed on a 62-year-old man with a bruit heard on the right side of the neck. He has had two episodes of **amaurosis fugax** affecting his right eye, each episode lasting less than 2 minutes. He has also had slight dizziness and dysphasia. Carotid ultrasound examination shows a minimal homogeneous thickening with no evidence of flow disturbance on the left. On the right, a heterogeneous plaque with irregular borders is noted in the proximal ICA. Doppler analysis shows a PSV of 180 cm/sec and an EDV of 90 cm/sec. Flow in the common carotid artery is a PSV of 90 cm/sec and an EDV of 35 cm/sec. What do these findings suggest?

2. A 59-year-old man with left arm pain has a carotid ultrasound. The study reveals normal flow velocities bilaterally in the carotid arteries. Interrogation of the vertebral arteries shows reversed flow in the left vertebral. Bilateral blood pressures are taken, with the systolic pressure in the left arm 86 mm Hg and the systolic pressure in the right arm 134 mm Hg. What is the most likely diagnosis?

3. Severe headaches have plagued this 32-year-old woman for years. She has had intermittent episodes of left-sided amaurosis fugax for 2 years. She has recently been diagnosed with hypertension. Carotid ultrasound identifies a distinctive peapod appearance of the ICAs bilaterally, although the left is more prominent. A 75% stenosis on the left and a 50% stenosis on the right are identified with Doppler. What do these findings suggest?

4. A 79-year-old woman is admitted to the hospital after having a stroke. She has right **hemiplegia** and **aphasia**. Carotid ultrasound on the right demonstrates a homogeneous plaque with smooth borders and a Doppler spectrum, indicating a 40% to 59% stenosis. Imaging of the left internal carotid displays echogenic material within the entire lumen. No color or Doppler flow can be obtained. Doppler spectral analysis of the common carotid shows a low-velocity systolic thump. What do these findings indicate?

5. During a routine physical examination, the physician hears a left carotid bruit on a 72-year-old woman. Carotid ultrasound reveals a PSV of 300 cm/sec and an EDV of 178 cm/sec in the left ICA. Left common PSV is 79 cm/sec, and EDV is 30 cm/sec. Color imaging indicates a decrease in lumen patency. A homogeneous, smooth-bordered plaque is noted within the lumen. What percentage of stenosis is suspected?

STUDY QUESTIONS

1. A 56-year-old man is seen with dizziness and bilateral visual disturbances. Carotid ultrasound reveals bilateral mild plaque. Examination of the vertebral vessels shows blue color on the left and flow below baseline when compared with antegrade flow in the common carotid. These findings suggest:
   a. internal carotid artery dissection
   b. stenotic external carotid artery
   c. subclavian steal syndrome
   d. fibromuscular dysplasia
   e. normal finding

2. A carotid ultrasound performed on a 75-year-old woman reveals a peak systolic velocity in the right internal carotid artery of 140 cm/sec and an end diastolic velocity of 50 cm/sec. This would indicate a stenosis in the range of:
   a. 0% to 39%
   b. 40% to 49%
   c. 50% to 79%

   d. 80% to 99%
   e. 100%

3. A patient with an 80% reduction in vessel patency on the right most likely has symptoms affecting the:
   a. contralateral side of head
   b. contralateral side of body
   c. ipsilateral side of body
   d. contralateral side of body and head
   e. ipsilateral side of body and head

4. An 89-year-old man with a long history of smoking and hypertension is sent for a carotid ultrasound. With ultrasound, the anteromedial vessel appears to have a cervical branch indicating the external carotid artery. Doppler analysis shows this vessel to be a low-resistance waveform. What could be the cause?
   a. this is a normal finding
   b. stenotic external carotid artery
   c. 80% stenosis in the internal carotid artery

d. low resistance from collateral branch
e. internalized external carotid artery from occluded internal carotid artery

5. The optimal obtainable Doppler angle for spectral analysis is:
   a. 0 degrees
   b. 30 to 50 degrees
   c. 45 to 60 degrees
   d. 60 to 75 degrees
   e. 90 degrees

6. A 69-year-old woman is sent for carotid ultrasound after her physician hears a bilateral bruit. The patient states she has a history of aortic valve disease. Carotid ultrasound shows only minimal bilateral plaque. What would be the most likely cause of the bruit?
   a. aortic stenosis
   b. fibromuscular dysplasia
   c. tight stenosis not detected with imaging or Doppler
   d. thrombus from heart
   e. subclavian steal syndrome

7. A 36-year-old woman is sent for a carotid ultrasound after multiple transient ischemic attacks (TIAs). She states that her mother also had TIAs at a young age and had some surgery performed, but she could not supply any further details. During scanning of the carotid, the sonographer will most likely identify which of the following?
   a. 50% to 79% stenosis from plaque in the internal carotid arteries
   b. carotid dissection
   c. peapod appearance of internal carotid arteries
   d. intimal flap
   e. right carotid steal

8. A 32-year-old man has relatively sudden onset of left-sided weakness and numbness. Before the onset of symptoms, he was very active and played multiple weekend sports. During the taking of his history, it is discovered that he sees a chiropractor every 6 weeks. Symptoms began after his last visit. What will the carotid ultrasound most likely reveal?
   a. fibromuscular dysplasia
   b. plaque formation
   c. left subclavian steal
   d. intimal flap
   e. thrombus

9. During a carotid ultrasound, which method is most accurate for determination of percent stenosis?
   a. internal carotid/common carotid artery ratios only
   b. peak systolic and end diastolic velocities taken from Doppler spectral waveforms
   c. area measurements
   d. diameter measurement
   e. color-flow analysis

10. Characteristics of fibromuscular dysplasia include all of the following except:
    a. provides environment for embolic events
    b. more often affects women 30 to 50 years old
    c. may affect systemic vessels
    d. may have a hereditary factor
    e. is atherosclerotic in origin

ACKNOWLEDGMENT

Special thanks to Ruben Martinez, James Graven, and especially Leslie Youngman for their assistance.

REFERENCES

1. *2002 Heart and stroke statistical update.* Dallas, 2001, American Heart Association.
2. Biller J, Thies WH: When to operate in carotid artery disease, *Am Fam Physician* 61:400-406, 2000.
3. Henderson SO, Kilaghbian T: Dissection, carotid artery, *eMedicine J* 2; 2001.
4. Finster J, Strassegger J, Haymerle A et al: Bilateral stenting of symptomatic and asymptomatic internal carotid artery stenosis due to fibromuscular dysplasia, *J Neurol Neurosurg Psychiatry* 69:683-686, 2000.

BIBLIOGRAPHY

Anderson KN, Anderson LE, Glanze WD: *Mosby's medical, nursing & allied health dictionary*, ed 5, St Louis, 1998, Mosby.
Brophy DP: Subclavian steal syndrome, *eMedicine J* 2; 2001.
Zwiebel WJ: *Introduction to vascular ultrasonography*, vol 1, ed 4, Philadelphia, 1999, WB Saunders.
Rumwell C, McPharlin M: *Vascular technology: an illustrated review*, ed 2, Pasadena, Calif, 2000, Davies Publishing.
Kelly-Hayes M, Robertson JT, Broderick JP et al: The American Heart Association stroke outcome classification: executive summary, *Circulation* 97:2474-2478, 1998.

34

Leg Pain

LEIF PENROSE

CLINICAL SCENARIO

◼ A venous leg ultrasound is ordered for a 24-year-old male patient in the intensive care unit. The patient was involved in a motor vehicle accident 2 days ago and has fractures of the distal right tibia and fibula, pelvis, and ribs. In addition to the fractures, the patient also has a chest tube for a collapsed left lung. The patient underwent a closed reduction procedure in the operating suite 1 day previously and is enclosed from the knee to the foot in a fiberglass cast. The patient now has swelling greater than expected in the right leg, which is also red and warm to the touch. The contralateral leg is normal in size and color. The ordering physician wants to know whether the right leg swelling is caused by an infection or from thrombus within the veins of the right leg.

The sonographer finds that the common femoral vein is larger than the pulsatile common femoral artery. No flow is seen within the common femoral vein, but flow is entering from the saphenous vein. In some views, low-level echoes are seen within the saphenous system (Fig. 34-1; see Color Plate 25). The sonographer applies external pressure in a transverse plane but is unable to get the vein walls to coapt, even though the common femoral artery is deforming with the amount of pressure applied. Further examination down the leg shows the same findings in the superficial femoral vein. The popliteal and calf vessels cannot be evaluated because of the cast. The contralateral leg shows normal flow within the arterial and venous system, and the walls of the veins easily coapt with slight to moderate transducer pressure. What is the most likely diagnosis?

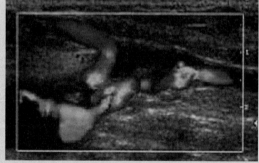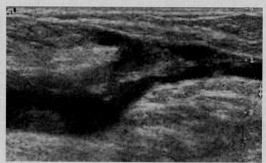

Fig. 34-1 **A,** Color flow is used to show flow in saphenofemoral junction. **B,** Low-level echoes are identified within vessel walls.

OBJECTIVES

◼ Differentiate between the various causes of leg pain.
◼ Describe the sonographic appearance of thrombosis of the deep venous system.
◼ Describe the duplex and indirect studies that can be used to detect arterial disease of the lower extremity.
◼ Describe the physiologic changes to the venous system that help in the diagnosis of deep vein thrombosis.

◼ Differentiate between acute and chronic venous thrombosis.
◼ Define the various types of aneurysms and aneurysmal defects.

GLOSSARY OF TERMS

Aneurysm: a bulging that results from weakened walls of a vessel; predisposing factors include arteriosclerosis, syphilis, and cystic medial necrosis

Ankle brachial index: a comparison of the blood pressure of the ankle and arms; the ratio of those pressures is called an ankle brachial index; normal ratios are greater than 1

Atherosclerosis: a disease of the linings of a vessel; plaque material builds up within the tunica media; as the plaque builds within the walls, the tunica intima bulges inward and decreases the internal diameter of the vessel

Augmentation: external compression of the distal extremity with squeezing of the lower leg/ankle in an attempt to increase proximal venous flow

Baker's cyst: a communication between the synovial fluid of the knee joint and the tissue spaces of the popliteal fossa

Buerger's disease, or thromboangiitis obliterans: as described by Buerger in 1908, an inflammatory and occlusive disease of the extremity arteries, veins, and nerves, with most symptoms occurring in the distal lower extremity

Coapt: when the vessel is subjected to pressure from an outside source (transducer or fingers), the opposite walls of the vessel touch together

Collateral circulation: the flow of blood through an alternative pathway

Compartment syndrome: a painful condition that occurs when swelling is confined within muscle and connective tissue sheets; if the swelling continues or worsens, the pressure may occlude the vascular system

Deep vein thrombosis: thrombosis located within the deep veins of the extremity; the major concern with deep vein thrombosis is that it can lead to pulmonary embolism, which is a potentially fatal disease

Emboli: any object floating along with the flow of blood that is capable of blocking a vessel; venous emboli arising from the lower extremity flow towards and through the heart and then occlude the flow of blood into the lungs

Entrapment syndrome: occurs from external compression of the popliteal artery, most often by the medial head of the gastrocnemius muscle; the occlusion of the popliteal artery and the subsequent ischemia causes intermittent pain, which may be exacerbated by extremity position or exercise

Intermittent claudication: pain that occurs in the extremity after exercise for a given period; the pain diminishes once exercise has ended and the muscle is no longer working with a deficit flow

Plethysmography: an indirect technique for assessment of arterial blood flow; as an extremity receives blood, it increases in girth and then becomes smaller as venous flow drains the extremity; any method that measures and records this girth change may be considered plethysmographic; air plethysmography (pneumoplethysmography, pulse volume recording) and strain gauge plethysmography are two true plethysmographic techniques; photoplethysmography is not a true plethysmographic technique

Photoplethysmography: uses an infrared light attached to a digit to measure the number of red blood cells in a capillary bed; it is not considered a true plethysmographic technique because it does not measure limb volume

Pseudoaneurysm, or false aneurysm: a tear in the arterial wall that allows blood to leak from the vessel; the ectopic blood is then confined within the surrounding tissues

Raynaud's disease: a disease that causes the distal vessels to spasm and obstructs the flow of blood to the extremities

Segmental pressures: blood pressures that are obtained with the color-flow Doppler unit at either the dorsalis pedis or posterior tibial arteries; a cuff is placed higher up the leg, and the cuff is inflated past the point of stopping flow to the dorsalis pedis/posterior tibial arteries; the cuff is slowly deflated until flow resumes; the pressure at which flow returned is recorded

Superficial vein thrombosis: thrombosis located in the superficial veins of the extremity; the thrombosed vein appears as a cord just below the surface of the skin and on ultrasound examination has the characteristics of a thrombosed vessel; patients with thrombosis localized to the superficial system undergo conservative management but may be monitored to ensure that the thrombus does not progress to the deep system

Thrombosis: clotted blood within a vessel

GLOSSARY OF TERMS—cont'd

Valsalva maneuver: a maneuver performed by the patient in an effort to momentarily stop venous flow to the heart; the patient is asked to take a breath and bear down as though trying to have a bowel movement and then hold that pressure; the subsequent increase in abdominal pressure causes a cessation of antegrade venous flow and an increase in distal vein size; once the patient releases the pressure, the backed-up venous blood is able to rapidly flow antegrade again

Varicose veins: dilated and tortuous veins of the superficial venous system

Venous insufficiency: refers to a vein in which the valves are no longer functioning correctly, allowing blood to flow in a retrograde fashion; the tissues distal to chronic venous insufficiency may become hyperpigmented, indurated, and ulcerative

Virchow's triad: a set of three causative factors described by Rudolph Virchow in 1862; damage to the venous wall, decrease in flow (stasis), and increase in coagulability increase the probability of venous thrombosis; damage to the vessel wall may be through surgery, trauma, or indwelling lines; decrease in flow may be through immobility, external pressure, varicose veins, congestive heart failure, or other causes; increased incoagulability may be caused by a release of factor III in surgical patients who are healing, by malignant tissues of cancer patients, or by burned damaged tissue

Yin Yang sign: a color Doppler pattern in which a vessel examined in a transverse plane shows the swirling pattern flow; the blood coming toward the transducer is color encoded red, and the flow away from the transducer is color encoded blue

This chapter describes a variety of causes of leg pain and the role of ultrasound in diagnosis of these diseases. Protocols may vary depending on whether these examinations are performed in a radiology-based ultrasound department versus a dedicated vascular laboratory. This chapter focuses more on the protocols followed in a radiology department. A brief explanation of normal anatomy is included, but the focus is on the pathology and diseases that lead to leg pain.

For the lower extremity arterial system, the vascular-based ultrasound department has a variety of duplex and indirect physiologic tests that can narrow the diagnosis in patients with leg pain. The radiology-based ultrasound department concentrates primarily on the diagnosis of **deep vein thrombosis (DVT)**, **pseudoaneurysm,** and posterior knee masses.

B-mode Doppler ultrasound and the indirect tests of the vascular laboratory can be quite useful in diagnosis of vascular causes of leg pain. Although bony fractures, tendinous sprains, ligamental ruptures/tears, muscle strains, tears and ruptures, nerve impingement, and trauma are the most common sources of lower extremity pain, these diagnoses are left to plain film radiograph, computed tomography (CT), and magnetic resonance imaging (MRI). Fig. 34-2 shows how a physician would decide which imaging examination would best assess the patient's condition based on history, symptoms, and physical examination.

NORMAL VASCULAR ANATOMY

In most instances with a single vein, an artery is found with the same name. Exceptions to this rule are that the veins of the calf distal to the popliteal vein are normally paired and an artery does not accompany the superficial saphenous vessels. The veins of the leg can be divided into those that are superficial and those that are deep. Although they are called deep veins, they are actually superficial enough to be well visualized on most patients with 5- to 7-MHz linear transducers.

Starting at the iliac bifurcation, the veins are listed in a retrograde order (Figs. 34-3 and 34-4; see Color Plates 26 and 27) and the arteries are listed in an antegrade order. The two common iliac vessels branch into the inferior vena cava (IVC) and from the aorta at the level of the umbilicus. They continue until the level of the sacroiliac joints before the internal iliac (hypogastric) vessels angle steeply into the pelvis feeding/draining the rectum, sigmoid, and genitals. After the internal iliacs have departed, the external iliac vessels proceed along the lateral wall of the pelvis before leaving the pelvis at the inguinal canal. After passing the inguinal ligament, the vessels are called the common femoral vessels. After about 4 cm, the common femoral vein (CFV) is joined by the saphenous vein (SV) from an anterior medial direction. Within a few centimeters of the SV/CFV junction, the common femorals branch into the superficial femorals and the deep femorals. The deep femorals are also called the *profunda femoris* or simply the *profunda*. The profunda serves the upper thigh. The

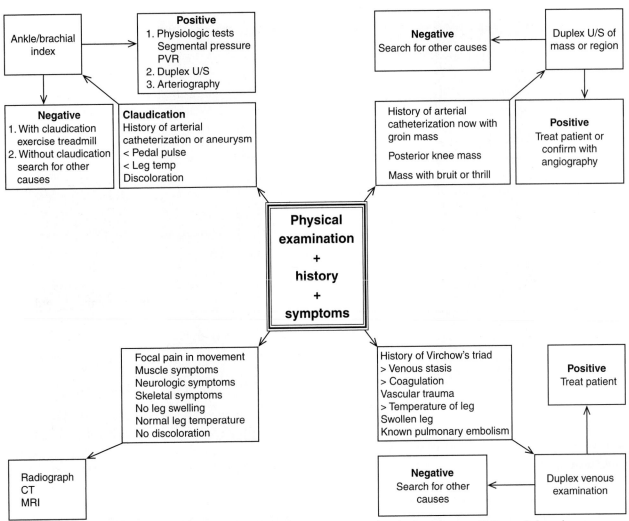

Fig. 34-2 Leg pain examination selection protocol. *Hx,* History; *PVR,* peripheral vascular resistance; *U/S,* ultrasound.

superficial femorals continue along the anterior medial leg until they dive deep through the ligaments of the adductor muscles, known as the *adductor hiatus* or the *Hunter's Canal.*

Once the superficial vessels pass through the adductor hiatus, they can be located posterior to the knee and are termed the *popliteal vessels.* The popliteal vessels quickly start branching into other vessels of various sizes. The anterior tibial vessels branch off anterior and lateral, passing through the space formed between the tibia and fibula then lateral to the tibial shaft with a single artery and paired veins. The popliteal continues for a few centimeters before the peroneal (fibular vessels) and posterior tibial vessels branch off. The peroneal vessels run deeper and more lateral with a single artery and paired veins, and the posterior tibials (one artery and two paired veins) continue more medial

and superficial down to the area just posterior to the medial malleolus.

Arteries of the ankle/foot that are commonly used for continuous wave Doppler samples or pulses include the posterior tibial, which can be found about 1 inch posterior to the medial malleolus, and the dorsal pedis, which is found in the anterior midfoot just over the proximal third metatarsal.

A superficial vein that is routinely visualized is the greater SV, which travels, without an accompanying artery, along the superficial medial aspect of the leg, starting near the ankle and continuing up to its insertion into the CFV just inferior to the groin crease.

Artery or Vein?

A number of assessments are useful in determination of whether an extremity vessel is an artery or a vein.

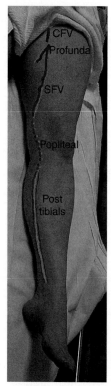

Fig. 34-3 Vascular anatomy identified at anterior and medial aspect of leg.

- The arteries maintain a round shape when viewed in cross section.
- The veins are ovoid unless distended.
- The arteries pulsate with each heartbeat.
- The veins dilate during Valsalva maneuver or when the patient's trunk is elevated in relation to the extremity.
- The vein has the potential of being larger than the accompanying artery. In a thrombus-filled state, it is larger; but in the healthy patient, it may appear slightly smaller.

ARTERIAL DISEASE
Atherosclerosis

Most of the tissue of the lower extremity is composed of muscle. Muscle tissue creates pain stimuli whenever there is inadequate blood supply. During clinical histories, much can be learned with questioning of the patient concerning the amount of pain and its frequency. In cases of severe **atherosclerosis** or when an embolic event has occurred, the extremity receives inadequate blood supply even when the patient is resting. Patients with less severe atherosclerosis or well-developed collateral circulation only have symptoms during times of higher demand (during exercise). Patients with a decreased arterial blood supply may

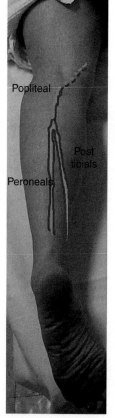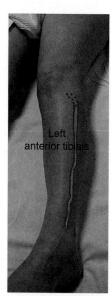

Fig. 34-4 Vascular anatomy identified at posterior *(left)* and lateral *(right)* aspects of lower leg.

have decreased function and, in severe cases, increased risk of tissue necrosis and gangrene.

Intermittent Claudication

Pain that occurs during exercise and diminishes after resting is termed *intermittent claudication.* Testing to assess this symptom usually occurs in a vascular laboratory. The goal is documentation of the onset of this pain in a controlled setting and, with confirmation, location of the area of constriction. Unlike venous extremity disease, in which thrombus is seen within the lumen of the veins, this disease is atherosclerotic in nature, with the plaque located within the walls of the vessel and bulging the tunica intima into the lumen. The confirmation of the symptoms is usually performed with indirect testing methods of **ankle brachial index** (ABI) and localized with **segmental pressures.** Once localization to a specific region is complete, a careful duplex examination of the arteries within that area can be performed.

Bilateral ankle and brachial blood pressures are taken before having the patient walk on a constant-load treadmill. The bilateral ankle pressures are recorded from the posterior tibial artery (PTA) or the dorsalis pedis artery, and the brachial pressures are recorded from the antecubital fossa (both brachials are measured, but the higher reading is used for the ABI). The ratio of those pressures is the ABI. If the ABI is normal (1 or more), the patient may go on to a treadmill examination. Treadmill protocols vary but are designed to increase demand on the muscles of the leg, thus inducing symptoms in patients whose symptoms are produced only with exercise. After walking, the ankle pressures are repeated every minute for a specific time period and the pressures are graphed. If the pressures remain normal or are slightly elevated, the test is considered within normal limits. If the pressure drops immediately after exercise, the test is considered positive and the source of occlusion is sought with either lower extremity angiography or duplex ultrasound of the arterial system. The extent of disease can be estimated on the basis of the severity of the pressure decrease and the length of time for recovery.

If the ABI is less than 1, it is considered abnormal and segmental blood pressures are taken to localize the area of occlusion. Any drop of greater than 20 to 30 mm Hg from one level to the next or from one side to the other is an indication of atherosclerosis proximal to or at the level of the cuff.

It must be noted that cuff pressure changes with width. Before they occlude the flow, narrow cuffs must be inflated to a higher pressure compared with the pressure necessary for wide cuffs. For this reason, the width of the cuff should be 20% wider than limb diameter. With a four-cuff technique, an artificial elevation of the high thigh measurement is seen from the use of a narrow cuff.

Popliteal Entrapment Syndrome

External compression of the popliteal artery, most often by the medial head of the gastrocnemius muscle, can cause intermittent calf claudication. This compression can occur with an abnormal location of the medial head laterally, an abnormal location of the popliteal artery medially, or development of the gastrocnemius muscle in athletes. The occlusion of the popliteal artery and the subsequent ischemia cause intermittent pain. This pain may be exacerbated by the extremity position or exercise. The sonographer assesses posterior tibial flow with the patient's ankle in multiple positions. The knee should be extended without flexion, then PTA pulses in neutral and dorsiflexed positions should be recorded. In addition, if consistent claudication is seen with exercise, examination after exercise treadmill may

be useful. **Entrapment syndrome** can be documented when a decrease in flow to the calf/foot from exercise or position can be identified. Various types of classifications have been assigned on the basis of the anatomic cause. In some patients, an increase in muscle mass of the leg can cause a previously silent anatomic anomaly to become clinically significant.

Constant Resting Pain and Foot Pain

Resting pain occurs when the patient has either severe or multilevel atherosclerosis or has had an embolic event. Severe atherosclerosis shows vascular compromise with ABIs of 0.25 and less.

Distal foot pain can occur from arterial **emboli** arising from the abdomen, pelvis, or upper femoral regions. In these instances, the emboli occlude flow distal to the occlusion. Embolism has a random pattern of distribution of tissue affected, with some toes or regions being affected while others are normal. The foot or toes may be cold and pulseless distal to the occlusion. Spectral and color Doppler and **photoplethysmography** (PPG) should show decreased or absent flow when compared with the contralateral normal foot.

Aneurysm

Soft Tissue Mass on Posterior Knee. The most common posterior knee mass is a **Baker's cyst.** The sonographer's role in this examination is to differentiate a Baker's cyst from a popliteal artery **aneurysm.** A Baker's cyst (Fig. 34-5) is a communication between the synovial fluid of the knee joint and the tissue spaces of the popliteal fossa. B-mode ultrasound should show an anechoic sac with or without septations or low-level echogenic debris (see Fig. 34-5). A Baker's cyst should not communicate with the popliteal artery or have pulsatile flow. Popliteal aneurysms (Fig. 34-6) have pulsatile flow within the lumen, connect to the popliteal artery, and may have clot within the aneurysm. A popliteal artery aneurysm may show the classic **Yin Yang sign** (Fig. 34-7; see Color Plate 28). Patients with a popliteal artery aneurysm are at increased risk for aneurysms in the abdomen or contralateral knee.

Pseudoaneurysm

Patients who have recently undergone angiographic procedures that required a femoral artery stick may have a painful leg in the groin area with an associated mass effect. These studies require that the mass be examined with B-mode and color Doppler. A sacular defect adjacent to the femoral artery is visualized in positive studies. If the pseudoaneurysm (Fig. 34-8; see Color

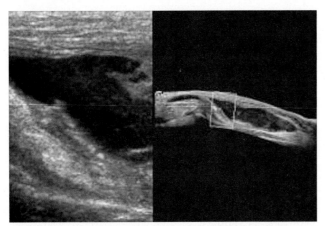

Fig. 34-5 Baker's cyst does not show evidence of blood flow.

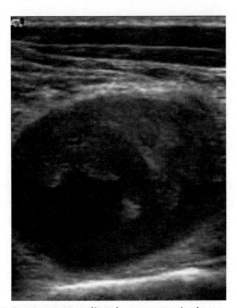

Fig. 34-6 Large popliteal aneurysm is shown.

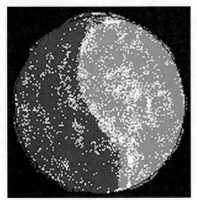

Fig. 34-7 Yin Yang sign shows swirling blood flow pattern.

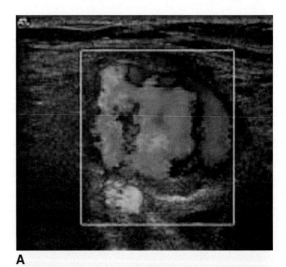

A

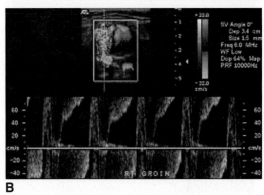

B

Fig. 34-8 **A,** Pseudoaneurysm shows Yin Yang sign with color flow Doppler. **B,** Spectral analysis also shows turbulent flow.

Plate 29) has not spontaneously occluded, the sonographer sees flow within the sac. Color Doppler shows a Yin Yang flow pattern with a neck that connects directly to the femoral artery. Compression with the probe decreases the size of the aneurysm. With sufficient probe pressure and sufficient time, the sonographer may be able to produce clotting within the aneurysm, thus "curing" the patient. A growing number of facilities use ultrasound guidance and monitoring during and after the injection of thrombin (Fig. 34-9; see Color Plate 30) into these defects.

Trauma

Patients who have had trauma that disrupts the normal flow of blood to distal tissues have pain in the oxygen-starved, downstream tissues. Unless precluded by the wound, the ABI may show arterial flow to the foot. If the ABI is equivocal or more detailed information is needed, duplex scanning may be a means of rapid assessment of the vascular system. Angiography remains

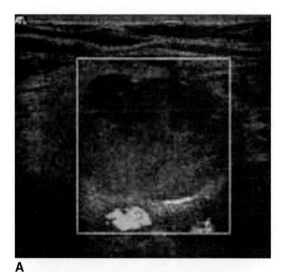

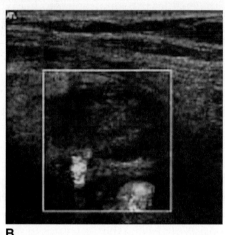

Fig. 34-9 Ultrasound may be used to, **A,** guide injection of thrombin and, **B,** monitor follow-up.

the gold standard for vascular injury, but the length of time necessary to obtain an angiogram is sometimes unacceptable for a patient with vascular compromise from trauma.

Compartment Syndrome

Patients who have had recent trauma or other history of extremity tissue swelling can have **compartment syndrome.** This painful condition occurs when swelling is confined within muscle and connective tissue sheets. The buildup of fluid is unable to find release through the compartmental fascia, and the pressure can cause occlusion of the vascular system. Without relief, tissue necrosis results. Sonographic evaluation can show a decrease in distal pressures with ABI and compression of the vessels with duplex examination. The treatment for compartment syndrome involves a fasciotomy to relieve the pressure.

OTHER ARTERIAL OCCLUSIVE DISEASES
Raynaud's Disease

A patient with **Raynaud's disease** has distal extremity vasospasms, which obstruct the flow of blood to the hands and digits. This spasm can be brought on by either exposure to cold stimulus or by emotions. Symptoms more often are noted in the upper extremity, and the extremity becomes pale or blue and cold. Secondary Raynaud's phenomenon is related to an autoimmune disorder or vascular occlusion, and primary Raynaud's disease does not have an underlying cause.

A variety of protocols are used to confirm Raynaud's disease. The goal of the sonographer is to determine whether the cause of the vasospasm is cold. Duplex examination, segmental pressures, and PPG may first be performed to rule out occlusive disease. If these results prove normal, then a cold immersion test can be performed. A baseline PPG is performed, and the hand is then immersed in ice-cold water for 3 minutes or as long as the patient can tolerate. Subsequent PPGs are performed on each digit for 10 minutes. A normal examination shows a return to baseline within 5 minutes, and patients with Raynaud's disease do not have a return to normal until after 10 minutes.

Buerger's Disease

Thromboangiitis obliterans, also known as *Buerger's disease,* is relatively rare. It is an inflammation of the arteries, veins, and nerves of the hands and feet that leads to restricted arterial flow. Buerger's disease is found almost exclusively in smokers and predominantly in men ages 20 to 40 years. Progression of the disease may be halted by cessation of smoking. Symptoms in the lower extremity include resting pain, especially in the arch of the foot, and ischemia in the digits. Documentation of decreased peripheral flow to the digits can be accomplished with PPGs. In advanced disease, the tissue may be necrosed so that PPG cannot be performed.

VENOUS DISEASE
Deep Vein Thrombosis

Pulmonary embolism has a high rate of morbidity (600,000 hospitalizations and 200,000 deaths each year). The primary source of pulmonary embolism is **thrombosis** of the deep venous system (Fig. 34-10; see Color Plate 31) in the lower extremities (90%). The primary symptom of DVT of the lower extremity is a painful swollen leg. Duplex sonography is accurate in determination of the presence or absence of venous

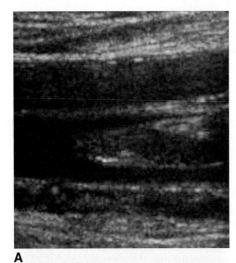

A

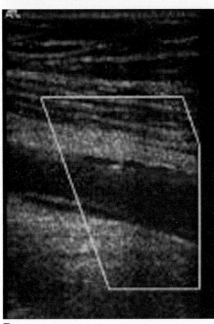

B

Fig. 34-10 **A,** Deep vein thrombosis (DVT) of femoral vein may show tongue of intraluminal material that may move within vessel. **B,** Acute DVT shows homogeneous, low-level echoes.

venous **insufficiency,** progression of **superficial vein thrombosis** [SVT]), increases a patient's coagulability (oral contraceptive use, coagulation disorders, recent surgery, cancer), or decreases natural flow pressures (congestive heart failure) increases the possibility of venous thrombosis. The three primary factors that lead to venous thrombosis—vessel damage, flow stasis, and hypercoagulability—are known as *Virchow's triad.*

Leg pain can arise from a number of areas other than the venous system: arterial, muscle, connective tissue, nerve, trauma, infection, or skeletal. The role of the sonographer is as much to rule out different possible causes as to determine what the exact cause may be. Clinical history is as critical to successful diagnosis as is the sonographic study itself. Nevertheless, adherence to strict criteria enables the sonographer to help diagnose venous occlusion.

Beyond the discovery of venous thrombosis, the clinical course can be significantly altered by the determination of the age of a clot. Chronic clot is not treated aggressively, and acute clot may respond favorably to aggressive use of antiembolytic/antithrombolytic therapy. Ultrasound findings can strongly suggest whether a clot is acute or chronic, ensuring that the patient receives appropriate treatment.

Patients with DVT may have symptoms directly related to the leg (acutely swollen, painful leg) or symptoms of pulmonary embolism (shortness of breath). The examination consists of viewing the deep veins of the leg with B-mode ultrasound, compressing the vessels to assess for coaptation, and documenting the changes in the spectral Doppler waveform during **Valsalva maneuver** or distal **augmentation.**

The patient should be positioned with the trunk slightly elevated and the lower extremity slightly rotated outward. Some experts suggest having the patient dangle the affected leg during examination of the calf vessels. The sonographer should start high in the groin crease, documenting the common femoral artery and vein. Spectral Doppler of the veins should demonstrate phasic flow that varies with respiration, augmentation, and Valsalva maneuver. If the patient's trunk is elevated, the vein appears distended, but there should be no evidence of thrombus within the vein. When moderate probe pressure is increased, the walls of the vein should **coapt.** Probe pressure is adequate if the accompanying artery begins to deform. (It should be noted that this maneuver must be done in a transverse plane and should not be done with the transducer in a longitudinal plane because it is too easy to slide off the side of the vessel in longitudinal plane).

clot. Its advantages over venography include better patient tolerance, similar accuracy, lower risk, and lower cost.

Certain patient populations are at increased risk for development of thrombosis in the legs. Blood that is not moving tends to clot. The combined factors of muscle contraction and venous valve action and the effects of respiration propel venous blood in the extremities. Any event that immobilizes the leg (trauma, surgery, advanced age, obesity, prolonged sitting), damages the deep venous valves (**varicose veins,**

The sonographer should begin moving down the leg at close intervals and show the absence of echogenic intraluminal material, the continuation of phasic flow that varies with respiration, and coaptation of the vein walls. Doppler analysis can be helpful in documenting thrombus that has progressed to a size that can interrupt flow. Doppler signals that show a continuous flow pattern or lack of increased flow during distal augmentation suggest flow-restricting thrombus.

The vessels that should be interrogated include the CFV, SV, profunda, superficial femoral vein (SFV), and popliteal veins (Fig. 34-11, *A*) to the popliteal trifurcation. Controversy exists as to the value of continuing through the calf vessels. Most dedicated vascular laboratories also interrogate the anterior tibials, posterior tibials, and peroneals, but many radiology-based ultrasound department protocols do not include these venous trees. In addition, when DVT is identified, the sonographer should interrogate cephalad to document the extent of the thrombus, which may include imaging of the iliac vessels (Fig. 34-11, *B*).

Imaging hints include:
- Keeping the focal zone at the level of the vessel being viewed
- Imaging the vessel from an approach that is closest to the skin for that vessel at that level
- Keeping the vessel in the middle of the transducer face
- Carefully adjusting the gain so that soft internal plaque is visualized and not "blacked out" by incorrect gain settings

The study is considered positive for DVT if the walls of the vein do not coapt when the artery has begun to deform or if thrombus can be documented within the vein. The spectral Doppler proximal to the thrombus is continuous with distal augmentation, having little or no effect on the proximal waveform.

When thrombus is found, analysis of the clot is important to determine whether the thrombus appears acute or chronic. The sonographic findings for acute and chronic thrombus are listed subsequently.

Acute thrombus:
- Is uniform in texture, with low level echoes
- Is soft or slightly compressible
- Is poorly attached; may sometimes "flap about" within the vessel
- Distends the vessel

Chronic thrombus:
- Is heterogeneous, with bright echoes
- Does not compress
- Is rigidly attached

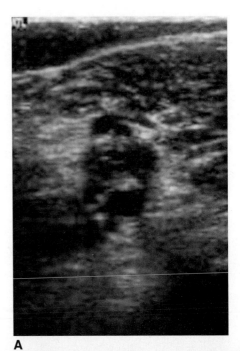

A

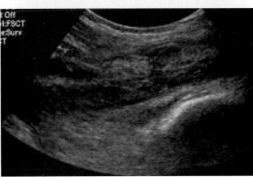

B

Fig. 34-11 Thrombus may be identified in, **A,** popliteal veins or, **B,** iliac veins.

- Tends to contract the vessel and may show a partial recanalization of the vein with a tortuous flow channel with well-developed collateral circulation

Superficial Vein Thrombosis

Superficial vein thrombosis is usually diagnosed clinically with a painful superficial cord with surrounding erythema. The condition is treated with anticoagulation therapy or ligation of the offending vessel at its proximal attachment to the deep system. Ultrasound can be useful to ensure that the swelling, pain, and redness are not caused by other underlying causes, such as soft-tissue infection or hematoma. Ultrasound is also valuable in determination of the extent of the thrombosis (Fig. 34-12) and monitoring of progression or regression with therapy.[1]

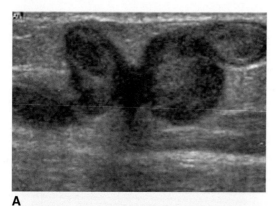

A

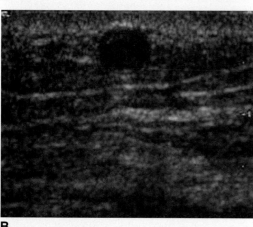

B

Fig. 34-12 Superficial venous thrombosis is seen as palpable, tender cord. **A** and **B,** Low-level echoes are shown within affected vessels.

Venous Insufficiency

The superficial venous system is a common site of valvular insufficiency that leads to varicose veins. Superficial veins that have increased pressure from failure of downstream valves tend to enlarge and shift to a superficial location. They can become infected and are unsightly. If the venous insufficiency occurs because

of DVT, it is termed *secondary,* whereas if venous insufficiency exists without DVT, it is termed *primary.* High-frequency linear transducers can be used to document the valves in motion on B-mode. Spectral Doppler shows reversed flow during Valsalva maneuver and after augmentation.

SUMMARY

Vascular leg pain is a serious symptom. Arterial vascular compromise can rapidly lead to limb loss, and venous vascular disease has a high mortality rate from pulmonary embolism. A complete and thorough patient history is crucial in effective sequencing of examinations. When sequenced properly, ultrasound is a quick and effective method of determining vascular causes of leg pain. Ultrasound of the veins of the leg has proven to be an effective method of determining not only the presence but also the age of thrombus within the deep venous system. Ultrasound and the indirect testing have made a major impact in decreasing the number of invasive procedures previously necessary to document arterial disease.

CLINICAL SCENARIO—DIAGNOSIS

▨ This patient has the classic signs of DVT. The immobilization necessary from the motor vehicle accident makes this patient susceptible to clotting of the slow-moving venous return system. The fact that the end of the clot is not shown in the CFV means the sonographer should evaluate higher into the iliac vein, although compression would be difficult, especially in this patient with a fractured pelvis. Careful transducer manipulation reveals clot extending into the iliac vessel.

CASE STUDIES FOR DISCUSSION

1. A 55-year-old female with a swollen and painful right leg for the past 36 hours is seen. During scanning of the common femoral vein, a moveable tongue of echogenic intraluminal material is identified. The superficial femoral and popliteal veins are dilated and do not compress. The thrombus is relatively homogeneous in echogenicity. What is the most likely diagnosis?

2. A 39-year-old male patient is seen with a palpable mass in the left popliteal fossa. Duplex examination of the posterior surface of the left knee shows a large fluid collection. Flow is seen, and the popliteal arteries/veins are shown as separate structures. With movement of the leg and external pressure from the transducer, the cystic mass is shown to increase and decrease in size. What is the most likely diagnosis?

3. A 59-year-old woman had a coronary catheterization procedure 3 days ago and has a pulsatile groin mass. B-mode shows a 3-cm cystic mass immediately adjacent to the common femoral artery. With external probe pressure, the mass decreases in size. Color Doppler shows flow towards the transducer on one side of the cyst, with flow away from the transducer on the other. What is the most likely diagnosis?

4. A 49-year-old man with distal leg pain is seen. The lower leg is swollen and painful. The upper leg is normal, as is the contralateral leg. The veins of the affected upper leg compress and demonstrate phasic flow in the common femoral vein. The superficial femoral vein (SFV) compresses from the groin to the point where it dives through the adductor hiatus. However, as flow in the SFV is checked further down the thigh, the flow changes to a continuous low-velocity pattern. In addition, a peaking of flow on the spectral waveform does not occur during distal augmentation. When the sonographer examines the popliteal system, a dilated vein filled with low-level echoes is shown. Flow is not demonstrated within the vein but is seen in the accompanying popliteal artery. What is the most likely diagnosis?

5. A 52-year-old woman is seen with a painful left leg by her physician. Physical examination finds a red swollen leg with "tough cords" running just below the skin surface. B-mode examination shows dilated, superficial vessels filled with low-level echoes. These vessels are identified as superficial in that their course lies within the first fascial plane. The deep veins of the upper and lower leg are compressible and show normal flow without evidence of internal thrombus. What is the most likely diagnosis?

STUDY QUESTIONS

1. A 45-year-old man has a patent and compressible superficial femoral vein for most of the distance through the leg. Doppler signals show normal respiratory phasicity, and distal augmentation shows normal increased flow. In the lower third of the femur, the vein becomes harder to compress. The sonographer compresses but is unable to cause the femoral vein or artery to collapse before the patient has pain. Examination below the knee and in the calf veins appears normal. The findings are consistent with which of the following?
   a. chronic deep vein thrombosis of the distal superficial femoral vein
   b. acute deep vein thrombosis of the distal superficial femoral vein
   c. interference by the ligaments of the adductor muscles
   d. compartment syndrome
   e. entrapment syndrome

2. A 65-year-old woman is seen in the ultrasound department 1 day after coronary angiography. The patient had no leg symptoms before the angiogram. The patient has proximal leg and groin pain. On physical examination, a pulsatile soft tissue mass in the groin area is discovered. Ultrasound shows a compressible fluid sac anterior to the common femoral vein. Color Doppler shows a Yin Yang flow pattern. What is the most likely diagnosis for this ultrasound finding?
   a. femoral artery pseudoaneurysm
   b. Baker's cyst
   c. arteriovenous fistula of the femoral system
   d. deep vein thrombosis
   e. intermittent claudication of the arterial system

3. A 34-year-old obese woman who is an inpatient in the trauma intensive care unit (ICU) has shortness of breath, leg pain, and swelling of the right lower extremity. The portable ultrasound in the ICU shows

an enlarged common femoral vein with walls that do not coapt with extrinsic transducer pressure. The lumen of the vessel is a low-level homogeneous gray. Which of the following is the most likely diagnosis?

a. femoral artery pseudoaneurysm
b. Baker's cyst
c. acute deep vein thrombosis
d. chronic deep vein thrombosis
e. atherosclerosis

4. A 55-year-old woman is seen with long-term varicose veins. She states that her legs have been painful for the past 5 years from the varicosities. She now has gradual swelling in her left leg for the past month. Ultrasound evaluation shows a small contracted superficial femoral vein that is brightly echogenic, inhomogeneous, and noncompressible. Color Doppler shows flow that is following a tortuous path within the central lumen. What is the most likely diagnosis?

a. Buerger's disease
b. Raynaud's disease
c. acute deep vein thrombosis
d. chronic deep vein thrombosis
e. atherosclerosis

5. A venous ultrasound is ordered for a 40-year-old inpatient to rule out deep vein thrombosis. The patient had a renal arteriogram 2 days previously and now has a painful distal lower extremity. On physical examination, the leg is not swollen, the distal lower leg is pale, and the foot has decreased pulses. The skin of the foot and ankle shows a mottled pattern. Ultrasound finds the deep veins of the femur, knee, and lower leg to be patent and compressible without evidence of internal thrombus. What is a likely explanation of the patient's symptoms?

a. Buerger's disease
b. Raynaud's disease
c. embolization of the distal lower extremity arterial system
d. acute deep vein thrombosis
e. chronic deep vein thrombosis

6. A 47-year-old man with diabetes is seen with a painful swollen lower leg. The patient is a salesperson who returned home 2 days ago from a weeklong series of business meetings on the opposite coast. He had no symptoms until the morning after his return flight. His common femoral and superficial femoral veins are normal in size, and the walls coapt completely. The Doppler signal in the superficial femoral vein (SFV) is continuous without phasicity. Distal augmentation does not show a change in the SFV waveform. The popliteal vein is normal in size but does not coapt completely. Which of the following is the most likely diagnosis?

a. Buerger's disease
b. Raynaud's disease
c. embolization of the distal lower extremity arterial system
d. acute deep vein thrombosis
e. chronic deep vein thrombosis

7. A 25-year-old man is seen with a gradual onset of leg claudication. The common femoral and superficial femoral veins are normal in size, and the walls coapt completely. Distal augmentation does not show a change in the superficial femoral vein waveform. Although compression is difficult because of the patients well-developed leg musculature, the popliteal vein is normal in size and coapts completely. The ankle brachial index (ABI) shows variation based on the patient's leg and ankle position. The ABI is normal when the foot is in neutral position but decreases when the foot is plantar flexed. What is the most likely diagnosis?

a. chronic deep vein thrombosis of the distal superficial femoral vein
b. acute deep vein thrombosis of the distal superficial femoral vein
c. interference of compression by the ligaments of the adductor muscles
d. compartment syndrome
e. entrapment syndrome

8. A 62-year-old woman has a painful leg, and an ultrasound evaluation is ordered. The pain is intermittent although severe enough at times that she must stop walking, at which time the pain subsides. The ultrasound examination of the venous system shows common femoral and superficial femoral veins that are normal in size and the walls coapt completely. The Doppler signal in the superficial femoral vein (SFV) shows respiratory phasicity. Distal augmentation causes a normal change in the SFV waveform. The popliteal vein is normal in size and coapts completely. The veins of the lower calf appear normal. Ankle brachial index (ABI) of the affected leg is 0.50, and the contralateral leg has an ABI of 0.98. What is the most likely diagnosis?

a. Buerger's disease
b. Raynaud's disease
c. acute deep vein thrombosis
d. chronic deep vein thrombosis
e. atherosclerosis causing intermittent claudication

9. A 71-year-old woman with multiple prior events of deep vein thrombosis is seen with a red swollen leg that is warm to the touch. Physical examination reveals serpiginous enlarged tough "cords" just below the skin surface. The ultrasound evaluation shows that the greater saphenous vein is enlarged and noncompressible. The common femoral vein is enlarged and does not coapt. The superficial femoral vein is difficult to visualize and appears small and tortuous. What is the most likely diagnosis?
   a. primary superficial vein thrombosis
   b. secondary superficial vein thrombosis with acute deep vein thrombosis
   c. primary superficial vein thrombosis with chronic deep vein thrombosis
   d. secondary superficial vein thrombosis with recurrent deep vein thrombosis and collateral replacement of the superficial femoral vein
   e. atherosclerosis

10. A 9-year-old boy was admitted to the intensive care unit 1 day ago. The patient was riding a bicycle when he was struck from the side by a slow-moving car. The patient has a broken arm and a large hematoma on the right mid thigh but no leg fractures. The right knee and calf are now swelling, and lower leg pain is increasing. Ultrasound examination of the high thigh shows normal veins that coapt completely. The veins in the region near the hematoma are collapsed. The veins distal to the hematoma are enlarged and coapt completely but need more pressure than expected. The spectral Doppler waveform shows continuous flow in the common femoral vein (CFV) and minimal continuous flow that has an elevated velocity in the veins of the knee and lower leg. Augmentation produces no effect in the CFV. What is the most likely cause for these findings?
   a. chronic deep vein thrombosis of the distal superficial femoral vein
   b. acute deep vein thrombosis of the distal superficial femoral vein
   c. pseudoaneurysm compression of the distal superficial femoral vein
   d. compartment syndrome
   e. entrapment syndrome

ACKNOWLEDGEMENT

The author thanks Phillips Medical Systems for providing images for this chapter.

REFERENCES

1. Zweibel WJ: *Introduction to vascular ultrasonography*, ed 4, Philadelphia, 2000, WB Saunders.

BIBLIOGRAPHY

Ridgway DP: *Introduction to vascular scanning*, ed 2, Pasadena, 1998, Davies Publishing.

Hagen-Ansert S: *Textbook of diagnostic medical sonography*, ed 5, St Louis, 2001, Mosby.

Curry R, Bates-Tempkin B: *Ultrasonography: an introduction to normal structure and functional anatomy*, Philadelphia, 1995, WB Saunders.

Daigle R: *Techniques in noninvasive vascular diagnosis*, Littleton, 2002, Summer Publishing.

ANSWERS TO CASE STUDIES

Chapter 1

1. The diagnosis of gastritis explains the symptoms. Multiple small polyps would be consistent with cholesterolosis, which in this case is most likely an incidental finding.
2. The gallbladder findings are consistent with cholelithiasis and sludge. The findings in the duct are consistent with ductal dilatation explained by choledocholithiasis.
3. Acute cholecystitis.
4. Amebic abscess.
5. Polycystic disease of the liver.

Chapter 2

1. Metastatic disease to the liver.
2. A logical response is liver metastasis with a history of endometrial carcinoma. However, the ultrasound appearance is consistent with a hemangioma, confirmed with ab-dominal computed tomographic scan.
3. Ultrasound-guided biopsy is used to confirm the diagnosis of focal nodular hyperplasia.
4. Computed tomographic scan is used to confirm the infiltrating nature of the lesion along with the nodular cirrhotic liver and gallstones. In addition, computed tomographic scan is used to identify a small left pleural effusion and varicosities in the abdomen. The diagnosis of hepatocellular carcinoma is made with biopsy.
5. Computed tomographic scan–guided biopsy is performed. The specimen is sent to the pathology laboratory and reveals metastatic disease. The patient also has a bone scan that reveals multiple metastatic lesions.

Chapter 3

1. Fatty liver disease.
2. Acute hepatitis.
3. Hepatocellular carcinoma.
4. Cirrhosis.
5. Patent TIPS catheter with hepatopetal flow noted.

Chapter 4

1. Surgical biopsy confirms the diagnosis of insulinoma, a type of islet cell tumor.
2. If the patient does not have a hormone imbalance, a nonfunctioning islet cell tumor is possible. A solid cystadenoma/cystadenocarcinoma or squamous cell carcinoma should be considered. A solid pseudocyst is unlikely without evidence of inflammation. Although this lesion is located in the pancreatic tail, CT scan–guided biopsy reveals adenocarcinoma.
3. Alcoholism is one of the major causes of pancreatitis. Because of the echogenicity and heterogeneity of the pancreas, this case is diagnosed with sonography as chronic pancreatitis. The presence of pancreatic duct stones is also strongly suggestive of chronic pancreatitis.
4. Benign microcystic cystadenoma.
5. Acute focal pancreatitis.

Chapter 5

1. Whenever a solid renal mass is identified, vascular involvement should be investigated. Benign renal masses and stage 1 renal malignant diseases both have the same sonographic characteristics and may have the same clinical presentation. This mass is diagnosed as RCC, the clear cell type.
2. Congenital anomalies of the kidneys can cause hematuria with no other clinical symptoms. The diagnosis is cross-fused ectopic kidneys versus horseshoe configuration in the pelvis.
3. TCC. When an irregular shape mass is identified in the urinary bladder, a malignant mass should be considered. The most common malignant bladder tumor is a TCC, which typically appears as an echogenic, irregularly shaped mass in the lumen of the urinary bladder. Metastatic disease to the urinary bladder can be from direct extension of a rectum carcinoma or from the upper urinary system.
4. The large mass is confirmed to be an AML. AMLs are typically located in the renal cortex and do not cause disruption of the renal sinus. AMLs can grow large and cause hematuria and flank pain. Disruption of the diaphragm was noted.
5. TCC. TCC is usually seen as painless hematuria and is more common in elderly men. On ultrasound, a TCC will appear either as a complex mass or as a hypoechoic mass located in the central portion of the kidney. The mass may interrupt the echogenic renal sinus and cause hydronephrosis. No hydronephrosis is noted on the ultrasound. A CT scan of the abdomen is performed to identify the presence of any extension of the malignant disease. No other pathology is found.

Chapter 6

1. The mass in the left kidney is sonographically undistinguishable from renal cell carcinoma. The mass is most likely xanthogranulomatous pyelonephritis because of the findings of the staghorn calculi in the renal pelvis, the laboratory finding of infection, the enlarged kidney, and the long history of obstruction. Biopsy of the mass is necessary for positive identification.

2. The thinned parenchyma, the decreased renal size, and the abnormal laboratory values coupled with the history of diabetes mellitus lead to a finding of chronic renal failure.

3. Patients with immunosuppression (e.g., AIDS) are at risk for progression from obstructive hydronephrosis to pyonephrosis. The diagnosis of pyonephrosis is confirmed with sonographic presence of the echogenic fluid-debris levels and laboratory results that show pyuria.

4. This patient shows clinical signs of acute glomerulonephritis. The young patient's sore throat and foggy urine are strong clues that aid the sonographic indicators (renal enlargement and irregular cortical echotexture) in a diagnosis of acute glomerulonephritis.

5. This patient shows sonographic (enlarged kidney, echogenic foci, and dirty shadows) and clinical (extreme illness, flank pain, and laboratory findings of *E. coli* bacteria) signs of emphysematous pyelonephritis.

Chapter 7

1. The renal findings are consistent with ADPKD. Subsequent laboratory tests suggest pancreatitis, and computed tomography of the abdomen is ordered because of the suboptimal visualization of the pancreas with ultrasound. The computed tomographic scan confirms the renal findings of ADPKD, the associated hepatic cyst, and three additional small liver cysts that were not seen on the ultrasound examination. The pancreas appears normal, and the acute pancreas was self limiting without further complication.

2. Multiple simple cysts, which are an insignificant finding in this 79-year-old patient.

3. This patient has a simple cyst on the right kidney and a parapelvic cyst on the left kidney. The additional finding of an enlarged prostate suggests benign prostatic hypertrophy, although neoplasm cannot be ruled out. The radiologist recommends follow-up with digital rectal examination and prostatic specific antigen.

4. ADPKD. This patient has a computed tomographic scan subsequent to the ultrasound examination that confirms the presence of ADPKD with multiple calcifications. The complex appearance of the cysts could be the result of previous hemorrhage or infection. The multiple small calcifications arising from the cyst walls may also represent the resolution of infection or hemorrhage. The computed tomographic scan also shows multiple cysts in the liver.

5. The sonographic findings are consistent with a calcified cyst. Minimal calcifications in a cyst wall are usually insignificant, but thick calcifications and ring calcifications may be associated with malignant disease and necessitate further testing.

Chapter 8

1. The lesion is similar in echogenicity to that of the spleen, which suggests an accessory spleen. A retrospective review of the CT scan confirms the diagnosis.

2. Splenomegaly as the result of underlying cirrhosis from chronic disease.

3. The extensive amount of fluid in the left upper quadrant with extension of fluid on the right side of the abdomen is consistent with splenic rupture, which is confirmed with CT scan.

4. Because lymphoma is the most common malignant disease to affect the spleen and can be a diffuse process, it is the most likely diagnosis.

5. Splenomegaly from alcoholic-induced cirrhosis with portal hypertension.

Chapter 9

1. Choledochal cyst. In addition, no evidence is seen of intrahepatic ductal dilatation associated with this finding.

2. A CT scan of the abdomen is suggested in the ultrasound report and confirms a high likelihood of Wilms' tumors. Bilateral Wilms' tumors are confirmed at surgery.

3. The right kidney reveals moderate hydronephrosis without visualization of the ureter, which is consistent with a UPJ obstruction. The left renal bed shows the presence of a left adrenal gland and the absence of the left kidney; however, an ectopic kidney is identified posterior to the bladder. The diagnosis of a pelvic kidney with contralateral UPJ obstruction is confirmed.

4. An adrenal hemorrhage that resolved.

5. Contrast studies of the kidney are performed and confirm severe right-sided hydronephrosis consistent with a UPJ obstruction and non-functioning left kidney with multiple noncommunicating cysts consistent with MCDK.

Chapter 10

1. Aortic aneurysm with thrombus. The patient is referred to a vascular surgeon because of the increased risk of rupture from the size of the dilation.

2. Aortic aneurysm that measures 5.58 cm.

3. An aortic aneurysm that has ruptured.

4. Aortic dissection.

5. The current recommendation is to follow an aortic aneurysm that is less than 4 cm on an annual basis.

Chapter 11

1. The patient returns to the operating room 9 days later for a scheduled D&C for a missed abortion and a post-appendectomy pelvic abscess drainage. The surgeon requests ultrasound assistance in the operating room for

both procedures. Transabdominal scanning reveals a missed abortion, and the D&C is performed (Figs. 11-33, 11-34, and 11-35). The endocavitary probe with needle guide is then used to guide transrectal drainage of the pelvic abscess (Fig. 11-36).

2. Pyloric stenosis is diagnosed with ultrasound (Fig. 11-37), and pyloromyotomy is performed. The jaundice clears within 3 days, and the infant is discharged.

3. An abdominal radiograph is ordered, but the results are unremarkable. A BE then reveals an ileocecal intussusception that extends to the hepatic flexure, and hydrostatic reduction is attempted without success (Fig. 11-38). The intussusception is reduced surgically without complications, and the child is discharged on the third postoperative day.

4. The sonographer performs graded-compression sonogram over the area of the appendix and finds an inflamed tubular structure in the right lower quadrant that contains a 1-cm echogenic shadowing mass. The structure is tender and does not compress with pressure. The AP wall thickness measures 3.3 mm, with a diameter of 1.8 cm and a channel length of 2 cm. Appendicitis with an appendicolith is confirmed by the pediatric radiologist, and the patient is scheduled for surgery the same afternoon.

5. A sonogram of the abdomen reveals a complex soft tissue mass in the region of the pylorus and a small amount of ascites in the pelvis. The abdomen is so distended and gassy that the ultrasound of the pylorus is inconclusive. The subsequent KUB radiograph suggests distal distended small bowel loops rather than pyloric stenosis. A BE is performed and shows intussusception at the transverse colon, presumably representing the midabdominal mass seen with sonographic examination. The patient is sent to surgery for intraoperative reduction.

Chapter 12

1. Adrenal cyst.
2. Pheochromocytoma.
3. Functioning adrenal adenoma.
4. Multiple enlarged lymph nodes (lymphadenopathy) are identified. The underlying cause is unknown.
5. Metastatic disease to the adrenal gland.

Chapter 13

1. Adenomyosis. This patient may benefit from oral contraceptive therapy, a course of GnRH agonists, hysteroscopic endometrial resolution, or hysterectomy.
2. Either sonohysterography, hysteroscopy, or endometrial biopsy. Because the endometrium is greater than 5 mm in thickness and is focally thickened, the gynecologist

orders a sonohysterogram, which reveals a small polyp. The gynecologist removes the polyp with outpatient hysteroscopy.

3. Either endometrial biopsy or hysteroscopy. The gynecologist performs an office endometrial biopsy because the endometrium is globally thickened, and the results reveal simple hyperplasia without atypia. The gynecologist prescribes progesterone and performs an endometrial biopsy 6 months later, the results of which are normal. The patient stops the progesterone therapy and is currently asymptomatic.

4. The patient has choices such as expectant management, GnRH agonist therapy, myomectomy, or hysterectomy. The physician suggests GnRH agonist therapy over the next 4 to 6 months to help shrink the fibroid while the patient starts a weight loss program to decrease the chance of surgical complications, such as wound breakdown. At the end of 6 months, a pelvic sonogram reveals that the fibroid is now 7 cm. The patient undergoes successful myomectomy and recovers uneventfully.

5. The sonographic findings and pathology report confirm a submucosal fibroid. After the removal of the fibroid, the patient reports resolution of symptoms.

Chapter 14

1. The IUD is located lateral to the gestational sac. The lack of a heart beat suggests embryonic death.
2. An endocervical IUD with cul-de-sac fluid.
3. The IUD is shown on the radiograph but is not noted within the uterus on endovaginal ultrasound, which suggests that the IUD has perforated the uterus.
4. An intrauterine gestational sac is identified. The yolk sac is shown within the sac, and a IUD is identified inferior to the sac within the uterus. A fetal heart beat is also shown with endovaginal technique; however, with a history of bleeding, the patient may still have spontaneous abortion of the pregnancy.
5. The IUD is identified within the uterus. The strings have most likely become detached or broken or have migrated up into the cervix.

Chapter 15

1. Possible TOA. The patient is referred for a surgical consult. Laparotomy reveals TOA in the left adnexa with extension into the cul-de-sac.
2. Unresolved PID that has progressed to TOA and possible peritonitis.
3. PID probably related to IUCD. The patient is placed on antibiotic therapy, and the IUCD is removed.
4. Endometritis.
5. Bilateral pyosalpinx.

Chapter 16

1. Localized endometriosis, endometrioma, or chocolate cyst.
2. Because the uterus only has a slight fundal notch, septate uterus is the most likely diagnosis.
3. PCOD.
4. Bicornuate uterus. Correlation with the last menstrual period and a quantitative pregnancy test are needed to determine the course of this pregnancy.
5. Endometrioma or chocolate cyst.

Chapter 17

1. Paraovarian cyst with a cystadenoma.
2. The sonographic appearance suggests abscesses, but that diagnosis is unlikely because the patient does not have symptoms of systemic illness. Hemorrhagic cysts are another possibility, but again, this diagnosis is not supported by the patient's clinical history. In the absence of intratumoral vascularity, an ovarian neoplasm is unlikely. Consequently, these masses are most likely endometriomas.
3. The appearance of the mass suggests either a serous or a mucinous cystic mass. Diarrhea and hypogastric pain, however, are symptomatic of Zollinger-Ellison syndrome, which supports the diagnosis of a gastrin-secreting mucinous cystadenoma or cystadenocarcinoma. Papillary projections are more common in mucinous cystadenocarcinomas.
4. Fibroma, thecoma, and Brenner tumors are all solid tumors that may occur at this patient's age, and they all may be associated with ascites. In this case, further diagnostic evaluation reveals the additional finding of a pleural effusion, establishing a diagnosis of Meigs' syndrome. The mass, along with the affected ovary, is resected and, with pathologic evaluation, is diagnosed as a Brenner tumor. The ascites and pleural effusion resolve after surgery.
5. Acute pain often occurs with rupture and hemorrhage into a cyst. Given the patient's age and menstrual status, a hemorrhagic follicular cyst is the most likely diagnosis. Absence of neovascularity in the mass suggests clot rather than ovarian neoplasm, further supporting the diagnosis.

Chapter 18

1. Measurements of all extremity long bones and the binocular distance may be performed. The BPD and HC should not be included in estimation of gestational age because of the pathologic condition that affects head shape and size. Close follow-up examinations should be performed for evaluation of the ventriculomegaly in addition to fetal growth progression.
2. The TCD and the binocular distance may be used.
3. The gestational age at the examination should be considered 33 weeks and 3 days based on the first ultrasound examination. The current measurements should be interpreted as a fetal size that indicates a growth restriction.
4. The patient most likely had ovulation later in the menstrual cycle than typically seen, and the finding is a normally progressing gestational sac. Until the gestational sac measures greater than 8 mm, the yolk sac or embryo may not be visualized. The patient should return in 5 to 10 days for a follow-up examination for evaluation of the continued progression of the pregnancy and the presence of a live embryo.
5. Ultrasound imaging and biometric measurements are still relatively accurate at this gestational age. The gestational age should be interpreted as 21 weeks and 5 days, and the AFP value should be recalculated for this age. The patient may have interpreted some vaginal bleeding associated with implantation as a menstrual period. The estimated due date will most likely be changed, but a follow-up examination later in the pregnancy may be performed to assess the correlation of fetal size and the estimated gestational age.

Chapter 19

1. Hydrops fetalis and placentamegaly are the most likely contributing factors associated with the increased fundal height. The hydrops is the result of the diaphragmatic hernia. These findings combined carry a poor prognosis.
2. Beckwith-Wiedemann syndrome.
3. A calcified uterine leiomyoma.
4. The ultrasound reveals a twin gestation with two placentas and a thick separating membrane consistent with diamniotic/dichorionic twins. This explains the increased fundal height. Skin edema and absent fetal heart motion are also noted in one of the twins.
5. The single pocket measurement of amniotic fluid greater than 8 cm is consistent with polyhydramnios. The increased fluid is most likely the result of anencephaly, which is often associated with polyhydramnios from poor fetal shallowing.

Chapter 20

1. PROM.
2. Anhydramnios is identified. The ultrasound examination also fails to identify the fetal bladder. Power Doppler shows the absence of renal arteries, confirming a diagnosis of renal agenesis.
3. Unilateral MCDK is identified in the right renal bed. The normal left kidney and amniotic fluid reassure that this fetus has renal function. The MCDK can be managed expectantly after birth.

4. Because the gestational age was established with a first-trimester ultrasound, the growth discrepancy would indicate severe IUGR. The failure for identification of fetal anomalies would suggest the growth restriction is the result of the multiple fibroids that includes a large retroplacental fibroid. The Doppler shows absence of diastolic flow, which coupled with the fact that the fetus did not move during the examination would indicate fetal distress. The patient is immediately admitted to the hospital and given steroids to promote fetal lung maturity. The infant male is delivered by cesarean section at 30 weeks' gestation.

5. Bilateral hydronephrosis with a grossly distended bladder suggests a bladder outlet obstruction. PUV is most likely because it is the most common and is more prevalent in males. After further testing to ensure fetal renal function, the patient consents to having a pigtail stent placed in the fetal bladder to allow drainage into the amniotic cavity, promoting fetal lung development. The patient is followed closely throughout the pregnancy. On subsequent examinations, fetal bladder decompression is noted and redundant abdominal skin folds are identified. At 38 weeks' gestation, the infant is delivered by cesarean section. PUV is confirmed, in addition to prune-belly syndrome. In addition to surgical correction of the bladder outlet obstruction, the male infant will eventually have surgery for cryptorchism and to improve abdominal wall laxity.

Chapter 21

1. Complete placenta previa is shown in the ultrasound image of the lower uterine segment. Because of the history of prior cesarean sections, the obstetrician should also be alerted to the possibility of placenta accreta, which is identified in this patient at the time of delivery.

2. The ultrasound findings are consistent with retained products of conception from an incomplete abortion. A D&C is subsequently performed in addition to a follow-up ultrasound of the uterus, which was within normal limits.

3. Ectopic pregnancy.

4. SAB.

5. A subchorionic hemorrhage that resolved as did the bleeding.

Chapter 22

1. This is a dizygotic gestation in which an obvious discordance is seen in the fetal size. Twin A's abdominal circumference is 52 mm smaller than twin B's, and a 4-week discordance is found in the estimated gestational age. Because this is a dichorionic gestation, twin-twin transfusion syndrome is not suspected. Twin B is considered to have growth restriction, and careful screening for fetal anomalies should be performed.

2. This is an early monozygotic twin gestation that is monochorionic and diamniotic.

3. This is an early monozygotic twin gestation that is monochorionic. The gestation is most likely monoamniotic because only one yolk sac is observed. This pregnancy should be closely monitored for indications of growth discordance, twin-twin transfusion syndrome, TRAP sequence, possible cord entanglement, and fetal anomalies.

4. Twin B appears to be an acardiac twin. Follow-up ultrasound examinations are performed later that week and 4 weeks after the finding of the acardiac twin to check the viability of each fetus. An amniocentesis is suggested, but the patient refuses the procedure. Both twins die in utero. A postmortem examination documents a male acardiac, acephalic twin with no heart or upper torso development. All the abdominal and urogenital organs are absent. The fetus shows rudimentary development of the lower half of the body. The placenta is monochorionic and monoamniotic. The umbilical cords of both fetuses are seen interconnected by a direct anastomosis. Postmortem examination of the male "pump" twin shows a normal fetus. The fetus has normal abdominal and urogenital organs. The fetal heart is normal in size, but the right atrium appears to be more prominent. No other abnormalities are seen in the "pump" twin.

5. This is a monozygotic twin gestation that is monochorionic and diamniotic. Twin B is normal, and twin A has a Dandy-Walker malformation. Because this is a monochorionic gestation, the pregnancy should be closely monitored for indications of growth discordance, twin-twin transfusion syndrome, TRAP sequence, possible cord entanglement, and fetal anomalies.

Chapter 23

1. Anencephaly.

2. Omphalocele. A thorough survey of the cardiac structures should ensue because of the increased risk of cardiac anomalies; however, in this instance, the fetal heart appears within normal limits. The patient consents to amniocentesis, which reveals a normal karyotype.

3. May recalculate AFP because gestational age is less than 21 weeks.

4. Posterior encephalocele.

5. LBWC, which is considered lethal.

Chapter 24

1. In isolation, choroid plexus cysts are insignificant. With any other positive marker, such as the abnormal triple test results, trisomy 18 should be considered and amniocentesis offered.

2. Although cystic hygroma can be associated with a variety of chro-mosomal anomalies, it is most specifically linked with Turner's syndrome.

3. The findings of persistently clinched hands is associated with trisomy 18. Micrognathia, polyhydramnios, intra-uterine growth restriction, and decreased movement are also iden-tified in this examination, all of which are associated with trisomy 18.

4. Nuchal fold thickening is most specific for trisomy 21, which is the diagnosis with the amniocentesis.

5. The amniocentesis reveals a male fetus with trisomy 13, which is consistent with the finding of holo-prosencephaly.

Chapter 25

1. Isolated bilateral talipes. The patient is referred to a maternal fetal center for a targeted sonographic evaluation, which concurs with the previous findings. Bilateral talipes without evidence of other anomalies is confirmed at delivery.

2. DWM. Because of the large head size, the patient is counseled that delivery with cesarean section is likely.

3. The patient is counseled that the mass is most likely a hemorrhagic cyst. The female infant undergoes a sonographic evaluation of the abdomen at the age of 3 months that reveals no evidence of any pathology. The ovarian cyst is postulated to have spontaneously resolved.

4. OI type II. The fetus dies during delivery.

5. An isolated unilateral cleft lip.

Chapter 26

1. AVSD. An incomplete AVSD may result in a cleft mitral valve (the anterior part of the leaflet is divided into two parts—medial and lateral). When the leaflet closes, blood leaks through this hole into the left atrial cavity. The leaflet is usually somewhat malformed, causing further regurgitation into the atrium. A complete AVSD may have several variations in valve abnormalities. One of these variations has a single, undivided, free-floating AV leaflet stretching across both ventricles. The anterior and posterior leaflets are on both sides of the interventricular septum, causing the valve to override or straddle the septum. This is a more complex abnormality to repair because the defect is larger and the single AV valve is more difficult to clinically manage, depending on the amount of regurgitation present.

2. This is suggestive of Ebstein's anomaly of the tricuspid valve. The septal leaflet has apical displacement; as a result, massive tricuspid regurgitation is present, causing the right atrial cavity to enlarge. If the regurgitation is severe in the early gestational period, the prognosis is poor. The sonographer should look for signs of cardiac failure: decreased contractility, pericardial effusion, and fetal hydrops.

3. These findings suggest tetralogy of Fallot, which is best shown on the parasternal long-axis view. The large aorta overrides the ventricular septum. If the override is greater than 50%, the condition is called a double-outlet right ventricle (both great vessels arise from the right heart). A septal defect is present, and the size may vary from small to large. The short-axis view shows the small, hyper-trophied right ventricle (if significant pulmonary stenosis is present). The pulmonary artery is usually small, and the cusps may be thickened and domed or difficult to image well. Doppler evaluation should be made in the high parasternal short-axis view to determine the turbulence of the right ventricular outflow tract and pulmonary valve stenosis. Color flow is helpful in this condition to actually delineate the abnormal high-velocity pattern and to direct the sample volume into the proper jet flow. If the ventricular septal defect is large, increased flow is seen in the right heart (increased tricuspid velocity, right ventricular outflow tract velocity, and also increased pulmonic velocity). A large septal defect with mild to moderate pulmonary stenosis is classified as acyanotic disease, whereas a large septal defect with severe pulmonary stenosis is considered cyanotic disease.

4. The hypertrophied left ventricle and aorta would be compatible with the hypoplastic left heart syndrome. Thickening and immobility (atresia) of the mitral valve or aortic valve may be seen.

5. The great vessels should normally arise in a criss cross from their respective ventricles. The aorta is the most posterior, and the pulmonary artery anterior. In trans-position of the great vessels, the great vessels arise in parallel, with the aorta anterior (from the right ventricle) and the pulmonary arising from the left ventricle. A ventricular septal defect is often present with this lesion.

Chapter 27

1. The patient returns $2^1/_2$ weeks later for an aspiration. At that time, the skin has a 4-cm moderately severe red wheal with mild induration. A central skin eruption with some drainage is also noted. The aspirate pathology confirms a diagnosis of abscess. The patient is referred to a surgeon for consultation and probable removal of the area because antibiotic treatment has been ineffective.

2. Breast biopsy confirms the diagnosis of galactocele.

3. An ultrasound-guided breast core biopsy is positive for a well-differentiated infiltrating ductal tubular carcinoma with associated lobular neoplasia and ductal carcinoma in situ. No evidence of metastases is found.

4. An ultrasound-guided breast core biopsy is performed of both lesions. The lesions are diagnosed as poorly differentiated in situ and invasive ductal carcinoma. The patient has an ultrasound-guided lymphoscintigraphy at the time of the right modified radical mastectomy. Two of the three lymph nodes removed are positive for metastatic disease.

5. An ultrasound-guided breast core biopsy confirms the diagnosis of invasive poorly differentiated carcinoma, predominantly lobular type. The patient has an ultrasound-guided needle localization and lymphoscintigraphy before surgical removal of the mass. No metastatic disease is identified.

Chapter 28
1. Lymphoma of the left testicle.
2. Hematoma of the right testicle.
3. Torsion.
4. The enlargement of the epididymis surrounded by a loculated hydrocele is consistent with epididymitis. The increased perfusion noted in the testicle with color Doppler evaluation suggests that the inflammation may extend to the testis, which is consistent with epididymoorchitis.
5. Scrotal hernia.

Chapter 29
1. Benign, hyperplastic thyroid nodule.
2. Papillary thyroid cancer.
3. Papillary thyroid cancer.
4. Parathyroid adenoma.
5. Benign hyperplastic thyroid nodule.

Chapter 30
1. BPH.
2. Prostate cancer.
3. Prostate length (cm) × width (cm) × AP (cm) × 0.523 × 0.12 PSAD (2 × 4.1 × 3.9 = 83.148; 83.148 × 0.523 = 43.49; 43.49 × 0.12 = 5.2).
4. Acute prostatitis.
5. BPH/chronic prostatitis.

Chapter 31
1. The finding is most likely the result of physiologic laxity often identified in the immediate newborn period. No treatment is necessary at this time, but the infant should be followed between 4 to 6 weeks of age to document that the laxity has resolved.
2. The Pavlik harness would not be an appropriate treatment option for this infant because the hip is irreducible with stress maneuvers. A closed reduction may be attempted, and a fixed abduction device (brace or cast)

secured. Open reduction is reserved for infants in whom a stable reduction cannot be achieved.
3. There is greater than 50% coverage, which indicates a normal hip. No additional follow-up is necessary.
4. The iliac line inclines rather than being perfectly parallel with the transducer. Although this appears to be a normal hip, the reliability of hip ultrasound can be affected by images that do not meet specific guidelines.
5. In the initial treatment period, the purpose of the ultrasound examination is to ensure that the Pavlik harness is keeping the femoral head in the acetabulum. The Pavlik harness should be kept in place unless otherwise specifically directed by the treating physician.

Chapter 32
1. A grade I bleed on the right side.
2. The conus medullaris is identified at the level of L1, which is consistent with a normal examination. The sonographer also notes pulsations in the nerve roots and documents that no sinus tract leads to the dimple.
3. The prenatal ultrasound and postnatal CT scan confirm hydranencephaly. The infant did breath spontaneously at birth but continually has difficulty controlling temperature. The mother is counseled that the baby will not survive for long. The mother and baby go home with hospice care.
4. Intraventricular hemorrhage and ventricular enlargement are noted bilaterally and are consistent with a grade III hemorrhage.
5. PVL.

Chapter 33
1. A 50% to 79% stenosis in the right ICA.
2. Left SSS.
3. Fibromuscular dysplasia.
4. Left ICA occlusion.
5. An 80% to 99% stenosis.

Chapter 34
1. Acute DVT.
2. Baker's cyst.
3. A Yin Yang sign is shown, which is classic in a pseudoaneurysm arising after angiography. Sonography has proven to be helpful in the treatment and diagnosis of this finding. Two methods are currently used. Extended external compression and ultrasound-guided/monitored injection of thrombin into the pseudoaneurysm have both been proven effective. The patient is successfully treated with extended external compression.
4. The patient has DVT of the popliteal vein.
5. The patient has primary SVT.

ANSWERS TO STUDY QUESTIONS

Chapter 1

1. b	5. e	8. e
2. e	6. e	9. d
3. d	7. a	10. c
4. c		

Chapter 2

1. c	5. c	8. d
2. a	6. e	9. d
3. b	7. b	10. e
4. d		

Chapter 3

1. d	5. e	8. a
2. e	6. a	9. d
3. a	7. f	10. d
4. b		

Chapter 4

1. e	5. c	8. b
2. b	6. b	9. d
3. d	7. d	10. a
4. c		

Chapter 5

1. d	5. d	8. c
2. b	6. b	9. d
3. a	7. e	10. a
4. c		

Chapter 6

1. e	5. a	8. d
2. b	6. d	9. b
3. c	7. b	10. a
4. d		

Chapter 7

1. e	5. b	8. a
2. b	6. a	9. e
3. c	7. c	10. b
4. d		

Chapter 8

1. e	5. e	8. d
2. b	6. b	9. e
3. d	7. a	10. c
4. a		

Chapter 9

1. d	5. a	8. c

2. a	6. d	9. e
3. c	7. b	10. b
4. e		

Chapter 10

1. a	5. b	8. b
2. c	6. c	9. c
3. b	7. c	10. a
4. a		

Chapter 11

1. c	5. d	8. b
2. b	6. c	9. c
3. d	7. a	10. a
4. b		

Chapter 12

1. e	5. d	8. e
2. b	6. c	9. b
3. e	7. d	10. b
4. b		

Chapter 13

1. d	5. e	8. c
2. a	6. b	9. b
3. c	7. a	10. b
4. d		

Chapter 14

1. b	5. d	8. a
2. a	6. a	9. c
3. e	7. a	10. a
4. b		

Chapter 15

1. c	5. b	8. d
2. b	6. d	9. a
3. a	7. b	10. d
4. d		

Chapter 16

1. c	5. b	8. c
2. d	6. c	9. b
3. b	7. b	10. e
4. b		

Chapter 17

1. b	5. b	8. a
2. a	6. d	9. a
3. d	7. a	10. d
4. c		

Chapter 18
1. c
2. d
3. a
4. b

5. a
6. c
7. c

8. c
9. a
10. b

Chapter 19
1. c
2. d
3. a
4. b

5. a
6. e
7. c

8. d
9. c
10. b

Chapter 20
1. b
2. b
3. d
4. d

5. c
6. a
7. c

8. c
9. c
10. d

Chapter 21
1. a
2. c
3. c
4. d

5. b
6. c
7. a

8. d
9. c
10. b

Chapter 22
1. d
2. b
3. c
4. e

5. b
6. a
7. e

8. a
9. c
10. a

Chapter 23
1. b
2. b
3. d
4. c

5. d
6. c
7. b

8. c
9. e
10. b

Chapter 24
1. e
2. d
3. a
4. a

5. d
6. e
7. c

8. a
9. c
10. a

Chapter 25
1. d
2. d
3. c
4. e

5. c
6. a
7. d

8. e
9. c
10. d

Chapter 26
1. b

5. a

8. d

2. b
3. c
4. d

6. a
7. c

9. a
10. d

Chapter 27
1. e
2. b
3. b
4. c

5. e
6. d
7. a

8. b
9. d
10. a

Chapter 28
1. d
2. b
3. d
4. b

5. a
6. e
7. c

8. c
9. d
10. a

Chapter 29
1. c
2. a
3. c
4. b

5. c
6. b
7. a

8. b
9. b
10. a

Chapter 30
1. a
2. c
3. b
4. a

5. b
6. a
7. b

8. d
9. 44.4 cm^3; 5.33
10. Yes

Chapter 31
1. d
2. b
3. d
4. b

5. e
6. b
7. c

8. b
9. e
10. b

Chapter 32
1. a
2. b
3. b
4. a

5. a
6. e
7. c

8. b
9. a
10. e

Chapter 33
1. c
2. c
3. b
4. e

5. c
6. a
7. c

8. d
9. b
10. e

Chapter 34
1. c
2. a
3. c
4. d

5. c
6. d
7. e

8. e
9. d
10. d

ILLUSTRATION CREDITS

Anderhub B: General sonography: a clinical guide, St Louis, 1995, Mosby.
Figures 15-2, 15-10

Johnson PT, Kurtz AB: Case review obstetric and gynecologic ultrasound, Case review series, St Louis, 2001, Mosby.
Figure 15-6

Hagen-Ansert S: Textbook of diagnostic ultrasound, ed 5, St Louis, 2001, Mosby.
Figures 1-25 A&B; 1-26 A-C; 2-4 A&B; 2-6; 4-3; 7-3; 8-2 A&B; 11-17; 12-9; 16-12; 17-10; 19-4; 19-5; 19-7 A; 19-8 to 19-11; 19-14; 19-15; 20-2 B; 21-5 C; 21-6; 22-5; 22-6; 23-2 B; 23-5; 23-9; 24-1 B&C; 24-7; 24-8 B&D; 24-17 A; 24-18; 25-2 A, E, F; 25-9 A; 25-11; 25-12; 25-15; 25-23; 25-24 C; 25-26; 26-12; 28-2; 28-23; 29-10; 32-4 A; 32-7; 32-13 B; 32-15 A

Rumack C: Diagnostic ultrasound, ed 2, St Louis, 2001, Mosby.
Figures 1-18, 1-19 B, 1-24, 2-5, 2-7, 2-8, 7-6, 7-10, 8-5 to 8-11, 9-2, 9-6, 9-7, 10-6, 12-3, 12-7, 12-10, 20-2 C, 21-5 B, 22-7, 22-8, 23-8, 27-8, 31-5 C, 31-6, 31-7 B, 32-13 A, 32-14

Index

A

Abdominal aortic aneurysm (AAA)
  causing pulsatile abdominal mass, 135-136
  echogenicity of, 136f, 137f
  findings of, 139t
  ruptured
    causing pulsatile abdominal mass, 137
    echogenicity of, 134f, 138b
    findings of, 139t
Abdominal circumference (AC)
  in size greater than date, 267
  in uncertain LMP, 257, 257f
Abdominal cysts, fetal, 364-365
  echogenicity of, 365f
  sonographic findings of, 356t
Abdominal mass, pulsatile
  aortic disorders causing, 135-138
  case studies involving, 139-140
  clinical scenario of, 134, 138b
  references for diagnosing, 142
  study questions about, 141-142
Abdominal pain. *See* Pain.
Abdominal wall defects, 328-331
Abduction, hip, 461b, 463
Abnormal uterine bleeding (AUB). *See* Uterine
    bleeding.
Abortion
  bleeding with pregnancy due to, 293
  missed, 293, 302t
  spontaneous
    definition of, 198b
    due to subchorionic hemorrhage, 292
    sonographic findings of, 302t
    vs. threatened abortion, 293
Abruptio placenta
  bleeding with pregnancy due to, 298
  echogenicity of, 299f
  sonographic findings of, 302t
Abscess
  breast, 410, 411f
  definition of, 144b, 420b
  liver
    causing right upper quadrant pain, 11-13, 15t
    echogenicity of, 12f, 13f
  postappendectomy, 150f, 157f

prostatic, 454f
renal, 84-85, 87t
scrotal, 426, 433t
splenic, 107, 111t
tubo-ovarian
  definition of, 207b
  in pelvic inflammatory disease, 209, 211t
uterine, 157f
Acalculous cholecystitis (ACC), 6
Acardia, 308b
Acardiac twin, 316f
Accessory spleen, 105-106, 106f
Acholic, 117b
Achondrogenesis, fetal, 367, 369f
Achondroplasia
  definition of, 471b
  fetal anomalies in, 367
  sonographic findings of, 356t
Acini, 50b
Acquired cystic kidney disease (ACKD)
  echogenicity of, 97f
  renal mass due to, 97
  symptoms and findings of, 99t
Acute tubular necrosis. *See* Kidney tubular necrosis, acute.
Adduction, hip, 461b, 463
Adenocarcinoma
  epigastric (pancreatic) pain due to, 53
    echogenicity of, 49f, 54b
    location and findings of, 54t
  gallbladder (RUQ) pain due to, 9t
Adenoma
  adrenal mass due to, 162-164, 167t
  breast mass due to
    echogenicity of, 393f, 402f, 411b
    symptoms and findings of, 401, 414t
  definition of, 440b
  hematuria due to, 62, 70t
  liver mass due to, 23
    echogenicity of, 23f, 24f
    symptoms and findings of, 28t
  neck mass due to, 442, 444-445
    echogenicity of, 443f, 445f
    symptoms and findings of, 447t
Adenomatoid tumor
  causing scrotal mass, 429-430
  echogenicity of, 430f
  symptoms and findings of, 433t

Page numbers followed by f indicate figures; t, tables; b, boxes.

Adenomyoma
abnormal uterine bleeding due to, 181-183
echogenicity of, 181f, 182f
Adenomyomatosis
gallbladder (RUQ) pain due to, 8
symptoms and findings of, 9t
Adenomyosis
abnormal uterine bleeding due to, 180-181
definition of, 174b
echogenicity of, 182f
symptoms and findings of, 192t
Adenopathy
cervical
causing neck mass, 445
definition of, 440b
symptoms and findings of, 447t
glandular, 162b
Adrenal adenoma
adrenal mass due to, 162-165
symptoms and findings of, 167t
Adrenal cortical disease
adrenal mass due to, 163-165
echogenicity of, 164f, 165f, 166f
Adrenal cyst
adrenal mass due to, 162-163
echogenicity of, 164f
symptoms and findings of, 167t
Adrenal mass, 162-165
case studies involving, 168-169
echogenicity of, 161f, 166b, 167f, 168-169f
pediatric, 119-120
symptoms and findings of, 167t
Adrenal myelolipoma
adrenal mass due to, 162, 163-164
symptoms and findings of, 167t
Adrenocortical carcinoma
adrenal mass due to, 162, 164-165
symptoms and findings of, 167t
Aflatoxin, 21b
Agenesis of corpus callosum (ACC)
fetal anomalies in, 359
echogenicity of, 360f
sonographic findings of, 356t
infant anomalies in, 477
echogenicity of, 482f
sonographic findings of, 486t
Alanine aminotransferase (ALT) level, 34b, 37t
Albumin, 34b
Alcoholic hepatitis, 34b
Alkaline phosphatase (ALP) level, 36t, 37t
Alpha fetoprotein (AFP)
decreased, in fetal anomalies, 332t
defined, 34b, 308b
elevated
case studies involving, 333-334
clinical scenario of, 323, 333b
in diffuse liver disease, 37t

in fetal anomalies, 325-332, 332t
references for diagnosing, 335-337
study questions about, 334-335
testing maternal serum for, 324
Amaurosis fugax, 491b
Amebiasis, liver, 12-13
Amebic abscess, liver, 12-13, 13f
Amenorrhea, 217b
American Cancer Society
on ovarian cancer, 229
on prostate cancer, 452
Ammonia level, 36t
Amniocentesis, 250b, 341
Amnion, 250b, 308b
Amnionicity of pregnancy
definition of, 308b
determining, 310
echogenicity of, 314f
in embryology of twinning, 311-313, 312f, 313t
Amniotic band syndrome (ABS), 331
alpha fetoprotein level in, 332t
echogenicity of, 332f
Amylase level, 50b, 228b
Anastomosis, 308b
Anemia, 77b, 105b
Anencephaly, 325-326
alpha fetoprotein level in, 332t
echogenicity of, 325f
Aneuploid, 292b
Aneuploidy, fetal
definition of, 250b, 339b, 355b
echogenicity of, 348f
nuchal translucency and, 255
soft markers for, 343t
Aneurysm
aortic abdominal
echogenicity of, 136f
pulsatile abdominal mass due to, 135-136
symptoms and findings of, 139t
definition of, 503b
popliteal, 507, 508f
ruptured aortic
echogenicity of, 134f, 137f, 138b
pulsatile abdominal mass due to, 137, 139t
Angiitis, 4b
Angiogenesis, 228b
Angiomyolipoma (AML)
definition of, 21b
hematuria due to, 64, 64f, 71t
liver mass due to, 24
splenic (LUQ) pain due to, 109
Angiosarcoma
definition of, 21b
liver mass due to, 28
splenic (LUQ) pain due to, 109, 111t
Aniridia, 59b
Ankle brachial index, 503b

Anodontia, congenital familial, 93b
Anomalies. *See* Alpha fetoprotein (AFP); Chromosomal anomalies; Fetal anomalies; Heart anomalies; Uterine anomalies.
Anorexia, 4b, 21b
Anovulation, 217b
Antiinflammatory drugs, nonsteroidal, 277b
Antiradial imaging plane, 394b
Anuria, 77b, 117b
Aorta
    echogenicity of abnormal, 139-140f
    echogenicity of normal, 135f
    sonographic anatomy of normal, 135
Aortic aneurysm, abdominal
    pulsatile abdominal mass due to, 135-136
        echogenicity of, 136f, 137f
        symptoms and findings of, 139t
    ruptured
        echogenicity of, 134f, 138b
        pulsatile abdominal mass due to, 137
        symptoms and findings of, 139t
Aortic atresia. *See* Hypoplastic left heart syndrome.
Aortic dissection
    echogenicity of, 137f
    pulsatile abdominal mass due to, 137-138
    symptoms and findings of, 139t
Aortic graft, 137f
Aphasia, 491b
Appendicitis, 145-147
    echogenicity of, 149f
    sonographic findings of, 147-150
    symptoms and findings of, 156t
Appendicolith, 144b
Appendix
    atypical location/shapes of, 146f
    echogenicity of inflamed, 148f, 149f
    echogenicity of normal, 148f
    normal location/shape of, 145f, 146f
Appendix testis, 420b
Aqueductal stenosis, 355b, 471b
Arachnoid cysts, 355b
Arcuate uterus
    causing infertility, 222-223
    development and findings of, 223t
    echogenicity of, 223f
Areola, 394b
Arnold-Chiari malformation
    definition of, 324b
    fetal anomalies in, 323, 326, 333b
    infant anomalies in, 477, 481f, 486t
Arrhythmias, fetal cardiac, 378-380
Arsenic, 105b
Arterial disease, 506-509
Arteries, leg
    normal vascular anatomy of, 504-505, 506f
    vs. veins, 505-506
Ascites

definition of, 34b, 144b, 228b
echogenicity of
    in abdominal anomalies, 364f
    in appendicitis, 150f
    in cirrhosis, 33f, 44b
    in hepatoma, 42f
in fetal anomalies, 356t, 364
Aspartate aminotransferase (AST) level, 34b, 37t
Asphyxia, 471b
Aspiration, fine-needle. *See* Fine-needle aspiration (FNA).
Asymptomatic, 394b
Atherosclerosis
    definition of, 4b, 135b, 503b
    leg pain due to, 506
Atrial fibrillation/flutter, fetal, 377b
Atrial septal defect, 380-381
Atrialized chamber, 384
Atrioventricular block, fetal, 377b, 380, 380f
Atrioventricular canal malformation, 382
Atrioventricular node, 377b
Atrioventricular septal defects, 382-383, 382f, 383f
Atrium, left/right, 377b
Augmentation, 503b
Autosomal dominant polycystic kidney disease (ADPKD)
    fetal size less than date due to, 279-280, 285t
    liver cysts (RUQ pain) and, 13, 17f
    pediatric renal mass due to, 123-124, 127f
    renal mass due to, 96-97
        echogenicity of, 92f, 96f, 97f, 98b
        symptoms and findings of, 99t
Autosomal recessive polycystic kidney disease (ARPKD), 93b, 123-124
Avascular, 228b
Axilla, 394b
Azotemia, 77b

B
Bacteriuria, 77b
Baker's cyst, 503b, 507, 508f
Barium enema, 144b
Barlow maneuver, 464f
Beat-to-beat variability, 277b
Beckwith-Wiedemann syndrome, 59b, 117b, 265b
Beemer-Langer syndrome, 369
Benign, definition of, 452b
Benign prostatic hypertrophy (BPH)
    causing elevated PSA, 453, 454
    echogenicity of, 454f
    symptoms and findings of, 456t
beta-hCG. *See* Chorionic gonadotropin, beta human.
Bicornuate uterus
    causing infertility, 220-221
    development and findings of, 223t
    echogenicity of, 222f
Bile level, 36t
Biliary atresia, 117-118, 118f

Biliary tract diseases
case studies involving, 16f
pediatric mass due to, 117-118
right upper quadrant pain due to, 9-11, 11t
Bilirubin
direct
definition of, 34b
in diffuse liver disease, 37t
laboratory values for, 36t
indirect
definition of, 34b
in diffuse liver disease, 37t
laboratory values for, 36t
Binocular distance in uncertain LMP, 259, 259f
Biometry for estimating gestational age. *See also*
Measurements, fetal sonographic.
definition of, 250b
during first trimester, 250-255, 251b
during second/third trimester, 255-261, 256b
Biparietal diameter (BPD) in uncertain LMP, 256, 256f
Bleeding with pregnancy. *See also* Hemorrhage; Uterine
bleeding.
case studies involving, 302-303
causes of, 302t
clinical scenario of, 291, 301b
during first trimester, 292-297
references for diagnosing, 305-306
during second trimester, 297-301
study questions about, 304-305
Blood urea nitrogen level, 77b
"Blue baby", 383
Bone length, fetal. *See* Fetal bone length in uncertain LMP.
Bowel obstruction, fetal, 356t, 363, 364f
Brachial plexus injury, 265b
Brainstem, 471b
Branchial cleft cyst, 440b, 447t
Breast augmentation, 408
Breast, human
definition of, 394b
diseases of male, 411
shape of female, 398f
sonographic anatomy of, 397-398
tissue layers of, 398f
Breast mass
benign, 401-403, 414t
case studies involving, 415-417
clinical scenario of, 393, 411b
cystic, 398-400, 414t
hematoma causing, 410
implant-induced, 408, 409f
inflammation-induced, 408, 410
location of
annotation for, 395, 396f, 397f
with mammogram, 395, 397, 397f
scanning planes for, 395, 396f
malignant, 403-407, 414t
metastatic, 407-408

references for diagnosing, 418
study questions about, 417-418
Brenner tumor. *See also* Transitional cell carcinoma (TCC).
causing ovarian mass, 239-240
echogenicity of, 240f
symptoms and findings of, 242t
Budd-Chiari syndrome, 21b
Buerger's disease, 503b, 509
Bulbus cordis, 377b
Bull's-eye appearance, 148

C
Calcifications
carotid plaque, 496f
cyst vs. renal mass, 95
prostate, 455, 455f, 456t
scrotum, 424-426
thyroid nodule, 443f
Calcium, serum, 440b
Calculi, hematuria due to, 60-62, 62f
Camptomelic dysplasia, 355b
Cancer, definition of, 452b
Candida albicans in renal failure, 85f
Candle sign, 59b, 62f
Capsule, definition of, 452b
Carcinoembryonic antigen, 4b, 10
Carcinoma. *See also* Neoplasms.
adrenal gland
echogenicity of, 164f, 166f
symptoms and findings of, 164, 167t
biliary tract
echogenicity of, 10f
epigastric pain due to, 49f, 54b
right upper quadrant pain due to, 10, 11t
breast
echogenicity of, 404-407f
in male, 411, 414f
symptoms and findings of, 403-407, 415t
gallbladder
echogenicity of, 3f, 15b
right upper quadrant pain due to, 9, 9t
liver
echogenicity of, 3f, 15b, 26f, 27f
fibrolamellar, 21b, 28
liver function tests for, 37t
symptoms and findings of, 24-26, 28t, 42-43, 44t
ovarian
causing mass, 234-237
echogenicity of, 237f
findings and occurrence of, 241t, 242t
pancreatic
causing epigastric pain, 53
echogenicity of, 49f
location and findings of, 54t
testicular
scrotal mass due to, 427, 428, 428f
symptoms and findings of, 433t

thyroid, neck mass due to, 440b
uterine
abnormal uterine bleeding due to, 183-186
bleeding with pregnancy due to, 297
definition of, 174b
echogenicity of, 187f
symptoms and findings of, 192t
Caroli's disease, 93b, 98
Carotid arteries
branches of, 492f
Doppler imaging of
color, 494-495
spectral analysis, 494, 495f
normal anatomy of, 492
occlusion of, 497, 498f
sonographic imaging of
techniques for, 492-495
views of, 493-494f
ulceration of, 496f
Carotid artery disease, 495-497
case studies involving, 500
clinical scenario of, 491, 499b
imaging techniques for, 492-495
references for diagnosing, 501
study questions about, 500-501
Carotid artery stenosis, 495-497
Doppler analysis of, 497f
echogenicity of, 495f
measuring, 487t, 496f
Carotid bruit, 491b
Carotid dissection, 498
clinical scenario of, 491, 499b
Doppler analysis of, 499f
echogenicity of, 498f
Catecholamine, 117b, 162b
Caudothalamic notch/groove, 471b, 472
Cebocephaly, 355b, 471b
Cerebral edema, 475, 478f, 486t
Cerebral palsy, 471b, 474
Cerebrovascular accident (CVA), 491b, 492
Cerebrovascular anatomy, 492f
Cervical incompetence
causing bleeding with pregnancy, 300-301
echogenicity of, 300f
resolved, echogenicity of, 301f
Cervix sign, 144b
Cesarean section, 250b
Chiari II malformation. *See* Arnold-Chiari malformation.
Chlamydia
definition of, 420b
epididymitis due to, 425
pelvic inflammatory disease due to, 207
Chocolate cyst, 217
Cholangiocarcinoma
echogenicity of, 10f
right upper quadrant pain due to, 10
symptoms and findings of, 11t

Cholangitis
echogenicity of, 11f
right upper quadrant pain due to, 11
symptoms and findings of, 11t
Cholecystitis
right upper quadrant pain due to, 5-8
symptoms and findings of, 9t
Choledochal cyst
definition of, 355b
echogenicity of, 118f
pediatric biliary mass due to, 118
Choledocholithiasis
definition of, 50b
right upper quadrant pain due to, 9-10
symptoms and findings of, 11t
Cholelithiasis
definition of, 21b, 50b
right upper quadrant pain due to, 4-5
symptoms and findings of, 9t
Cholesterol levels, 36t
Cholesterolosis
right upper quadrant pain due to, 8
symptoms and findings of, 9t
Chorioadenoma destruens, 297
Chorioamnionitis, 277b
Choriocarcinoma
bleeding with pregnancy due to, 297
definition of, 420b
scrotal mass due to, 428
echogenicity of, 428f
symptoms and findings of, 433t
Chorion, 250b, 308b
Chorionic gonadotropin, beta human
definition of, 250b, 308b, 420b
maternal serum screening for, 340
Chorionic villus sampling, 250b, 341
Chorionicity of pregnancy
definition of, 308b
determining, 310
in embryology of twinning, 311-312, 312f, 313t
Choroid plexus cysts, fetal
chromosomal anomalies with, 343, 343t
echogenicity of, 343f, 350f
Chromosomal analysis, 342f
Chromosomal anomalies, 341-342. *See also* Fetal anomalies.
case studies involving, 350-351
controversial findings of, 342-344
genetic testing for, 340-341
maternal serum screening for, 339-340
references for diagnosing, 353
sonographic findings of, 340t
study questions about, 352
Chromosomes, 339b
Ciliated cells, 228b
Cirrhosis
case studies involving, 30f

Cirrhosis—cont'd
  definition of, 34b
  diffuse liver disease due to, 39-40, 44b
  echogenicity of, 33f, 40f
  liver function tests for, 37t
  splenomegaly and, 107f
  summary of findings with, 44t
Cisterna magna in uncertain LMP, 259, 259f, 261b
Cleavage, 308b, 312
Cleft lip
  fetal, 359-360
    echogenicity of, 348f, 358f, 360f
    sonographic findings of, 356t
  infant, 482f
Clinodactyly, 339b
Clubfoot/hand, 347f, 370-371, 371f
Coapt, 503b
Collateral circulation, 503b
Colocolic intussusception, 153f
Colon, ascending, 147f
Comet-tail artifact
  in emphysematous cholecystitis, 7f
  in hyperplastic cholecystosis, 8f
  in nephrolithiasis, 62f
Compartment syndrome, 503b, 509
Congenital cystic adenomatoid malformation (CCAM), 361, 362f, 371b
Congenital diaphragmatic hernia (CDH), 360-361
  definition of, 339b
  echogenicity of, 347f, 361f
  nuchal translucency and, 342
  sonographic findings of, 356t
Congenital liver cysts, 13
Conjoined twins, 312, 315
  etiology and findings of, 317t
  increased fundal height of, 268f
Conn's syndrome, 162b
Contrast agents
  intravenous, 42-43
  oral, 50b, 52f
Conus medullaris, 471b, 482, 485f
Cooper's ligament, 394b
Copper T IUD, 198, 200f
Corpora amylacea, 455
Corpus callosum, agenesis of. *See* Agenesis of corpus callosum (ACC).
Corpus luteum cyst, 236-237
  echogenicity of, 231f
  findings and occurrence of, 241t
  ovarian mass due to, 230-232
Cortex, kidney, 77b
Cortex of organ, 228b
Courvoisier's gallbladder
  definition of, 50b
  epigastric pain due to, 49f, 54b
Craniopagus twins, 315
Creatinine level, 77b

Crenulated, 228b
Cruveilhier-Baumgarten syndrome, 34b
Cryptorchidism, 432
  definition of, 394b, 420b
  echogenicity of, 432f
  findings of, 433t
  male breast cancer and, 411
Cushing's syndrome, 162b
Cutaneous dimple, 471b, 485
Cyanotic heart disease, 277b, 383
Cyclopia
  definition of, 339b, 355b, 471b
  echogenicity of, 348f
Cystadenocarcinoma
  definition of, 228b
  liver mass due to, 28
  ovarian mass due to
    echogenicity of, 227f, 237f, 242b
    findings and occurrence of, 241t, 242t
    mucinous, 236-237
    serous, 234-235
  splenic (LUQ) pain due to, 110
Cystadenoma
  definition of, 21b, 228b, 265b
  liver mass due to, 24
  ovarian mass due to
    echogenicity of, 134f, 138b
    mucinous, 236-237
    serous, 234-235
  pancreatic (epigastric) pain due to, 53-54, 54t
Cystic adenomatoid malformation, congenital, 361, 362f, 371b
Cystic fibrosis
  definition of, 50b
  possible soft markers for, 343t
Cystic follicular adenoma, thyroid, 442-443, 443f
Cystic hygroma, 339b, 349f, 350f
Cystic teratoma, benign
  causing ovarian mass, 232-233
  echogenicity of, 233-234f
  findings and occurrence of, 241t
Cystosarcoma phylloides
  breast mass due to, 401-402
  echogenicity of, 402-403f
  symptoms and findings of, 414t
Cystoscopy, 59b
Cysts
  abdominal
    echogenicity of, 365f
    in fetal anomalies, 364-365
    sonographic findings of, 356t
  adrenal gland
    causing mass, 162-163
    echogenicity of, 164f
    symptoms and findings of, 167t
  arachnoid, 355b
  biliary tract, pediatric mass due to, 118

branchial cleft, 440b
breast
  causing mass, 398-400
  echogenicity of, 399f, 400f
  symptoms and findings of, 414t
cerebral fossa, 483f
chocolate, 217
choledochal, 355b
definition of, 394b
liver
  causing right upper quadrant pain, 13
  echogenicity of, 12f, 14f
  vs. lymphoma, 43f
  symptoms and findings of, 15t
"moth-eaten" formation of, 228b
ovarian
  bleeding with pregnancy due to, 291f, 301b
  mass due to, 229-232, 230-232f, 241t
  size greater than date due to, 269-270
prostate
  causing elevated PSA, 454-455
  echogenicity of, 455f
  symptoms and findings of, 456t
renal mass vs., 93-96
  case studies involving, 99-101
  echogenicity of, 94f, 98f
  symptoms and findings of, 99t
scrotal
  causing mass, 421-424
  echogenicity of, 422f
  symptoms and findings of, 433t
splenic
  causing left upper quadrant pain, 107, 111t
  echogenicity of, 104f, 110f, 111b
thyroid
  causing neck mass, 446
  echogenicity of, 446f
  symptoms and findings of, 447t
urachal, 355b
Cytomegalovirus, 105b, 277b
Cytomegalovirus (CMV) infection, 339b, 479f

D
Dalkin Shield, 198
Dandy-Walker malformation
  fetal anomalies in, 358-359
    echogenicity of, 347f, 349f, 357f, 359f
    sonographic findings of, 356t
  infant anomalies in, 477-479
    echogenicity of, 483f
    sonographic findings of, 486t
Decidua, 250b
Decidua capsularis, 250b
Decidual parietalis, 250b
Deep vein thrombosis
  causing leg pain, 509-511
  color Doppler evaluation of, 502f, 512b

  definition of, 503b
  echogenicity of, 510f
Definity, 43
Developmental dysplasia of hip (DDH), 462-463
Diabetes, gestational, 264, 265b, 271b
Diabetes mellitus
  definition of, 77b, 277b
  fetal size and, 269f, 276, 284b
  liver mass in, 21b
  right upper quadrant pain in, 4b
Diamniotic pregnancy
  definition of, 308b
  echogenicity of, 314f, 320f
  embryology of, 311f
  sonographic findings of, 313t
Diaphragmatic hernia, congenital. See Congenital
    diaphragmatic hernia (CDH).
Diastrophic dysplasia, 355b
Dichorionic pregnancy
  definition of, 308b
  echogenicity of, 318f
  embryology of, 311f
  sonographic findings of, 313t
Didelphic uterus
  causing infertility, 219-220
  clinical scenario of, 216, 223b
  development and findings of, 223t
  echogenicity of, 216f, 220f, 223b
Digital rectal examination (DRE), 453
Diplegia, 471b
Discordant growth, 308b
Diverticulitis, 50b
Diverticulum, 144b
Dizygotic twins, 312, 313t
Down syndrome. See also Trisomy 21.
  alpha fetoprotein level in, 332t
  echogenicity associated with, 357f
Duodenal atresia, fetal, 362-363
  definition of, 339b
  echogenicity of, 345f, 363f
  sonographic findings of, 356t
Dwarfism, non-lethal. See Achondroplasia.
Dysfunctional uterine bleeding. See Uterine bleeding.
Dysmenorrhea, 217b
Dyspareunia, 207b
Dyspnea, 292b
Dysraphism, 324b
Dysuria, 59b, 77b, 93b

E
Ebstein's anomaly, 377b, 384, 385f
Echinococcus
  adrenal mass due to, 163
  right upper quadrant pain due to, 11-12
Echocardiography
  abnormal fetal
    case studies involving, 388

Echocardiography—*cont'd*
  abnormal fetal—*cont'd*
    clinical scenario of, 376, 387b
    references for diagnosing, 389
    risk factors that indicate, 377-378
    study questions about, 388-389
   transesophageal, 138
Echogenic bile. *See* Sludge.
Echogenic bowel, fetal
  chromosomal anomalies with, 343-344, 343t
  echogenicity of, 344f
Echogenic intracardiac focus (EIF), fetal
  chromosomal anomalies with, 343, 343t
  echogenicity of, 343f
Ectoderm, 228b
Ectopia, 217b
Ectopia cordis, 332
  alpha fetoprotein level in, 332t
  echogenicity of, 332f
Ectopic pregnancy
  causing bleeding, 293-294
    echogenicity of, 295f
    sonographic findings of, 302t
  definition of, 198b, 250b
  with use of IUD, 200-201
    echogenicity of, 201f
    symptoms and findings of, 202t
Ectopic spleen, 106
Edema. *See* Cerebral edema; Hydrops.
Edwards' syndrome. *See* Trisomy 18.
Ehlers-Danlos syndrome, 93b
Eklund maneuver, 394b
Emboli, 503b
Embolization, uterine artery, 179
Embryo in uncertain LMP
  crown-rump length (CRL) of, 252-254, 253f, 254f
  gestational sac diameter of, 251-252, 251f
  nuchal translucency thickness of, 254-255, 255f
  yolk sac diameter of, 252, 252f
Embryonal cell carcinoma
  causing scrotal mass, 427
  echogenicity of, 428f
  symptoms and findings of, 433t
Embryonic heart rate (EHR), 253f
Emphysematous cholecystitis, 6-7, 7f
Emphysematous pyelonephritis
  echogenicity of, 84f
  in renal failure, 83
  symptoms and findings of, 86t
Encapsulated, 228b
Encephalocele, 326, 328
  alpha fetoprotein level in, 332t
  echogenicity of, 328f
Endarterectomy, 491b, 496
Endocardial cushion defect, 382
Endoderm, 228b
Endometrial carcinoma

abnormal uterine bleeding due to, 183-186
  definition of, 174b
  echogenicity of, 187f
  specimen of, 184f
  symptoms and findings of, 192t
Endometrial hyperplasia
  abnormal uterine bleeding due to, 183-186
  Brenner tumor causing, 239
  definition of, 174b, 228b
  echogenicity of, 187f
  specimen of, 184f
  symptoms and findings of, 192t
Endometrial polyp
  abnormal uterine bleeding due to, 186-188
  clinical scenario of, 173, 191b
  definition of, 174b
  echogenicity of, 188f
  sonohysterography of, 191f
  symptoms and findings of, 192t
Endometrioid
  causing ovarian mass, 237-238
  echogenicity of, 238-239f
  findings and occurrence of, 242t
Endometrioma
  causing ovarian mass, 232
  echogenicity of, 233f
  findings and occurrence of, 241t
Endometriosis, 217, 218f
Endometritis, 210, 211t
Endometrium
  definition of, 174b, 198b
  after dilation and curettage, 157f
  normal menstrual
    echogenicity of, 185f
    thickness of, 185t
  postmenopausal
    anomalies of, 186t
    thickness of, 186t, 187f
Endomyometritis, 198b
Endoscopic retrograde cholangiopancreatogram, 50b
Endotoxemia, 207b
Endovaginal imaging, 179, 250b
Enema, hydrostatic, 144b
Entamoeba histolytica, 12
Entrapment syndrome, 503b
Epicanthal fold, 339b
Epidermoid, 420b
Epididymis, 420b
Epididymis cyst, 422, 423f
Epididymitis
  causing scrotal mass, 425
  definition of, 420b
  echogenicity of, 426f
  symptoms and findings of, 433t
Epididymoorchitis, 420b, 426f
Epigastric pain
  case studies involving, 55-56

clinical scenario of, 49, 54b
diseases causing, 52-54
references for diagnosing, 57
study questions about, 56-57
Epithelioid hemangioendothelioma, 21b, 28
Epithelium, 228b
Erythrocyte sedimentation rate, 207b
Erythropoietin, 59b
Escherichia coli, 12, 83
Esophageal atresia, fetal, 363, 363f
Esophageal veins, 34b
Esophagitis, 50b
Estrogen, 228b
Ethmocephaly, 355b, 471b
European Carotid Surgery Trial (ECST), 496
Exsanguination, 292b, 298
Extravasation, 59b
Exudate, 4b

F
Facial palsies, 265b
Fallopian tubes in PID, 208
False aneurysm. *See* Pseudoaneurysm.
Falx cerebri, 471b
Familial adenomatous polyposis, 117b
Fat sparing areas, 34b, 44t
Fatty acids level, 36t
Fatty infiltration, 50b
Fecalith, 144b
Femoral epiphysis, distal, 250b, 258
Femur length (FL) in uncertain LMP, 257-258,
    258f
Fertilization, in vitro, 308b
Fetal anomalies. *See also* Alpha fetoprotein (AFP);
    Chromosomal anomalies.
  of abdomen, 362-365
  of brain, 355, 357-359
  case studies involving, 372-373
  clinical scenario of, 354, 371b
  of face, 358f, 359-360
  of limbs, 370-371, 371f
  references for diagnosing, 374-375
  of skeleton, 365-370
  study questions about, 373-374
  of thorax, 360-362
Fetal bone length in uncertain LMP
  femur, 257-258
  long, 260-261, 261b
Fetal death
  in multifetal gestation, 315f
  in triploidy, 350f
  in trisomy 21, 338f, 348b
Fetal echocardiography. *See* Echocardiography, abnormal
    fetal.
Fetal gender, evaluation of, 310
Fetal growth, excessive, 265-266
Fetal hydrops. *See* Hydrops fetalis.

Fetal measurements
  in size greater than dates
    case studies involving, 271-273
    clinical scenario of, 264, 271b
    conditions causing, 266-270
    references for, 274-275
    study questions about, 273-274
  in size less than dates, 277
    case studies involving, 285-287
    clinical scenario of, 276, 284b
    conditions causing, 277-284, 285t
    references about, 289-290
    study questions about, 288-289
  in uncertain LMP. *See also* Biometry; Embryo in
      uncertain LMP
    during second/third trimester, 259-261, 261b
Fetal rhythm irregularities, 378-380
Fetal weight, estimation of, 266
Fetus papyraceus, 315, 317t
Fibroadenomas
  breast mass due to, 401
  definition of, 394b
  echogenicity of, 393f, 402f, 411b
  symptoms and findings of, 414t
Fibroid, uterine. *See* Leiomyoma.
Fibrolamellar carcinoma, 21b, 28
Fibroma
  hematuria due to, 65
  ovarian mass due to, 240, 242t
Fibromuscular dysplasia, 499, 499f
Fibrosarcoma, splenic, 110
Fibrous histiocytoma, malignant splenic, 110
Fine-needle aspiration (FNA), 440b, 444
"Fish in fishbowl" appearance, 269
Fitz-Hugh–Curtis syndrome, 207b
Focal nodular hyperplasia (FNH)
  causing liver mass, 24, 28t
  echogenicity of, 20f, 24f, 25f, 28b
Follicular cancer
  definition of, 440b
  neck mass due to, 447t
Follicular cysts
  causing ovarian mass, 229-230
  echogenicity of, 230f
  findings and occurrence of, 241t
Food and Drug Administration, U.S., IUD approval by,
    198
Foot pain, constant, 507
Foramen ovale, 377b
Forceps, 198b
Forebrain, 471b
Fossa cyst, 483f
Fossa ovalis, 377b
Fraternal twins, 312
Fredet-Ramstedt operation, 144b
Fungal balls, 85f
Fungal infection, kidney, 85, 87t

G

Galactocele
  breast mass due to, 399-400
  echogenicity of, 400f
  symptoms and findings of, 414t
Gallbladder. *See also* Gallstones; Sludge.
  contracted, 6f
  normal sonographic anatomy of, 4, 4f
  perforation of, 7-8
  polyp of, 4b
  porcelain, 4b
  strawberry, 8
Gallbladder diseases
  case studies involving, 15f, 16f
  causing right upper quadrant pain, 4-9, 9t
Gallstones, 4, 5f
Gamma-glutamyl transpeptidase, 34b
Gangrenous cholecystitis
  epigastric pain due to, 7f, 8f
  right upper quadrant pain due to, 7
Gastric reflux, 50b
Gastrin, 228b
Gastrinoma, 54t
Gastrointestinal diseases, echogenic
  case studies involving, 157-158
  clinical scenario involving, 143, 156b
  references for diagnosing, 159-160
  study questions about, 159
  symptoms and findings of, 145-156, 156t
Gastroschisis, 329-330
  alpha fetoprotein level in, 332t
  echogenicity of, 329f
Genetic testing, 340-341. *See also* Chromosomal
    anomalies.
  anomalies confirmed by, 344-348
  case studies involving, 350-351
  clinical scenario about, 338, 348b
  maternal serum screening in, 339-340
  references for using, 353
  soft markers in, 342-344
  study questions about, 352
Genitourinary system, normal, 60, 61f
Genotype, 93b
Germ cell, 228b
Gestation, multifetal
  abnormal twinning in, 314-316
  alpha fetoprotein level in, 324, 332t
  case studies involving, 318-321
  clinical scenario of, 307, 317b
  complications of, 313-314
  fundal height of, 268f
  imaging protocol (evaluation) of,
    310-311
  maternal complications with, 316
  references for diagnosing, 322
  size greater than date due to, 270t
  study questions about, 321

Gestational age
  definition of, 250b, 308b
  estimating
    case studies involving, 262
    clinical scenario of, 249, 261b
    during first trimester, 250-255
    references for, 263
    during second/third trimester, 255-261
    study questions about, 262-263
  size greater than
    case studies involving, 271-273
    clinical scenario of, 264, 271b
    fetal growth causing, 265-266
    fundal height causing, 267-270
    references about, 274-275
    study questions about, 273-274
  size less than
    case studies involving, 285-287
    clinical scenario of, 276, 284b
    conditions causing, 277-284, 285t
    references about, 289-290
    study questions about, 288-289
Gestational sac in uncertain LMP, 251-252, 251f
Gestational trophoblastic disease, 294-296
Glomerulonephritis, acute, 78-79, 86t
Glucose level, 36t
Goiter, 440b, 441, 447t
Goldstein catheter, 189
Gonorrhea, 207, 207b
Graafian follicle, 228b
Granuloma, breast, 394b, 409f
Granulosa, 228b
Graves' disease
  definition of, 440b
  neck mass due to, 441
  symptoms and findings of, 447t
Gunshot wound to testis, 430f
Gynecomastia
  causing male breast mass, 411
  definition of, 394b
  echogenicity of, 413f

H

Hamartoma. *See* Angiomyolipoma (AML).
Haploid, 228b
Harmonics
  definition of, 50b
  of pancreas, 52, 52f
Hashimoto's disease, 440b
  causing neck mass, 441-442
  echogenicity of, 442f
  symptoms and findings of, 447t
Head circumference (HC) in uncertain LMP, 257,
    257f
Heart anomalies, 380-387
Heart block, atrioventricular (fetal), 377b, 380, 380f
Heart rhythm irregularities, fetal, 378-380

Heart septal defects
  echogenicity of, 347f
  types of, 377b, 380-382
Heart ventricle, double-outlet right, 384
Hemangioendothelioma
  pediatric liver mass due to, 118-119
    echogenicity of, 119f, 121f
    symptoms and findings of, 129t
  splenic LUQ pain due to, 109
Hemangioma
  definition of, 59b
  hematuria due to, 62, 70t
  liver mass due to, 21-22
    echogenicity of, 20f, 22f, 28b
    pediatric, 120f
    symptoms and findings of, 28t
  splenic LUQ pain due to, 108-109
    echogenicity of, 104f, 111b
    symptoms and findings of, 111t
Hemangiopericytoma, splenic, 109
Hematocele, 420b
Hematocolpos, 217b
Hematocrit
  definition of, 105b, 471b
  laboratory values for, 36t
Hematoma
  breast mass due to, 411, 412f
  definition of, 59b, 420b
  hematuria due to, 63, 70t
  hepatic RUQ pain due to, 13
    echogenicity of, 14f
    symptoms and findings of, 15t
  scrotal mass due to, 430f
  splenic LUQ pain due to, 110, 110f
  uterine, 301f
Hematometra
  abnormal uterine bleeding due to, 185
  definition of, 174b
  echogenicity of, 186f
Hematometracolpos, 217b
Hematuria, 59-60
  benign neoplasms causing, 62-65, 70-71t
  case studies involving, 71-73
  clinical scenario of, 58, 69b
  definition of, 59b, 77b, 93b
  gross, 59b
  malignant neoplasms causing, 65-68,
    70-71t
  microscopic, 59b
  nephrolithiasis causing, 60-62, 70t
  references for diagnosing, 75
  study questions about, 74-75
Hemianopia, 491b
Hemihypertrophy, 59b, 93b, 117b
Hemiplegia, 491b
Hemoglobin, 36t
Hemoperitoneum, 135b

Hemorrhage
  bleeding with pregnancy due to, 292-293
    echogenicity of, 292f
    sonographic findings of, 302t
  carotid intraplaque, 495f
  intracranial, 472, 474
    echogenicity of, 475f, 480f
    sonographic findings of, 486t
  intraventricular
    echogenicity of, 470f, 486b
    grades III & IV, 476f
  pediatric adrenal mass due to, 119
    echogenicity of, 122f, 123f
Hemorrhagic adenoma, hepatic, 24f
Hemorrhagic cyst, renal, 95, 99t
Hepatic artery, 121f
Hepatic cysts. See Cysts.
Hepatic echinococcosis, 11-12
Hepatic lipoma, 24, 25f
Hepatitis
  acute/chronic
    compared, 38t
    definition of, 34b
    echogenicity of, 39f
    summary of findings with, 44t
  A-G, 38t
  alcoholic, 34b
  definition of, 34b
  diffuse liver disease due to, 39
  liver function tests for, 37t
Hepatoblastoma
  causing pediatric liver mass, 119
  echogenicity of, 122f
  symptoms and findings of, 129t
Hepatocellular adenoma. See Liver cell adenoma.
Hepatocellular carcinoma (HCC). See also
    Hepatoma.
  causing liver mass, 24-26, 28t
  in diffuse liver disease, 42-43, 44t
  echogenicity of, 26f, 27f
  liver function tests for, 37t
Hepatocellular disease
  definition of, 34b
  in diffuse liver disease, 35-36
  laboratory tests for, 35, 36t
Hepatocytes, 21b
Hepatofugal portal vein blood flow, 34b, 40f
Hepatoma, 34b, 42-43, 43f
Hepatopetal portal vein blood flow, 34b, 40f
Hernia
  causing scrotal mass, 424
  definition of, 420b
  echogenicity of, 425f
  symptoms and findings of, 433t
Heterotopic pregnancy, 292b
Heterozygous, 355b
Hip anatomy, infant, 462, 462f, 465f

Hip dysplasia, infant
  case studies involving, 468
  clinical scenario of, 461, 467b
  developmental, 462-463
  dislocated hip in, 461f, 465f, 466f, 467b
  references for diagnosing, 469
  risk factors for, 463
  sonographic evaluation of infant for, 463-464
    coronal/flexion view, 465, 466f
    coronal/neutral view, 464, 465f, 468f
    transverse/flexion view, 465-466, 466f
  study questions about, 468-469
  treatment (Pavlik harness) for, 467
Hippel-Lindau disease, 50b, 93b
Hirsutism, 217b, 228b
Hodgkin's lymphoma/disease
  definition of, 34b, 105b
  in diffuse liver disease, 43
  left upper quadrant pain due to, 109
"Hole sign," 7-8
Holoprosencephaly
  fetal, 357
    definition of, 339b
    echogenicity of, 348f, 350f, 358f
    sonographic findings of, 356t
  infant, 479-480
    echogenicity of, 482f, 484f
    sonographic findings of, 486t
Homozygous, 355b
Hormone replacement therapy, 394b
Hydatidiform mole
  causing bleeding with pregnancy, 294-296, 297
  definition of, 265b
  echogenicity of, 296f
  sonographic findings of, 302t
  in triploidy, 350f
Hydramnios, 308b, 313-314
Hydranencephaly
  fetal, 357-358
    echogenicity of, 359f
    sonographic findings of, 356t
  infant, 480
    echogenicity of, 484f
    sonographic findings of, 486t
Hydrocele
  causing scrotal mass, 421
  definition of, 420b
  echogenicity of, 422f
  findings of, 433t
Hydrocephalus
  fetal, 355, 356t
  infant, 476-477
    echogenicity of, 479f, 483f
    after shunt, 480f
    sonographic findings of, 486t
Hydronephrosis
  definition of, 339b

fetal size less than date due to, 280-282
    echogenicity of, 282f
    sonographic findings of, 285t
  pediatric renal mass due to, 120-122
    echogenicity of, 125f, 126f
  renal failure in, 77-78
    echogenicity of, 78f
    symptoms and findings of, 86t
Hydrops, 339b, 355b
Hydrops fetalis
  in congenital diaphragmatic hernia, 361
  definition of, 265b, 308b
  echogenicity of, 354f, 371b
  nuchal translucency and, 342
  size greater than date due to, 267, 270t
  in twin-twin transfusion syndrome, 315
Hydrosalpinx, 208-209, 211t
Hydroureter, 59b
Hygroma, cystic
  causing neck mass, 446
  definition of, 440b
  symptoms and findings of, 447t
Hyperemesis gravidarum, 308b, 316
Hyperkalemia, 77b
Hyperparathyroidism
  causing neck mass, 444, 445
  primary/secondary, 440b
Hyperplasia
  adrenal mass vs., 164
  definition of, 162b, 452b
  neck mass due to, 445
Hyperplastic cholecystosis, 8-9, 8f
Hyperplastic nodules of neck, 440b,
    442-443
Hypertelorism, 250b
Hypertension, chronic, 277b
Hyperthyroidism, 440b, 441
Hypertrophic pyloric stenosis, 150
Hypogastric, 228b
Hypoglycemic episode, 50b
Hypophosphatasia, 440b
Hypoplastic left heart syndrome, fetal, 384
  clinical scenario of, 376, 387b
  definition of, 377b
  echocardiography of, 385f
Hypotelorism, 250b, 339b, =55b
Hypotension, 135b
Hypovolemia, 77b
Hypoxia, 471b
Hysterosalpingography (HSG)
  definition of, 174b, 217b
  vs. sonohysterography, 188
Hysteroscopy
  biopsy and polyp removal by, 187f,
    192f
  definition of, 174b, 198b, 217b
  vs. endovaginal imaging, 179

I

Iatrogenic, 135b
Icteric, 144b
Identical twins, 312
Idiopathic, 59b, 292b
Ileocolic intussusception, 154f, 155f
In vitro fertilization, 308b
Incarcerated, 420b
Incidentaloma, 162
Infant
    head
        pathology of, 472, 474-480, 486t
        sonographic views of, 473-474f
        techniques for imaging, 471-472
    hip
        developmental dysplasia of, 462-463
        sonographic evaluation of, 463-466
        treatment for abnormal, 467
    spine
        sonographic appearance of, 485f
        sonographic evaluation of, 482-486
Infantile hypertrophic pyloric stenosis (IHPS), 150-152
    clinical scenario of, 143f, 156b
    echogenicity of, 151f, 152f
Infarction
    definition of, 105b
    of scrotum, 433t
    of spleen, 108, 111t
Infection
    cytomegalovirus (CMV), 339b, 479f
    fungal, of kidney, 85, 87t
    with IUD use, 199-200, 202t
    renal, 82-85, 86-87t
    TORCH, of fetus, 339b
    urinary tract
        causing elevated PSA, 453
        causing hematuria, 59-60
        in renal failure, 77
Inferior vena cava, 377b
Infertility
    case studies involving, 224-225
    clinical scenario of, 216, 223b
    definition of, 198b
    references for diagnosing, 226
    study questions about, 225-226
Inflammation. *See also* Pelvic inflammatory disease.
    breast mass due to, 408, 410, 415t
    elevated PSA due to, 454
Infundibulum, 59b
Inguinal canal, 420b, 432
Inspissated, 394b
Insulinoma, 54t
Interhemispheric fissure, 471b
Intermenstrual bleeding, 174b
Intermittent claudication, 503b, 506-507
Intracapsular rupture, 394b
Intraperitoneal, 144b

Intrauterine device (IUD)
    complications with use of, 199-200,
        202t
    definition of, 198b
    ectopic, 200, 201f
    lost
        case studies involving, 202-203f
        clinical scenario of, 197, 201b
        references about, 205
        study questions about, 204-205
    perforation by, 200
    radiograph of, 200f
    sonographic appearance of, 198-199
    types of, 198, 199f
    use of, in PID, 207
Intrauterine growth restriction (IUGR)
    definition of, 308b
    fetal size less than date due to, 282-283
        echogenicity of, 284f
        sonographic findings of, 285t
    maternal diseases associated with, 283-284
    in multifetal gestation, 314, 314f
Intussusception, 153-156
    echogenicity of, 154-156f, 158f
    symptoms and findings of, 156t
Involute, 228b
Ipsilateral, 228b
Iron level, serum, 36t
Ischemia, 77b
Islet cell tumors
    epigastric (pancreatic) pain due to, 54
    location and findings of, 54t
Islets of Langerhans, 50b
Isthmus, 440b

J

Jaundice, 50b, 144b
Juxtaglomerular tumor, renal, 65

K

Kaposi's sarcoma, splenic, 110
Karyotype, 228b, 277b, 292b, 339b
Kasai operation, 117b
Kidney, echogenicity of
    compared to adrenal gland, 168-169f
    compared to liver, 12f, 61f
Kidney tubular necrosis, acute
    echogenicity of, 81f
    renal failure in, 81-82
    symptoms and findings of, 86t
Klebsiella pneumoniae, 12
Klinefelter's syndrome, 394b
Klippel-Trénaunay-Weber syndrome, 105b
Knee mass, 507
Krukenberg's tumor
    causing ovarian mass, 238-239
        Doppler evaluation of, 229f, 239f

Krukenberg's tumor—*cont'd*
   echogenicity of, 238-239f
   findings and occurrence of, 242t
Kupffer's cells, 21b

L
Lactic dehydrogenase (LDH) level, 36t
Large for gestational age (LGA), 265, 270t
Leg pain
   arterial diseases causing, 506-509
   case studies involving, 513
   clinical scenario of, 502, 512b
   protocol for, 505f
   references for diagnosing, 515
   study questions about, 513-515
   venous diseases causing, 509-512
Leiomyoma
   abnormal uterine bleeding due to, 176-180
      echogenicity of, 180f, 181f
      locations of, 177f
      pathology specimen of, 179f
      sonohysterography of, 191f
      symptoms and findings of, 192t
   vs. adenomyomas, 179, 181
   definition of, 174b, 228b
   vs. endometrial carcinoma, 184f
   hematuria due to, 65
   methods for identifying, 179
   predicting myomas from, 179
   size greater than date due to, 269, 270f, 270t
Leiomyomata, 21b
Leiomyosarcoma, splenic, 110
Lesions, definition of, 452b
Leukocytosis, definition of, 4b, 50b, 77b, 105b, 207b
Leukoplakia, 59b
Levovist, 34b, 43
Leydig's cell tumors, scrotal, 429, 433t
Limb-body wall complex, 331
   alpha fetoprotein level in, 332t
   echogenicity of, 331f
Lipase, 50b
Lipids, total, 36t
Lipoma
   breast mass due to, 403
      echogenicity of, 403f
      symptoms and findings of, 414t
   hematuria due to, 63, 70t
   liver mass due to, 24
      echogenicity of, 25f
      symptoms and findings of, 28t
   splenic (LUQ) pain due to, 109
Lithotripsy, 59b
Littoral cell angioma, splenic, 109, 110
Liver
   lesions of
      liver mass due to, 28t
      right upper quadrant pain due to, 11-15, 15t

   mass in
      benign neoplasms causing, 21-24
      case studies involving, 29-30
      causing elevated MSAFP levels, 332t
      clinical scenario of, 20, 28b
      echogenicity of, 20f, 28b
      lesions causing pediatric, 118-119
      malignant neoplasms causing, 24-28
      references for diagnosing, 32
      study questions about, 31-32
   normal sonographic anatomy of, 21, 22f
      compared to kidney, 12f, 61f
Liver cell adenoma
   causing liver mass, 23
   echogenicity of, 20f, 23f, 28b
Liver diseases
   diffuse
      case studies involving, 45-46
      clinical scenario of, 33, 45b
      laboratory tests for, 35, 36t, 37t
      references for diagnosing, 48
      study questions about, 47-48
      summary of findings with, 44t
   fatty, 37
      definition of, 34b
      echogenicity of, 37f
      summary of findings with, 44t
   metastatic
      causing liver mass, 26, 28
      echogenicity of, 27f
Liver function tests. *See* Hepatocellular disease.
LMP. *See* Menstrual period.
Loculation, 228b
Locus, 93b
Longus colli muscles, 440b
Low birth weight, 314
Luteinization, 228b
Lymph nodes
   normal sonographic anatomy of, 445, 445f
   sonography of abnormal, 445-446, 446f
Lymphadenopathy
   breast mass and, 410f
   definition of, 34b
   in retroperitoneal disease, 162
      echogenicity of, 161f, 163f, 166b
Lymphangioma
   capillary/cavernous, 440b, 446
   definition of, 21b
   hematuria due to, 68
   liver mass due to, 24
   splenic LUQ pain due to, 109, 111t
Lymphoma
   definition of, 21b, 34b, 50b, 162b, 420b
   diffuse liver disease due to, 43
      echogenicity of, 43f
      summary of findings with, 44t
   hematuria due to, 68, 69f

liver mass due to, 28
scrotal mass due to, 428
echogenicity of, 429f
symptoms and findings of, 433t
splenic LUQ pain due to, 109
Lymphosarcoma, 34b
Lymphoscintigraphy, 394b

M

Macroglossia, 59b, 117b
Macrosomia
clinical scenario of, 264, 271b
echogenicity of, 267f, 268f
size greater than date due to, 266-267
sonographic findings of, 270t
Magnetic resonance imaging (MRI), 105b
Majewski syndrome, 369
Malaise, 162b
Malaria, 105b
Malignant, definition of, 452b
Mammary layer, 394b
Mandibular frenulum, 144b
Marfan syndrome, 93b, 135b
Marker screening, multiple
for aneuploidy, 343t
in first trimester of pregnancy, 340
Marshall-Smith syndrome, 265b
Masculinization, 162b
Mastitis
breast mass due to, 408, 410
echogenicity of, 410f
malignancy of, 410, 415t
Maternal serum alpha fetoprotein (MSAFP). *See* Alpha
fetoprotein (AFP).
Maternal serum screening, 339-340
McBurney's sign, 144b
Measurements, fetal sonographic, 259-261
Measurements, sonographic fetal, 261b. *See also* Biometry.
Meckel-Gruber syndrome, 324b
Meckel's diverticulum, 144b
Meconium, 324b
Meconium ileus, 144b
Meconium peritonitis, 363-364
echogenicity of, 364f
sonographic findings of, 356t
Mediastinum testis, 420b
Medulla of organ, 228b
Medullary sponge kidney vs. renal mass, 98, 99t
Meigs' syndrome, 228b
Membranous septal defect, 381-382
Meningoencephaloceles, 328
Meningomyelocele, 326, 339b
Menometrorrhagia, 174b, 198b
Menorrhagia, 174b, 217b
Menstrual cycle
echogenicity of phases in, 178f, 185f
thickness of endometrium during, 183-184, 185t

Menstrual period
last, pregnancy dating after, 266
uncertain last
case studies involving, 262
clinical scenario of, 249, 261b
estimating due date after, 250, 266. *See also* Biometry
references about, 263
study questions about, 262-263
Mesoblastic nephroma, pediatric, 125, 129t
Mesocaval shunt, 34b
Mesoderm, 228b
Mesothelial cells, 228b
Metabolic alkalosis, 144b
Metanephrine, 162b
Metastases, neoplasm
adrenal mass due to, 165
clinical scenario of, 161f, 166b
echogenicity of, 167f
breast mass due to, 407-408
echogenicity of, 408f
symptoms and findings of, 415t
hematuria due to
clinical scenario of, 58, 69b
echogenicity of, 68f
liver mass due to, 26, 28
echogenicity of, 27f
symptoms and findings of, 28t
splenic LUQ pain due to, 109-110, 110f
Methysergide, 162b
Metrorrhagia, 228b
Microcalcifications, 440b
Micrognathia
anomalies of, 360
definition of, 292b, 339b
echogenicity of, 350f, 361f
sonographic findings of, 356t
Microlithiasis
definition of, 420b
echogenicity of, 425f, 432f
scrotal mass due to, 424
Microphthalmia, 339b
Mid gut, 324b
Milk of calcium cyst vs. renal mass, 95, 95f, 99t
Mirror artifacts with hemangioma, 22f
Missed abortion (MAB), 293, 302t
Mitral valve, 377b
Mole, hydatidiform. *See* Hydatidiform mole.
Monoamniotic pregnancy
definition of, 308b
echogenicity of, 320f
embryology of, 311f
sonographic findings of, 313t
Monochorionic pregnancy
definition of, 308b
echogenicity of, 320f
embryology of, 311f
sonographic findings of, 313t

Mononucleosis, 105b
Monozygotic twins, 312, 313t
Morbidity, 117b, 265b
Morison's pouch, 34b
Mortality, 117b, 265b
Mosaicism, 339b
"Moth-eaten" cyst formation, 228b, 239f
Mucin, 228b
Mucinous cystadenoma
    ovarian mass due to, 235-237
        echogenicity of, 237f
        findings and occurrence of, 241t
    size greater than date due to, 270f
Multicystic dysplastic kidney (MCDK)
    definition of, 93b
    fetal size less than date due to, 280
        echogenicity of, 281f
        sonographic findings of, 285t
    pediatric renal mass due to, 122-123, 127f
Multifetal, 309b
Multiocular cyst, 95
Multiparous, 292b
Multiples of the median/mean, 324b
Murphy's sign, 4b
Muscles around thyroid, 440b
Muscular septal defect, 382
Myelolipoma, adrenal, 165f
Myoma. *See* Leiomyoma.
Myometrium, 198b
Myxoma, renal, 65

N
Nägele's rule, 250
Neck mass
    benign nodules causing, 442-443
    case studies involving, 448
    clinical scenario of, 439, 447b
    diseases causing, 440-441
    malignant nodules causing, 443-444
    references for diagnosing, 449-450
    study questions about, 448-449
    symptoms and findings of, 447-448t
Necrosis, 144b
Neonatal neurosonography. *See* Neurosonography, neonatal.
Neonate, 117b
Neoplasms. *See also* Metastases, neoplasm.
    benign
        of adrenal cortex, 163-164
        of breast, 401-403, 414t
        of genitourinary system, 62-65
        of liver, 21-24
        of ovaries, 239-242, 241t
        of pancreas, 53-54
        of scrotum, 421
        of spleen, 108-109
        of thyroid, 442-443

    cystic
        of breast, 398-400
        of ovaries, 232-239
        of scrotum, 421-424
        of thyroid, 446
    definition of, 21b, 77b, 162b, 228b
    malignant
        of adrenal gland, 164-165
        of breast, 403-407
        of genitourinary system, 65-68
        of liver, 20f, 24-28, 28b
        of ovaries, 236-237, 241t, 242t
        of pancreas, 53-54
        of prostate, 455-456, 456f
        of scrotum, 426-430
        of spleen, 109-110
        of thyroid, 443-444
    pediatric, 129t
Nephroblastoma. *See also* Uterine bleeding.
    hematuria due to, 65-67, 68
        echogenicity of, 66f
        symptoms and findings of, 71t
    pediatric renal mass due to, 124-125
        echogenicity of, 128-129f
        symptoms and findings of, 129t
Nephrocalcinosis, 93b, 98f
Nephrolithiasis
    causing hematuria, 60-62
    definition of, 59b
    echogenicity of, 62f
    symptoms and findings of, 70t
Nephroma, pediatric mesoblastic, 125
Neural tube, 324b
Neural tube defects (NTDs), 325
Neuroblastoma
    pediatric adrenal mass due to, 119-120
        clinical scenario of, 116f, 128b
        echogenicity of, 124f
        symptoms and findings of, 129t
    pediatric renal mass due to, 124-125, 129t
Neurosonography, neonatal
    case studies involving, 487-488
    clinical scenario of, 470, 486b
    of head pathologies, 472-481
    references for evaluating, 490
    sonographic findings of, 486t
    of spinal pathologies, 482-485
    study questions about, 489-490
    techniques for, 471-472
"Nipple" sign, 455
Nodular regenerative hyperplasia, 21b, 24
Nodule, definition of, 228b, 452b
Non-Hodgkin's lymphoma
    definition of, 34b, 105b
    in diffuse liver disease, 43, 44t
    splenic LUQ pain due to, 109
Nonsteroidal antiinflammatory drugs, 277b

North American Symptomatic Carotid Endarterectomy Trial (NASCET), 496
Nuchal fold in uncertain LMP, 260, 260f, 261b
Nuchal translucency (NT)
  in chromosomal anomalies, 341-342, 342f, 349f
  in uncertain LMP, 254-255, 255f
Nuclear medicine, 144b

O

Obstetrician, 250b
Occipitofrontal diameter (OFD) in uncertain LMP, 258-259, 258f
Occupational Safety and Health Administration (OSHA) on hepatitis B, 39
Oil cyst
  causing breast mass, 399
  echogenicity of, 400f
  symptoms and findings of, 414t
Oligohydramnios
  definition of, 250b, 309b, 339b, 461b
  fetal size less than date due to, 277-278
    echogenicity of, 278f
    sonographic findings of, 285t
  hip dysplasia associated with, 463
  in multifetal gestation, 313-314
Oligomenorrhea, 217b
Oliguria, 77b, 117b
Omentum, 420b
Omphalocele, 330-331
  alpha fetoprotein level in, 332t
  definition of, 339b
  echogenicity of, 330f, 346f, 347f
Omphalopagus twins, 268f, 315f
Oncocytoma, renal, 63, 64f, 70t
Oocyte, 228b
Optison, 34b, 43
Orchiectomy, 420b
Orchitis
  definition of, 420b
  scrotal mass due to, 425-426
  symptoms and findings of, 433t
Ortolani maneuver, 463f
Ossification, 250b
Osteogenesis imperfecta
  echogenicity of, 370f
  fetal anomalies in, 370-371
  radiograph of, 370f
  sonographic findings of, 356t
Ostium primum atrial septal defect, 382
Ovarian mass
  case studies involving, 243-244
  clinical scenario of, 227, 242b
  cystic/complex neoplasms causing, 232-239
  in endometriosis, 217
  lesions causing, 241-242t
  ovarian cysts causing, 229-232
  references for diagnosing, 245

solid neoplasms causing, 239-241
  study questions about, 244-245
Ovaries normal anatomy of, 229
Ovulation induction, 309b
Ovum, blighted, 292b

P

Pain
  epigastric
    case studies involving, 55-56
    clinical scenario of, 49, 54b
    diseases causing, 52-54
    references for diagnosing, 57
    study questions about, 56-57
  left upper quadrant
    case studies involving, 111-113
    clinical scenario of, 104, 111b
    references for diagnosing, 115
    spleen disorders causing, 105-108, 110
    spleen neoplasms causing, 108-110, 111t
    study questions about, 114-115
  leg
    arterial diseases causing, 506-509
    case studies involving, 513
    clinical scenario of, 502, 512b
    protocol for, 505f
    references for diagnosing, 515
    study questions about, 513-515
    venous diseases causing, 509-512
  right upper quadrant
    biliary tract diseases causing, 9-11
    case studies involving, 15-17
    clinical scenario of, 3, 15b
    gallbladder diseases causing, 4-9
    liver diseases causing, 11-15
    references for diagnosing, 18-19
    study questions about, 17-18
Palliative treatment, 4b
Palpable, 394b
Pancreas
  conventional vs. harmonic imaging of, 52f
  echogenicity of normal, 51f
  normal sonographic anatomy of, 51-52
  relationship of, to other GI parts, 51f
Pancreatic neoplasms
  case studies involving, 55-56
  echogenicity of, 49, 54b
  epigastric pain due to, 53-54
  location and findings of, 54t
Pancreatitis, 52-53, 55f
Papillary necrosis, renal, 79, 86t
Papilloma
  intraductal
    causing breast mass, 402-403, 414t
    echogenicity of removed, 403f
  renal, 65

Parapelvic cyst
  echogenicity of, 96f
  vs. renal mass, 95
  symptoms and findings of, 99t
Parathyroid gland
  adenoma of, 444-445
    echogenicity of, 445f
    symptoms and findings of, 447t
  hyperplasia of, 445
    definition of, 440b
    symptoms and findings of, 447t
  normal sonographic anatomy of, 444
Parathyroid hormone, 440b
Parenchyma of organ, 228b
Parovarian cyst
  echogenicity of, 232f
  findings and occurrence of, 241t
  ovarian mass due to, 232
Patau's syndrome. *See* Trisomy 13.
Pathology, 250b
Pavlik harness, 467f
Peau d'orange, 394b
Pediatric mass
  adrenal diseases causing, 119-120
  biliary tract diseases causing, 117-118
  case studies involving, 130-131
  clinical scenario of, 116, 128b
  liver diseases causing, 118-119
  references for diagnosing, 133
  renal diseases causing, 120-125
  study questions about, 132-133
Pedunculated, 228b
Pelvic anatomy, 176f
Pelvic inflammatory disease, 207-208
  case studies involving, 212-213
  clinical scenario of, 206, 210b
  definition of, 198b
  references for diagnosing, 215
  study questions about, 214-215
  symptoms and findings of, 208-210, 211t
  with use of IUD, 198
Pentalogy of Cantrell, 324b, 328
Periportal cuffing, 34b
Peritoneum
  definition of, 144b
  mass in, 432
  pseudomyxoma, 228b
Peritonitis
  definition of, 144b
  echogenicity of, 150f
  meconium, 363-364
    echogenicity of, 364f
    sonographic findings of, 356t
Periventricular leukomalacia (PVL), 474-475
  echogenicity of, 477f
  sonographic findings of, 486t
Pharyngitis, 77b

Pheochromocytoma, adrenal, 163, 167t
Phospholipids level, 36t
Photoplethysmography, 503b
Placenta
  evaluation of, 311f
  in multifetal gestation, 310-311
  in size greater than date, 267f
Placenta accreta, 298-300, 298f
Placenta previa
  bleeding with pregnancy due to, 297-298
    echogenicity of, 298f, 299f
    sonographic findings of, 302t
    types of, 297f
  definition of, 309b
  in multifetal gestation, 316
Placental abruption
  definition of, 309b, 324b
  in multifetal gestation, 316
Placental insufficiency, 309b
Placentation, 309b
Platelet count, 36t
Plethysmography, 503b
Pleural effusion, 362
  echogenicity of, 362f
  sonographic findings of, 356t
Polycystic disease
  kidney
    definition of, 93b
    echogenicity of, 17f, 96f, 97f, 98b
    fetal size less than date due to, 279-280, 285t
    liver cysts and, 13
    pediatric renal mass due to, 123-124, 127f
    renal mass due to, 96-97
    symptoms and findings of, 99t
  pancreatic, 50b, 53-54
Polycystic ovarian disease
  echogenicity of, 219f
  infertility due to, 217, 219
Polydactyly
  definition of, 339b
  echogenicity of, 349f, 350f
  sonographic findings of, 356t
  syndrome with, 367, 369
    echogenicity of, 369f, 371f
Polyhydramnios
  causing size greater than date, 269f, 270t
  in congenital diaphragmatic hernia, 361
  definition of, 308b, 339b, 355b
  echogenicity of, 363f, 366f
Polyp, 144b
Polysplenia, 106, 117b
Polyuria, 77b
Popliteal entrapment syndrome, 507
Popliteal vessels
  anatomy of, 505, 506f
  aneurysm of, 507, 508f
Portacaval shunt, 34b

Portal hypertension
    definition of, 34b
    in diffuse liver disease, 40-41
        echogenicity of, 42f
        summary of findings with, 44t
    in splenomegaly, 107f
Portal vein
    cavernous transformation of, 40
    in hepatoma, 42f
    hepatopetal/fugal blood flow of, 24b, 40f
Postmenopausal women, endometrial anomalies
        in, 186t
Postpartum bleeding, 301, 301f
Precocious puberty, 117b, 162b
Preeclampsia
    definition of, 277b, 309b, 324b
    during multifetal gestation, 316
    with size less than dates, 276, 284b
Pregnancy
    anembryonic, 292b, 293f, 296
    bleeding with. See Bleeding with pregnancy
    dating beginning of. See also Biometry; Gestational age
        calculation software for, 266
        during first trimester, 250-255
        during second/third trimester, 255-261
    ectopic. See Ectopic pregnancy
    gallstones and, 5f
    heterotopic, 292b, 294
    high-order multiple, 308b
    induction of, 250b
    with IUD, 200, 201f, 202t
    maternal complications during, 316
    misdated, 324, 332t
    molar
        bleeding due to, 294-295, 296f
        size greater than date due to, 269f, 270t
    multifetal. See Gestation, multifetal
    postpartum bleeding after, 301
    prognosis milestones for, 293
    serum screening during, 339-340. See also Alpha
        fetoprotein (AFP)
Pregnancy-associated plasma protein A (PAPP-A),
        339-340
Premature atrial/ventricular contractions (fetal),
        378-379
    definition of, 377b
    M-mode tracing of, 378f
Premature labor in multifetal gestation, 314
Premature rupture of membranes (PROM)
    definition of, 277b
    fetal size less than date due to, 284
    sonographic findings of, 285t
Primigravida
    definition of, 461b
    hip dysplasia associated with, 463
Proboscis, 355b
Progesterone, 228b

Prosencephalon, 471b
Prostate
    normal sonographic anatomy of, 452, 453f
    pathology of, 456t
    sonographic evaluation of, 453f
    zonal anatomy of, 452f
Prostate cancer
    clinical scenario of, 451f, 456b
    echogenicity of, 455f
    elevated PSA due to, 455
    symptoms and findings of, 456t
Prostate specific antigen (PSA), elevated
    case studies involving, 457
    clinical scenario of, 451, 456b
    conditions causing, 454-456
    methods for evaluating, 453-454
    references for diagnosing, 458
    screening for, 452-453
    study questions about, 457-458
Prostatitis
    causing elevated PSA, 453, 454
    symptoms and findings of, 456t
Proteinuria, 77b
Prothrombin time, 34b
Prune-belly syndrome, 277b
Pruritus, 4b, 77b
Psammoma bodies, 440b, 443f
Pseudoaneurysm, 507-508
    definition of, 503b
    echogenicity of, 508f
Pseudocyst
    definition of, 50b
    epigastric pain due to, 53
    location and findings of, 54t
Pseudomyxoma peritoneum, 228b
Pulmonary artery, 377b
Pulmonary embolism, 509
Pulmonary sequestration, 356t, 361-362
Pulmonary stenosis, 377b
Pulmonary veins, 377b
Pyelectasis, 277b, 339b. See also Hydronephrosis.
Pyelogram, intravenous, 59b
Pyelonephritis
    echogenicity of, 83f
    renal failure in, 82-84
    symptoms and findings of, 86t
Pyloric canal, 144b
Pyloric stenosis, 150-152
    clinical scenario of, 143f, 156b
    echogenicity of, 151f, 152f, 158f
    symptoms and findings of, 156t
Pyloromyotomy, 144b
Pylorus, echogenicity of, 151f
Pyogenic abscess, liver, 12
Pyonephrosis, 82, 86t
Pyosalpinx, 208, 211t
Pyuria, 77b

Q
Quadriplegia, 471b
Quadruple screen, 340

R
Radial, 394b
Radial ray defect, 339b
Raynaud's disease, 503b, 509
Rebound tenderness, 207b
Regression models, 265b
Renal abscess, 84-85, 87t
Renal agenesis
    echogenicity of, 279f
    fetal size less than date due to, 278-279
    sonographic findings of, 285t
Renal artery stenosis, 80-81
    clinical scenario of, 76f, 85b
    echogenicity of, 81f
    symptoms and findings of, 86t
Renal cell carcinoma (RCC)
    causing hematuria, 65
    echogenicity of, 65f, 66f
    symptoms and findings of, 71t
Renal colic, 59b
Renal cystic disease
    causing pediatric renal mass, 122-124
    vs. renal mass, 96-98
Renal cysts vs. renal mass, 93-96
Renal failure
    acute/chronic, 79-80
        echogenicity of, 80f
        pathology associated with, 86t
    ruling out
        case studies involving, 87-88
        clinical scenario of, 76, 85b
        pathology associated with, 77-79, 80-85,
            86t
        references for diagnosing, 90-91
        study questions about, 89-90
Renal infection
    pathology associated with, 86-87t
    renal failure in, 82-85
Renal mass. *See also* Neoplasms.
    cystic vs. solid
        case studies involving, 99-101
        clinical scenario of, 92, 98
        references for diagnosing, 103
        study questions about, 102-103
    pediatric diseases causing, 120-125
Renal parenchyma, 77b
Renal pyelectasis, fetal
    chromosomal anomalies with, 343, 343t
    echogenicity of, 344f
Renal pyramids, 77b
Renal sarcoma, 68, 69f, 70f
Reninoma. *See* Juxtaglomerular tumor.
Resting pain, constant, 507

Retroareolar, 395b
Retromammary layer, 395b
Retroperitoneal diseases, echogenic
    case studies involving, 168-169
    clinical scenario of, 161, 166b
    references for diagnosing, 170
    study questions about, 169-170
    symptoms and findings of, 162-167
Retroperitoneal fibrosis, 165-166, 167f
Rhabdoid tumor, renal, 68
Rhizomelia, 355b
Rokitansky-Aschoff sinuses, 8
Ruvalcaba-Myhre syndrome, 265b

S
Sacrococcygeal teratoma (SCT), 365
    echogenicity of, 366f
    sonographic findings of, 356t
Saldino-Noonan syndrome, 369
Salpingitis
    definition of, 207b
    in pelvic inflammatory disease, 208
    symptoms and findings of, 211t
Sarcoma
    benign
        breast mass due to, 401-402
        echogenicity of, 402-403f
        symptoms and findings of, 414t
    causing hematuria. *See* Renal sarcoma
    definition of, 34b
    splenic LUQ pain due to, 110, 111t
Schizencephaly, 480, 482
    echogenicity of, 485f
    sonographic findings of, 486t
Scrotal mass
    calcifications causing, 424-426
    case studies involving, 434-435
    clinical scenario of, 419, 432b
    cysts causing, 421-424
    extratesticular, 421
    intratesticular, 426-430
    references for diagnosing, 437-438
    study questions about, 436-437
    trauma causing, 430-432
Scrotal pearls, 424
Scrotum. *See also* Testicle.
    definition of, 420b
    hernia of
        causing scrotal mass, 424
        echogenicity of, 425f
        symptoms and findings of, 433t
    normal sonographic appearance of, 420-421
    pathology and findings of, 433t
Sebaceous cyst
    causing breast mass, 400
    echogenicity of, 401f
    symptoms and findings of, 414t

Sebum, 228b
Secundum atrial septal defect, 381, 381f
Segmental pressures, 503b
Seminal vessels, normal vs. abnormal, 456f
Seminoma
    causing scrotal mass, 427
    clinical scenario of, 419f, 432b
    echogenicity of, 427f
    symptoms and findings of, 433t
Seminomas, 420b
Sensitivity, definition of, 174b
Sentinel node mapping, 394b
Septate uterus
    causing infertility, 222
    development and findings of, 223t
    echogenicity of, 222f
Septations, 228b
Septum primum, 377b
Septum secundum, 377b
Seroma
    breast mass due to, 412f
    vs. hematoma, 411
Serous, 228b
Sertoli-Leydig cell tumor (SLCT), ovarian, 240-241, 242t
Sexually transmitted disease (STD) in PID, 207
Shock, 135b
Short rib–polydactyl syndrome (SRPS)
    anomalies of, 367, 369
    echogenicity of, 370-371
    sonographic findings of, 356t
Shoulder dystocia, 265b, 267f
Sickle cell anemia, 277b
Signet-ring cell, 228b
Sinoatrial code, 377b
Sinus venosus septal defect, 381
Situs, 105b
Sludge, gallbladder, 5, 10
Snowstorm sign
    in breast implant rupture, 408
    definition of, 395b
    echogenicity of, 409f
Sonazoid, 43
Sonography, saline-infusion, 174b
Sonohysterography
    definition of, 174b
    equipment used for, 189b, 189f
    to evaluate abnormal uterine bleeding, 188-190
    indications and contraindications for, 188t
    views of normal/abnormal, 190f, 191f
Sonologist, 250b
SonoVue, 43
Sotos' syndrome, 265b
Soules catheter, 189
"Spacesuit" hydrops, 342
Specificity, 174b
Sperm, 420b
Spermatocele

causing scrotal mass, 423
    definition of, 420b
    echogenicity of, 424f
    findings of, 433t
Spina bifida
    aperta/occulta, 326, 471b, 482
    definition of, 324b
    fetal
        alpha fetoprotein level in, 326, 332t
        echogenicity of, 327f, 328f
    infant
        echogenicity of, 479f, 481f
        neurosonography of, 482-484
Spleen
    case studies involving, 111-113
    congenital variants of, 105-106
    lesions of, 111t
    normal sonographic anatomy of, 105, 106f
Splenia ectopia, 106
Splenic infarction, 108
Splenomegaly
    echogenicity of, 107f
    left upper quadrant pain due to, 106-107
    liver mass and, 30f
Splenorenal shunt, 34b
Spontaneous abortion (SAB)
    defined, 198b
    due to subchorionic hemorrhage, 292
    sonographic findings of, 302t
    vs. threatened abortion, 293
Squamous cell carcinoma (SCC)
    causing hematuria, 68
    echogenicity of, 68f
    symptoms and findings of, 71t
Stein-Leventhal syndrome, 217b
Stepladder sign
    in breast implant rupture, 408
    definition of, 395b
    echogenicity of, 409f
Sternocleidomastoid muscles, 440b
Strap muscles, 440b
Strawberry gallbladder, 8
Stroma, definition of, 452b
Stuck twin, 309b, 314
Subchorionic hemorrhage
    bleeding with pregnancy due to, 292-293
    echogenicity of, 292f
    sonographic findings of, 302t
Subclavian steal syndrome (SSS), 498
Subcutaneous layer, 395b
Subphrenic spaces, 34b
Superficial vein thrombosis
    causing leg pain, 511-512
    definition of, 503b
    echogenicity of, 512f
Superior vena cava, 377b
Syncope, 105b

Syndactyly
 definition of, 292b, 339b
 in triploidy, 348
Systemic lupus erythematosus, 277b

T

Tachyarrhythmias, supraventricular (fetal), 379-380
 definition of, 377b
 M-mode tracing of, 379f
Talipes, 339b
Tapeworm in liver abscess, 11-12
"Target" sign, 148
Teratologic, 461b
Teratoma
 definition of, 228b
 sacrococcygeal
 causing fetal anomaly, 365
 echogenicity of, 366f
 sonographic findings of, 356t
 scrotal
 causing mass, 428
 echogenicity of, 428f
 symptoms and findings of, 433t
 splenic LUQ pain due to, 110
Teratomas, 420b
Terminal ductal-lobular unit, 395b
Testicle. *See also* Testis.
 abscess of
 causing scrotal mass, 426
 symptoms and findings of, 433t
 definition of, 420b
 malignant mass of, 426-430
 ruptured
 causing scrotal mass, 431
 echogenicity of, 431f
 symptoms and findings of, 433t
 torsion of
 causing scrotal mass, 431
 echogenicity of, 432f
 symptoms and findings of, 433t
 trauma to
 causing scrotal mass, 430-431
 echogenicity of, 430f
 undescended, 432, 433t
Testis, anatomy of, 421f
Tethered cord (spinal), 484-485, 485f
Tetralogy of Fallot, 383-384
 definition of, 324b, 377b
 echocardiography of, 383f
 echogenicity of, 345f
Thanatophoric dysplasia
 anomaly of, 367
 echogenicity of, 368f
 sonographic findings of, 356t
Theca, 228b
Theca lutein cysts, 291f, 301b
Thecoma

causing ovarian mass, 240
 echogenicity of, 240f
 findings and occurrence of, 242t
Thoracic circumference in uncertain LMP, 260, 260f, 261b
Thoracopagus twins, 315
Thorium dioxide, 105b
Threatened abortion (TAB), 293
Thrombin injection, ultrasound guidance during, 509f
Thromboangiitis obliterans. *See* Buerger's disease.
Thrombocytopenia, 105b
Thrombocytopenia–absent radius syndrome, 355b, 366-367
Thrombosis, 503b, 511f. *See also* Deep vein thrombosis; Superficial vein thrombosis.
Thyroglossal duct cyst, 446f
Thyroid cancer
 anaplastic, 440b, 447t
 medullary, 440b, 448t
 papillary
 clinical scenario of, 439, 447b
 definition of, 440b
 echogenicity of, 443f
 symptoms and findings of, 448t
Thyroid gland
 benign nodules of, 442-443
 diffuse disease of, 441-442
 malignant nodules of, 443-444
 normal sonographic anatomy of, 440-441, 441f
Thyroid inferno
 color Doppler of, 442f
 definition of, 440b
 in hyperthyroidism, 441
"Tip-of-iceberg" sign, 234f
Tomography, computed, 105b, 144b
TORCH infections, 339b
Torsion
 definition of, 420b
 testicular
 causing scrotal mass, 431
 echogenicity of, 432f
 symptoms and findings of, 433t
Torticollis
 definition of, 461b
 hip dysplasia associated with, 463
Total parenteral nutrition (TPN)*, 4b
Transaminase level, 36t
Transcerebellar diameter (TCD) in uncertain LMP, 258, 259f
Transient ischemic attack (TIA), 491b, 492
Transitional cell carcinoma (TCC)
 causing hematuria, 67-68
 echogenicity of, 67f
 symptoms and findings of, 71t
Transjugular intrahepatic portosystemic shunt (TIPS)
 definition of, 34b
 echogenicity of, 42f
 for portal hypertension, 41

Translocation, 339b
Transposition of great arteries
　anomaly of, 385-386
　definition of, 377b
　echocardiography of, 386f
Transrectal ultrasound (TRUS), 453
Trauma
　carotid dissection due to, 491, 499b
　hematoma due to, 14f, 110
　leg pain due to, 508-509
　scrotal mass due to, 430-431, 430f
　splenic cyst after, 104f, 111b
Tricuspid valve, 377b
Triglycerides level, 36t
Triple screen, 309b, 340
Triploidy
　description and findings of, 347-348
　echogenicity of, 350f
　sonographic findings of, 340t
Trisomy 13
　chromosomal analysis of, 342f
　description and findings of, 345-346
　echogenicity associated with, 349f
　soft markers for, 343t
　sonographic findings of, 340t
Trisomy 18
　alpha fetoprotein level in, 332t
　description and findings of, 344-345
　echogenicity associated with, 346f, 347f
　soft markers for, 343t
　sonographic findings of, 340t
Trisomy 21
　clinical scenario of, 338f, 348b
　description and findings of, 344
　echogenicity associated with, 345f, 346f
　soft markers for, 343t
　sonographic findings of, 340t
Trophoblast, 292b, 339b
Trophoblastic disease, gestational
　bleeding with pregnancy due to, 294-296
　definition of, 265b
　size greater than date due to, 269
Truncus arteriosus, 377b, 386-387
Tuberous sclerosis, 21b, 59b, 93b
Tuboovarian abscess
　definition of, 207b
　in pelvic inflammatory disease
　　sonographic findings of, 209
　　symptoms and findings of, 211t
Tubular necrosis, acute. See Kidney tubular necrosis, acute.
Tunica albuginea, 420b, 422
Tunica vaginalis, 420b
Turner's syndrome
　chromosomal anomalies with, 346-347
　echogenicity of, 349f
　sonographic findings of, 340t
Twin, death of, 315f

Twin embolization, 309b, 313
Twin gestation. See Gestation, multifetal.
Twin reversed arterial perfusion (TRAP) sequence, 316, 317t
Twinkle sign
　definition of, 59b
　in nephrolithiasis, 62f
　in urolithiasis, 63f
Twinning
　abnormal, 314-316, 317t
　embryology of, 311-313, 313t
　evaluation of, 309-311
Twin-twin transfusion syndrome
　clinical scenario of, 307f, 317b
　etiology and findings of, 317t
　in multifetal gestation, 315-316

U
Ulceration of carotid artery, 496f
Ultrasound, saline-infusion, 174b
Umbilical vein, recanalized, 34b
Upper gastrointestinal, 144b
Urachal cysts, 355b
Urea, blood level of, 36t
Uremia, 77b
Ureteropelvic junction, 59b
Ureteropelvic junction obstruction
　size less than date due to, 281
　sonographic findings of, 285t
Ureterovesical junction obstruction
　echogenicity of, 282f
　fetal size less than date due to, 281
　sonographic findings of, 285t
Urethral valves, obstruction of posterior
　size less than date due to, 281-282
　sonographic findings of, 285t
Urinary tract infection (UTI)
　causing elevated PSA, 453
　causing hematuria, 59-60
　in renal failure, 77
Urogram, intravenous, 59b
Urolithiasis
　causing hematuria, 60-62
　definition of, 59b
　echogenicity of, 62f, 63f
Uterine anatomy, 175-176, 176f
Uterine anomalies, congenital
　causing infertility, 219-223
　clinical scenario of, 216f, 223b
　development and findings of, 223t
　diagrams of, 220f
　echogenicity of, 220-223f
Uterine artery embolization, 179
Uterine bleeding
　abnormal
　　anatomic causes of, 192t
　　case studies involving, 192

Uterine bleeding—*cont'd*
  abnormal—*cont'd*
    causes of, 175b
    clinical scenario of, 173, 191b
    definition of, 174b
    references for diagnosing, 194-195
    study questions about, 193-194
    types of, 174
  dysfunctional, 174b
Uterus
  broad ligament of, 228b
  during dilation and curettage, 157f
  enlarged, 179-180, 182
  increased fundal height of, 267-270
  retroverted, 198b
  sonographic evaluation of, 177f

V
VACTERL association, 370-371
Vaginal sonography. *See* Endovaginal imaging.
Valsalva maneuver, 504b
Vanillylmandelic acid, 162b
Vanishing twin, 314-315, 317t
Varicocele
  causing scrotal mass, 422-423
  definition of, 420b
  echogenicity of, 424f
  findings of, 433t
Varicose veins, 504b
Vas deferens, 420b, 423
Vasa previa
  bleeding with pregnancy due to, 298
  echogenicity of, 298f
  sonographic findings of, 302t
VATER association, 370
Veins, leg
  vs. arteries, 505-506
  normal vascular anatomy of, 504-505, 506f
Venereal disease, 207b
Venous collateral flow, 34b
Venous disease, leg pain due to, 509-512

Venous insufficiency, 504b, 512
Ventricle, left/right, 377b
Ventricular septal defect (VSD), 347f, 381, 387f
Ventriculomegaly, 471b, 472
Verma-Naumoff syndrome, 369
Vertebral artery, 494f
Vinyl chloride, 105b
Virchow's triad, 504b
Virilization, 162b
Volvulus, 355b
Von Gierke's disease, 21b
von Hippel-Lindau disease, 59b

W
Wandering spleen, 106
Weaver syndrome, 265b
WES sign (Wall, Echo, Shadow), 6
Wharton's jelly, 324b
Wilms' tumor. *See* Nephroblastoma.
Wolffian, 228b
Wolff-Parkinson-White (WPW) syndrome, 379

X
Xanthogranulomatous pyelonephritis, 83-84, 87t
X-linked anomalies, 355b

Y
Yin Yang sign
  definition of, 504b
  in popliteal aneurysm, 507, 508f
Yolk sac, secondary
  biometry of, for due date, 252
  definition of, 309b
  echogenicity of
    for estimating gestational age, 252f
    to locate embryo, 253f

Z
Zollinger-Ellison syndrome, 228b
Zygosity, 309b, 312f
Zygote, 309b